Essential Urologic Laparoscopy

Second Edition

Current Clinical Urology

Eric A. Klein, MD, Series Editor

For other titles in this series, go to
www.springer.com/series/7635

Essential Urologic Laparoscopy

The Complete Clinical Guide

Second Edition

Edited by

Stephen Y. Nakada

The University of Wisconsin Medical School
Madison, WI

Sean P. Hedican

The University of Wisconsin Medical School
Madison, WI

Humana Press

Editors
Stephen Y. Nakada
Department of Urology
University of Wisconsin-Madison
School of Medicine & Public Health
600 Highland Ave.
Madison WI 53792-3236
USA

Sean P. Hedican
Department of Urology
University of Wisconsin-Madison
School of Medicine & Public Health
600 Highland Avenue
Madison WI 53792
USA

ISBN 978-1-60327-819-5 e-ISBN 978-1-60327-820-1
DOI 10.1007/978-1-60327-820-1

Library of Congress Control Number: 2009929374

Printed on acid-free paper

springer.com

We dedicate this book to our spouses,
Deanna and Catigan,
and our children, Sarah, Schuyler, and Ian,
who bring so much joy to our lives.

Preface

The last six years since the publication of the first edition of *Essential Urologic Laparoscopy: The Complete Clinical Guide* have marked continued improvements in technology and further refinement of techniques that have gained popularity in the field of urology. The most noteworthy technological advance since the first edition of this book is the use of the da Vinci robot to assist in surgical dissection and laparoscopic suturing in the pelvis and retroperitoneum. A wealth of literature confirming the benefits of the laparoscopic approach in urology and easy access to this information via the Internet have created an even greater demand for acquiring the knowledge and expertise to perform these operations. This has further accentuated the educational burden to provide training and resources for practicing urologists who wish to offer these procedures to their patients.

The purpose of the second edition of *Essential Urologic Laparoscopy* is to provide a practical, updated, step-by-step guide for initiating, maintaining, and expanding a successful practice in urologic laparoscopy and robotic surgery. In this edition, we have also added full descriptive sections on robotic-assisted laparoscopic prostatectomy and pyeloplasty. Three new chapters providing concise, yet rich descriptions of the techniques of laparoscopic retroperitoneal lymph node dissection, renal ablation, and the hand-assisted approach to laparoscopic cystectomy have also been added. Once again, each chapter is organized into pre- and postoperative care, key surgical steps, common pitfalls, and take home messages. Each contributing author was specifically selected for his or her expertise in performing the described procedure.

An updated chapter on starting a laparoscopic as well as a robotic practice including establishing institutional privileges is also provided. The popular cross-referenced instrumentation chapter and individualized procedural instrumentation lists are once again included to enable the second edition of *Essential Urologic Laparoscopy* to serve as a reference guide for surgeons and their operating room personnel. The book concludes with a chapter on complications including informed consent and the more common complications occurring during robotic-assisted laparoscopic procedures.

It is our hope that the second edition of *Essential Urologic Laparoscopy* will provide a step-by-step manual to create and maintain a successful urologic laparoscopic and robot-assisted laparoscopic practice. The updated and new chapters as well as the sections on robotics are written as a clear and concise reference guide that should remain applicable for many years to come.

Sean P. Hedican, MD, and Stephen Y. Nakada, MD
The University of Wisconsin Medical School,
Madison, Wisconsin
July 2009

Contents

DVD Contents

Contributors

J. KYLE ANDERSON, MD • *Assistant Professor of Urologic Surgery, Department of Urologic Surgery, University of Minnesota, Minneapolis, MN*

MURALI K. ANKEM, MD • *Assistant Professor, Division of Urology, Department of Surgery, Robert Wood Johnson Medical School, University of Medicine and Dentistry of New Jersey, New Brunswick, NJ*

GAURAV BANDI, MD • *Assistant Professor, Department of Urology, Thomas Jefferson University Hospital, Jefferson Medical College, Philadelphia, PA*

ANDRE BERGER, MD • *Department of Urology, Center for Laparoscopic and Robotic Surgery, Glickman Urological and Kidney Institute, Cleveland Clinic, Cleveland, OH*

VINCENT G. BIRD, MD • *Assistant Professor of Clinical Urology, Department of Urology, University of Miami Leonard Miller School of Medicine, Miami, FL*

JEFFREY A. CADEDDU, MD • *Department of Urology, The University of Texas Southwestern Medical Center, Dallas, TX*

DAVID CANES, MD • *Department of Urology, Center for Laparoscopic and Robotic Surgery, Glickman Urological and Kidney Institute, Cleveland Clinic, Cleveland, OH*

SIDNEY CASTRO DE ABREU, MD • *Section of Laparoscopy and Endourology, ANDROS, Hospital Urológico de Brasília, Brasilia, Brazil*

RALPH V. CLAYMAN, MD • *Professor and Chair, Department of Urology, University of California at Irvine, Orange, CA*

LESLIE A. DEANE, MBBS, FRCSC • *Department of Urology, University of California, Irvine, Orange, CA*

GRANT I.S. DISICK, MD • *Department of Urology, Hackensack University Medical Center, Hackensack, NJ*

JOSEPH J. DEL PIZZO, MD • *Director, Laparoscopic and Minimally Invasive Surgery, Department of Urology, The New York Presbyterian Hospital and Weill Cornell Medical Center, New York, NY*

INDERBIR S. GILL, MD, MCh • *Head, Section of Laparoscopic and Robotic Surgery, Glickman Urological Institute, Cleveland Clinic Foundation, Cleveland, OH*

CARL K. GJERTSON, MD • *Division of Urology, University of Connecticut Health Center, Farmington, CT*

TRICIA D. GREENE, MD • *Departmental Fellow and Senior Instructor in Robotics and Minimally Invasive Surgery, Department of Urology, University of Rochester Medical Center, Rochester, NY*

SEAN P. HEDICAN, MD • *Associate Professor, Department of Urology, University of Wisconsin-Madison, Madison, WI*

DAVID J. HERNANDEZ, MD • *Senior Assistant Resident, James Buchanan Brady Urological Institute, Johns Hopkins Medical Institutions, Baltimore, MD*

ELIAS S. HYAMS, MD • *Department of Urology, New York University School of Medicine and Langone Medical Center, New York, NY*

MARKLYN J. JONES, MD • *The Urology Center of Colorado, Denver, CO*

LOUIS KAVOUSSI, MD • *Smith Institute for Urology, North Shore-Long Island Jewish Health System, New Hyde Park, NY*

STUART S. KESLER, MD • *Department of Urology, Hackensack University Medical Center, Hackensack, NJ*

MICHAEL O. KOCH, MD • *Professor and Chairman, Department of Urology, Indiana University Simon Cancer Center, Indianapolis, IN*

KENNETH S. KOENEMAN, MD • *Associate Professor, Department of Urologic Surgery, University of Minnesota, Minneapolis, MN*

JAIME LANDMAN, MD • *Director of Minimally Invasive Urology, Department of Urology, Columbia University Medical Center, New York, NY*

DAVID I. LEE, MD • *Chief of the Division of Urology at Penn Presbyterian Medical Center, Assistant Professor of Surgery, Division of Urology, University of Pennsylvania School of Medicine, Philadelphia, PA*

ADAM W. LEVINSON, MD, MS • *James Buchanan Brady Urological Institute, Johns Hopkins Medical Institutions, Baltimore, MD*

YAIR LOTAN, MD • *Assistant Professor of Surgery, Department of Urology, University of Texas Southwestern Medical Center, Dallas, TX*

PATRICK S. LOWRY, MD • *Assistant Professor of Surgery, Texas A&M Health Science Center College of Medicine, Scott & White Clinic, Temple, TX*

TIMOTHY D. MOON, MD • *Department of Urology, University of Wisconsin Medical School, Madison, WI*

RAVI MUNVER, MD • *Associate Professor of Urology; Chief, Minimally Invasive Urologic Surgery, Department of Urology, Hackensack University Medical Center, Hackensack, NJ*

EDWARD G. MYER, MD • *Department of Urology, University of Connecticut Health Center, Farmington, CT and Hartford Hospital, Hartford, CT*

STEPHEN Y. NAKADA, MD • *The David T. Uehling Professor of Urology, Chairman of Urology, University of Wisconsin at Madison, Madison, WI*

GYAN PAREEK, MD • *Assistant Professor of Surgery, Department of Urology, Brown University Medical School and Rhode Island Hospital, Providence, RI*

ERNESTO REGGIO, MD • *Smith Institute for Urology, North Shore-Long Island Jewish Health System, New Hyde Park, New York*

STEVEN J. SHICHMAN, MD • *Connecticut Surgical Group, Senior Attending Urologist, Hartford Hospital, Associate Clinical Professor of Urology, University of Connecticut Health Center, Hartford, CT*

ARIEH L. SHALHAV, MD • *Professor of Surgery, Chief, Section of Urology, Director, Minimally Invasive Urology, University of Chicago Medical Center, Chicago, IL*

KEVIN SMITH • *Smith Institute for Urology, North Shore-Long Island Jewish Health System, New Hyde Park, NY*

JOSHUA M. STERN, MD • *Center for Minimally Invasive Urologic Cancer Treatment, Department of Urology, University of Texas, Southwestern Medical Center, Dallas, TX*

MICHAEL D. STIFELMAN, MD • *Assistant Professor, Department of Urology, New York University School of Medicine, New York, NY*

LI-MING SU, MD • *Associate Professor of Urology, Director of Robotic and Laparoscopic Urology, James Buchanan Brady Urological Institute, Johns Hopkins Medical Institutions, Baltimore, MD*

CHANDRU P. SUNDARAM, MD • *Associate Professor, Department of Urology, Indiana University School of Medicine, Indianapolis, IN*

INGOLF A. TUERK, MD, PhD • *Head, Section of Laparoscopy and Robotic Surgery, Department of Urology, Lahey Clinic Medical Center, Burlington, MA*

HOWARD N. WINFIELD, MD • *Professor, Director of Laparoscopic, Robotic and Minimally Invasive Urologic Surgery, University of Iowa, Iowa City, IA*

J. STUART WOLF, JR., MD • *Professor, Department of Urology, University of Michigan Health System, Ann Arbor, MI*

ILIA S. ZELTSER, MD • *Clinical Assistant Professor of Urology, Jefferson University, Philadelphia, PA*

KEVIN C. ZORN, MD • *Assistant Professor of Surgery, Co-Director, University of Chicago Minimally Invasive Urology Program, University of Chicago Hospitals and Weiss Memorial Hospital, Chicago, IL*

Getting Started in Laparoscopy

Joseph J. Del Pizzo

Laparoscopy was first performed by Kelling in 1901 *(1)*, as a method to view the abdomen of a dog. One hundred years later, this technique has gained global popularity and widespread use for many procedures in multiple specialities. The technique made a major advance in the early 1980s with the invention of the television-chip camera, which afforded advantages including a magnified image with a binocular view, easy observation of the procedure by the entire operating room, and the ability of the surgeon to operate with both hands. Soon after this, the first successful laparoscopic appendectomy was performed. This was followed in 1985 by the first laparoscopic cholecystectomy, performed by Muhe, for which he received the highest award of the German Surgical Society *(2)*. Laparoscopic cholecystectomy became the procedure to showcase the benefits of laparoscopic surgery: lower morbidity, better cosmesis, shorter hospitalization, and more rapid convalescence. With this, laparoscopy moved into the mainstream of accepted surgical practice for a variety of general surgical disorders.

The adaptation of laparoscopy into the urologic armamentarium has been a slower process. The laparoscope was initially used to locate cryptorchid testicles and to plan a subsequent open procedure. Schuessler was the first to present a laparoscopic approach to a common urologic procedure, the pelvic lymphadenectomy *(3)*. Although the initial excitement over this new technology waned after the staging pelvic lymphadenectomy fell out of favor, the impact of Schuessler's report remained monumental as there was a surge in the types of urologic procedures attempted laparoscopically as well as a deluge of reports and videos generated to document the progress. Clayman et al. *(4)* were the first to show that laparoscopic extirpative renal surgery was possible, describing the first laparoscopic total nephrectomy in 1991. This was soon followed by the initial laparoscopic radical nephrectomy in 1992, the first laparoscopic radical prostatectomy in 1992, the first laparoscopic partial nephrectomy in 1993, and the initial laparoscopic live donor nephrectomy in 1995. Since these initial cases, the popularity of these procedures has steadily increased and they have been adopted by most major medical centers *(5)*.

Until recently, the overwhelming majority of extirpative urologic surgery was done via an open technique. The main reason for this is the relatively steep learning curve that exists in performing laparoscopic cases safely and efficiently. Novice laparoscopists must learn to overcome several constraints in performing procedures that they have done with little difficulty for years via an open approach. The three-dimensional operative field is viewed in two dimensions. There is a loss of the tactile sensation that the surgeon has long relied upon as a dissector, retractor, and hemostatic instrument. Other challenges arise from the inherent difficulty of laparoscopic suturing and knot tying. Another dissuasive factor is that, relative to our general surgical colleagues, there are few urologic interventions that are candidates for the laparoscopic approach. The level of difficulty of a laparoscopic nephrectomy far

From: *Current Clinical Urology: Essential Urologic Laparoscopy*
Edited by: S. Y. Nakada and S. P. Hedican, DOI 10.1007/978-1-60327-820-1_1

exceeds that of a laparoscopic cholecystectomy. In addition, most urologists do not see the volume of radical nephrectomies necessary not only to maintain the laparoscopic skills that they have acquired, but also to improve them to a point where more challenging procedures can be attempted, such as laparoscopic radical prostatectomy or laparoscopic radical cystoprostatectomy.

With this being said, the enthusiasm for laparoscopy as a defining tool for the urologist remained at a high level throughout the first half of this decade. Many urologists in practice remained interested in incorporating laparoscopy into their daily practice. More physicians attended introductory training courses, worked in training laboratories, observed experienced laparoscopic surgeons, and learned about requirements for attainment of laparoscopic privileges at their hospital.

The introduction of robotic technology earlier this decade has delivered minimally invasive surgery to the forefront of our specialty. It has helped to optimize three-dimensional surgical magnification and technical refinement to allow complex manipulation and reconstruction within a limited operative space. This expensive technology has allowed shortening of the learning curve and the inclusion of more and more conventional open surgeons into the domain of minimally invasive surgery. These advancements, coupled with the modern-day patient having access to unlimited medical information from the cyber-media, have increased the demands on our colleagues to incorporate laparoscopy and robotics into their clinical practice.

This chapter will review the basic steps necessary for the urologist to bring laparoscopy into his/her everyday practice.

THE SURGEON

The prospective laparoscopic surgeon is the centerpiece of the project. Any urologist who wishes to incorporate laparoscopy into his/her practice must be dedicated to learn the skills and, just as important, to maintain and develop them over time. To learn the skills, the surgeon has many options available. There are many introductory, hands-on laparoscopy courses given throughout the year. These courses include both didactic lectures and time in a dedicated, hands-on animate laboratory. The evolution of the hand-assisted technique for laparoscopic extirpative renal surgery has increased the number of training courses available and has shortened the learning curve for many urologists, allowing them to combine their open surgical skills with the laparoscopic approach *(6)*. Upon completion of a course, the surgeon is encouraged to continue training through use of an inanimate laboratory or other laparoscopic training device. Before attempting his/her first laparoscopic case, which is most likely to be a simple or radical nephrectomy, the surgeon is encouraged to watch an experienced laparoscopic surgeon perform a case, preferentially another urologist performing a laparoscopic nephrectomy. Laparoscopic pelvic surgeries (prostatectomy, cystectomy/urinary diversion) are extremely complex procedures that require an advanced level of laparoscopic skills to perform safely. It is not recommended that the novice laparoscopic surgeon attempt these until a significant amount of experience in renal surgery has been attained.

The prospective surgeon must think ahead before scheduling his/her first laparoscopic case. This includes understanding and meeting the hospital's requirement for securing and maintaining laparoscopic privileges. In addition, the surgeon must secure the support of not only the hospital, but also his/her practice, ensuring that the partners in the practice will commit to support laparoscopy. This includes not only financial support, but also education of potential patients and referring physicians. Next, the surgeon should construct a dedicated laparoscopy team including an experienced laparoscopist, a dedicated assistant, preferably a partner who has also completed a laparoscopic training course, an anesthesiologist familiar with the physiology of laparoscopy, and a dedicated operating room ancillary staff. Finally, the surgeon must become familiar with the basic instruments needed to safely perform the initial laparoscopic procedures.

"TEAM LAPAROSCOPY"

Experienced Laparoscopist

Taking a team approach to getting started in laparoscopy is the safest and most efficient way to adopt this technologically advanced procedure. The novice laparoscopic urologist will need an experienced laparoscopic surgeon available to assist on the first few cases. At many large centers, this is often another urologist. In many smaller community settings, the urologist often is more likely to know a general surgeon with significant laparoscopic experience. The experienced general surgeon represents an excellent source of knowledge for the novice laparoscopic urologist in terms of introduction of trocars, instrument set-up, and basic laparoscopic dissection technique. The urologist is encouraged, however, to rely on his/her expertise in open urologic surgery in performing the steps of the procedure (i.e., radical nephrectomy), as well as to draw on what was learned during introductory courses in terms of trocar placement and selection of instruments to use. When performing these initial cases, it is recommended that the pair take turns assisting each other. This will afford the novice surgeon the opportunity to become comfortable as the primary surgeon and as an assistant. Learning to operate the laparoscopic camera and becoming a good assistant are critical in the development and maintenance of laparoscopic surgical skills. If an experienced laparoscopic surgeon is not available in the community, the practice has the option of inviting one to proctor the initial cases.

Designated Assistant

The next component of the team to be assembled is a dedicated assistant. Ideally, this would be another urologist in the group who also has an interest in learning and supporting the influx of laparoscopy into the practice. It is recommended that the surgeons take any introductory courses together. This assistant should be available, if possible, for all of the initial cases. This will allow the pair to become comfortable operating with each other laparoscopically, to learn how to communicate with each other, and to anticipate each other's steps during the procedure. In addition, it will allow the novice surgeons to become familiar with the instruments together, and perhaps most importantly, to learn to troubleshoot problems when they arise. All of these facets of the team approach are important in shortening the learning curve and increasing the safety of the procedure in a novice surgeon's hands. This learning process should continue outside the operating room, as beginning surgeons should also practice together in animate and inanimate laparoscopic laboratories to maintain and improve their developing skills.

Anesthesiologist

The anesthetic care of the patient during laparoscopy is largely determined by the alterations in physiology associated with the pneumoperitoneum. With peritoneal insufflation, significant alterations in hemodynamics, pulmonary function, acid–base balance, urinary output, and hormonal secretion can occur. The anesthesiologist working these initial cases should have experience in monitoring these intraoperative parameters. With rapid systemic absorption of carbon dioxide, the peritoneal insufflation may result in hypercapnia with concomitant pulmonary hypertension and systemic vasodilatation. An increase in peak airway pressures can be a manifestation of the positive intraperitoneal pressure. Other potential problems include extensive subcutaneous emphysema, pneumothorax, and gas embolism *(7)*. Also very important is the fluid management of a patient with an induced pneumoperitoneum. A decrease in glomerular filtration rate (GFR) is seen, resulting in a relative oliguria during the course of the procedure. The anesthesiologist may be tempted to aggressively hydrate the patient based on this finding, which may lead to a fluid overload status postoperatively. Avoidance of nitrous oxide during the case is recommended, as it usually causes bowel distention and may impede the surgical dissection or increase the likelihood of an intraoperative bowel injury. An anesthesiologist with an understanding of the physiology of laparoscopy and the potential physiologic compromises will be able to easily recognize and correct complications or prevent them from occurring in the first place. This is a critical part of the novice laparoscopist's learning curve as he/she begins to take care of patients via a minimally invasive approach.

Operating Room Staff

The importance of the operating room and ancillary staff to the novice laparoscopist cannot be understated. The surgeon depends upon this staff to keep the operating room organized and to have the equipment available and working properly. Dedicated scrub and circulating nurses should be made part of the team. This continuity will allow the nurses to become familiar with the instrumentation, including retractors and dissectors, reloading stapling devices, troubleshooting malfunctions, and organizing the operative field. In addition, the scrub nurse will learn the operative steps and be able to anticipate what instruments the surgeon prefers to use at distinct parts of the procedure. This will help the surgeon operate more efficiently and reduce avoidable delays in operative time. The circulating nurse is responsible for the room set-up including monitors, laparoscopic towers, and all the equipment, including having back-up equipment available. Also, the circulator should always have an open instrument tray available in the operating room in anticipation of possible urgent or elective open conversion.

Instrumentation

A multitude of forceps, grasping instruments, dissectors, hemostatic agents, and trocars are available for use in a laparoscopic urologic procedure. A detailed account of laparoscopic instrumentation is given in the following chapter. Table 1 includes a list of the basic laparoscopic instruments recommended for the novice laparoscopist, presumably for a laparoscopic nephrectomy. With experience, each surgeon will develop his/her preferences for certain instrumentation and should modify the list over time.

Table 1
Basic operative laparoscopic instrumentation

• Laparoscopic cart	• Scissors
Television monitor	• Harmonic scalpel
Color video chip camera	• Endovascular stapler
High-intensity light sourc	• Port closure device
High-flow CO_2 insufflator	• Endoscopic specimen bag
• Laparoscope	• Hemostatic agent
10 mm 30, 45°	Surgicel, avitene
• Clip applicators	• Suction irrigator
5 mm, 11 mm	• Grasping forceps
• Trocars	Maryland, right angle
(2) 12 mm, (2) 5 mm, (1) 15 mm	• Hand access device (optional)

Patient Selection

With a dedicated team in place, the novice laparoscopist must choose a patient for his/her initial case. As stated, the urologist interested in learning laparoscopy will most likely apply it initially to radical nephrectomy in hopes of avoiding a flank incision and its attendant morbidity. More complex cases such as live donor nephrectomy, radical prostatectomy, and radical cystectomy should not be attempted by the inexperienced laparoscopist, regardless of how adept that surgeon may be at the open procedures.

When selecting an appropriate initial case, the surgeon should make every effort to maximize the chance of completing the case laparoscopically. This will provide the most benefit for the patient and will help the surgeon with his/her confidence level for future cases. Favorable renal tumors that can be approached laparoscopically by the novice surgeon include small tumors, lower pole tumors, and tumors away from the hilum. These cases are typically not associated with friable, parasitic vessels and will afford the surgeon the opportunity to approach the case systematically and most closely simulate the animate laboratory experience. On the contrary, initial cases to avoid include tumors near the hilum, tumors with a venous thrombosis, and large upper pole tumors, especially on the right side, where the lesion may be close to the inferior vena cava.

Another key component to initial case selection involves avoiding cases in patients who have undergone extensive prior intra-abdominal surgery. This may significantly prolong operative time and increase the chance of injury to other intra-abdominal injury. In addition, very thin patients with tight abdominal musculature often prove a challenge, as their abdominal cavity does not expand much with insufflation, thereby limiting the working space for the surgeon. This will especially hinder the novice laparoscopist performing a hand-assisted nephrectomy, as the surgeon's hand will occupy much of the working space in this patient. Also, patients who are morbidly obese do not represent good initial cases, as these procedures are often long and require a much more laborious dissection through extensive perinephric fat.

A complete patient evaluation is recommended for any patient undergoing a laparoscopic nephrectomy. In preparation for initial cases, the novice surgeon will benefit from an advanced radiologic evaluation of the kidney, such as a computerized tomography angiogram, preferably with three-dimensional reconstructed images. This will detail the vascular anatomy for the surgeon and allow careful preoperative planning of the hilar dissection.

Another important component of patient preparation is the surgeon's preoperative discussion with the patient about the laparoscopic approach. The rationale for electing to use a laparoscopic approach should be detailed, including less postoperative pain, better cosmesis, and a shorter hospitalization. In addition, if indicated, assure the patient that the procedure adheres to all oncological principles of extirpative surgery. Most importantly, the novice laparoscopist should be honest with the patient about his/her experience with this new technique. If it is the initial case, the patient must know this and be reassured that the first priority is to complete the surgery safely, even if this entails converting to an open procedure, if necessary. Patients' consent should always be obtained for a possible open procedure, regardless of the experience of the operating surgeon. It is important for all parties to understand that an open conversion is not a failed procedure. Conversion to an open procedure is part of the learning curve for any laparoscopic procedure and remains a safe option for any laparoscopic case that fails to progress.

THE ROBOT

The field of robotics has emerged as an invaluable tool to the practicing urologist. The *da Vinci* Surgical System is the most successful and widely used surgeon-driven robot used to date. Since its introduction in Europe in 2000 by cardiovascular surgeons, its applications have evolved to include surgical procedures in general, gynecologic, and urologic surgery. Urologists have been leaders in its continued development and expansion. As a result, its application in our field encompasses a wide variety of surgical procedures including radical prostatectomy, radical cystectomy, pyeloplasty, partial nephrectomy, and vasovasostomy.

COST

This new technology has a number of implications for patients, health care providers, hospitals, quality of care, and society as a whole. One important consequence is in the allocation of resources. There have been numerous studies examining the "cost effectiveness" of laparoscopy versus open surgery *(8–10)*. The evidence is not conclusive about whether laparoscopic surgery results in lower costs for the health care system. Laparoscopy does bring savings in a reduced hospital stay, and indirectly as a result of a reduced period of sick leave. From the point of view of the hospital, laparoscopic operations cost more than open operations because of the initial investment in instruments and initial longer duration of operating and anesthesia time. Due to these direct costs, some novice surgeons may encounter resistance from their hospitals regarding these start-up expenses (Table 2). However, as laparoscopic skills are learned, operating times decrease and more patients are recruited to the hospital rather than away to seek minimally invasive treatment elsewhere. In addition, with a steady increase in the number of cases performed, investment in reusable instrumentation and trocars may be an opportunity for cost savings per case for the hospital. Also, capital equipment that is multipurpose (monitors, cameras) and is used by different specialities contributes minimal added expense on a per case basis.

Table 2
Direct costs of basic laparoscopy set-up

• Laparoscopic cart	$47,000
• Laparoscopes (3)	$15,500
• Trocars (reposable)	$1,000
• Instruments	$12,000
• Harmonic scalpel	$24,000
Generator	
Hand pieces	
• Hand access device (2)	$1,000
Total	$100,500

The purchase of the *da Vinci* Surgical System represents a significant and sometimes daunting financial investment for a hospital. The system costs over $1.4 million with a $100,000 yearly service contract. Such costs are not reimbursed to the hospital on a case basis, and if the system is underutilized, it can represent a significant financial burden. On the other hand, use of the system can add over $1,000 per case if utilized for 300 cases per year and amortized over 7 years *(11)*.

The cost to the novice surgeon is primarily indirect. Initially, the surgeon will experience longer operative times, which translates into less revenue from time lost in the office and doing other procedures. With time, as skills are improved and maintained, the technology offers opportunities to expand the scope of the urologic practice and increase the referral base. Once again, this project begins with a prospective urologist who is dedicated to developing laparoscopic skills and incorporating a safe and effective treatment option to open surgery into his/her armamentarium.

CONCLUSIONS

Laparoscopic and robotic surgeries are part of the rapidly growing field of minimally invasive therapy that has moved to the forefront in many urologic extirpative procedures, especially simple and radical nephrectomy. The adoption of laparoscopic surgery as a new therapy necessitates a considerable commitment by the prospective surgeon to endure the steep learning curve that exists in acquiring and maintaining basic laparoscopic skills. In addition, there is a significant financial commitment to be made by the hospital and the members of the practice.

There are several *take home points* from this chapter for the prospective laparoscopic surgeon. They include the following: (1) take an introductory course featuring didactic lectures and training in an animate laboratory; (2) work with an experienced laparoscopic surgeon during the initial cases; (3) take a team approach to getting started in laparoscopy by designing a dedicated operating room team including a camera operator, anesthesiologist, and nursing staff; (4) choose a "beginner-friendly" case to develop skills and build confidence; and (5) educate patients and referring physicians about laparoscopy in order to advance and maintain laparoscopic skills. These concepts will help the novice laparoscopist develop the safest and most efficient way to adopt this technologically advanced procedure.

REFERENCES

1. Kelling, G.U.: Uber Oesophagoskopie, gastroskopie and zolioskopie. Munchene Med. Wochenschrift, **49**: 21, 1902.
2. Reynolds, W.: The fist laparoscopic cholecystectomy. JSLS, **5**: 89, 2001.
3. Schuessler, W.W., Vancaillie, T.G., Reich, H., Griffith, D.P.: Transperitoneal endosurgical lymphadenectomy in patients with localized prostate cancer. J Urol, **145**: 988, 1991.
4. Clayman, R.V., Kavoussi, L.R., Soper, N.J., et al.: Laparoscopic nephrectomy: Initial case report. J Urol, **146**: 278, 1991.
5. Hagood, P.G.: History and evolution of laparoscopic surgery. In: Urologic Laparoscopic Surgery. Edited by Raul O. Parra. New York: McGraw-Hill, chapt 1, p.3, 1996.
6. Sosa, R.E., Seiba, M., Shichman, S.J.: Hand-assisted laparoscopic surgery. In: Seminars in Laparoscopic Surgery. Edited by Raph V. Clayman. Philadelphia: W.B. Saunders Company, **7(3)**, p.185, 2000.
7. Richard, H.M., Stancato-Pasik, A., Salky, B.A., et al.: Pneumothorax and Pneumomediastinum after laparoscopic surgery. Clin Imag, **21**: 337, 1997.
8. Jonsson, B., Zethraeus, N.: Costs and benefits of laparoscopic surgery – a review of the literature. Eur J Surg, **585**: 48, 2000.
9. Brazier, J.E., Johnson, A.G.: Economics of surgery. Lancet, **358**: 1077, 2001.
10. Kenyon, T.A., Lenker, M.P., Bax, T.W., Swanstrom, L.L.: Cost and benefit of the trained laparoscopic team. Surg Endosc, **11(8):** 812, 1997.
11. Patel, V., Cadeddu, J.A., Gettman, M.T.: The new economics of radical prostatectomy: cost comparison of open, laparoscopic and robot-assisted techniques. J Urol, **172**: 1431, 2004.

Laparoscopic Instrumentation

Patrick S. Lowry

INTRODUCTION

Laparoscopic instrumentation continues to evolve towards smaller, more reliable, and better ergonomic devices, with a larger variety of choices. Since the first edition of this textbook, subtle improvements are readily apparent in existing devices as first-generation instruments progress towards later-generation models. New technology exists to allow procedures to be performed with fewer complications. Combined with refinements in techniques, new and improved instrumentation provides urologic surgeons the opportunity to safely perform more challenging procedures by a laparoscopic approach.

CAMERA SYSTEMS

Camera systems still have three integral parts: the camera head, the camera system control unit, and the monitor. These systems have progressed from analog to digital to advanced applications of digital technology *(1)*.

Most cameras attach to the end of the scope to capture the image coming through the lens. This image is then captured as a digital signal and transferred by the control unit to the monitor. Newer monitors are flat screen panels. Early flat screens did not provide adequate imaging, but by increasing pixel concentration and subsequently progressing into high-definition (HD) imaging, current monitors surpass previously available picture quality. To achieve this, significant improvement was required in the transfer of the digital signal to the monitor. Early-generation digital units suffered from a millisecond lag time between what was performed surgically and what was seen on the screen. This delay can be distracting, due to the subtle disconnect between surgeon and image. The current units process the signal to an image with increased speed, making any delay imperceptible.

Some systems, videolaparoscopes, employ a single camera/scope unit. These units have a charged coupled device (CCD), which is a minute digital chip attached to the tip of the scope *(2)*. Their advantage is improved picture clarity, due to the capability to capture the picture digitally at the scope tip, rather than capturing the image of the picture after it has passed through the lens of the scope. Since the picture travels via wire instead of through a lens, some scopes have been developed with the capability to flex at the tip (see "Scopes"). Additionally, HD videolaparoscopes are now being released, further enhancing the picture clarity. Regarding HD systems, one must realize that to visualize a true HD image, the camera, the camera system control unit, and the monitor must all be HD capable.

From: *Current Clinical Urology: Essential Urologic Laparoscopy*
Edited by: S. Y. Nakada and S. P. Hedican, DOI 10.1007/978-1-60327-820-1_2

A 3D viewing system (Viking Systems) gives the surgeon a 3D view of the operative field with either standard or HD technology *(3)*. This unit requires a type of helmet to be worn by the surgeon in order to visualize the 3D picture.

Laparoscopy has enjoyed rapid advancements in picture quality. Interestingly, although the images are significantly improved, as are costs, surgical outcome is unlikely to be affected.

SCOPES

Basic laparoscopes are 5 or 10 mm in diameter. The lens at the tip of the scope is generally fixed at 0, 30, or 45° of angulation. Larger scopes present a better image with a larger field of view, but smaller scopes may be used through smaller, less invasive, trocars. Videolaparoscopes may employ a deflectable tip (Fig. 1, Olympus), allowing the same scope to be used from 0 to 90° without the need to change scopes. The flexible tip allows significant flexibility, yet the camera holder must remain cognizant of the scope tip and keep the surgeon aware of the angle in use. A 10 mm scope with a traditional lens that rotates on an axis from 0 to 45° is currently in the prototype stage of development (Storz).

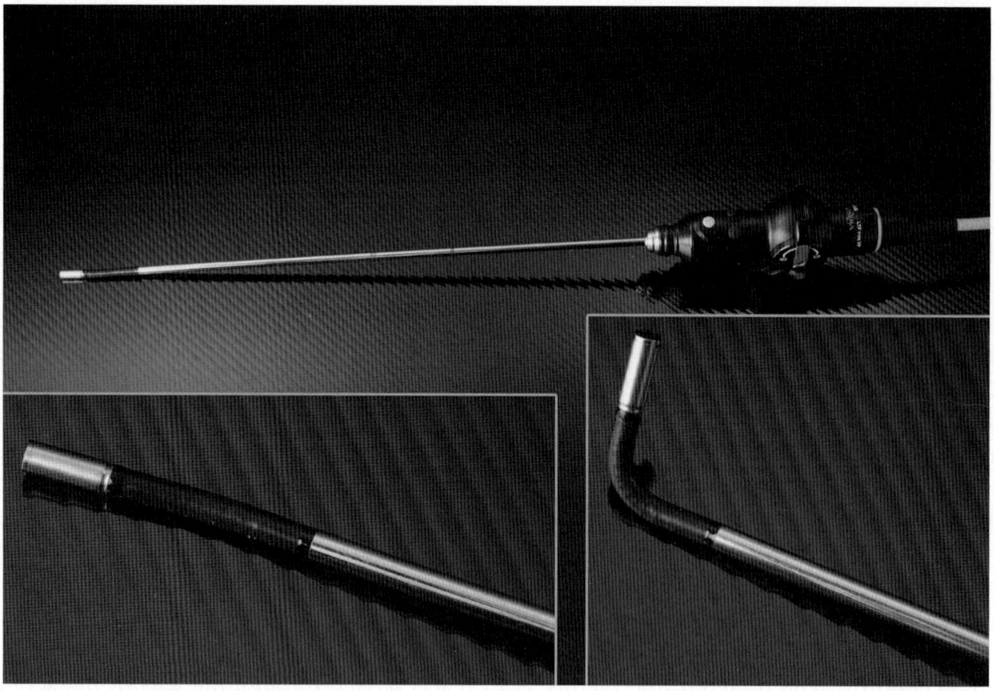

Fig. 1. 5-mm Videolaparoscope with flexible tip (Olympus). *Insets* show scope flexed at 0 and 90°.

Three-dimensional scopes, such as those used in the Viking or DaVinci systems, utilize two parallel lenses in the scope. The tips of these are fixed in a slightly different orientation, which provides 3D viewing when seen through the appropriate viewing system *(4)*.

Laparoscope fogging may be kept to a minimum by keeping the scopes at body temperature. When not in use, the end of the scope should be submerged in a heating thermos or water bath. Alternatively, a disposable heating pad (Stryker) may be wrapped around the end of the scope to keep it at the appropriate temperature. Additionally, anti-fogging solution should be used at the tip of the scope.

INSUFFLATION

The rate and pressure of the gas flow into the abdominal cavity is controlled by the insufflator, which acts as an adjustable interface between the pressurized gas bottle and the abdomen. The role of the insufflator is to control the flow of insufflant into the body in such a manner that the pressure stays very close to predetermined parameters that may be chosen by the surgeon.

Carbon dioxide (CO_2) is the most commonly used insufflant since it is inert, inexpensive, and very soluble in blood, which decreases the risk of gas embolus. Due to its solubility into the bloodstream, CO_2 may cause a mild respiratory acidosis, which should not be an issue during a general endotracheal anesthesia. Helium is also inert and may be safely used. Argon is not easily absorbed into the bloodstream, and consequently should not be used due to the risk of air embolus. Nitrous oxide can support combustion in combination with cautery or laser and should not be used as either an insufflant or an anesthetic.

ACCESS

Designed for access into the peritoneal cavity, the Veress needle is a 14-guage needle with a spring loaded blunt tip inner stylet which springs out to protect the abdominal contents after the needle is placed through the fascia. After adequate insufflation pressure is achieved, a trocar with a scope in the sheath may be used to visualize placement of the initial trocar. Subsequent trocars are then placed under vision.

Alternatively, a direct vision cutdown through the fascia may be performed with placement of the Hasson trocar. The abdomen is then inflated after the initial port placement so the remaining trocars may be placed under vision.

For retroperitoneal access, the working space may be created with a retroperitoneal balloon (US Surgical). The scope may be placed through the trocar into the balloon to allow visualization of the retroperitoneal structures through the balloon.

TROCARS

Trocars may be categorized as either bladed or non-bladed trocars (Fig. 2). Bladed trocars cut through the fascia, whereas non-bladed use different mechanisms to spread the fascia. Reusable bladed trocars have a sharp trocar to pierce the fascia and disposable bladed trocars use a spring mechanism to retract the blade after it has cut completely through the fascia and entered the peritoneum (Fig. 2). A novel trocar uses a cutting blade with a protective tip to protect the abdominal contents (Passport Trocar, Patton Surgical). The blade has a protective tip that springs out over the sharp tip immediately upon entry of the tip of the blade into the abdomen, allowing the remainder of the blade to cut through fascia with the tip covered to help prevent inadvertent visceral or vascular injury. Since all bladed trocars cut the fascia, 5 and 10-mm sites must undergo fascial closure to prevent incisional hernia formation *(5)*.

Non-bladed trocars dilate the fascia rather than cut them. This creates a smaller fascial defect, which reduces the risk of postoperative hernia formation *(6)*. Some centers believe that closure of the fascia is unnecessary for 10-mm dilating trocars *(7)*. Although the incidence is rare, one must note that trocar site hernia has been described when the fascia is not closed, even with dilating trocars *(5)*. In all children, 5- and 10-mm port sites must be closed.

Several types of dilating trocars exist. One design advances a cone-shaped plastic tip through the fascia in a twisting motion (Ethicon, Applied Medical). Another style, the Step trocar, places a sheath through the abdominal wall with the Veress needle (Tyco). Five or 10-mm trocars are placed through the sheath, which radially dilate the fascia in a stretching manner (Fig. 3) *(8)*. This system allows the surgeon to quickly replace a 5-mm trocar with a larger 10-mm size through the existing sheath.

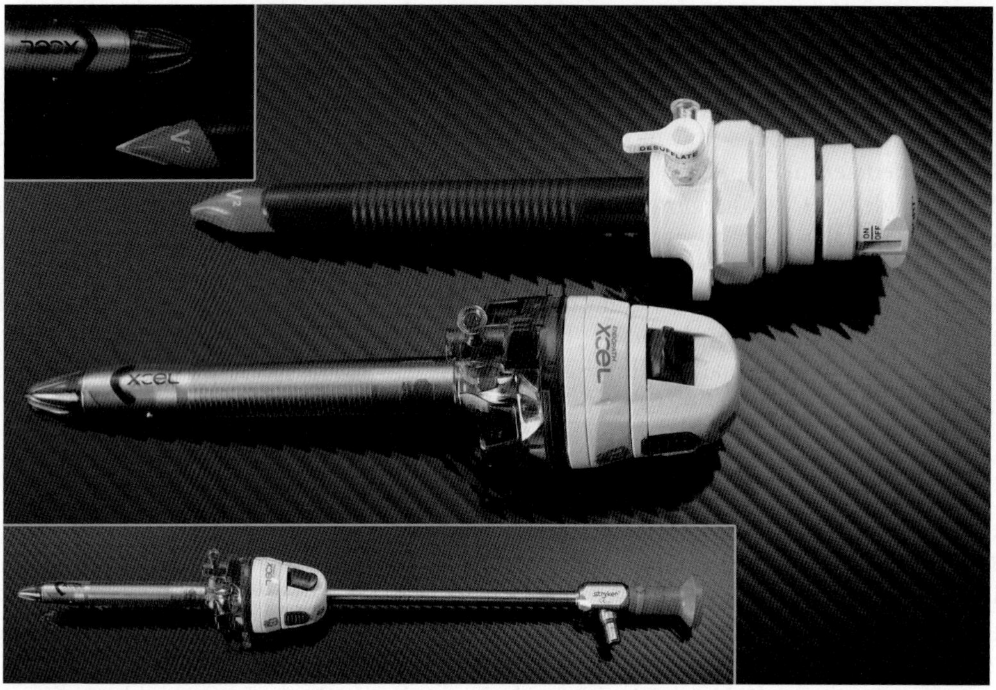

Fig. 2. 10-mm trocars. Upper trocar is bladed (Versaport plus V2, Autosuture); lower trocar is non-bladed (Endopath Xcel, Ethicon). *Upper inset* shows non-bladed tip and bladed tip with sharp edge exposed. *Lower inset* illustrates how a 10-mm scope fits into trocar for visual placement.

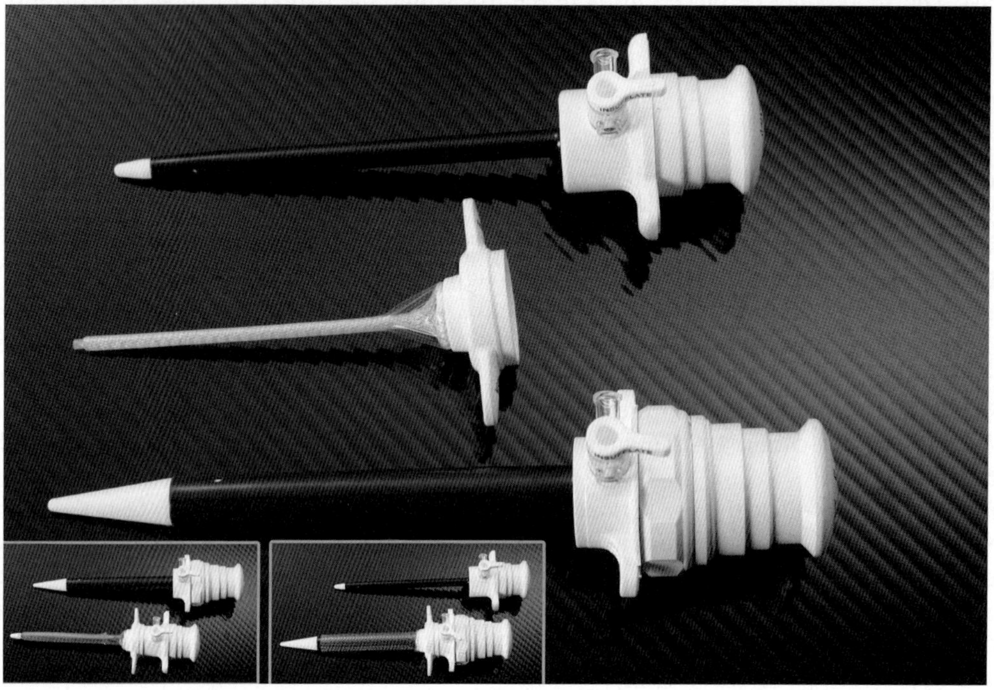

Fig. 3. Step trocar system (Tyco) with 5- and 10-mm trocar, and sheath. *Insets* show 5- and 10-mm trocars placed through the sheath.

Initial trocar placement must be done by the Hasson technique under direct vision, or using a visual device after Veress needle insufflation *(9)*. Two visual devices exist. The Optiview Excel (Ethicon) is a dilating trocar that allows the scope to be placed inside the trocar (Fig. 2). This allows visualization of the trocar entry through the layers of the abdomen through the clear dilating tip. A similar system, the Visiport (US Surgical) uses an optical system with a small trigger activated blade that snaps only 2 mm into and then immediately back out of the tissue, to protect against inadvertent injury of abdominal contents. By activating this blade repeatedly, one can watch the careful progress through the various layers of the abdomen until the peritoneum is entered. Care must be made not to apply too much pressure, or injury of abdominal contents immediately below the fascia can occur.

A novel port with multi-channel access that allows three instruments through one trocar that requires only a 3–4 mm incision *(10)*. For nephrectomy, this results in one extraction incision through the single larger port site, as compared to current nephrectomy with the extraction incision and 2–3 additional port sites.

HAND-ASSIST DEVICES

The first-generation hand-assist ports have given way to the Omniport (Tyco), the Gelport (Applied Medical), and the LapDisc (Ethicon). The Omniport is a one piece device that is inflated around the wrist to create an airtight seal. The LapDisc is comprised of two parts; the airtight seal is created by an adjustable iris type system that is tightened around the wrist. The most recent Gelport employs two pieces and has a soft gel cap that gently stretches around the wrist to create a seal. The Gelport allows an instrument to be placed through the gel adjacent to the hand, allowing another instrument without requiring another port placement. The Gelport also allows exchange of surgeon's and assistant's hands without loss of pneumoperitoneum.

The various ports have been directly compared and characterized by ease of device insertion, ease of hand insertion, and exertion of forearm compression forces *(11)*. The devices are all safe and effective, and surgeon preference will vary.

Recently, small finger mounted dissecting devices (Ethicon) have been developed to potentially improve the usefulness of the intra-abdominal hand. Currently, these are not yet available for clinical use and their utility remains to be proven.

HEMOSTASIS

Energy-Based Dissectors

Early energy-based dissection was performed with the hook monopolar cautery, which still has widespread usage today. Monopolar energy may also be used with shears and graspers. The monopolar current spreads out in all directions for several millimeters from the tips of monopolar devices, and great care must be taken to avoid cautery injury to nearby organs.

Bipolar cautery allows the current to travel from one jaw of an instrument to the other jaw, which focuses the energy between the jaws, decreasing energy dispersion. Bipolar graspers may be used to cauterize a structure, which may then be divided. The Ligasure system (Valleylab) uses bipolar energy combined with controlled pressure to seal vessels up to 7-mm in diameter. The Ligasure compresses the tissue to be treated until it "clicks" into the proper pressure, after which the bipolar is delivered. This device has a feedback mechanism that automatically stops the energy when the vessel is appropriately sealed. After creating a wide seal, an integral blade is then manually activated to cut through the treated tissue (Fig. 4).

The Harmonic Scalpel (Ethicon) and the Auto-Sonix (US Surgical) are ultrasonic devices which use ultrasound energy. Compared to the Auto-Sonix, the Harmonic Scalpel has a superior dissecting

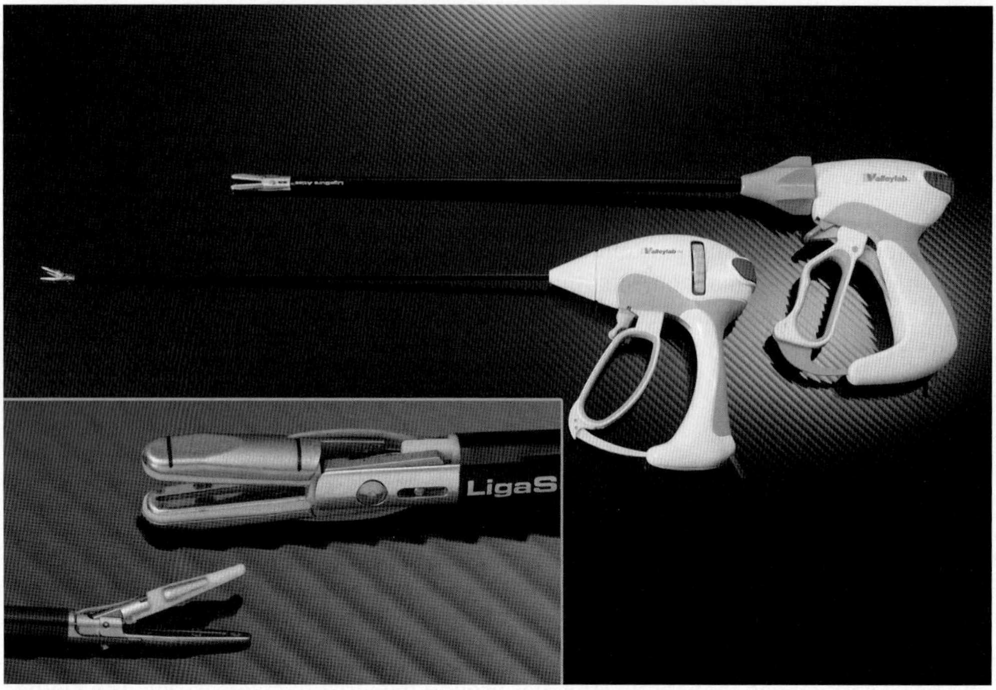

Fig. 4. Ligasure (Valleylab). 5- and 10-mm devices. *Inset* illustrates close-up view of the instrument tips.

tip, as well as the choice of either a straight or curved tip. Tissue is grasped between an active blade and a passive blade with a protective Teflon backing. The active blade vibrates at 55,000 Hz, which denatures and coagulates proteins in the vessel walls, resulting in a protein coagulum that reliably seals small vessels. No electricity is used and the vessels are controlled at lower temperatures (50–100°C) than electrocautery (150–200°C). Ultrasonic energy has very little thermal spread, less than 1 mm *(12)*, decreasing the chance for damage to adjacent organs. The Auto-Sonix and the Harmonic Scalpel can both safely divide vessels 3–4-mm in diameter. The newer Harmonic ACE is approved for division of vessels up to 5 mm, albeit with higher temperatures. All instrument tips, especially the ACE, are hot immediately after use, and contact with abdominal structures must be avoided to prevent inadvertent thermal damage *(13)*.

The argon beam coagulator employs a flow of argon gas by an electrode. When activated, the electrode produces a stream of electrons to the tissue surface. Superficial bleeding is controlled without deep dispersal of energy into the tissue. As the high flow of argon gas causes buildup of pressure, ports should be opened and insufflation pressures must be closely monitored to avoid air embolus or pneumothorax.

Mechanical Vascular Control

While energy-based dissectors control most potential bleeding encountered during surgery, they may not be effective during active bleeding and cannot safely divide larger vessels. Energy may need to be avoided to prevent damage to nearby nerves through thermal spread. In these instances, bleeding may be controlled and prevented by mechanically sealing vessels.

Clips will control almost all vessels. Titanium clips are available in a disposable applier, which rotate to simplify deployment. These are available in 5- and 10-mm sizes, with staples in line or at right angles to the applier (Fig. 5). Hem-O-Lok clips (Weck) are made of a non-absorbable polymer

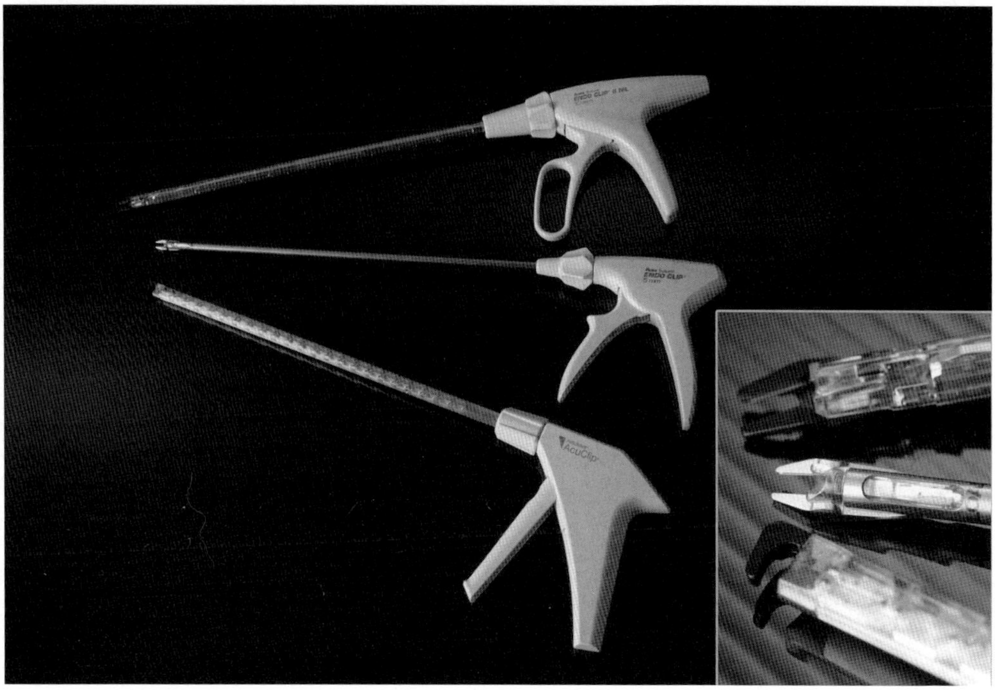

Fig. 5. Disposable titanium clip appliers (Autosuture). 5-mm straight, 10-mm straight, and 10-mm right angle devices. *Inset* magnifies the instrument tips.

and are less easily dislodged than titanium clips due to a locking mechanism. Four sizes exist for controlling tissue from 2 to 16-mm.

Staplers will simultaneously divide and mechanically seal arteries and veins of any size. Six layers of staples are deployed, and a blade cuts through the center. One must note that different types of staples are available for different uses and *vascular* loads must be used for division of vessels. Staplers rotate and some have articulating tips that deflect to help present better angles for usage.

Vascular clamps atraumatically control the renal artery and vein during partial nephrectomy. Small hand-held bulldog clamps may be placed via hand-assist technique (Fig. 6) and laparoscopic appliers place clamps through 10-mm ports (Fig. 7).

Biologic Hemostasis

The final method for achieving hemostasis is through the use of agents that augment the human coagulation cascade. Surgicel (Ethicon) and oxidized cellulose formulation may be held with pressure to assist with clot formation which helps control minor bleeding in locations that are not amenable to other means. Bolsters and rolls of Surgicel also assist with renal reconstruction during laparoscopic partial nephrectomy. Three types of Surgicel with varying thickness and texture are available.

Fibrin sealant (Tisseel, Baxter) can be applied via a needle-type applicator or a spray-type applicator. This sealant contains concentrated fibrinogen and creates a physiologic type fibrin clot to achieve hemostasis. Tisseel contains a bovine protein, and consequently should not be used in patients with known hypersensitivity to bovine products. Recently, another fibrin sealant was introduced, Evicel (Johnson and Johnson). Although not yet studied in urologic treatments, it has no bovine component and may have future application.

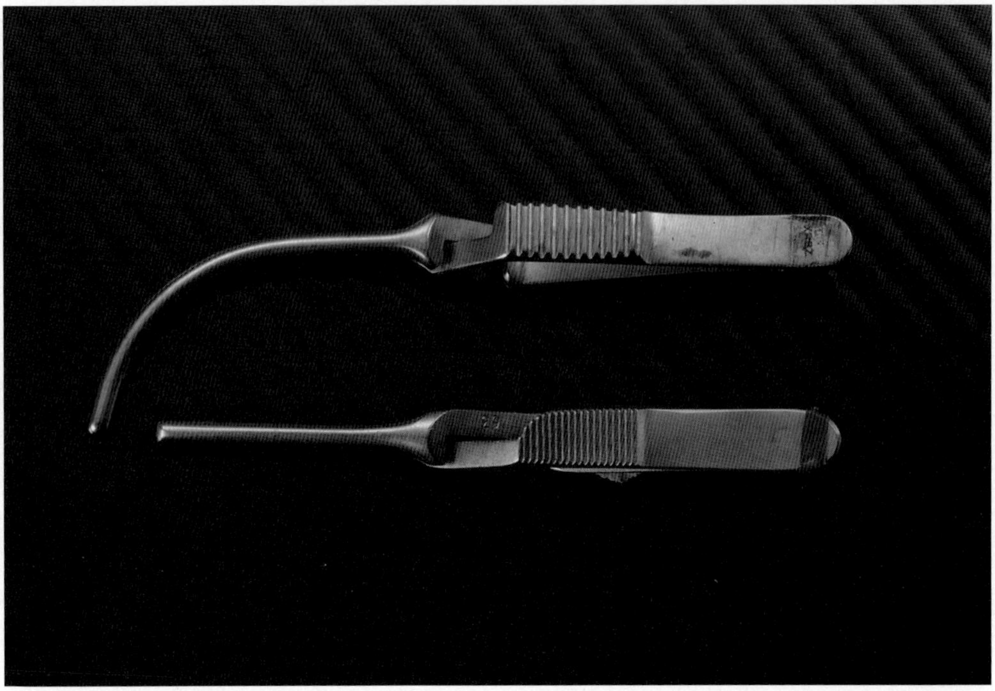

Fig. 6. Hand-held bulldog clamps (*curved and straight*) for hand-assist placement.

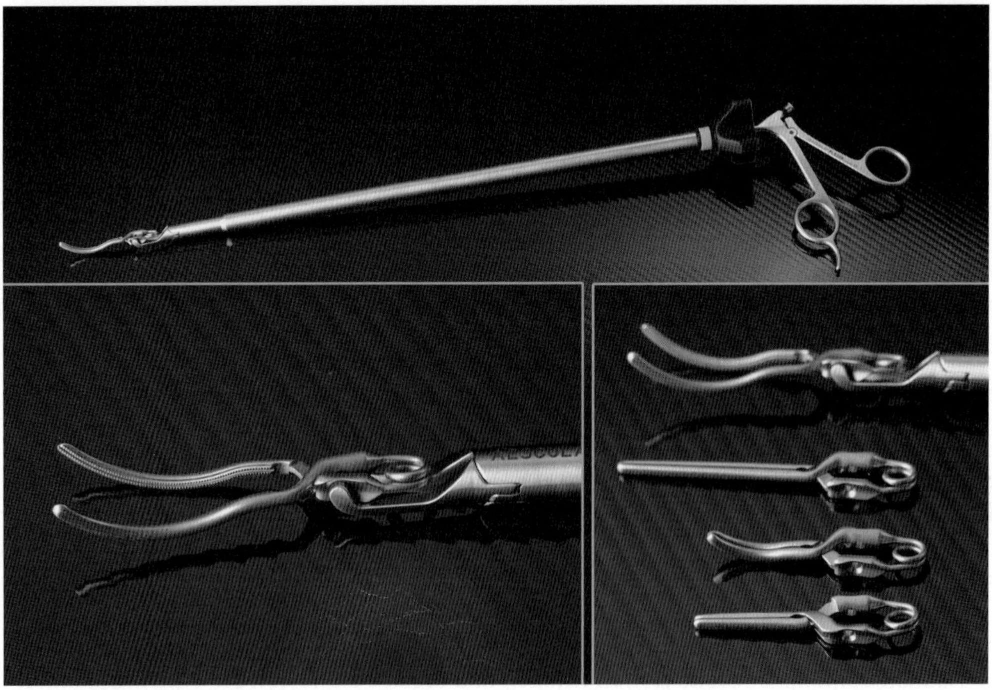

Fig. 7. 10-mm Laparoscopic vascular clamps (Aesculap). *Inset* shows close-ups of tips as well as various sizes.

Floseal (Baxter), a thrombin-infused gelatin matrix, may be applied onto bleeding sites and held with pressure. The Floseal material swells up to 20%, helping with tampanode into irregular areas of the bleeding surface. The fibrin in the gelatin granules activates the fibrinogen in the latter steps in the intrinsic coagulation pathway to form a fibrin clot. Whereas fibrin sealants (i.e., Tisseel) form a clot with the applied fibrinogen, Floseal assists the patient to create a naturally formed clot by activating the patient's own fibrinogen. In addition to helping with control of intraoperative bleeding, Floseal has been shown to decrease bleeding and bleeding complications associated with laparoscopic partial nephrectomy *(14)*. A newer gelatin thrombin product, Surgiflo (Johnson and Johnson), did not initially have FDA approval for urologic use. That has recently changed, and if studies show effectiveness, Surgiflo may also have future use. Both Floseal and Surgiflo have bovine components and should not be given to patients with known sensitivities.

DISSECTING INSTRUMENTS

A wide variety of options exist for fine dissection (Fig. 8). A Maryland dissector or a similar fine tipped instrument is most commonly used in combination with some type of energy-based dissector for the majority of the dissection. Many options exist to facilitate particular situations including Babcock graspers, Allis clamps, atraumatic bowel graspers, right angle dissectors, and dolphin-tipped graspers, just to name a few. Almost all are available as a 5-mm instrument, which have become much more durable. All instruments rotate 360°, and many can be obtained with locking mechanisms, if desired. The option of disposable versus reusable instruments has tilted towards reusable, as their durability has progressed. A possible exception may be scissors, as reusable types require frequent attention (sharpening, etc.). A newer type of shears utilizes a reusable hand piece, and a blade and action that may be

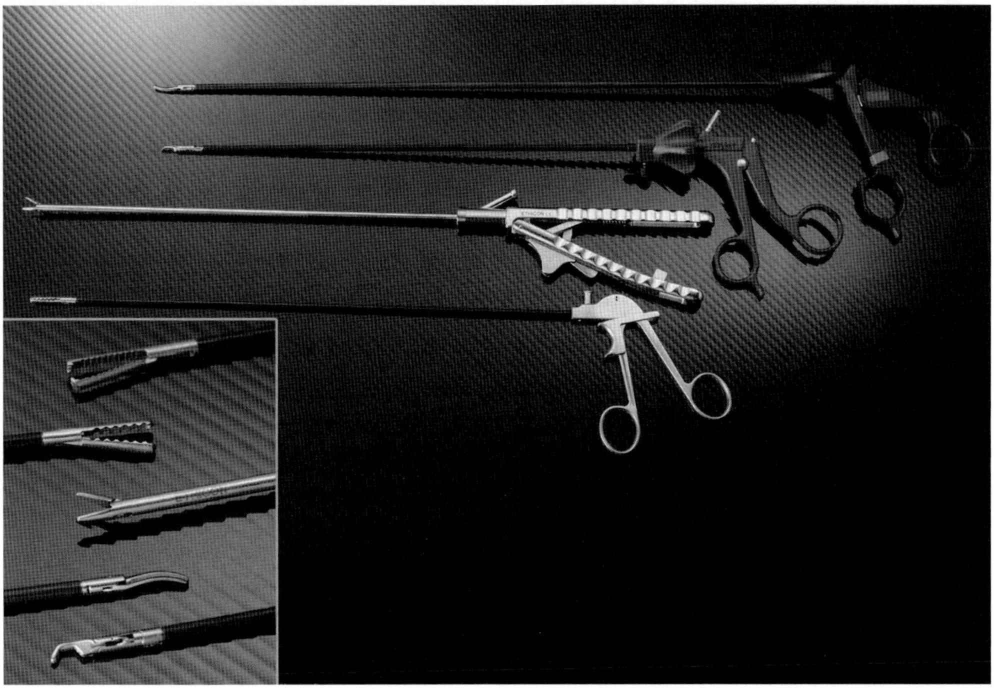

Fig. 8. Various 5-mm instruments. From *top down*, Maryland dissector, right angle dissector, needle holder, and mother-in-law. *Inset* shows close-up views of mother-in-law with teeth, mother-in-law without teeth, needle driver, scissors, and right angle dissector.

disposed of when it wears out. The disposable portion has similar durability to older reusable scissors and better quality than disposable ones, yet improves cost effectiveness by requiring replacement of only a portion of the instrument.

A new type of instrument with a deflectable distal tip offers additional degrees of freedom, similar to that seen with the DaVinci robotic system. The Autonomy Laparo-Angle (Cambridge Endoscopic) is equipped with a hand piece that allows flexion at the tip while simultaneously twisting the instrument or opening its jaws. Designed for creating the urethrovesical anastamosis in laparoscopic prostatectomy, this line of instruments may increase the capabilities of dissectors, scissors, and needle drivers.

An irrigation/aspiration instrument, or "sucker," is a mandatory instrument for complex procedures, and also functions well as a dissector. These are especially useful in longer lengths to allow for aspiration of irrigant in the farthest reaches (deep pelvis, above liver, etc.)

RETRACTORS

For retraction, the diamond flex retractor (Snowden-Pencer/Cardinal Health) provides excellent retraction with a blunt, atraumatic with a large surface through only a 5-mm port (Fig. 9). A disposable fan retractor inflates a fan-shaped end which is pliable enough to avoid damage during retraction. The Peer retractor (Jarit) works well and exists in 5- and 10-mm sizes. As it is more rigid and less forgiving, care must be used not to damage organs with overaggressive retraction.

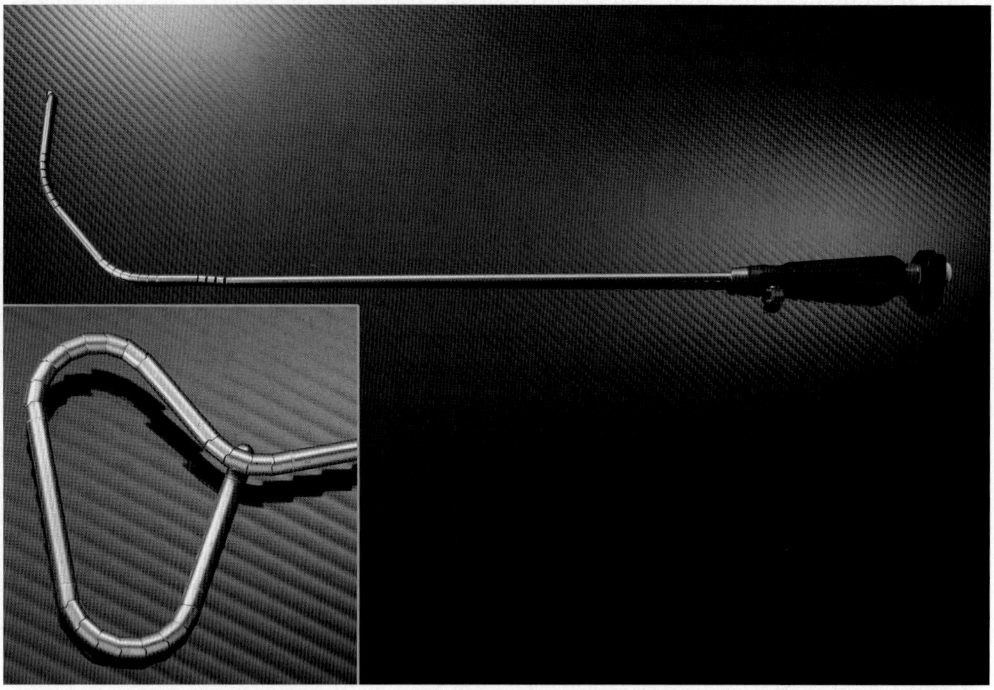

Fig. 9. 5-mm diamond flex liver retractor (Snowden-Pencer/Cardinal Health). *Inset* illustrates deployed tip.

SUTURING

Freehand intracorporeal knot tying is a tedious process that requires time and patience to perform, and a significant time investment to learn. The Endostitch (Autosuture) device is an automated stitching device that uses a double pointed with the stitch secured in the center *(15)*. The stitch can be passed back and forth between the two jaws of the needle holder. This facilitates throwing stitches as well as simplifics knot tying.

The Lapra-Ty (Johnson and Johnson) often eliminates the need for intracorporeal knot tying, which will save significant time for most surgeons. The Lapra-Ty is a vicryl clip that secures to the back of a stitch, securing the stitch where a knot would usually be required (Fig. 10). The Lapra-Ty is only approved for use with vicryl stitches. This device avoids the cost of the Endostitch, increases the choice of needles, and significantly decreases suturing time, especially helpful for partial nephrectomy reconstruction time (ischemic clamp time).

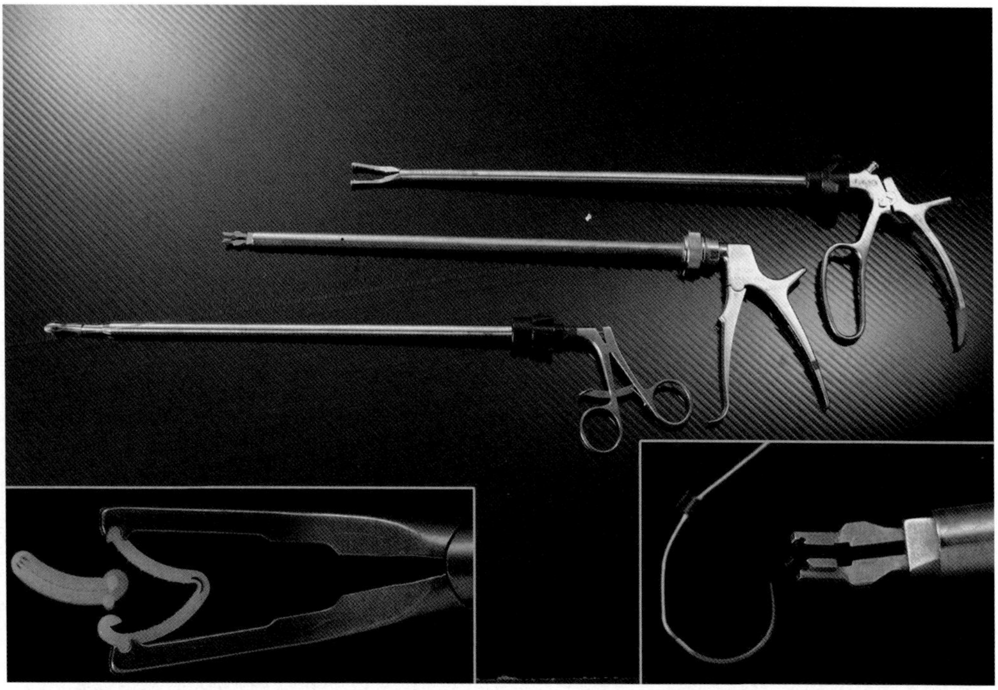

Fig. 10. 10-mm reusable instruments. Hem-O-Lock clip applier (Weck), Lapra-Ty applier (Johnson and Johnson), and an Allis clamp. *Lower right inset* shows the Hem-O-Lock clip with one clip deployed. The *lower left inset* illustrates a Lapra-Ty placed onto a polyglactin suture.

MORCELLATION

Morcellation must be performed in an impermeable entrapment bag. Instruments such as a ring forcep or heavy hemostats are used to break up and remove the specimen piecemeal until the entrapment sac can be extracted. Alternatively, electric powered devices can be pressed against the specimen to pull out 10-mm cores until the specimen is small enough to remove.

ADJUNCT INSTRUMENTS

Laparoscopic ultrasound probes are necessary during laparoscopic partial nephrectomy for evaluating the depth of tumor, as well as for excluding synchronous tumors. They are also needed to monitor the progression of the ice ball during cryotherapy.

The Carter–Thomason (Inlet Medical) fascial closure device assists placement of suture for closure of trocar sites *(16)*.

For specimen removal, the organ is captured in the retrieval bag and pulled toward the port for removal. One must understand that not all bags are impermeable to tumor cells and if morcellation is planned, it should only be performed in an impermeable bag. Currently, the LapSac (Cook Urological) is the only bag impermeable to tumor cells. It must be placed through a port or hand-assist incision and manually opened up to place the specimen inside (Fig. 11). A glidewire may be woven through the holes for the drawstring to assist with opening the Lapsac. The Endocatch (Tyco) extraction device is another option for specimen removal. It has a sheath through which the bag opens via a spring mechanism (Fig. 11).

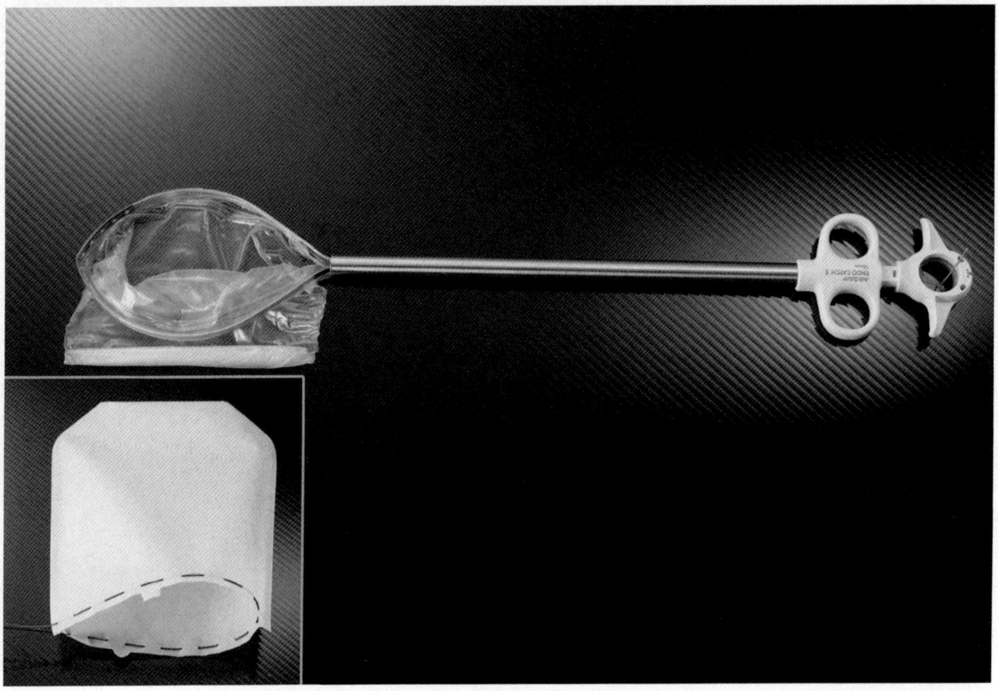

Fig. 11. 10-mm endocatch (Autosuture) specimen retrieval bag. *Inset* shows LapSac (Cook) with a 0.035-mm Hi-Wire (Cook) weaved through the eyelets.

ROBOTIC SYSTEMS

The DaVinci Robot (Intuitive Surgical) revolutionized laparoscopic prostatectomy and is currently the only available robotic surgical system. Specialized instrumentation allows for additional degrees of freedom not previously achieved. The tips of the 8-mm instruments move in a wrist-like manner, facilitating fine movements and suturing (Fig. 12). Additionally, the instruments are controlled by the surgeon, who is at the console, via the DaVinci robot which receives the input from the surgeon. Since the robot holds the instruments, no tremor exists. The surgeon has the ability to control two dissecting arms, the 3D camera, and a fourth retraction arm (on some units). Each instrument has approximately ten lives, which are monitored by the system, and after the tenth life, the instrument will not be recognized by the robot. Each instrument costs approximately \$2,000, making each instrument's per case usage about \$200. Generally, a case requires five instruments, sometimes more.

The newer DaVinci S system incorporates a number of advancements. The arms have more freedom, increasing the potential field of dissection. The visualization is enhanced with HD technology, and a

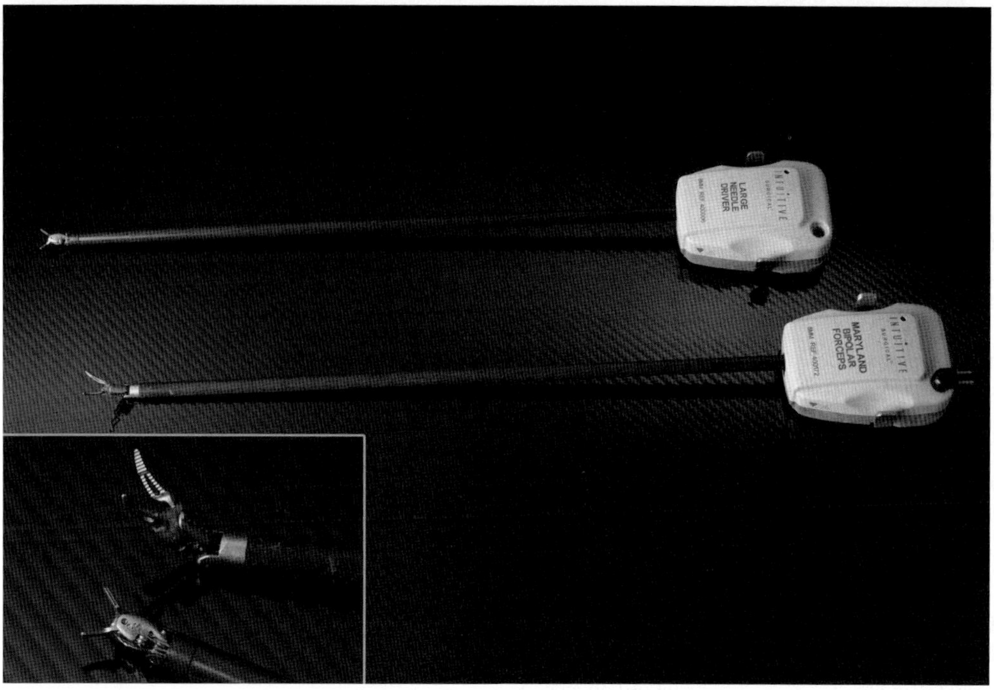

Fig. 12. Robotic instruments (intuitive surgical) needle driver above, Maryland Bipolar forceps below. *Inset* illustrates tips of instruments open with wrist-like motion flexed.

teaching screen allows notes to be drawn so that the surgeon may see the notes in the console. This improves the ability of an assistant to teach, by allowing for visual cues and directions to be given to the surgeon. Although improved, no difference in clinical outcome is appreciated. Currently, the list price for a DaVinci S system is 1.6 million dollars, with additional startup money required for instruments, camera lenses, and adjunct equipment that may total over 120,000 additional dollars.

FUTURE ADVANCEMENTS

Technological advancements will likely allow for an integration of radiologic imaging superimposed on a visual screen to help guide tumor removal in a precise manner.

Natural Orifice Transluminal Endoscopic Surgery continues to grow and will undoubtedly bring parallel progress in instrumentation, sealants, and camera systems.

Small robotic camera systems and arms have also been described that are deployed inside the patient on a type of platform to reduce the number of trocars *(17)*. As this technology progresses, it too, may bring further advancements.

CONCLUSION

Current advancements have provided the urologists with better and more durable instruments. Imaging has improved significantly, especially with smaller caliber scopes. Hemostatic agents have allowed more challenging surgery without an increase in morbidity. Laparoscopy should continue the trend toward providing equivalent outcomes through fewer, smaller, and less painful incisions.

Table 1
Instrumentation for urologic laparoscopy

Name of device[a]	General description	Company	Chapter references
Camera systems			
Camera head	Imaging	[b]	*(1, 3, 16)*
3D camera	Imaging	[b]	*(3)*
5-mm 0^0 laparoscope	Imaging	[b]	*(3, 6, 8, 14)*
5-mm 30^0 laparoscope	Imaging	[b]	*(3, 6–9, 14, 18)*
10-mm 0^0 laparoscope	Imaging	[b]	*(1, 3, 6, 8, 12–14, 16–18)*
10-mm 30^0 laparoscope	Imaging	[b]	*(1, 3, 6, 8, 9, 1118)*
DaVinci robot	Imaging	Intuitive surgical	*(1, 4, 13, 18)*
Access/trocars			
Veress needle	Access	[b]	*(1, 3, 4, 6, 8, 10–16, 20)*
Visiport trocar	Access	US surgical	*(5, 12)*
Optiview Xcel	Access	Ethicon	*(6, 13)*
		US surgical	
Passport trocar	Access	Patton surgical	
Trocar mounted balloon	Access (retroperitoneal)		*(3, 5–7, 10, 20)*
Bladed trocars	Access	[b]	*(3)*
Non-bladed (blunt) trocars	Access	[b]	*(3, 6–8, 13, 17, 18, 20)*
Hand-assist devices	Hand access		
Gelport	Hand access	Applied medical	*(1, 3, 6, 9, 11, 17)*
Lapdisc	Hand access	Ethicon	*(1, 3, 6, 9, 11, 17)*
Omniport	Hand access	Tyco	*(1, 3, 6, 9)*
Energy-based dissectors			
Harmonic scalpel	Ultrasonic energy	Ethicon	*(1, 6, 8–14, 16, 18)*
Autosonix	Ultrasonic energy	Tyco	
Ligasure	Bipolar energy	Valleylab	*(3, 8, 12, 17)*
Argon beam coagulator	Hemostasis	[b]	*(3, 5, 6, 8, 10)*
Mechanical vascular control			
Titanium clip applier (disposable)	Hemostasis	[b]	*(1, 5, 7, 8, 11, 12, 14, 16, 17)*
Hem-O-lock clip	Hemostasis	Weck	*(6, 7, 10, 12, 14–17)*
Vascular staplers	Hemostasis	[b]	*(6–9, 11, 12, 14, 16, 17)*
Laparoscopic vascular clamps	Hemostasis	[b]	*(8, 10)*
Biologic hemostasis			
Floseal	Hemostasis	Baxter	*(10, 20)*
Tisseal	Hemostasis/Sealant	Baxter	*(6, 10)*
Dissecting instruments			
Babcock graspers	Dissecting instruments	[b]	*(4)*
Allis clamps	Dissecting instruments	[b]	
Atraumatic bowel graspers	Dissecting instruments	[b]	*(4, 6–8, 14, 15, 17, 18)*
Right angle dissectors	Dissecting instruments	[b]	*(1, 6–9, 11, 13, 14, 17)*
Dolphin tipped graspers	Dissecting instruments	[b]	*(4)*
Needle drivers	Dissecting instruments	[b]	*(6, 8–10, 17, 18)*
Maryland dissector	Dissecting instruments	[b]	*(1, 6, 8, 9, 11–14)*
Autonomy laparo-angle	Dissecting instruments	Cambridge endoscopic	

Table 1
(continued)

Name of device[a]	General description	Company	Chapter references
Retractors			
Diamond flex retractor	Retraction	Snowden-Pencer/ Cardinal Health	*(13)*
Fan retractor (Disposable)	Retraction	[b]	*(4, 7, 16)*
Peer retractor	Retraction	Jarit	*(8, 11)*
Suturing			
Endostitch	Suturing	Autosuture	*(6, 8, 13)*
Needle driver	Suturing	[b]	*(6, 9, 10, 13, 15–18)*
Lapra-Ty	Suturing	Johnson and Johnson	*(6, 8, 10, 15)*
Adjunct instruments			
Laparoscopic ultrasound	Imaging	B-K Medical	*(5, 10, 14)*
Carter–Thomason fascial closure device	Closure	Inlet medical	*(1, 4, 8, 12, 13, 16, 18)*
DaVinci robotic system	Imaging/dissection	Intuitive surgical	*(1, 4, 13, 18)*

[a]Note that this list is not all encompassing, but it is useful to identify items that are mentioned by multiple experts.
[b]Available from several vendors.

Take Home Messages

1. Optics and camera systems for laparoscopy have undergone significant improvement with advances in digital and HD imaging.
2. Better durability and design have improved cost effectiveness by reducing the need for disposable instruments.
3. Hemostatic agents help prevent morbidity secondary to surgical bleeding.

Laparoscopic instrumentation companies and website information*

Applied Medical (Santa Margarita, CA)	www.appliedmed.com
Autosuture (Mansfield, MA)	www.autosuture.com
Baxter (Hayward, CA)	www.baxterbiosurgery.com
Cambridge Endoscopic (Framingham, MA)	www.cambridgeendo.com
Cook Urological (Bloomington, IN)	www.cookmedical.com
Ethicon (Cincinatti, OH)	www.ethicon.com
Inlet Medical (Trumball, CT)	www.inletmedical.com
Intuitive Surgical (Sunnyvale, CA)	www.intuitivesurgical.com
Jarit (Hawthorne, NY)	www.jarit.com
John son and Johnson (OH)	www.jnjgateway.com
Olympus (Center Valley, PA)	www.olympus.com
Patton Surgical (Austin, TX)	www.pattonsurgical.com
Snowden-Pencer (GA)	www.cardinal.com
Storz (Tuttlingen, Germany)	www.karlstorz.com
Stryker (Kalamazoo, MI)	www.stryker.com
Tyco (Mansfield, MA)	www.covidien.com
Valleylab (Boulder, CO)	www.valleylab.com
Weck (Markham, ON)	www.teleflex.com

*As of publication date

REFERENCES

1. Aslan P, Kuo RL, Hazel K, Babayan RK, Preminger GM. Advances in digital imaging during endoscopic surgery. J Endourol 1999; 13(4):251–255.
2. Amory SE, Forde KA, Tsai JL. A new flexible videoendoscope for minimal access surgery. Surg Endosc 1993; 7(3):200–202.
3. Bhayani SB, Andriole GL. Three-dimensional (3D) vision: Does it improve laparoscopic skills? An assessment of a 3D head-mounted visualization system. Rev Urol. 2005 Fall; 7(4):211–214.
4. Kourambas J, Preminger GM. Advances in camera, video, and imaging technologies in laparoscopy. Urol Clin North Am 2001; 28(1):5–14 Review.
5. Lowry PS, D'Alessandro AM, Moon TD, Nakada SY. Port site hernia associated with a non-bladed trocar following laparoscopic live donor nephrectomy. J Endourol 2003; 17(7):493–494.
6. Shekarriz B, Gholami SS, Rudnick DM, Duh QY, Stoller ML. Radially expanding laparoscopic access for renal/adrenal surgery. Urology 2001; 58(5):683–687.
7. Shalhav AL, Barret E, Lifshitz DA, Stevens LH, Gardner TA, Lingeman JE. Transperitoneal laparoscopic renal surgery using blunt 12-mm trocar without fascial closure. J Endourol 2002; 16(1): 43–46.
8. PG Schulam, SP Hedican, SG Docimo. Radially dialing trocar system for open laparoscopic access. Urology 1999; 54: 727–729.
9. McKernan JB, Finley CR. Experience with optical trocar in performing laparoscopic procedures. Surg Laparosc Endosc Percutan Tech 2002; 12(2):96–99.
10. Rane A, Rao P, Bonadio F, Rao P. Single port laparoscopic nephrectomy using a novel laparoscopic port (R-Port) and evolution of a single laparoscopic port procedure. J Endourol 2007; 21(suppl 1):V18–11 (abstract).
11. Monga M, Premoli J, Skemp N, Durfee W. Forearm compression by laparoscopic hand-assist devices. J Endourol 2004 Sep; 18(7): 654–656.
12. Landman J, Kerbl K, Rehman J, Andreoni C, Humphrey PA, Collyer W, Olweny E, Sundaram C, Clayman RV. Evaluation of a vessel sealing system, bipolar electrosurgery, harmonic scalpel, titanium clips, endoscopic gastrointestinal anastomosis vascular staples and sutures for arterial and venous ligation in a porcine model. J Urol. 2003 Feb; 169(2): 697–700.
13. Kim FJ, Chammas Jr. MF, Gewehr E, Morihisa M, Caldas F, Hayacibara E, et al. Temperature safety profile of laparoscopic devices: Harmonic ACE (ACE), Ligasure V (LV), and plasma trisector (PT) Surgical Endoscopy 2007 Nov 20 (epub ahead of print).
14. Gill IS, Ramani AP, Spaliviero M, Xu M, Finelli A, Kaouk JH, Desai MM. Improved hemostasis during laparoscopic partial nephrectomy using gelatin matrix thrombin sealant. Urology. 2005 Mar; 65(3):463–466.
15. Adams JB, Schulam PG, Moore RG, Partin AW, Kavoussi LR. New laparoscopic suturing device: initial clinic experience. Urology 1195; 46(2): 242–245.
16. Elashry OM, Nakada SY, Wolf JS Jr, Figenshau RS, McDougall EM, Clayman RV. Comparative clinical study of port-closure techniques following laparoscopic surgery. J Am Coll Surg 1996; 183(4): 335–344.
17. Zeltser IS, Bergs R, Fernandez R, Baker L, Eberhart R, Cadeddu JA. Single trocar laparoscopic nephrectomy using magnetic anchoring and guidance system in the porcine model. J Urol. 2007 Jul; 178(1):288–291.

Laparoscopic Access

Elias S. Hyams and Michael D. Stifelman

INTRODUCTION

A laparoscopic procedure is similar to flying a commercial plane. There is the captain (surgeon), co-pilot (assistant), and crew (anesthesia, scrub nurse, and circulator). Each works simultaneously performing distinct tasks leading to one goal. Both rely heavily on technology and require careful and thorough preparation prior to embarking. Similarly, like the captain of a plane, the surgeon is ultimately responsible for the outcome.

It is imperative that the surgeon arrive at the operating theatre with sufficient time to ensure all the equipment is present and functioning, similar to a pilot before take off. The time to realize that the nurse opened the wrong endoscopic linear stapler is not while ligating the renal vein, it is during the set-up of the procedure. Arriving early also allows the surgeon to position the many different pieces of equipment to his or her liking and ensure ease of traffic throughout the room. The operating room has a tendency to become very tight with two or more monitors, an argon beam coagulator, cautery generator, ultrasonic generator, compression stocking insufflator, and warming blanket as well as numerous power cords, cables, and foot pedals.

ROOM AND EQUIPMENT SET-UP

In an attempt to organize the preparation we created a checklist (Table 1). It is separated into four components: (1) imaging system; (2) insufflation; (3) hemostatic generators; and (4) instrumentation. Not every laparoscopic case requires all of the equipment listed; however, we made it comprehensive to provide a starting point. Subsequent chapters will deal specifically with each of these topics in greater detail.

Room arrangement depends upon the surgical procedure to be performed. However, there are some general principals that pertain to all cases. The surgeon, operative field, and monitor should be in a straight line (Fig. 1). This ensures the surgeon is optically correct, not in mirror image. The insufflator should be just below the main monitor or next to the main monitor so that the surgeon may have a constant and direct view. The surgeon should always be cognizant of the insufflation pressure, flow rate, volume used, and tank status. Typically, the camera and light source are also stored on the main monitor in direct view of the surgeon.

In addition to "lines" for insufflation tubing, camera and light cord, many other "lines" must enter the operative field including suction, irrigation, bovie, harmonic scalpel, etc. It is important to secure all "lines" to the operative field in a way that minimizes tangling and allows all devices including

From: *Current Clinical Urology: Essential Urologic Laparoscopy*
Edited by: S. Y. Nakada and S. P. Hedican, DOI 10.1007/978-1-60327-820-1_3

Table 1
OR set-up check list

Video equipment:
- Main monitor and slave monitor
- Camera box with three-chip camera or better
- Fiber optic light cord and xenon light source. Note: Check quality of light cord by holding end, which connects to xenon light source, up to fluorescent light. Look at the cord that connects to the laparoscope; each black dot represents a broken fiber optic fiber. There should be less than 15% of areas blacked out
- Laparoscope – 0 and 30°, diameter (3, 5, and 10 mm) is surgeon's preference
- Sterile camera bag
- +/– Video recorder. Note: a digital camcorder can easily be connected to the camera box via an S Video cable
- Connect all equipment, white balance and focus

Insufflation:
- High-flow insufflator, max flow $\geq$ 18 l/min, positioned on main monitor (especially useful for hand-assisted laparoscopy)
- Full CO_2 tank, connected without leak and turned on. Check level of tank on insufflation unit.
- Full spare CO_2 tank in room
- Insufflator tubing
- Set flow to 15 mmHg, check flow shut-off mechanism

Hemostatic generators:
- Electrocautery
  - o Grounding pad in place
  - o Cord on table and settings selected
  - o If using bipolar, cord is on table with bipolar instrumentation
  - o Foot pedal is on surgeon's side of table
- Harmonic scalpel/ligasure
  - o Laparoscopic handle assembled and connected
  - o Test function by activating on moist sponge
  - o Foot pedal is on surgeon's side of table
- Argon beam coagulator
  - o Laparoscopic handle on field and connected
  - o Argon gas tank is full, connected without leak, and turned on
  - o Test function by activating on moist sponge
  - o Foot pedal is on surgeon's side of table

Laparoscopic instruments:
- Veress needle
- Trocars
- Advanced laparoscopic set
- Basic surgical tray
- Laparotomy tray and self-retaining retractor unopened and in room

OR table:
- Electric motor which has capability of flexion, airplane tilt, and Trendelenberg

the laparoscope to be placed within any of the trocars. To facilitate this we recommend a specialized laparoscopy drape that has built in straps to secure lines and pockets to store and secure instruments. There are many available drapes on the market; one example designed by Allegiance is pictured in Fig. 2.

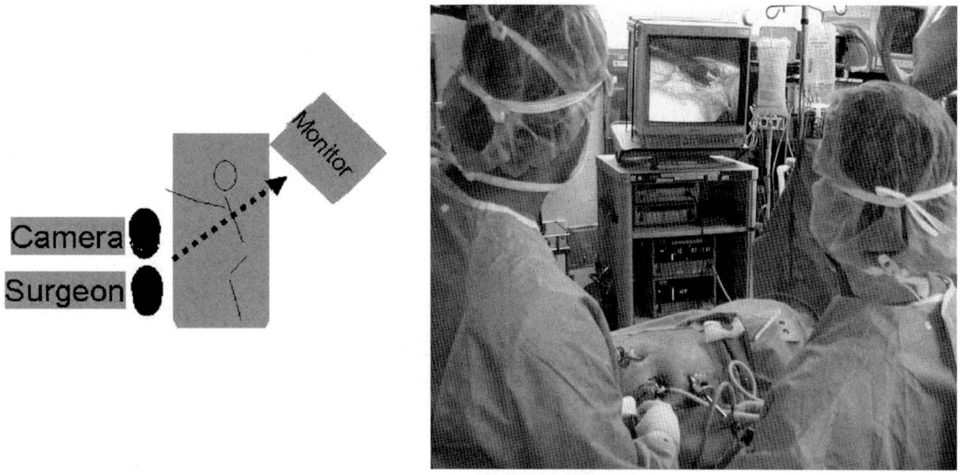

Fig. 1. Surgeon positioned to avoid mirror image.

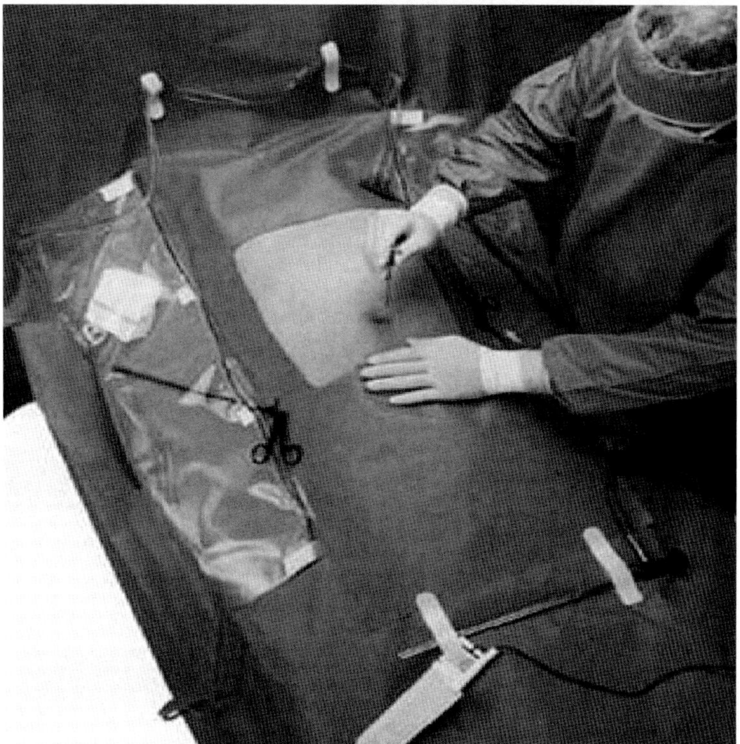

Fig. 2. Laparoscopy drape.

In terms of the scrub nurse and mayo stand, we suggest they be positioned opposite the surgeon so that instruments may be exchanged without having to turn one's head or lose eye contact with the monitor. This rule is less important in pelvic surgery where the nurse may stand on either side of the operative table as long as he or she is below the surgeon in line with the monitors. The hemostatic equipment should be placed at the foot of the bed, preventing the surgeon from becoming "entrapped" by cords or grounding pads.

We have outlined our preferred operating room set-up for transperitoneal, retroperitoneal, and pelvic procedures (Figs. 3–5).

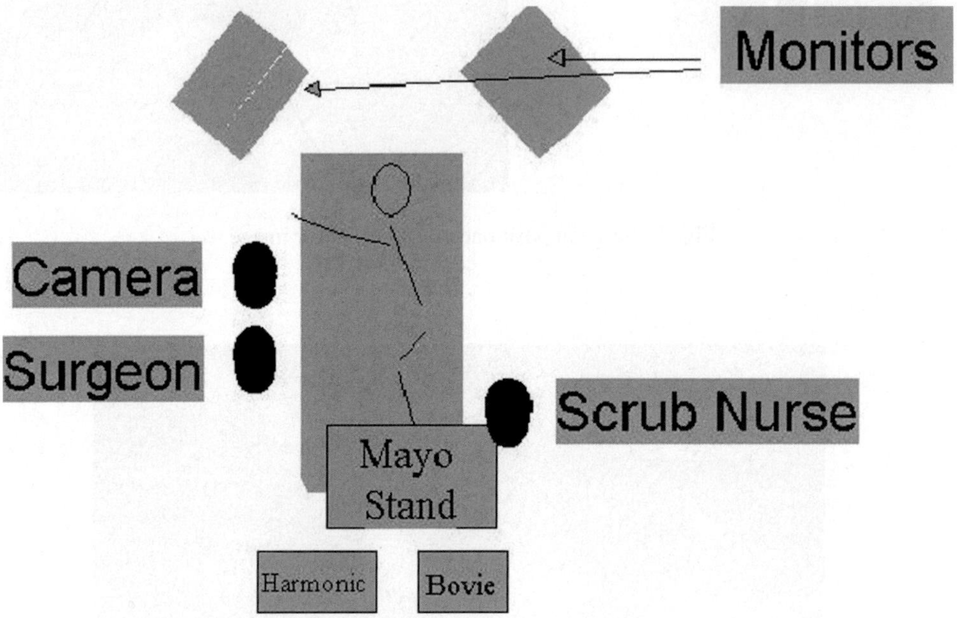

Fig. 3. Room set-up for transperitoneal procedure.

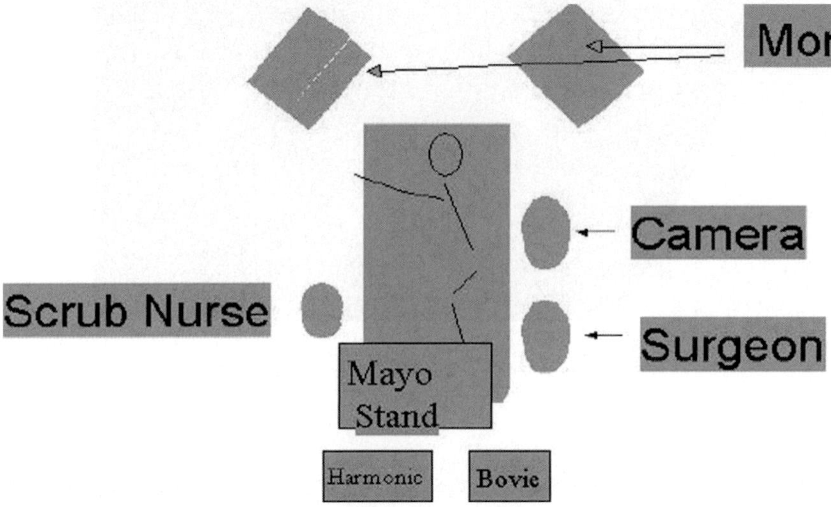

Fig. 4. Room set-up for retroperitoneal procedure.

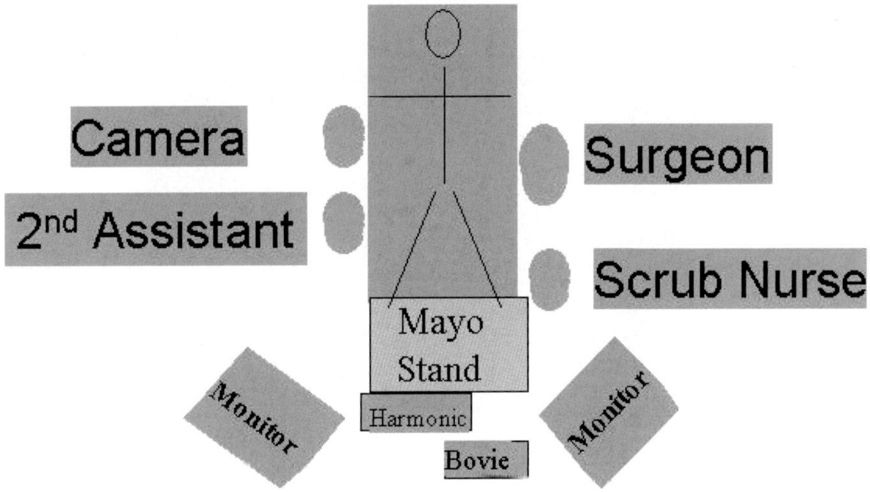

Fig. 5. Room set-up for pelvic procedure.

METHODS OF ACCESS

With the room set-up, checklist complete, patient intubated, positioned, prepped and draped it is time to begin. The first step requires obtaining access and establishing a pneumoperitoneum. This can be done either through an open or closed access technique. In either scenario it is important to use a foley catheter and oral gastric tube to decompress the bladder and stomach. In addition, it is recommended that the anesthesiologist avoid nitrous oxide to decrease bowel distention.

The closed technique has traditionally been performed using a Veress needle (Fig. 6). This specially designed needle measures 8 mm in length and 1.2 mm in diameter. The outer cannula has a beveled edge for cutting through tissue. The inner cannula has a blunt tip stylet that springs forward upon entering a space of low pressure such as the peritoneal cavity. This blunt stylet protects the abdominal contents from the sharp tipped outer cannula. On the opposite end of the needle is a stopcock, which is in continuity with the inner cannula allowing CO_2 to be insufflated into the abdomen.

When performing closed access the Veress needle is placed first. This allows the abdominal cavity to be insufflated separating the abdominal wall from the intra-abdominal viscera. A trocar is then placed blindly providing laparoscopic access. In theory the preliminary insufflation provided by the Veress needle decreases the risk of inadvertent injury to the abdominal viscera or vessels by separating the abdominal wall from the intra-abdominal viscera. Because this technique requires two blind "sticks" a thorough understanding of this approach as well as the checks and balances are required to minimize complications.

We prefer to obtain closed access at the level of the umbilicus. Here the abdominal wall is tethered to the fascia and the abdomen is most easily penetrated. If a midline scar is present we recommend using an alternate access site lateral to the rectus in the quadrant opposite the site of previous surgery. The skin incision is curvilinear when obtaining access peri-umbilically, vertical when placed anywhere else along the midline and horizontal for access obtained away from the midline. It is important to ensure the skin incision is large enough to accommodate the outer diameter of the trocar thus preventing excess force being placed on the trocar during insertion. One way to ensure this is to take the outer cannula of the trocar and make an impression on skin and use this as a guide for the length of the incision (Fig. 7).

After the incision is created it is important to lift the abdominal wall away from the underlying viscera with either towel clips placed just lateral to the edges of the incision or traction by the non-

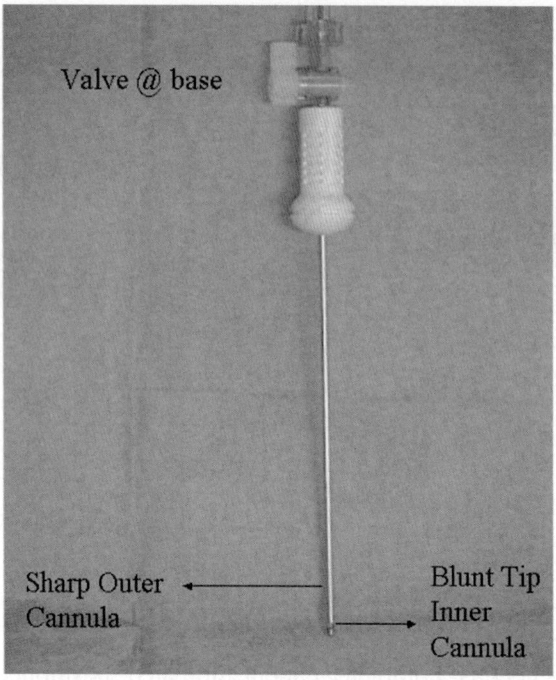

Fig. 6. Veress needle.

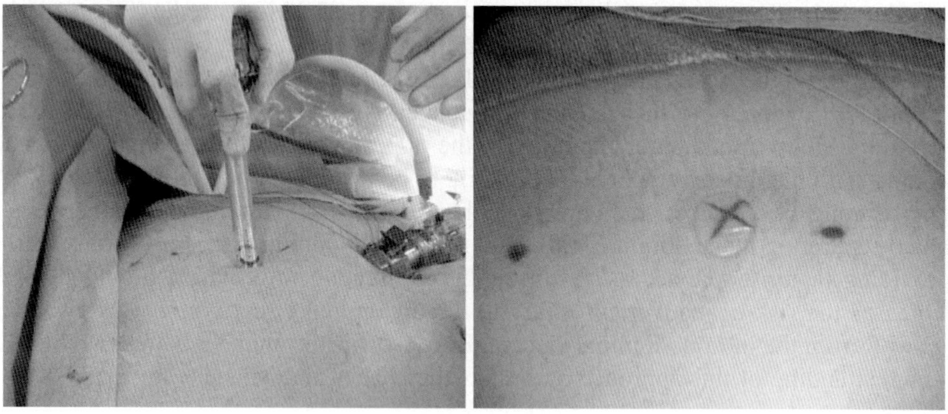

Fig. 7. Marking trocar incision.

dominant hand (Fig. 8). The Veress needle is then grasped like a dart and advanced at a right angle to the fascia. Elevation is maintained as the needle is advanced through the fascia and peritoneum. Two distinct pops may be felt as the abdominal wall is traversed and an audible click heard as the inner cannula springs forward upon entering the peritoneum. Deep penetration into the abdominal cavity should be avoided to minimize the risk of great vessel injury.

To ensure correct placement a 10 cc syringe with saline is attached to the needle and aspirated to look for blood, enteric contents or excessive air (Fig. 9). If blood is visualized, the Veress needle should

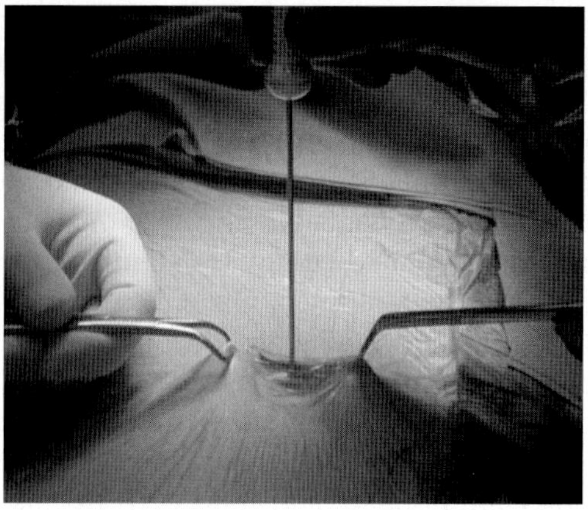

Fig. 8. Inserting Veress needle.

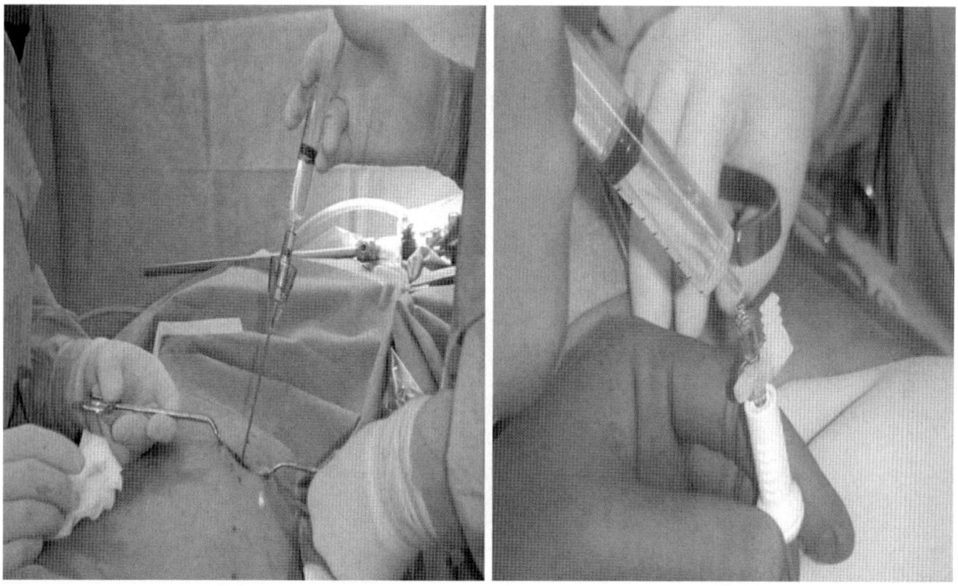

(a) (b)

Fig. 9. (**a**) and (**b**): Checking placement of Veress needle via aspiration and water test.

be removed. Secondary to the small diameter of the needle and blunt tip inner cannula, it is usually safe simply to remove the needle and replace it. Once access is obtained the initial puncture site should be inspected as well as the retroperitoneum for evidence of vascular injury or expanding hematoma. If the patient becomes hemodynamically unstable or vascular control is not feasible laparoscopically, emergent laparotomy should be performed. If enteric contents or excessive air is noticed then the needle should be left in place and a new access site should be chosen. Once laparoscopic access is obtained via the second site, the initial needle placement can be confirmed and any perforation repaired. The decision to repair the injury laparoscopically versus open is based on the experience and comfort of the surgeon. Though these complications are rare (0.05–0.2%), they do occur and vigilance is mandatory *(1–5)*.

Assuming no ill events have occurred, the next step is to inject 10 cc of saline through the needle and aspirate while maintaining elevation on the abdominal wall. No fluid should return. Next, a water droplet is placed at the hub of the needle and visually confirmed to pass freely into the abdominal cavity while elevating the abdominal wall. Inability to perform either of these steps suggests that the needle is not in the correct position and likely properitoneal. The needle should be removed, repassed and the steps listed above performed from the beginning. The final step is attaching the insufflator to the trocar. The initial pressure reading should be low (< 8 mmHg), the abdomen insufflated at a low flow rate (1–2 l/min), and no resistance confirmed. Once these steps have been completed, the flow rate may be increased and a four-quadrant pneumoperitoneum obtained.

Traditionally a sharp tip cone shaped trocar was used to penetrate the abdominal wall. Recently, newly designed disposable trocars have been introduced to further decrease the risk of inadvertent injury. These include trocars with flat blades that retract upon entering the abdominal cavity, blunt tip trocars that radially dilate as they are inserted, and "one step" trocars that utilize a mesh-like sleeve that is introduced with the Veress needle and serves as a tract through which a blunt tip radially dilating trocar may be placed (Fig. 10a, b). Advantages of radially dilating trocars are that they do not require closure of the fascia and may cause less pain than traditional cutting trocars *(6,7)*. Radially dilating trocars have also been shown to cause less abdominal wall bleeding *(8)*. Blunt versus sharp access, in general, uses muscle splitting (and subsequent muscle retraction) and has been shown to reduce the rate of incisional hernia and reduce the likelihood of trocar-related bleeding *(9, 10)*. Clear or optical access trocars, which allow a 0-degree laparoscope to be placed within the tip of the trocar, are being used with increasing frequency (Fig. 10a, b). These trocars allow the surgeon to visualize the different layers of the abdominal wall during placement into the peritoneal cavity. Some surgeons have used this

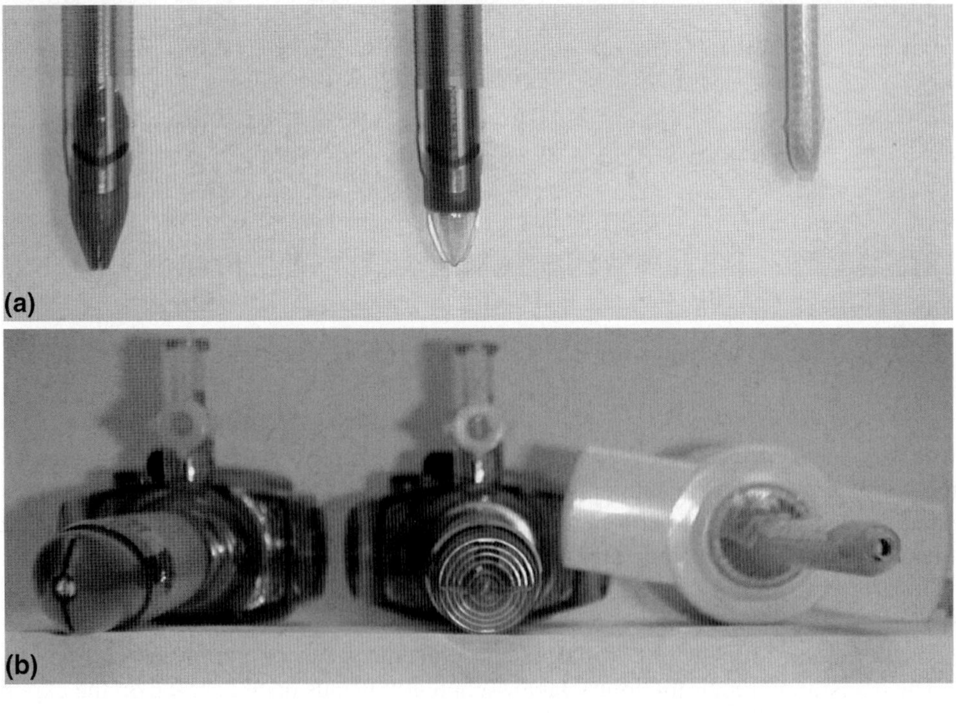

Fig. 10. Specialized trocar tips: (**a**) cutting flat blade, clear non-cutting blunt tip, radially expanding (*left to right*) and (**b**) tip perspective of prior trocars.

clear tip trocar to access the abdomen without prior insufflation *(11,12)*. No technique for obtaining access is completely safe, however, and injuries have been reported using clear trocars despite direct visualization *(13,14)*.

In general, trocars with a sharp tip, designed for cutting tissue, should be inserted without rotation. Trocars with a blunt tip, designed to dilate the tissues, should be inserted by rotating the trocar between the 10 and 2 o'clock position and applying a steady downward force. All trocars should be held in the palm of the hand with the index finger extended down the shaft to prevent inserting the trocar too far too quickly (Fig. 11). Once in position the inner cannula of the trocar is removed immediately and the laparoscope placed to ensure proper placement and inspect the viscera.

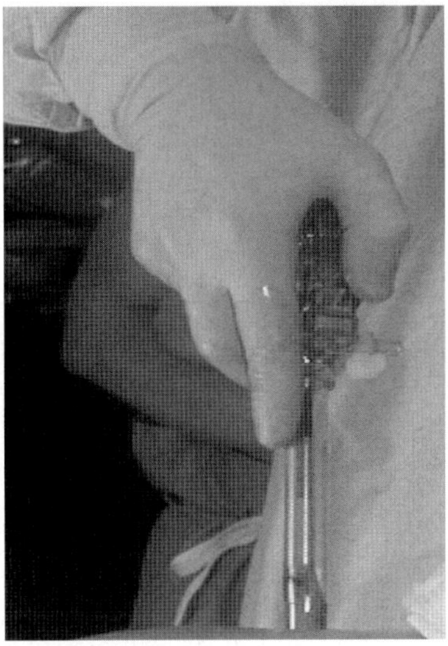

Fig. 11. Technique for inserting trocar.

Another option for laparoscopic access is the open or Hassan technique. Hassan introduced this method to minimize the risk of inadvertent injury thought to be associated with the closed technique *(15)*. Open access may eliminate the risk of major vascular injury and significantly reduce the rate of major visceral injury *(16)*. The open technique may be utilized during any transperitoneal approach and should be used in cases of previous intra-abdominal surgery, all retroperitoneal approaches, preperitoneal approaches, and when hand-assisted laparoscopy is to be performed. When performing a transperitoneal approach, a semi-circular incision is created either infra- or supra-umbilically (Fig. 12a). If there is a previous midline scar, the incision may be placed in an alternative position, usually lateral to the rectus and in a quadrant away from the previous surgery. The subcutaneous fat is cleared from the fascia using a combination of S retractors and a Kelly clamp. A 1.5 mm incision is created within the fascia, the peritoneum identified, grasped between two clamps and incised sharply (Fig. 12b). Entry into the abdominal cavity is confirmed visually or by placing a finger into the cavity and circumferentially palpating the smooth peritoneum lining the anterior abdominal wall (Fig. 12c).

For retroperitoneal access, a horizontal incision is placed 2 mm inferior to the tip of the 12th rib (Fig. 13a). The subcutaneous fat is cleared from the fascia using a combination of S retractors and a Kelly clamp. The lumbodorsal fascia is either incised or traversed bluntly with a Kelly clamp. Palpating the psoas muscle and/or visualization confirms entry into the retroperitoneum (Fig. 13b). A balloon dilator is inserted and expanded to increase the working space prior to placement of any trocars. The

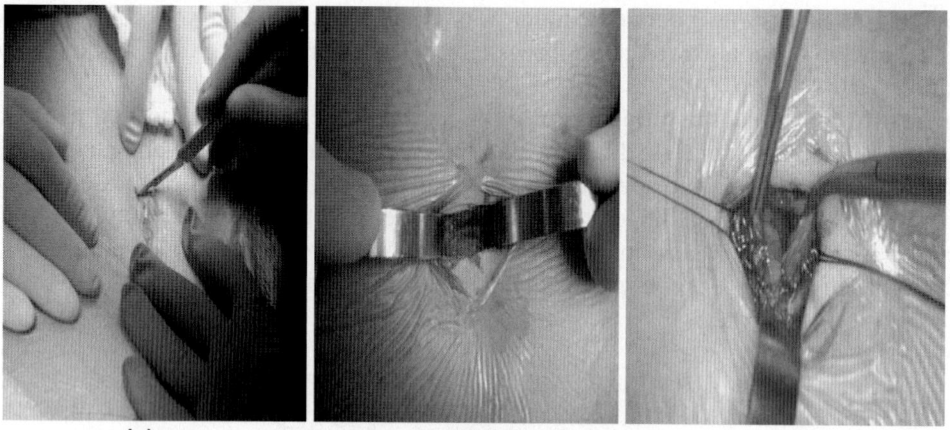

(a) (b) (c)

Fig. 12. (**a**), (**b**), and (**c**): Hassan technique transperitoneal.

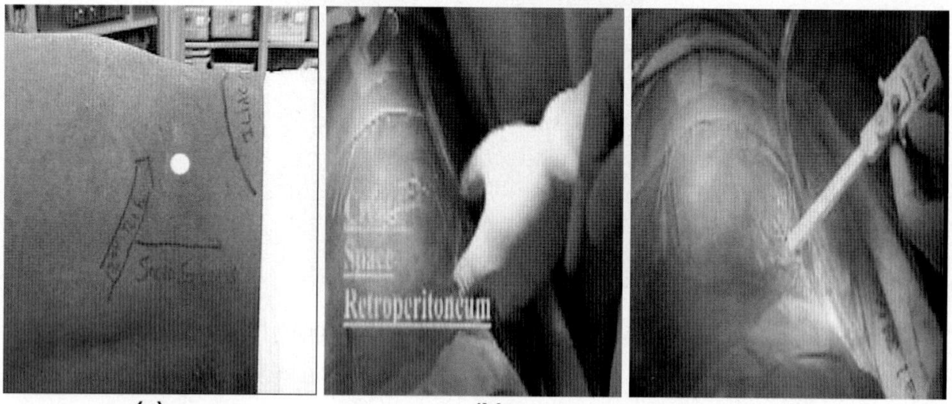

(a) (b) (c)

Fig. 13. (**a**), (**b**), and (**c**): Hassan technique retroperitoneal.

laparoscope may be inserted into the clear balloon dilator to confirm proper placement by identifying the psoas, ureter, and gonadal vessels (Fig. 13c, d).

For preperitoneal access (e.g., for laparoscopic radical prostatectomy or pelvic lymph node dissection), a trocar incision is made infra-umbilically or between the umbilicus and pubic symphysis *(17)*. Dissection is carried down to the rectus sheath which is incised and stay sutures are placed in the fascia. The rectus muscle is split, transversalis fascia incised, and blunt finger dissection is performed into the space of Retzius. A balloon dilator is inserted into this space and expanded. A blunt trocar is then inserted and secured with the previously placed stay sutures; visual confirmation of preperitoneal placement is made and the space is insufflated. Subsequent trocars are placed under direct visualization *(17)*.

Once access is confirmed, a Hassan trocar is placed. The Hassan has three parts: the outer sheath, blunt obturator, and cone that is movable along the sheath and may be locked into position. In addition the Hassan has wings or olives at the base of the trocar's outer sheath, where fascial sutures are wrapped and locked. The fascial sutures placed on each side of the incision help to wedge the trocar and cone

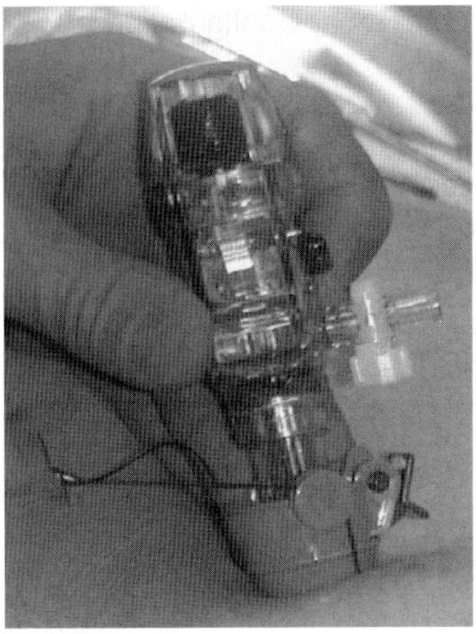

Fig. 14. Securing Hassan on olive.

tip firmly in the incision preventing CO_2 leakage (Fig. 14). Another option is to place a purse string suture within the fascia incision to prevent CO_2 leakage and lock these about the wings of the Hassan trocar. Recently, a new type of trocar has been introduced with an inflatable balloon at the tip. This may be used instead of a traditional cone shaped Hassan trocar and does not need fascial sutures. Once inserted, the balloon is inflated and the base of the trocar is pressed against the skin creating an airtight seal (Fig. 15). Crucial to all trocars used for open access is a tight secure fit that allows for movement of the trocar while also maintaining an airtight seal. Gas leak can be problematic by compromising exposure and prolonging operative time.

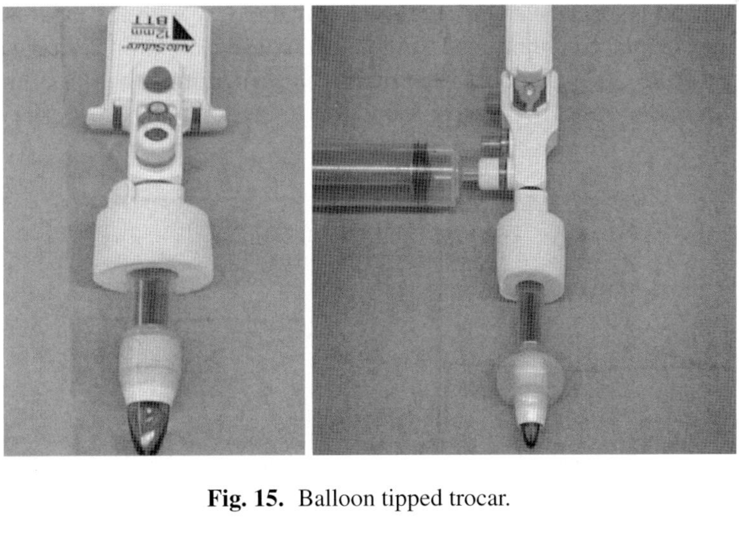

Fig. 15. Balloon tipped trocar.

Finally, in cases utilizing hand-assisted laparoscopy we recommend creating the hand incision initially to gain access to the peritoneal cavity. Our preferred hand incision sites for a nephrectomy are outlined in Fig. 16. The newer generation devices allow a trocar to be placed through the device

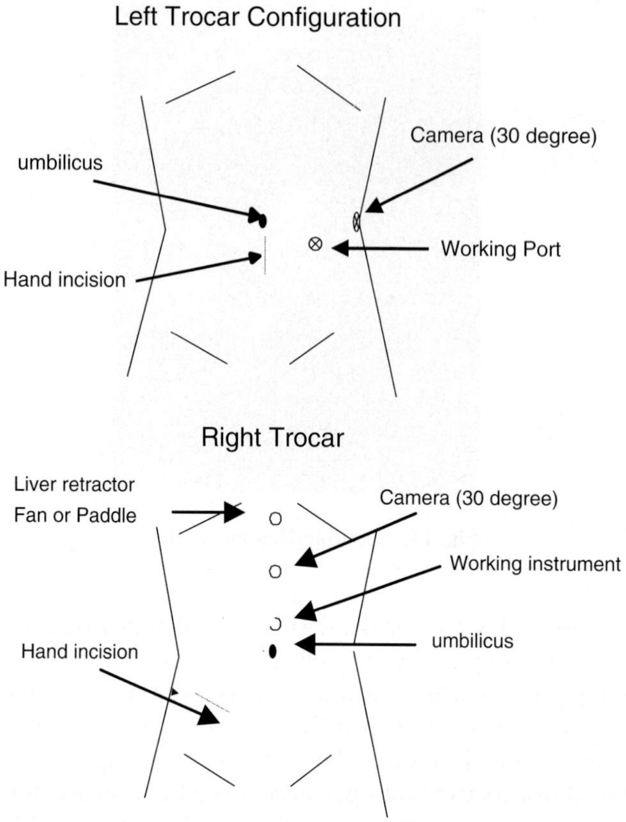

Fig. 16. HAL incision site for left and right nephrectomy.

allowing insufflation and inspection of the intra-abdominal cavity with the laparoscope (Fig. 17). The secondary trocars may be placed either under direct vision or by palpation with the non-dominant hand in the abdomen protecting the intra-abdominal organs. Insufflation is then performed with all trocars in place through a secondary trocar. We have found this approach to be most effective.

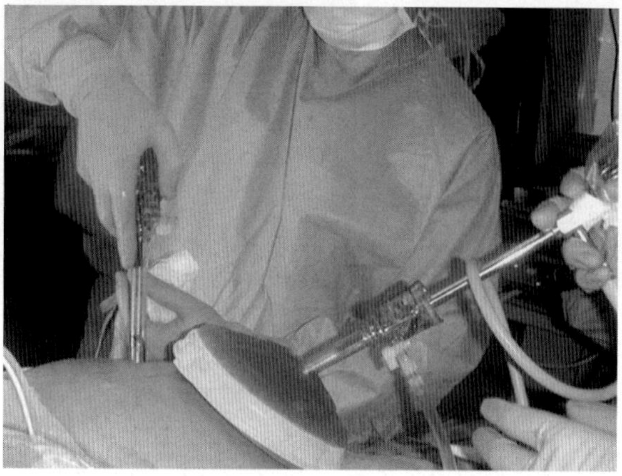

Fig. 17. Trocar inserted through hand device allowing placement of laparoscope and secondary trocars.

Exiting the abdomen should be performed with care. All port sites should be inspected for bleeding. Port sites >10 mm in adults should be closed with fascial sutures and in children all port sites should be closed regardless of size *(18)*.

ANATOMIC CONSIDERATIONS

Use of anatomic landmarks helps to ensure proper positioning of trocars and guide exposure of relevant structures. For transperitoneal access on the left side, structures that overlie the kidney and adrenal are the spleen, pancreas, left colon, and stomach. Mobilizing the splenic flexure medially and dividing the splenocolic ligament are initial steps to expose the left kidney *(17)*. On the right side, the hepatic flexure sits at a lower level, and mobilization is necessary to expose the kidney. For retroperitoneoscopy, the retroperitoneal space is developed with a balloon dissector and landmarks include the psoas posteriorly and the lower pole of the kidney superiorly. Other important landmarks are the peritoneal reflection, ureter and/or gonadal vein, aortic pulsation, renal artery pulsation, and the inferior vena cava *(19)*. Identifying at least four landmarks on entrance into the retroperitoneum can significantly accelerate hilar dissection *(19)*. For transperitoneal pelvic exposure, notable anatomic landmarks include the medial and lateral umbilical ligaments, as well as the vas deferens in males *(17)*.

COMPLICATIONS OF LAPAROSCOPIC ACCESS

During initial port placement, care should be taken to avoid injury to the epigastric vessels. Transillumination is useful to ensure avoidance of vessels on subsequent port placement. If a vessel is traumatized, the trocar alone may tamponade bleeding, or a foley catheter may be placed through the trocar site and pulled back for tamponade effect *(20)*. Deep sutures may be placed through the trocar site if necessary *(20)*.

Trocar-related complications are most commonly bowel and vascular injuries and can be catastrophic if recognition is delayed. Thin patients may be at increased risk for trocar injury to viscera or major vessels *(4)*. Open conversion is generally required to control bleeding from large vessels, though major venous injuries may be repaired laparoscopically. Laparoscopic repair is aided by increasing insufflation pressure to 15 mmHg, holding edges of venotomy/arteriotomy with atraumatic graspers and closing the vascular injury with running dissolvable suture *(4)*. Small arterial injuries may be sutured if possible but open conversion is generally required.

Visceral injury from trocar placement should be repaired at the time of injury. Delayed recognition can be devastating. Evidence of perforation post-operatively may be ileus or peritonitis *(20)*. Prior abdominal surgery, specifically an upper midline scar or ipsilateral upper quadrant scar, is associated with a higher access-related complication rate *(21)*. A retroperitoneal approach should be considered in patients with history of significant abdominal surgery.

Small bowel injuries can often be sutured or stapled laparoscopically. Large bowel injuries without spillage can also be repaired laparoscopically and the patient treated with intravenous antibiotics and drainage *(4)*. If spillage occurs, open repair and lavage with proximal diversion is generally necessary *(4)*.

Trocar-related bladder injuries should be carefully repaired if intraperitoneal injury has occurred, either laparoscopically or open, with foley catheter drainage post-operatively *(22)*. Foley catheter placement preoperatively decompresses the bladder and minimizes the likelihood of intraoperative bladder injury.

THE FUTURE OF LAPAROSCOPIC ACCESS

The future of laparoscopic access lies in further minimizing its invasiveness. For example, single trocar laparoscopic nephrectomy has been safely performed in the porcine model using magnetically anchored instrumentation *(23)*. Advantages of single "keyhole" surgery include further reducing wound morbidity and potential use of natural orifices. Also development of magnetic anchored instrumentation may help to overcome the limitations of fixed trocar technology.

REFERENCES

1. Crist DW, Gadacz TR. Complications of laparoscopic surgery. Surgery Clinics of North America. 73:265–289, 1993.
2. Baadsgaard SE, Bille S, Egebald K. Major vascular injuries during gynecologic surgery. ACATA Obstet Gynecol Scand. 68:283–285, 1989.
3. Champault G, Cazacu F, Taffinder N. Serious trocar accidents in laparoscopic surgery: a French survey of 103,852 operations. Surg Laparosc Endosc 6(5):367–370, 1996.
4. Pemberton RJ, Tolley DA, van Velthoven RF. Prevention and management of complications in urological laparoscopic port placement. Eur Urol. 50:958–968, 2006.
5. Vallancien G, Cathelineau X, Baumert H et al. Complications of transperitoneal laparoscopic surgery in urology: review of 1311 procedures at a single center. J Urol. 168(1):23–26, 2002 Jul.
6. Yim SF, Yuen PM. Randomized double-masked comparison of radially expanding access device and conventional cutting tip trocar in laparoscopy. Obstet Gynecol. 97(3):435–438, 2001.
7. Lam TY, Lee SW, So HS. Kwok SP. Radially expanding trocar: a less painful alternative for laparoscopic surgery. J Laparoendosc Adv Surg Tech A. 10(5):269–273, 2000.
8. Bhoyrul S, Payne J, Steffes B et al. A randomized prospective study of radially expanding trocars in laparoscopic surgery. J Gastrointest Surg. 4:392–397, 2000.
9. Shalhav AL, Barret E, Lifshitz DA et al. Transperitoneal laparoscopic renal surgery using blunt 12-mm trocar without fascial closure. J Endourol. 16(1):43–46, 2002.
10. Leibl BJ, Schmedt CG, Schwarz J et al. Laparoscopic surgery complications associated with trocar tip design: review of literature and own results. J Laparoendosc Adv Surg Tech A. 9:135–140, 1999.
11. String A, Berber E, Foroutani A, Macho JR, Pearl JM, Siperstein AE. Use of the optical trocar for safe and rapid entry in various laparoscopic procedures. Surg Endosc. 15(6):570–573, 2001.
12. Marcovich R, Del Terzo MA, Wolf JS Jr. Comparison of transperitoneal laparoscopic access technique: optiview visualizing trocar and Veress needle. J Endourol. 14(2):175–179, 2000.
13. Orvieto M, Breyer B, Sokoloff M et al. Aortic injury during initial blunt trocar laparoscopic access for renal surgery. J Urol. 171(349–350), 2004.
14. Thomas MA, Rha KH, Ong AM et al. Optical access trocar injuries in urological laparoscopic surgery. J Urol. 170: 61–63, 2003.
15. Hasson HM. Modified instrument and method for laparoscopy. Am J Obstet Gynecol, 110:886–887, 1971.
16. Larobina M, Nottle P. Complete evidence regarding major vascular injuries during laparoscopic access. Surg Laparosc Endosc Percutan Tech. 15:119–123, 2005.
17. Abdelmaksoud A, Biyani CS, Bagheri F et al. Laparoscopic approaches in urology. BJU Intl. 95:244–249, 2005.
18. Bloom DA, Ehrlich RM. Omental evisceration through small laparoscopy port sites. J Endourol. 7(1):31–32, 1993.
19. Sung GT, Gill IS. Anatomic landmarks and time management during retroperitoneoscopic radical nephrectomy. J Endourol. 16:165–169, 2002.
20. Madeb R, Koniaris LG, Patel HRH et al. Complications of laparoscopic urologic surgery. J Lap Adv Surg Tech. 14(5):287–301, 2004.
21. Seifman BD, Dunn RL, Wolf JS Jr. Transperitoneal laparoscopy into the previously operated abdomen: Effect on operative time, length of stay and complications. J Urol. 169:36–40, 2003.
22. Thomas R, Steele R, Ahuja S. Complications of urological laparoscopy: A standardized 1 institution experience. J Urol. 156:469–471, 1996.
23. Zeltser IS, Bergs R, Fernandez R et al. Single trocar laparoscopic nephrectomy using magnetic anchoring and guidance system in the porcine model. J Urol. 178:288–291, 2007.

Laparoscopic and Robotic Pelvic Lymphadenectomy

Vincent G. Bird and Howard N. Winfield

INTRODUCTION

In 1991, Schuessler et al. first reported the application of laparoscopic pelvic lymph node dissection (L-PLND) for staging of adenocarcinoma of the prostate *(1)*. Subsequently, laparoscopic-limited obturator PLND, and in select cases, extended obturator and iliopsoas node dissection, has become the primary initial application of urologic laparoscopic surgery as a diagnostic and therapeutic technique *(2)*. Follow-up studies on L-PLND clearly indicated that this procedure was comparable in accuracy and significantly less morbid than open PLND (Table 1) *(3–6)*. While early studies showed a longer operative time for L-PLND, they also demonstrated a significant reduction in postoperative pain, hospitalization, and convalescence compared with open PLND (3–5). As expected, L-PLND initially showed an increased overall cost. However, with gradual refinements of technique, reusable equipment, and a reduced need for specialized instrumentation, overall cost is now likely to be equivalent to or less than open PLND *(7–9)*. More recently, robot-assisted L-PLND has been performed in conjunction with robot-assisted laparoscopic radical prostatectomy, both by the transperitoneal and extraperitoneal routes. The cost effectiveness of this procedure is unclear in light of the need for significant capital investment in the robotic device, its maintenance, and the ongoing need for limited reusable accessories.

In the early 1990s L-PLND was predominantly used as a means of determining which patients with adenocarcinoma of the prostate were candidates for localized and potentially curative therapy in the form of surgery or radiation. Refinements in PSA testing such as percent free analysis and results from large-scale studies have led to earlier detection of prostate cancer and better defined which patients are candidates for curative procedures. Thus, indications for L-PLND have diminished. Possible indications today for this procedure are listed in Table 2.

Case-specific indications for L-PLND with respect to other forms of genitourinary malignancy also exist. Extended obturator node and iliopsoas node dissection have been applied for staging and evaluation of genitourinary malignancies such as bladder cancer, and other less common entities, such as penile and urethral cancer. These procedures generally require considerable laparoscopic experience and such extended dissections are obviously more time-consuming. However, the majority of these patients are still discharged home within 24 h. An extended L-PLND for adenocarcinoma of the prostate also has been shown to yield more positive nodes than limited PLND. However, the debate

From: *Current Clinical Urology: Essential Urologic Laparoscopy*
Edited by: S. Y. Nakada and S. P. Hedican, DOI 10.1007/978-1-60327-820-1_4

Table 1
Comparison between laparoscopic (L-PLND) and open pelvic lymph node dissection (O-PLND) for prostate cancer

	Study					
	Winfield et al. (3)		*Kerbl et al. (4)*		*Parra et al. (5)*	
Variable	L-PLND	O-PLND	L-PLND	O-PLND	L-PLND	O-PLND
No. of patients	89	26	30	16	12	12
Average age	68	65	69.7	65.5	67.0	67.9
Average Gleason score	6	7	–	–	7.5	5.25
Average no. of nodes removed	9	11	–	–	10.7	11
Average EBL (ml)	<100	215	100	212	<100	<100
Average OR time (min)	154	124	199	102	185	–
Average postoperative NPO (h)	9	24	14	67	–	–
Average parenteral narcotic (MS equivalent mg)	6.5	32.4	1.55	47	–	–
Average oral narcotic (codeine equivalent, mg)	26.5	67.0	–	–	–	–
Average postoperative time, hospitalization (days)	1.5	6.5	1.7	5.3	–	–
Average convalescence (days)	7	17	4.9	42.9	–	–

EBL, estimated blood loss; MS, morphine sulfate.

Table 2
Indications for obturator L-PLND in prostate cancer patients

- Clinical stage T2b–T3a
    - Whether surgery, radiation therapy, or hormonal manipulation is being considered; bone scan and CT are negative for metastatic disease
- Patients with stage T1b
    - With Gleason sums = 7 (4+3 more worrisome than 3+4)
- PSA <20 ng/mL
- Patients scheduled to undergo aperineal prostatectomy, brachytherapy, external beam radiotherapy or laparoscopic/robotic prostatectomy who have a risk of node positivity >25%
- Patients with suspicious lymph nodes visualized on CT that are not amenable to guided needle biopsy

continues as to whether the added morbidity of an extended dissection is worthy of node-positive detection with respect to long-term impact on patient survival *(10,11)*.

Complication rates for L-PLND have been relatively low (8 and 6% for major and minor complications, respectively) and have been reported as substantially lower with further experience *(12)*. The most common intraoperative complications are vascular, ureteral, bladder, bowel, and obturator nerve injury. The most common postoperative complications include urinary retention, prolonged ileus, lymphedema, and lymphocele formation. There have been no reported operative mortalities *(13,14)*. Clearly, L-PLND was the stepping-stone for urologists in gaining laparoscopic experience and proceeding to more advanced procedures. It has since allowed urologists to apply laparoscopic principles to other genitourinary disease entities, such as renal, bladder, and prostatic pathologies. Initial reports from robot-assisted series where PLND has been performed in conjunction with radical prostatectomy also demonstrate low complication rates with this evolving technique *(15)*.

PATIENTS

Selection and Assessment

As with open surgery, a complete assessment of the patient as an adequate candidate for L-PLND is necessary. Table 3 lists relative and absolute contraindications. Relative contraindications may become less of an issue as the surgeon gains laparoscopic experience. As with all laparoscopic procedures, the patient should always be informed that the potential for an open procedure exists should there be difficulty with complex anatomy or unforeseen complications.

Table 3
Relative and absolute contraindications to laparoscopic surgery *(11)*

Relative	
	Gross obesity
	Hiatal hernia
	Umbilical hernia
	Significant previous intraperitoneal surgery
	Abdominal wall infection
	Bowel obstruction
Absolute	
	Generalized peritonitis
	Severe obstructive airways disease
	Coagulopathy – uncorrectable
	Cardiac disease – inoperable
	Shock
	Morbid obesity

Preoperative Preparation

Specific preoperative preparation may involve clear fluids only the day prior. If the patient has certain preoperative features that may make bowel or other visceral organ injury more worrisome than normal, a limited bowel preparation of 1 gallon of Golytely® (Braintree Laboratories, Inc., Braintree, MA) or two bottles of magnesium citrate on the evening prior to surgery is suggested. A type and screen for blood products may be obtained depending on the surgeon's laparoscopic experience. A broad spectrum antibiotic should be administered on call to the operating room *(11)*.

Patients undergoing L-PLND in which the lymph nodes are negative on frozen section may be scheduled to proceed directly to radical prostatectomy in either an open, conventional laparoscopic, or robot-assisted laparoscopic approach.

OPERATING ROOM

Operating Room Set-Up

The operating room set-up for L-PLND is characterized in Fig. 1. The monitors are placed at the level of the hips of the patient on each side. The surgeon stands on the side of the table opposite the side of planned lymph node dissection. As one more routinely performs laparoscopic surgery it is quite helpful to have a regular operating room staff that is familiar with the dynamics and equipment needs of laparoscopic surgery.

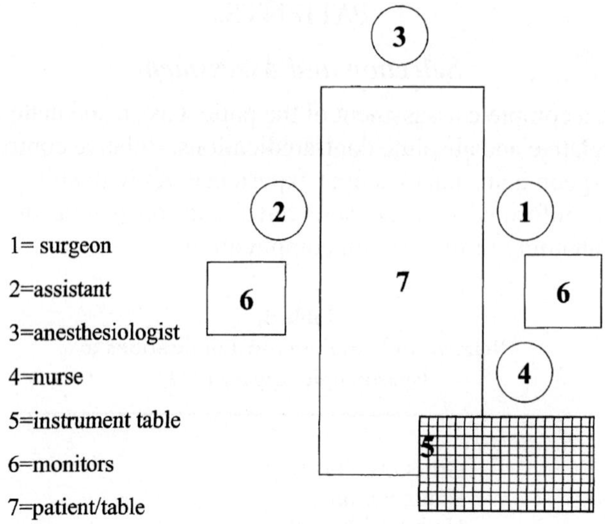

Fig. 1. Schematic of operating room set-up for L-PLND.

The operating room set-up for robot-assisted L-PLND follows standard room set-up and preparations for use of the surgical robot, which include the robotic operating device and the remote surgical console.

Patient Positioning and Preparation

The patient is placed in the supine position on an operating table capable of moving into Trendelenburg position and lateral rotation (Fig. 2). Pneumatic boots are then placed on the lower extremities. The patient is then given general anesthesia, preferably without the ongoing use of nitrous oxide, as this agent may cause gradual distention of the intestine resulting in possible compromise of the laparoscopic working space. An indwelling urethral catheter and orogastric tube are then placed for decompression of the bladder and stomach, respectively. The arms are padded and tucked in by the patient's sides. The lower extremities, including the heels of the feet, should also be well padded. Wide adhesive tape is then placed across the chest and thighs, which secures the patient and allows for table

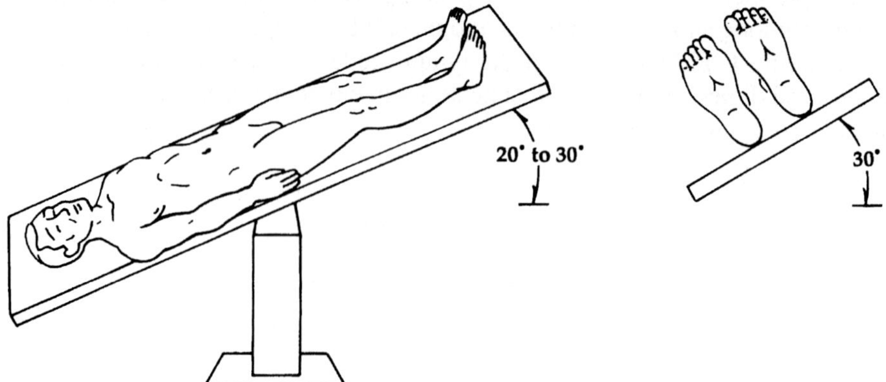

Fig. 2. Trendelenburg positioning and lateral rotation. (From Ref. *(11)*, permission granted.)

movement during the case as needed. The anesthesiologist must be informed that the patient is being secured across the chest to ensure that respiratory function is not compromised. The appearance of the properly positioned patient for standard L-PLND should appear as in Fig. 3. Patients undergoing robot-assisted PLND generally are positioned with the legs abducted on a Maquet split-leg table (Fig. 4) so that the legs are not flexed and there is less risk of lower extremity injury. The robot platform is then moved in between the patient's legs for docking. The use of leg stirrups is discouraged, due to patient sliding in the Trendelenburg position.

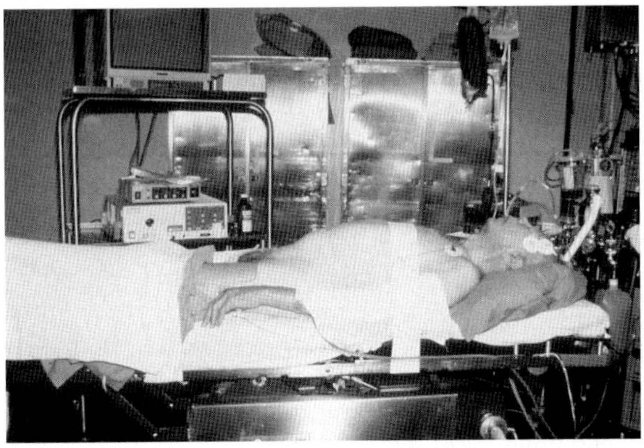

Fig. 3. Preparation of patient for L-PLND. With the patient well secured, the table can be safely placed in Trendelenburg, with lateral rotation as needed. (From Ref. *(11)*, permission granted.)

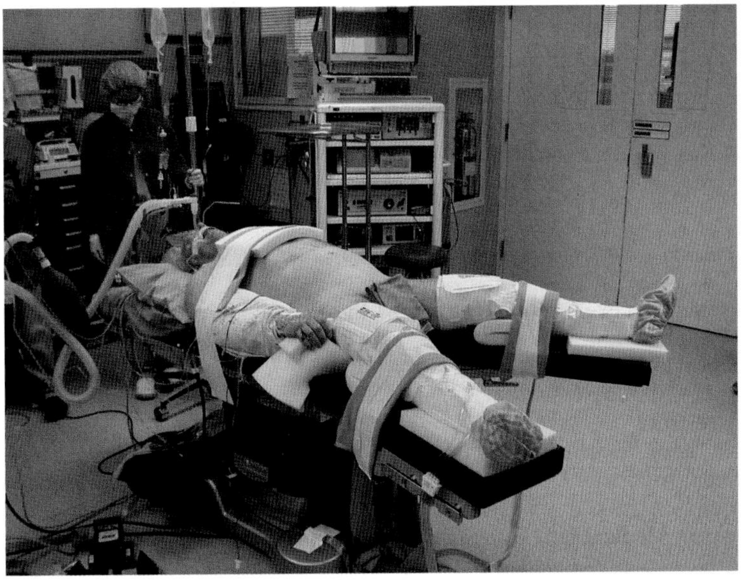

Fig. 4. Positioning on Maquet split-leg operating table for robotic or laparoscopic PLND.

Instrumentation

The continuing advancement of technology as it pertains to laparoscopic surgery results in a constant availability of new, high-quality equipment. Two television monitors, a three-chip camera, and use of both 0 and 30° lenses are sufficient for L-PLND. High-quality insufflators and light sources/cables are also readily available. A standard laparoscopy tray is also needed. For robot-assisted L-PLND, the surgical robot, its accompanying control tower, and robotic instrument accessories are all required. Our equipment tray includes the items listed in Table 4 *(10)*. All equipment is assembled, inspected, tested, and positioned before initiation of the procedure.

Table 4
Instrumentation for laparoscopic pelvic lymphadenectomy *(10)* and robot-assisted laparoscopic pelvic lymphadenectomy

Towel clips – to secure drapes/instrumentation
No. 15 surgical blade – for skin incision
14-gauge Veress needle – for initial entry
For possible initial entry by minilaparotomy
Hasson-type cannula
Two Sinn/S-type retractors
Two absorbable sutures
Trocars: standard – two 5 mm and two 10/11 mm
Obese patients – two 5 mm and three 10/11 mm
Trocar reducers
One 5 mm electrosurgical scissors
Two 5 mm atraumatic grasping forceps (spoon and dolphin types)
One 5 mm traumatic locking/grasping forceps (rat tooth)
One 5 mm fan-type retractor
One 10 mm traumatic grasping forceps (spoon type)
One 5 mm aspirator/irrigator (recommended: Nezhat–Dorsey irrigator/aspirator)
Two or three 0-absorbable sutures to close 10 mm ports
4-0 absorbable sutures to close port site skin incisions
Needle holder
Suture scissors
Two Kelly clamps
Other optional equipment:
Container for warm water to prevent scope fogging, or anti-fog solution (e.g., FRED)
Entrapment sacs for lymph nodes
10 mm multiload occlusive clip applier
One 5 mm Babcock
One 5 mm dissecting scissors
One 5 mm right-angle "hook" electrosurgical probe
One 5 mm straight fine tip dissector
One 5 mm bipolar equipped grasper
Carter–Thomason® (Inlet Medical Inc., Eden Prairie, MN) port closure set (consists of cone and suture passer)
Steri-strips
Tegaderm dressing
Equipment specific to robot-assisted laparoscopic pelvic lymphadenectomy
Monopolar hook cautery
Bipolar graspers
Roundtip or curved robotic scissors
deBakey or Cardier graspers

OPERATIVE APPROACH

Port Placement

Laparoscopic and robot-assisted PLND may be performed by a transperitoneal or extraperitoneal approach. Ports for robot-assisted L-PLND ports are generally placed in a fashion that accompanies preparation for robot-assisted radical prostatectomy.

Transperitoneal L-PLND

For the transperitoneal pure laparoscopic approach the patient is first placed in 10° Trendelenburg. The Veress needle is placed in the superior or inferior umbilical crease. When correct entry has been achieved, carbon dioxide insufflation is started and brought up to a pneumoperitoneal pressure of 20 mmHg. A 10/11 mm trocar/sheath unit is then inserted. Inspection of the abdominal cavity is then performed with the 10 mm laparoscope to ensure that no injury has occurred upon entry. A survey of the abdominal organs is also performed, with particular attention to the presence of abdominal adhesions. Additional ports are then placed under direct laparoscopic guidance. Our usual "diamond" shape arrangement of ports and sizes is shown in Fig. 5.

Obese patients with abundant fatty tissue may require additional retraction, and four working ports may be required, resulting in a "fan" or "inverted U" array (Fig. 6). Spatial arrangement of the ports may further vary in specific cases *(14)*. In addition, if laparoscopic radical prostatectomy is planned, the port placement may again vary to include five ports. When all ports have been placed, the surgeon may elect to secure them to the skin with 2–0 silk sutures to avoid potential dislodgement during the procedure. At this point abdominal pressure is lowered to 15 mmHg, the patient is placed in 30° Trendelenburg, and the table is laterally rotated to the left to allow the abdominal contents to fall away from the right-side field of dissection. The reverse would be required for left-sided PLND.

Port placement for the robot-assisted technique typically involves placement of five or six ports: one 12 mm umbilical or periumbilical port for the camera, two pararectal reusable 8 mm ports for

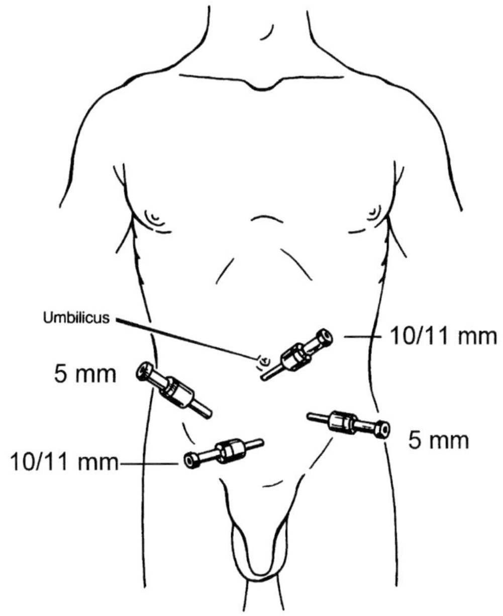

Fig. 5. Standard trocar arrangement for L-PLND. (From Ref. *(11)*, permission granted.)

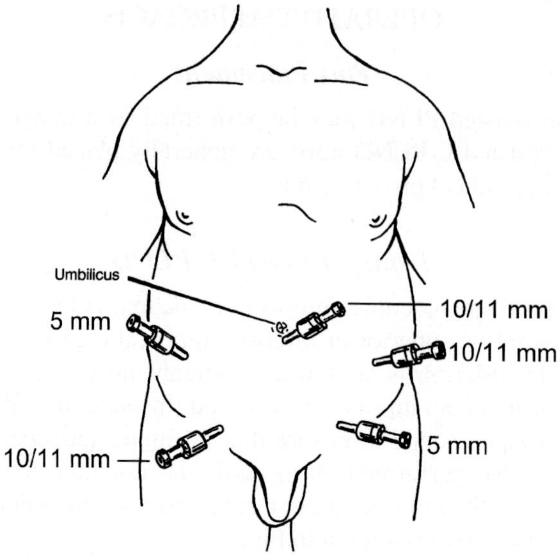

Fig. 6. Alternative trocar arrangement for L-PLND. (From Ref. *(11)*, permission granted.)

introduction of the robot instruments, and two working ports of variable size, dependent on surgeon preference. If a third robot arm is available for use, another trocar may be placed lateral to the right- or left-sided 8 mm robot port (Fig. 7). Precise placement of robot ports is essential to allow proper maneuverability of the robot arms.

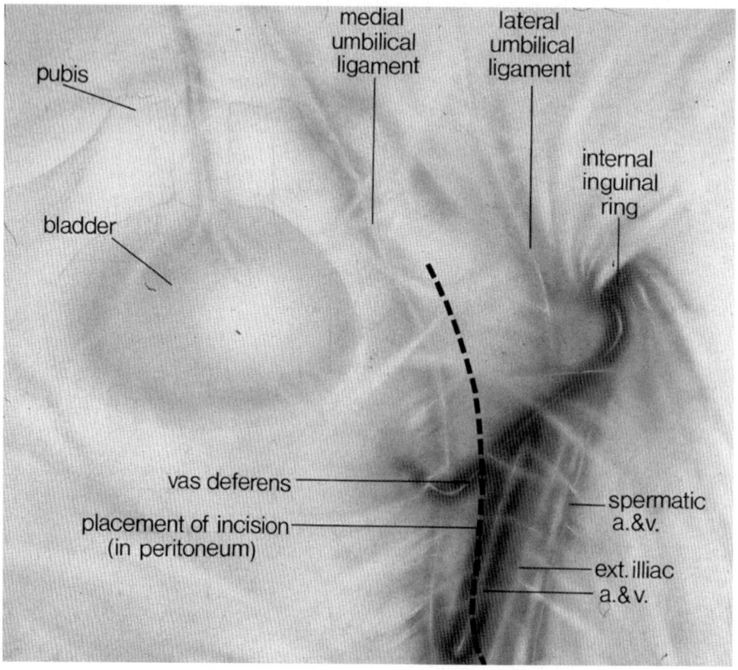

Fig. 7. Relationship of pelvic structures to peritoneal incision used for L-PLND.

Once ports have been placed the relevant pelvic anatomy must be identified. When one views the true pelvis from the umbilical region, the obliterated umbilical ligaments and testicular vessels should be identified. In thin patients the vas deferens can often be seen under the posterior peritoneum (Fig. 8). Dissection should normally be initiated on the side where most or all of the prostate tumor is present according to the prostate biopsy, or on the side where there is suspicious lymphadenopathy *(10)*.

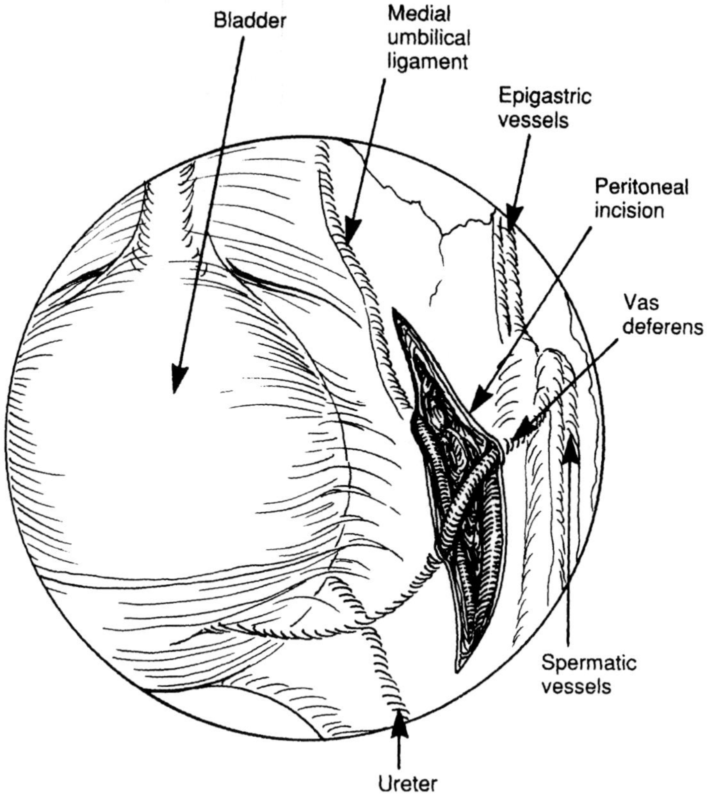

Fig. 8. The vas deferens is encountered after the peritoneal incision is made. (From Ref. *(11)*, permission granted.)

For conventional L-PLND, the surgeon uses the left lateral 5 mm port and the suprapubic 10 mm port when operating on the right pelvic lymph nodes. The assistant holds the camera through the umbilical port and retracts through the 5 mm right lateral port. For obese patients the surgeon would use the two lateral ports on his/her side. During robot-assisted procedures, the surgeon controls the camera and the two or three robotic arms. The assistant retracts and suctions as necessary. The initial incision is through the posterior peritoneum just lateral to the right obliterated (medial) umbilical ligament (Fig. 8). This incision is extended above the level of the internal inguinal ring anteriorly and is brought downwards, just medial to the pulsations of the right external iliac artery, which can usually be seen. This incision is completed posteriorly by continuing toward the level of the bifurcation of the common iliac vessels. This incision is best made by first scoring the line of incision with electrocautery and then grasping the edges to further open it with electrocautery scissors.

After the peritoneum has been opened, dissection through the immediate underlying fat will reveal the vas deferens (Fig. 9). The vas is safely and easily divided with cautery.

Dissection is then continued just inferior and medial to the pulsations of the external iliac artery until the external iliac artery is seen (Fig. 10). Our method of dissection used throughout this procedure generally involves gentle spreading of the tissue into packets and then slowly cauterizing and dividing

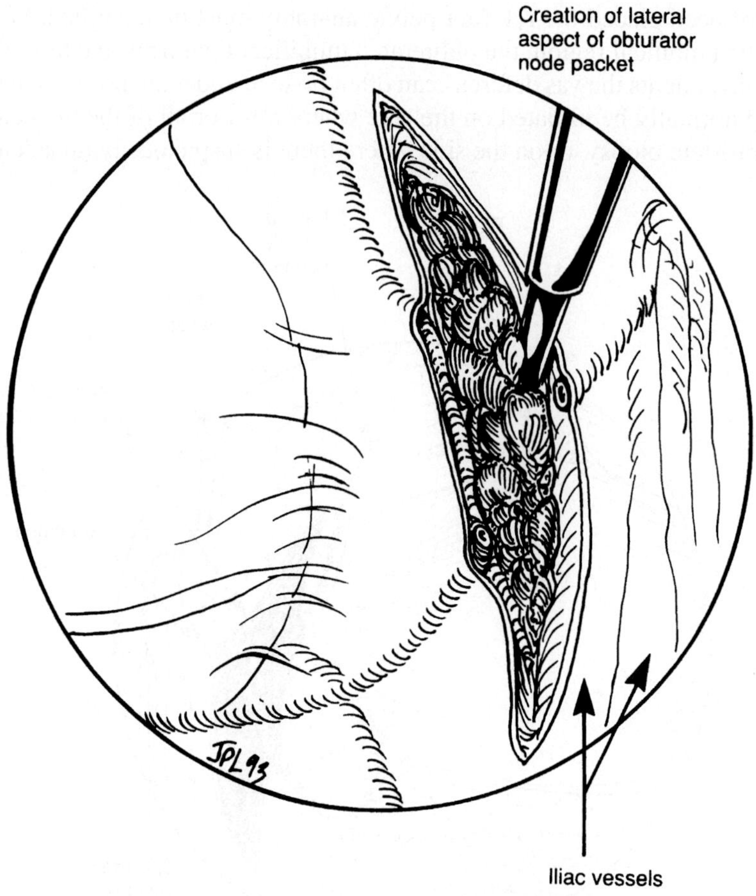

Fig. 9. The iliac vessels are identified. (From Ref. *(11)*, permission granted.)

them, being careful to note the absence of any other significant structures within. The assistant aids the surgeon with lateral retraction through the right lateral port. The fibrolymphatic tissue over the vein is cleared off the surface of the vein. This can be readily performed with a straight dissector. If the robot-assisted technique is being used, one of a variety of monopolar or bipolar instruments, as well as Debakey dissectors may be used. Once proper development of this layer has been initiated, it is continued down to the pelvic sidewall. This defines the lateral border of the lymph node dissection.

After the nodal tissue has been swept free of the pelvic sidewall, dissection is continued inferiorly to the level of the pubic bone (Fig. 11), which is usually easily identified visually as well as by tapping on it with one of the instruments. Proceeding inferiorly, the course of the obturator nerve and posterior vessels must be noted. Obturator vessels are prone to significant variations; thus, meticulous dissection is required. Posterior fat is carefully and slowly dissected through until these structures are identified. The nodal tissue is carefully swept off of these structures (Fig. 12).

The next step is to create the medial border of the lymph node package, by first retracting the obliterated umbilical ligament medially, and the identified lymph node package laterally (Fig. 13). This plane is developed with the same technique of carefully isolating packets of fibrofatty tissue, thinning them, and then proceeding with cautery. This dissection is continued inferiorly to the pubic bone. The lymph node package is then divided inferiorly right at the level of the pubic bone. This end of the package can then be retracted upwards and dissection is continued cranially toward the bifurcation

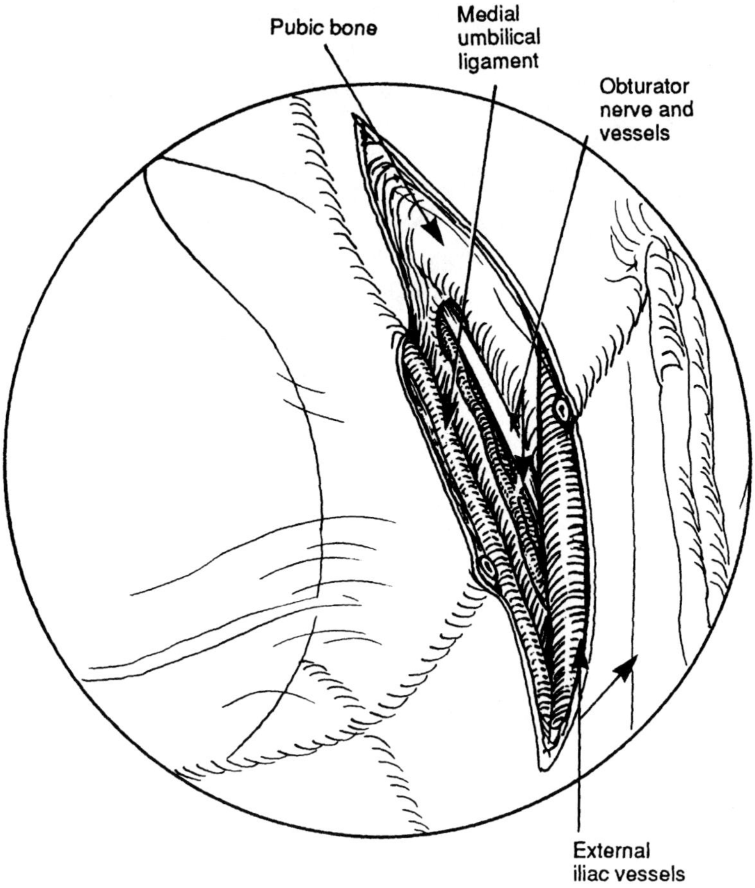

Fig. 10. The pubic bone is identified at the inferior aspect of the dissection. (From Ref. *(11)*, permission granted.)

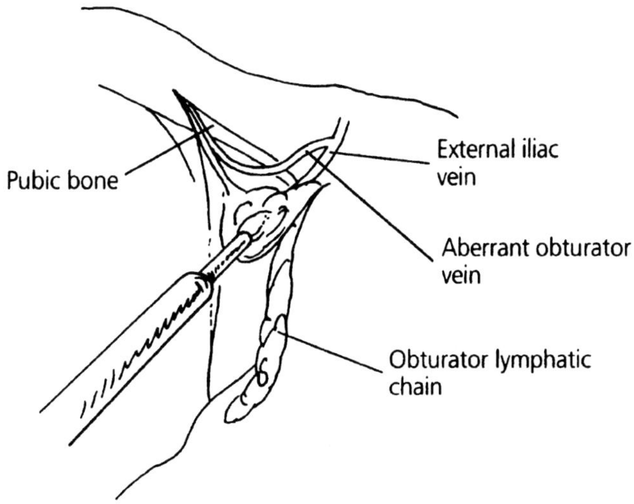

Fig. 11. The lymph node package is carefully freed from associated vessels. (From Ref. *(10)*, permission granted.)

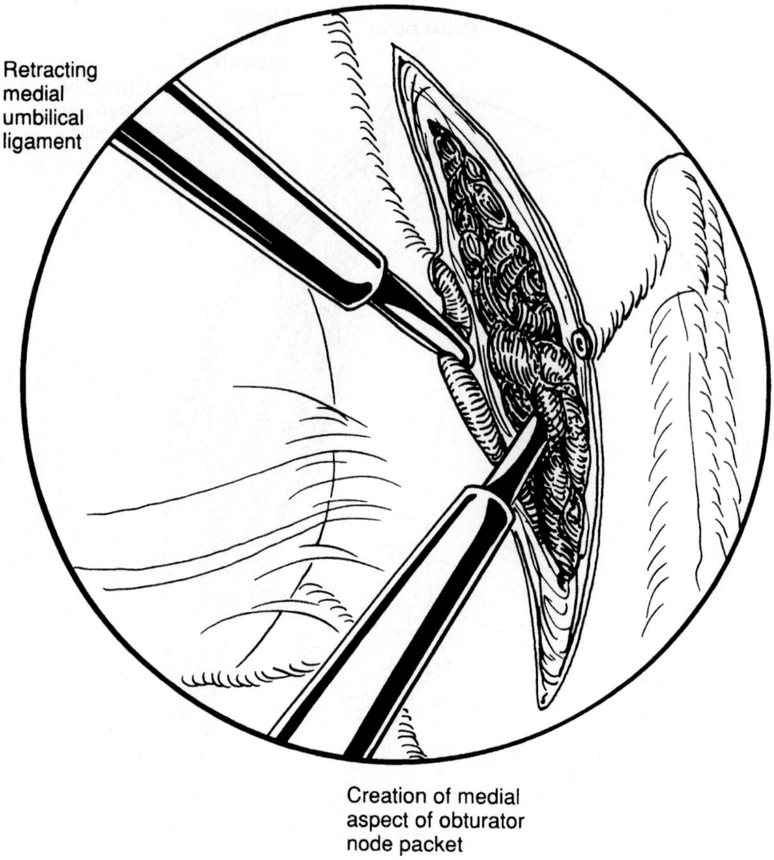

Fig. 12. The medial border of the dissection is then developed. (From Ref. *(11)*, permission granted.)

of the common iliac artery where the cranial end is divided (Fig. 14). The level of the obturator nerve is used as the posterior boundary for this portion of the dissection. Now that the lymph node package has been completely freed, it is removed using the 10 mm spoon shaped graspers through the inferior midline 10 mm port site. Alternatively, the package may be placed in an entrapment sac and pulled out of one of the port sites. The resection bed is then carefully inspected and any bleeding is controlled. Frozen section analysis is only performed if immediate radical prostatectomy is being considered, or if there is high suspicion of cancer that would preclude contralateral dissection.

Left-sided dissection is carried out when right-sided frozen section analysis is negative or when a bilateral procedure has been planned from the outset. Dissection is carried out in a similar fashion on the left side with only a few additional considerations and variations in technique. The patient is rotated now with the left side elevated. Often the sigmoid colon has a peritoneal attachment over the initial incision site (Fig. 15). Dissection of this attachment is performed by incising along the white line of Toldt, which will, with the aid of gravity, result in medial reflection needed prior to creation of an incision that is a mirror image of that made on the right (Fig. 16). Electrocautery should be used sparingly for this initial portion of the dissection so as to minimize the risk of bowel injury. In conventional left-sided L-PLND, it may also be beneficial for the surgeon to use the right and left lateral ports instead of the suprapubic trocar/sheath unit. For obese patients, the port configuration allows the surgeon the use of the two right-sided ports, and the assistant uses the two left-sided ports.

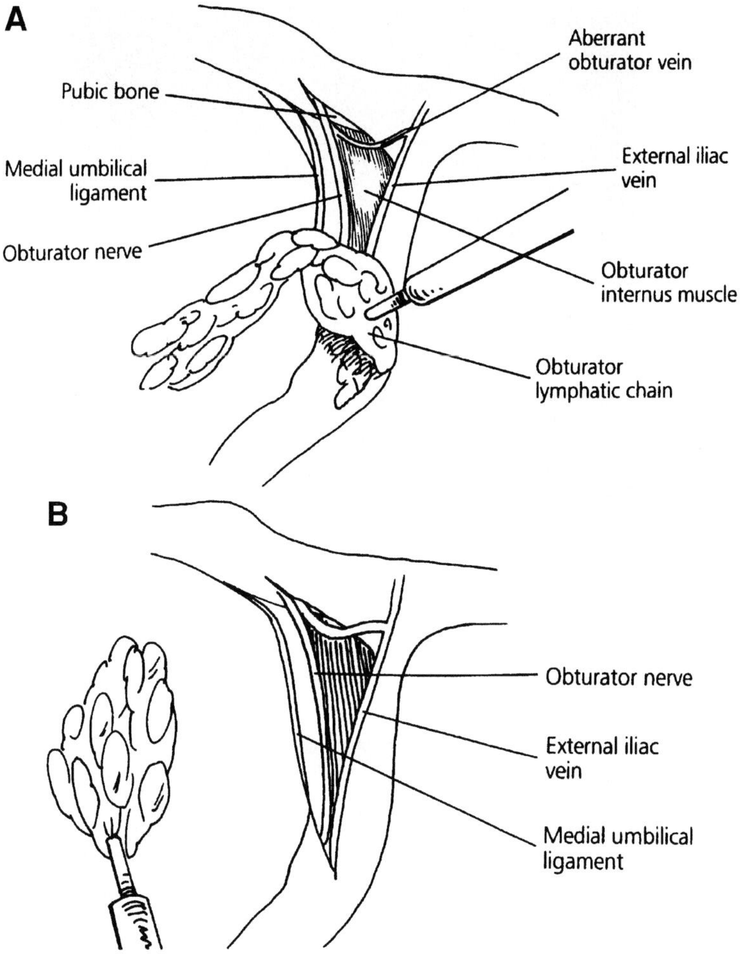

Fig. 13. **(A)** The lymph node package is retracted superiorly; **(B)** dissection is continued until the package is completely free. (From Ref. *(10)*, permission granted.)

Extraperitoneal L-PLND

The extraperitoneal approach is not used as commonly as the transperitoneal route, partly due to the need to open the retropubic space with balloon dissection, which creates a space not as well defined by natural planes, which may be confusing to the surgeon *(16)*. This procedure was developed after transperitoneal L-PLND with the belief that an extraperitoneal approach would, by maintaining the integrity of the peritoneal membrane, decrease the risks of visceral injury, preclude intraperitoneal spillage of potentially tumor-laden tissue, and prevent the potential postoperative development of intra-abdominal adhesions associated with instrumentation and manipulation of intraperitoneal contents. Such an approach may also preclude potentially time-consuming adhesiolysis in specific cases and bowel mobilization needed for extended lymph node dissection. The intact peritoneum may also aid in adequate exposure, which is at times difficult in the obese patient. However, the space developed by balloon dissection is small compared to the working space available for a transperitoneal approach. Furthermore, studies have revealed that patients undergoing the extraperitoneal approach appear to have higher postoperative analgesic requirements, possibly due to the stretching or tearing of nerve fibers during creation of a the retropubic space. Studies have also suggested that these patients appear

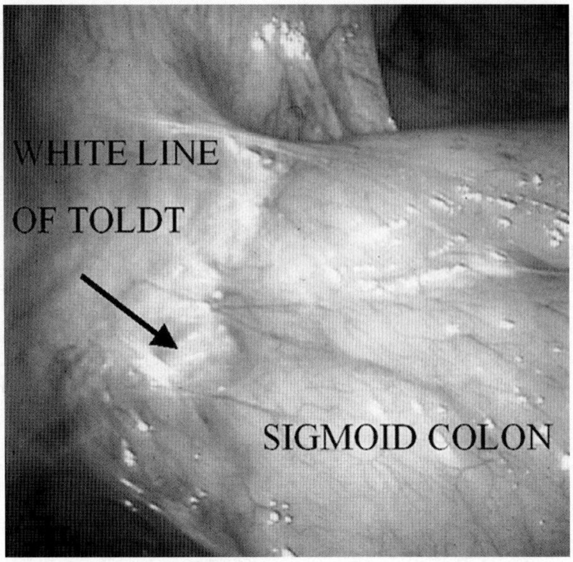

Fig. 14. The sigmoid colon must often be mobilized prior to initiation of left-sided L-PLND.

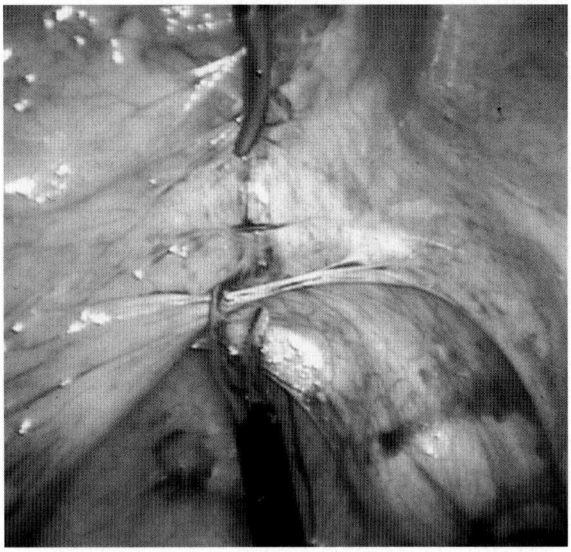

Fig. 15. The white line of Toldt is incised.

to have greater absorption of carbon dioxide, resulting in respiratory acidosis. Hypercarbia and acidosis have been associated with cardiac arrhythmias and cardiovascular compromise *(17)*. This technique may be contraindicated in patients with significant preexisting cardiopulmonary pathology. Patients who have undergone previous lower abdominal or inguinal surgery are also more prone to peritoneal membrane disruption during balloon dilation, which can further complicate the procedure.

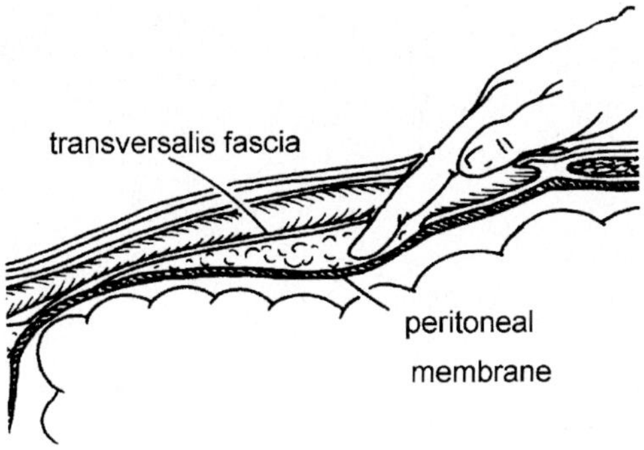

Fig. 16. Identification and development of the working space used in the extraperitoneal approach.

Extraperitoneal Operative Approach

This procedure is initiated with a subumbilical incision that is deepened down to the level of the rectus fascia. The fascia is divided in the midline, and creation of the properitoneal space is initiated with blunt finger dissection (Figs. 17 and 18) to the point at which a balloon inflation device may be inserted. Individually fashioned or specifically manufactured balloon inflation devices have both been used. We have previously described an easily fashionable device that consists of the finger cot of a transurethral resection drape tied to a 20 French red rubber (Robinson) urethral catheter *(18)*. Many commercial devices also exist. Whichever device is used, it is inserted and inflated with approximately 800–1,000 cc of saline to create an extraperitoneal working space. A Hasson-type cannula is then placed though the subumbilical incision, secured, and carbon dioxide insufflation up to 15 mmHg is begun. The laparoscope is then placed to completely survey the expanded space, with particular attention to any injury or peritoneal tears created by balloon inflation. It is important to recognize that this balloon dissection has created a space in which the pubic symphysis is already exposed. The obliterated umbilical ligaments are neither as apparent nor as necessary a landmark for dissection. The

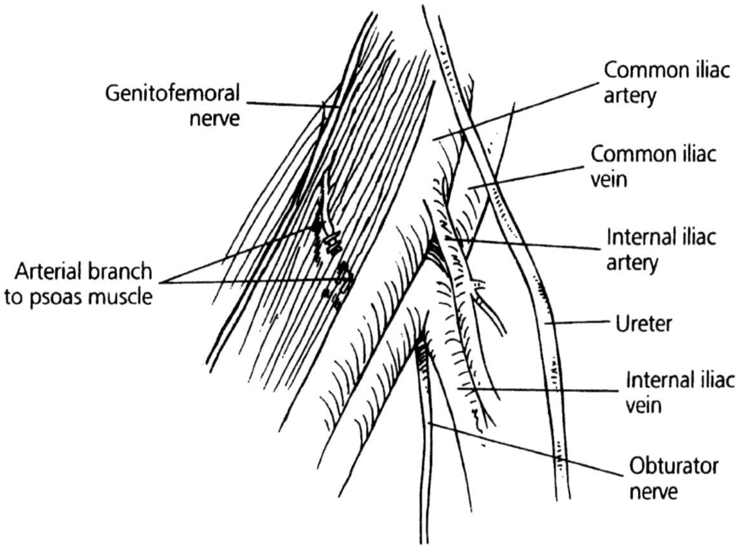

Fig. 17. Anatomy seen in extended L-PLND; if a small arterial branch going toward the psoas muscle is seen, it is usually clipped and ligated. (From Ref. *(10)*, permission granted.)

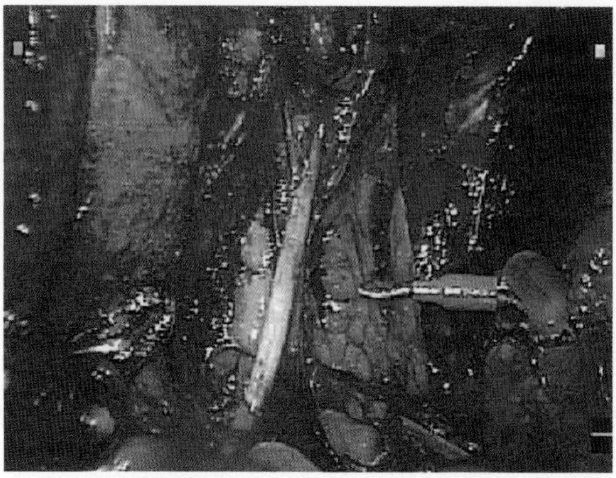

Fig. 18. Robotic dissection of left obturator fossa lymph nodes with exposure of obturator nerve.

vas deferens is now situated superiorly against the peritoneal membrane, and as such usually does not need to be transected.

Ports are placed in the same diamond configuration described for transperitoneal L-PLND. These ports must be placed into the properitoneal space under direct laparoscopic guidance so that they do not traverse the peritoneal membrane. Placement of ports for the extraperitoneal robotic approach is similar, which again, is a configuration used for concomitant radical prostatectomy. Proper mobilization of the peritoneum is required for all of extraperitoneal techniques. If the peritoneal membrane is violated, collapse of the properitoneal space will result. This may necessitate conversion to a transperitoneal procedure with subsequent intraperitoneal port placement.

The key to dissection in this procedure involves identifying the pulsations of the external iliac vessels. Dissection is begun by elevating the fibrofatty and adventitial tissue off the external iliac vein and continuing the procedure in a fashion similar to transperitoneal dissection.

Extended Lymph Node Dissection

Though obturator lymph node dissection is satisfactory for evaluation of prostate cancer, an extended lymph node dissection is required in cases of bladder, urethral, and penile cancer. An extended PLND may sometimes be carried out in patients with prostate cancer and negative obturator nodes that are highly suspected of having metastatic local disease (such as in cases of clinical T3 disease and/or markedly elevated PSA ($\geq$20) *(11)*.

For extended pelvic lymphadenectomy the "fan" or "inverted U" array as previously described is preferred as it allows for more assistance with retraction.

Lymph node dissection for these disease entities usually involves carrying the dissection out to the genitofemoral nerve laterally, to the bladder wall and ureter medially, the pubic bone caudally, and up to the bifurcation of the aorta cranially. This procedure has many similarities to standard PLND with a few modifications that account for inclusion of a larger lymph node package.

The initial peritoneal incision is made in a similar fashion, but now is extended along the white line of Toldt up toward the kidney. On the right-hand side, this extended dissection will require mobilization of ceco-appendiceal attachments, and on the left will require more extensive mobilization of the sigmoid colon. The vas is similarly then incised. This procedure then requires dissection and identification of the bifurcation of the iliac vessels and the ureter. After identifying the ureter, the tissue just lateral to the ureter is dissected. The assistant retracts tissue laterally, while the surgeon uses graspers and shears attached to cautery to retract medially and dissect. This dissection is continued caudally, staying lateral to the medial umbilical ligament and along the lateral sidewall of the bladder. When dissecting along the bladder wall it is important to stay in the fatty plane that easily partitions with blunt dissection. Bleeding and excessive sharp dissection in this area usually signifies that one is too close to the bladder wall. If there is any suspicion of bladder injury, the urinary catheter drainage bag should be inspected for blood, and the bladder should be filled with dye to delineate any inadvertent cystotomy, which should then be laparoscopically repaired with suturing. Dissection is continued to the pubic bone, which brings one to the caudal and medial border of the dissection.

Next, the lateral border of the package, which includes dissection from the pubic bone up to the level of the common iliac artery and medial to the external and internal iliac vessels, obturator internus muscle, and genitofemoral nerve. This is begun by dissecting the package off the anterior surface of the common iliac artery. As dissection takes place at this level, the genitofemoral nerve is located lateral to the common iliac artery. The nerve is swept lateral and the associated lymphatic tissue is swept medially. A lateral branch from the common iliac artery going toward the psoas muscle may be seen here. It should be clipped on both sides and ligated (Fig. 17). The package is divided cranially at this level. Clips may be placed on the cranial side to occlude any lymphatic channels located here. The package is then mobilized caudally. Dissection is continued caudally along the anterior surface of the external iliac artery down to the level of the circumflex iliac vein, which is the caudad lateral border of the dissection. At this point the common and external iliac arteries can be rolled medially, exposing the obturator internus muscle laterally and, posteriorly, the internal iliac vein and the obturator nerve running beneath it (Fig. 19). The lymphatic tissue in this area is carefully dissected out, being mindful of small vascular branches. Upon completion, the common and external iliac arteries are returned to their normal position. At this point the clearly identifiable lymphatic tissue lateral and anterior to the internal iliac vein is carefully dissected free. During this part of the procedure the assistant retracts the internal iliac vein laterally, while the surgeon retracts the tissue medial to the vein and pelvic sidewall medially. As described for obturator lymph node dissection, blunt dissection is initially used to free this tissue into packets that are then individually cauterized. The 5 mm hook electrode may be useful in dissecting tissue free from the internal iliac vein and pelvic sidewall. It is important to note that an aberrant obturator vein may be entering the medial wall of the external iliac vein just superior to the pubis (Fig. 20). Identification of this vessel may also aid in dissection toward the obturator fossa and nerve.

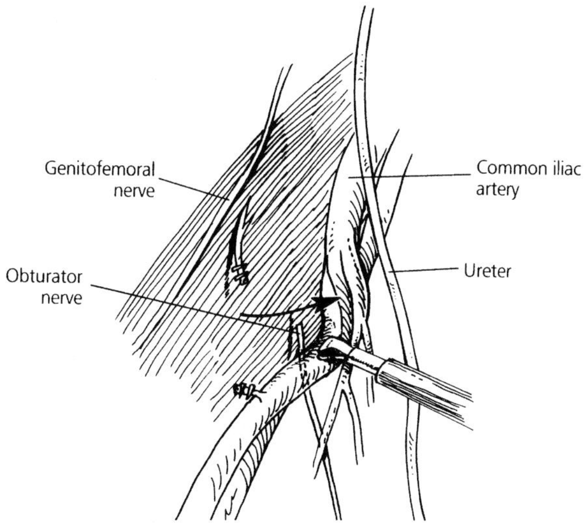

Fig. 19.

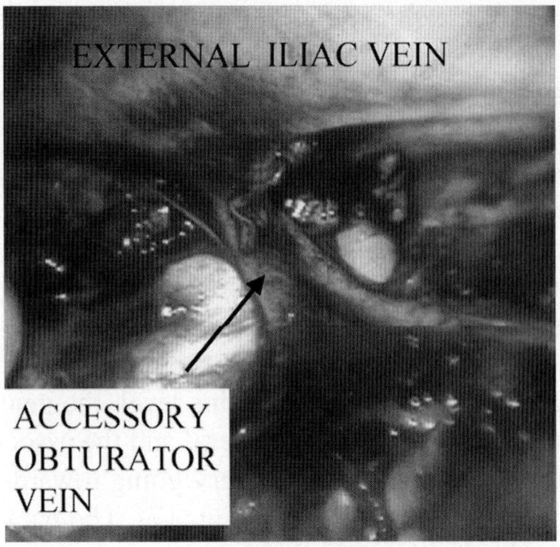

Fig. 20. Right acessory obturator vein joining posteromedial aspect of right external iliac vein

The caudal border of the packet may then be dissected off the pubic bone. This portion should be performed most meticulously, with cautery as necessary to avoid bleeding. Care should also be taken so that the dissection crosses the medial edge of the external iliac artery and the entire surface of the internal iliac vein. Also, at the lowest edge of the dissection, the superficial epigastric vein may be exiting from the femoral vein, traveling superomedially.

Now the packet can be retracted in the cephalad direction and posterior dissection carried out. This plane will free up with light retraction and blunt dissection, exposing the obturator nerve and the obturator vessels located inferomedial to the nerve. These vessels are dissected free and preserved. The obturator nerve is followed behind the internal iliac vein. Tissue deep to the obturator must be carefully teased free, as there are many small vessels here. It is important to include this tissue as the presciatic nodes are located here and may be the only positive nodes in the dissection *(19)*. Again, the hook electrode is useful in elevating this tissue off the obturator nerve and then carefully cauterizing through it. The assistant may also judiciously use the aspirator/irrigator in this region to retract the external iliac vessels laterally while keeping the operative field clear. Dissection is continued cephalad along the medial surface of the internal iliac artery until it gives rise to the obliterated umbilical artery. The notch at the junction of these two structures is completely dissected, thus freeing the package. The hook electrode is again used in lifting tissue off of the internal iliac artery and then cauterizing it in small portions. The cephalad border of the package may also be secured with clips and divided. The nodal packet is then removed either in pieces with the 10 mm spoon forceps, or removed in its entirety in an entrapment sac.

If the frozen section on the first side is negative or if bilateral dissection is planned from the outset, contralateral dissection is begun. This dissection is identical in every aspect to the contralateral side, with the exception that as this procedure is initiated adhesions between the colon and the side wall must be taken down prior to incision of the white line of Toldt. Again, electrocautery should be used carefully for this portion of the procedure.

Closure

Closure for all approaches is similar. Prior to closure the resection sites are again inspected under lower intra-abdominal pressure (5 mmHg) to ensure there is no active bleeding. The 10 mm laparoscopic ports can be easily and reliably closed with use of the Carter–Thomason® (Inlet Medical Inc., Eden Prairie, MN) closure set, which consists of an insertable cone and a pointed suture passer. Under direct vision the 10 mm trocar–sheath is removed, and the cone inserted with its holes for suture passage at 90° to the line that the fascial incision was made. Using the Carter–Thomason® suture passer, a 0-absorbable suture is passed through one hole of the cone, through the fascia into the abdomen under direct vision, and is held with a grasper inserted through another trocar port site. The passer is removed and inserted through the opposite hole and underlying fascia. The suture within the abdomen is grasped and brought out via this same hole. The cone is removed and the trocar–sheath can be replaced if more 10 mm sites need to be closed. When all 10 mm sites have sutures placed, the 5 mm ports are removed under direct vision, as are the 10 mm sites. The carbon dioxide is completely evacuated from the abdomen and then the last 10 mm port is removed. The fascial sutures on the sites are tied. The wounds are irrigated and the skin closed with a 4-0 absorbable stitch. Benzoin, Steri-strips, and Tegaderm may be then applied.

POSTOPERATIVELY

Following the procedure, regardless of technique, the patient is admitted to the short-stay ward. The nasogastric/orogastric tubes are removed in the operating room. The patient usually receives two more doses of antibiotics postoperatively. The urethral catheter is removed as soon as the patient is alert and oriented, and diet is advanced as tolerated.

The pneumatic boots are usually removed 4–6 h after the procedure and patients usually begin ambulation within hours following surgery. Most postoperative pain can be managed with oral analgesics. Intravenous narcotics are rarely necessary. Excessive pain immediately postoperatively is usually due to carbon dioxide diaphragmatic irritation. Nonsteroidal anti-inflammatory agents, such as ketorolac tromethamine, generally suffice. Postoperative monitoring is standard, with monitoring of vital signs for any evidence of bleeding or infection. Delayed abdominal pain that is constantly worsening and requiring narcotic analgesia may signify a significant complication, such as bowel perforation or retroperitoneal hematoma, and depending on the results of clinical evaluation of the patient, computerized tomography of the abdomen and pelvis may be required for evaluation. Most patients are discharged with 24 h and can resume normal activity within 1 week.

TAKE HOME MESSAGES

1. L-PLND is the initial urologic laparoscopic procedure in which urologists gained proficiency. Urologists having their first introduction to laparoscopy through performance of L-PLND can gain proficiency in this procedure without much difficulty, and use it as a "stepping-stone" for training toward more advanced urologic laparoscopic procedures.
2. L-PLND is as accurate a staging procedure as open PLND. With experience it requires only slightly more time to perform, and its cost may be reduced to that of open PLND. The robot-assisted form of this procedure is quite expeditious, though cost effectiveness is yet unclear. L-PLND in either form offers significant postoperative benefits including decreased hospitalization time, decreased postoperative pain, and decreased convalescence time compared to the open approach which may offset any increased operating room costs associated with this procedure.
3. L-PLND may also be considered for patients electing alternative minimally invasive treatments such as brachytherapy for treatment of localized prostate cancer.
4. L-PLND as a staging modality may also be applied to evaluation of urologic malignancies other than prostate cancer. However, extended L-PLND for the evaluation of such entities requires more laparoscopic experience and operative time. Again, postoperative benefits of this procedure compared to open surgery are significant.

REFERENCES

1. Schuessler WW, Vancaille TG, Reich H, et al.: Transperitoneal endosurgical lymphadenectomy in patients with localized prostate cancer. J Urol 145:988–991, 1991.
2. Griffith DP, Schuessler WW, Vancaille TH: Laparoscopic lymphadenectomy-a low morbidity alternative for staging pelvic malignancies. J Endourol 4 (Suppl 1):S-84, 1990.
3. Winfield HN, Donovan JF, See WA, et al.: Laparoscopic pelvic lymph node dissection for genitourinary malignancies: Indications, techniques, and results. J Endourol 6:103–111, 1992.
4. Kerbl K, Clayman RV, Petros J, et al.: Staging pelvic lymphadenectomy for prostate cancer: A comparison of laparoscopic and open techniques. J Urol 150:396–399, 1993.
5. Parra RO, Andrus C, Boullier J, et al.: Staging laparoscopic pelvic lymph node dissection: comparison of result with open pelvic lymphadenectomy. J Urol 147:875–878, 1992.
6. Winfield HN, See WA, Donovan JF, et al.: Comparative effectiveness and safety of laparoscopic vs open pelvic lymph node dissection for cancer of the prostate. J Urol 147:244A, 1992.
7. Winfield HN, Donovan JF, Troxel SA, et al.: Laparoscopic urologic surgery: the financial realities. Surg Oncol Clin North Am 4:307–314, 1995.
8. Troxel S, Winfield HN: Comparative financial analysis of laparoscopic versus open pelvic lymph node dissection for men with cancer of the prostate. J Urol 151:675–680, 1994.
9. Kozlowski PM, Winfield HN: Laparoscopic lymph node dissection: pelvic and retroperitoneal. Semin Laparosc Surg 7:150–159, 2000.
10. Winfield HN, Schuessler WW: Pelvic lymphadenectomy: limited and extended. In: Clayman RV, McDougall EM (eds): Laparoscopic Urology. St. Louis: Quality Medical Publishing, 1993; pp 225–259.
11. Winfield HN: Laparoscopic pelvic lymph node dissection for urologic pelvic malignancies. Atlas Urol Clin North Am 1:33–47, 1993.
12. Shackley DC, Irving SO, Brough WA, O′Reilly PH: Staging laparoscopic pelvic lymphadenectomy in prostate cancer. BJU Int 83: 260–264, 1999.
13. Kavoussi LR, Sosa E, Chandhoke P, et al.: Complications of laparoscopic pelvic lymph node dissection. J Urol 149:322–325, 1993.
14. Winfield HN: Laparoscopic pelvic lymph node dissection for urologic malignancies. In: Gomella LG, Kozminski M, Winfield HN, (eds): Laparoscopic Urologic Surgery. New York: Raven Press, 1994; pp 111–130.
15. Hua JC, Nelson RA, Wilson TG et al.: Perioerative complications of laparoscopic and robotic assisted laparoscopic radical prostatectomy. J Urol 175(2), 541–546, 2006.
16. Glascock JM, Winfield HN: Pelvic lymphadenectomy: intra- and extraperitineal access. In Smith AD, Badlani GH, Bagley DH, et al. (eds): Smith's Textbook of Endourology. St. Louis: Quality Medical Publishing, 1996; pp 870–893.
17. Glascock JM, Winfield HN, Lund GO, et al.: Carbon dioxide homeostasis during trans- or extraperitoneal laparoscopic pelvic lymphadenectomy: a real time intraoperative comparison. J Endourol 10:319–323, 1996.
18. Winfield HN, Lund GO: Extraperitoneal laparoscopic surgery: creating a working space. Contemp Urol 7:17–22, 1995.
19. Golimbu M, Morales P, Ali-Askari S, et al.: Extended pelvic lymphadenectomy for prostate cancer. J Urol 121: 617–620, 1979.

Laparoscopic Renal Cyst Decortication

Joshua M. Stern, Ilia S. Zeltser, Yair Lotan, and Jeffrey A. Cadeddu

INTRODUCTION

Renal cysts are the most common renal masses and occur in up to 50% of individuals over the age of 50 years *(1,2)*. Although renal cysts may be either congenital or acquired, most are simple, asymptomatic, and of unknown etiology. Intervention is needed when cysts are determined to be complex by radiographic criteria or when they are associated with pain, infection, hemorrhage, or urinary obstruction. Some congenital diseases such as autosomal dominant polycystic kidney disease (ADPKD), the most common form of renal cystic disease in the United States, are commonly associated with symptomatic cysts *(3)*. Other cystic diseases such as von-Hippel-Lindau (VHL), tuberous sclerosis, multilocular cystic nephroma, and acquired cystic disease have a predisposition toward malignant degeneration. The need for intervention in some cases of symptomatic or suspicious cysts has led to the development of less invasive strategies for renal cyst management *(4)*. This chapter will discuss the role of laparoscopy in evaluation and management of renal cysts.

PREOPERATIVE ASSESSMENT

The diagnosis of a renal cyst is made radiographically either as an incidental finding or during evaluation of symptoms such as flank or abdominal pain, early satiety, hematuria, hypertension, or urinary tract infection. Ultrasound or computed tomography (CT) provides the most reliable means of diagnosing renal cysts (Figs. 1 and 2). Intravenous urography (IVU) may suggest the presence of a cyst indirectly by demonstrating distortion of the collecting system, but in general IVU is not a reliable imaging modality for identification of renal cysts.

A history of ADPKD, VHL or tuberous sclerosis may prompt screening radiographic studies for monitoring the development or degeneration of renal cysts (Fig. 3). Likewise, patients with end-stage renal failure frequently develop renal cystic disease with a known potential for malignant degeneration and should be monitored radiographically.

Physical examination may reveal a palpable mass in rare cases but is usually not contributory in the diagnosis of renal cysts. Urinalysis is also generally non-diagnostic except to show proteinuria in cases of renal failure, pyuria, or hematuria in association with infection. Hypertension can occasionally lead to the diagnosis of a compressive renal cyst. Hypertension is thought to result from intra parenchymal renal ischemia and subsequent activation of the rennin–angiotensin–aldosterone system *(5)*. Relief of compression can result in blood pressure stabilization *(6)*.

From: *Current Clinical Urology: Essential Urologic Laparoscopy*
Edited by: S. Y. Nakada and S. P. Hedican, DOI 10.1007/978-1-60327-820-1_5

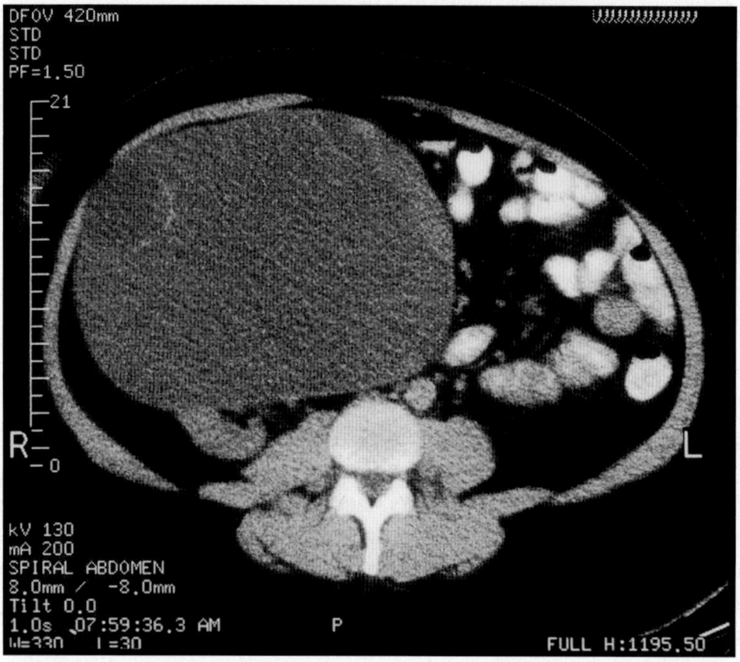

Fig. 1. Non-enhanced CT scan for patient with symptomatic right renal cyst.

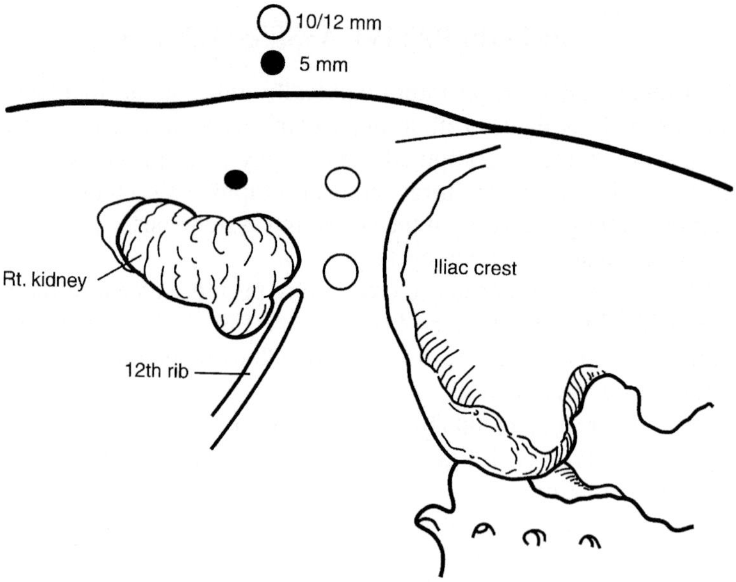

Fig. 2. Non-enhanced CT scan after laparoscopic cyst decortication.

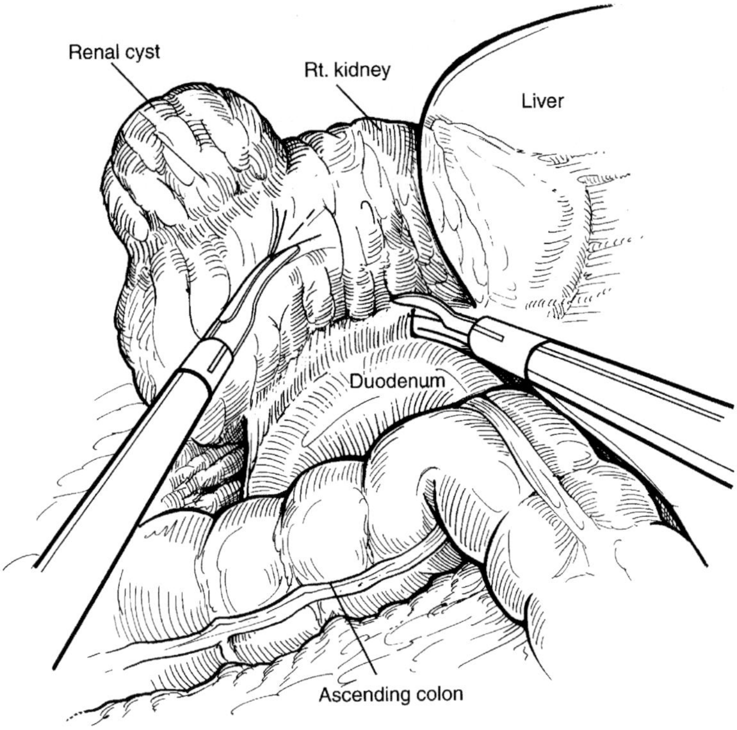

Fig. 3. Non-enhanced CT scan for patient with ADPKD.

MANAGEMENT ALGORITHMS

Complex Cysts

An attempt to predict the malignant potential of renal cysts has resulted in a classification scheme based on radiographic appearance. The Bosniak classification, first outlined in 1986, relies on CT criteria to categorize cysts into low, medium, or high risk groups (Table 1) *(4)*. In one meta-analysis, Bosniak Class II, III, and IV cysts were found to have malignancy risk of 24, 41, and 90%, respectively *(7)*. Harisinghani used CT guided biopsy to assess the rate of malignancy in 28 Bosniak III renal masses. Sixty-one percent were found to be malignant. Histology from these biopsies had 100%

Table 1
Bosniak criteria for renal cysts based on computer tomography *(4,9)*

Type	*Calcification*	*Septa*	*Wall*	*Enhancement*
I	None	None	Thin	None
II	Minimal	Few	Thin	None
IIF*	Yes	Multiple	Increased thickness	None
III	Extensive	Multiple	Increased thickness	None
IV	Significant, associated with a solid component	Numerous, very irregular	Thick	Yes

*Needs follow-up. Totally intrarenal non-enhancing high-attenuation renal lesions >3 mm are also included in this category.

concordance to final pathology *(8)*. Recently, category IIF has been added to the Bosniak classification to further delineate the malignant potential of the indeterminate renal cyst *(9)*.

Cytologic examination of the aspirated cyst fluid can help establish the cyst's malignant potential. A comprehensive meta-analysis by Wolf et al. found an overall sensitivity of cyst aspiration in diagnosing malignancy of 90%, a specificity of 92%, positive predictive value of 96%, and negative predictive value of 80% *(7)*. The risk of a false negative aspiration has been estimated at 20%, and the occurrence of tumor seeding along the needle tract has been reported *(10–16)*. Consequently, most groups forego diagnostic cyst aspiration believing that definitive management of complex cysts should include either open exploration and cyst excision or laparoscopic cyst decortication.

Symptomatic Simple Cysts

Although usually asymptomatic, renal cysts may cause pain, hypertension, or obstruction with dull flank pain as the most common symptom requiring intervention *(17)*. For symptomatic simple renal cysts, an initial attempt at conservative therapy with analgesics should be undertaken. If these measures fail, decompression can be performed via percutaneous aspiration with or without the injection of sclerosing agents, or via surgical decortication, either open or laparoscopically.

Cyst aspiration for simple, peripheral cysts can be performed using CT or ultrasound guidance and enables sampling of the cyst fluid for cytology. Unfortunately, simple percutaneous drainage is associated with a high rate of fluid reaccumulation resulting in the frequent addition of a sclerosing agent *(18,19)*. Multiple compounds have been used as sclerosing agents, including alcohol *(20–22)*, tetracycline *(23)*, minocycline *(18)*, and povodine–iodine *(24)*, with success rates ranging from 75 to 97% and complication rates from 1.3 to 20%. As such, if percutaneous aspiration is the management of choice, sclerosis should be used concomitantly. Interestingly, Okeke et al. *(25)* reported on 13 patients with symptomatic simple renal cysts that had previously undergone cyst aspiration with initial abatement of pain but subsequent symptomatic reaccumulation of cystic fluid. Patients were randomized to undergo either repeat aspiration with sclerotherapy using 95% ethanol or laparoscopic de-roofing. All of the patients in the sclerotherapy group had continued pain at a mean follow-up of 17 months. All patients in the laparoscopic group at a mean follow-up of 17.7 months were pain-free. Clearly a larger group is needed to validate this study, nevertheless, the polarity of these results are striking.

Endoscopic, open or laparoscopic cyst decortications provide alternative treatment options particularly if sclerosis fails. The role of endoscopic resection for management of renal cysts has been limited *(24, 26–28)*. Plas and Hübner reported only a 50% radiographic success rate at 46 months follow-up for percutaneous resection of renal cysts *(26)*. Though open cyst decortication has a high success rate, the procedure was associated with a high rate of perioperative complications *(29)*. As such, laparoscopic cyst decortication offers a less morbid, but equally efficacious approach for unroofing renal cysts as compared to open surgery *(30–32)*. The laparoscopic approach enables direct visualization of the cyst during aspiration, unroofing and biopsy of the cyst wall. Hemostasis can be easily obtained and the procedure performed with less morbidity than open procedures. Atug and colleagues reported their experience with 45 consecutive symptomatic patients treated with laparoscopic cyst decortication *(16)*. The mean cyst size was 9.7 mm with 53% failing percutaneous aspiration and sclerosing. Symptomatic and radiographic success was achieved in 91 and 95% of cases, respectively. Six of these cases included peripelvic cysts *(17)*.

Importantly, the management of peripelvic cysts differs from that of a simple peripheral renal cyst. These cysts present a special management challenge due to their proximity to the renal hilum and collecting system. Aspiration and sclerotherapy are associated with a high recurrence rate and the possibility of damage to the collecting system. While more technically challenging than a decortication of a peripheral cyst, laparoscopic decortication of a peripelvic cyst can be successful and is the preferred treatment approach *(17,33)*.

Adult Polycystic Kidney Disease

ADPKD is the most common renal cystic disease accounting for 9–10% of patients on chronic dialysis *(3)*. The disease typically presents in the third or fourth decade of life and is progressive in nature. The most common presenting symptoms are back, flank, or abdominal pain that are seen in up to 60% of patients *(3)*. Mutations in at least three genes thought to be responsible for the disease have been identified: PKD-1; PKD-2; and PKD-3, with a mutation in the PKD-1 gene on the short arm of chromosome 16 accounting for 85% of cases *(34,35)*. Despite increased understanding of the molecular biology of ADPKD, 45% of patients still develop end-stage renal disease by age 60 *(36)*. Additionally, hypertension affects 40–60% of patients and is thought to contribute to progressive loss of renal function *(37)*. While the primary management goal of ADPKD is control of hypertension and delay in loss of renal function, many patients suffer debilitating pain associated with expansion of renal cysts. Medical management with non-narcotic analgesics is the recommended initial therapy, although non-steroidal anti-inflammatory drugs may potentially exacerbate renal failure. Surgical management is reserved for those patients who fail conservative therapy. Percutaneous cyst aspiration has been used with variable success, but usually results in only transient relief due to cyst fluid reaccumulation and the limited ability to identify the symptomatic cysts in ADPKD *(38)*.

Open cyst decortication offers a more durable pain response especially when more aggressive cyst decortication is performed *(39,40)*. Ye and colleagues reported successful relief of pain at 1 year in 92% of patients, but at 5 years, success rates dropped to 81% *(40)*. Likewise, Elzinga and colleagues reported relief of pain in 80% of 26 patients at 1 year, but only 62% at 2 years *(39)*. Surgical decompression, either open or laparoscopically, of the renal cysts in ADPKD can also be associated with a reduction in hypertension and stabilization of renal function *(36,40,41)*.

As open cyst decortication has been associated with a 33% perioperative complication rate *(29)*, laparoscopic cyst decortication for ADPKD is considered an excellent option associated with equivalent outcomes to open surgery while decreasing surgical morbidity *(42)*. The use of a laparoscopic approach for cyst decortication in ADPKD was first described by Hulbert and associates in 1992 *(32)*. Early experiences report unroofing easily accessible large peripheral lesions. With increasing laparoscopic expertise, however, cysts of all sizes and locations can be approached laparoscopically *(36,43–47)*.

OPERATIVE TECHNIQUE

Patient Preparation

In preparation for surgery, all patients undergo routine laboratory studies such as serum creatinine, hematocrit, and urine culture. Confirmation of contralateral renal function is mandatory in cases in which the possibility of nephrectomy is present, such as in treatment of complex cystic disease. Similarly, the patient should be informed of the potential for conversion to an open procedure or the need for a nephrectomy in case of complications. A preoperative bowel preparation is not required but may be beneficial in cases of ADPKD or infected renal cysts.

Prior to initiating the procedure, it is important to determine that the necessary equipment is open or readily available. Table 2 lists the equipment recommended for laparoscopic renal cyst decortication.

Antibiotic prophylaxis with a cephalosporin or aminoglycoside is initiated prior to surgery. After induction of anesthesia, the stomach and bladder are decompressed with a nasogastric tube and bladder catheter, respectively. In patients with peripelvic cysts or deep parenchymal cysts with a potential for violation of the collecting system, an open-ended ureteral catheter may be placed at the start of the procedure for retrograde instillation of methylene blue to facilitate identification of an inadvertent collecting system injury. The ureteral catheter can be converted to an internal ureteral stent at the conclusion of the procedure if necessary.

Table 2
Instruments for laparoscopic cyst decortication

Cystoscopy equipment if planned
Veress needle
Direct vision access port (e.g., Visiport, U.S. Surgical Corporation)
Laparoscopic lens
Two–three 10/12 mm ports
Two 5 mm ports
Laparoscopic instruments including scissors, graspers, and suction-irrigator
Laparoscopic ultrasound
Argon beam coagulator
Retrieval bag
5- and 10-mm clip appliers
Oxidized cellulose
Laparoscopic aspiration needle

Patient Positioning

Anterior cysts are best approached transperitoneally, while isolated posterior cysts may be more easily approached retroperitoneally.

For the transperitoneal approach, the patient is placed in a 45-degree modified flank position with a roll under the back to support the scapula. The table may be slightly flexed. Sequential compression devices are applied to the legs, which are padded and secured, while the arms are folded over a pillow on the chest. The upper body and legs are then secured to the bed with wide tape. The table should be rotated in both directions to ensure the patient is secure prior to commencing the procedure. For obese patients, a more lateral position can be used to allow the pannus to fall medially.

For a retroperitoneal approach, a full flank position is utilized. After placing an axillary roll, the lower arm is positioned on an arm board and the upper arm is flexed across a pillow or an elevated support. The legs are well padded and both the upper and lower extremities are secured. The table is flexed and kidney rest elevated.

Trocar Placement

Transperitoneal Approach

Pneumoperitoneum is established using either the Veress needle or open canula technique. A 12 mm port is placed at the umbilicus, and the remaining ports are placed under laparoscopic vision as follows: on a left-sided cyst decortication, a 12 mm port is placed just below the umbilicus along the midclavicular line and a 5 mm port is placed midway between the xyphoid and the umbilicus along the midline;. for a right-sided procedure, a 5 mm upper midline is placed midway between the xyphoid and the umbilicus and a 12 mm port is placed just below the level of the umbilicus at the right midclavicular line. An optional 3 or 5 mm port may be placed in the upper midline to facilitate retraction of the liver or spleen (Fig. 4).

Retroperitoneal Approach

A 2 mm skin incision is made just at or posterior to the 12th rib at the superior lumbar triangle. Using blunt finger dissection a space is created anterior to the psoas muscle and outside Gerota's fascia to accommodate a balloon dilator. A commercially available trocar-mounted balloon or a modified Gaur

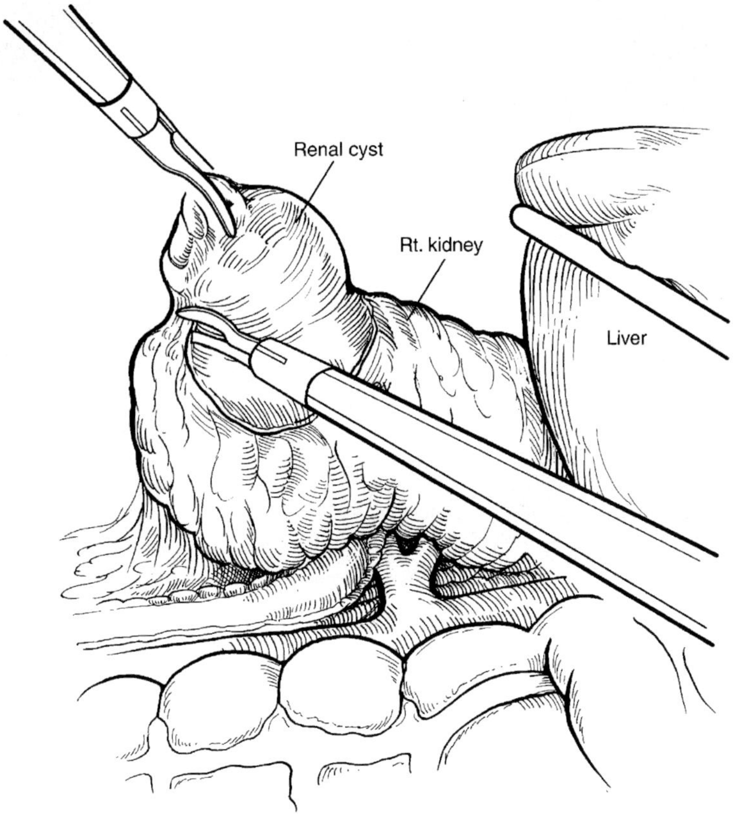

Fig. 4. Three ports are used for the transabdominal approach: the first 12 mm laparoscopic port is placed at the umbilicus, and the remaining ports are placed under laparoscopic vision as follows: a 12 mm port is placed just below the umbilicus along the midclavicular line and a 5 mm port is placed in the midline between the xyphoid and the umbilicus. (Reprinted by permission from Fabrizio MD: Laparoscopic evaluation and treatment of symptomatic and indeterminate renal cysts. *In* Bishoff JT, Kavoussi LR, ed: Atlas of Laparoscopic Retroperitoneal Surgery. Philadelphia, W. B. Saunders, 2000.)

balloon comprised of the middle finger of a size 8 latex surgeon's glove mounted on a 16F red rubber catheter is used to expand the retroperitoneal space to 800–1,000 cc. A 12 mm blunt-tipped cannula is placed at this site. A second 12 mm trocar is placed under laparoscopic vision along the anterior axillary line in line with the first trocar, taking care to avoid inadvertent injury to the peritoneum. A third 5-mm trocar is placed a few fingerbreadths posterior to the second trocar (at the lateral border of the paraspinous muscles) or superior to the12 mm trocar in the anterior axillary line (Fig. 5).

Procedure

Transperitoneal Approach

Once the trocars are secured, the line of Toldt is incised from the iliac vessels to the splenic or hepatic flexure and the colon is mobilized medially. On the left side, the splenicocolic and phrenicocolic ligaments are divided. The spleen should be lifted anteriorly as necessary to assist with this maneuver, which should provide access to the upper pole. On the right side, the hepatic flexure should be mobilized which may require an additional 3 or 5 mm trocar in order to elevate the liver. Additionally, it

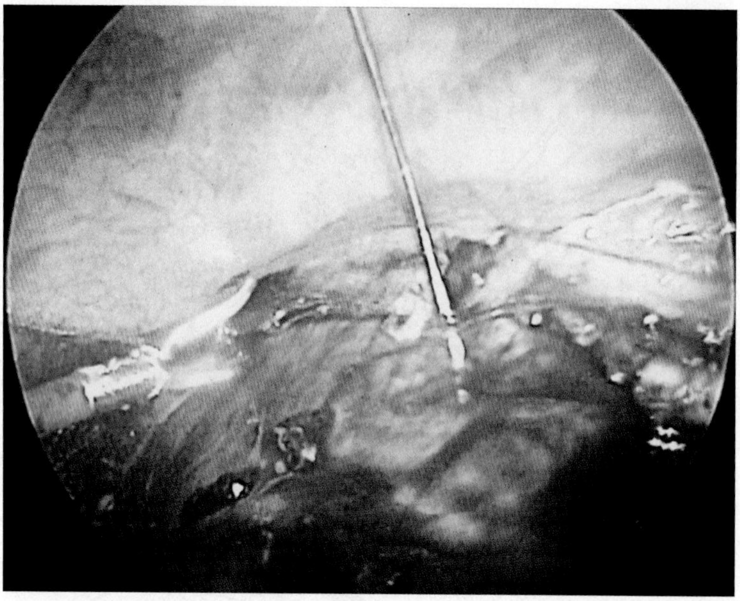

Fig. 5. In the retroperitoneal approach, a 12 mm blunt-tipped cannula is placed just at or posterior to the 12th rib at the superior lumbar triangle, and a second 12 mm trocar is placed in the anterior axillary line in line with the first trocar. This is placed under direct vision with care to avoid injury to the peritoneum, which can be swept medially as necessary. A third 5-mm trocar is placed a few fingerbreadths posterior (at the lateral border of the paraspinous muscles) under direct vision or superiorly above the 12 mm trocar in the anterior axillary line. (Reprinted by permission from Fabrizio MD: Laparoscopic evaluation and treatment of symptomatic and indeterminate renal cysts. *In* Bishoff JT, Kavoussi LR, ed: Atlas of Laparoscopic Retroperitoneal Surgery. Philadelphia, W. B. Saunders, 2000.)

may be necessary to mobilize the duodenum, particularly for treatment of medial and peripelvic cysts (Fig. 6). At this point, the portion of Gerota's fascia, where it overlies a solitary cyst, is opened. The kidney need not be mobilized in its entirety for unroofing of a single cyst. In contrast, the entire kidney is mobilized and the hilum exposed to provide optimal access to the maximum number of cysts in ADPDK.

Intraoperative ultrasonography with a laparoscopic transducer is invaluable in establishing the exact location of the cyst and its relationship to the collecting system and the hilum. It is also very helpful in visualizing septations, calcifications, thickening of the cyst wall, and complex debris that would alert the surgeon to the possibility of a malignancy. For a solitary cyst, the perinephric fat overlying the cyst is mobilized until a rim of normal renal parenchyma is exposed (Fig. 7). For large cysts, dissection may be facilitated by partially decompressing the cyst using an 18 gauge spinal needle placed percutaneously and guided by laparoscopic vision (Fig. 8). The cyst wall is then grasped and electrocautery scissors are used to excise the wall until it is flush with the renal capsule (Fig. 9). The specimen is then sent for histopathologic evaluation and the aspirated cyst fluid for cytology. The base of the cyst is inspected for suspicious nodules or irregularities that may be biopsied with cup biopsy forceps (Fig. 10). Hemostasis is obtained at the biopsy site and along the incised cyst wall with judicious use of electrocautery or the argon beam coagulator. Routine coagulation of the base of the cyst is discouraged due to the risk of collecting system injury *(48)*. Perirenal fat, a tongue of omentum, or a polytetrafluoroethylene (Gore-Tex) wick *(42)* may be placed into the cyst cavity to divert cyst fluid and prevent reaccumulation. For large cysts, a 7 mm suction drain may be placed through a lateral port and left for 1–2 days.

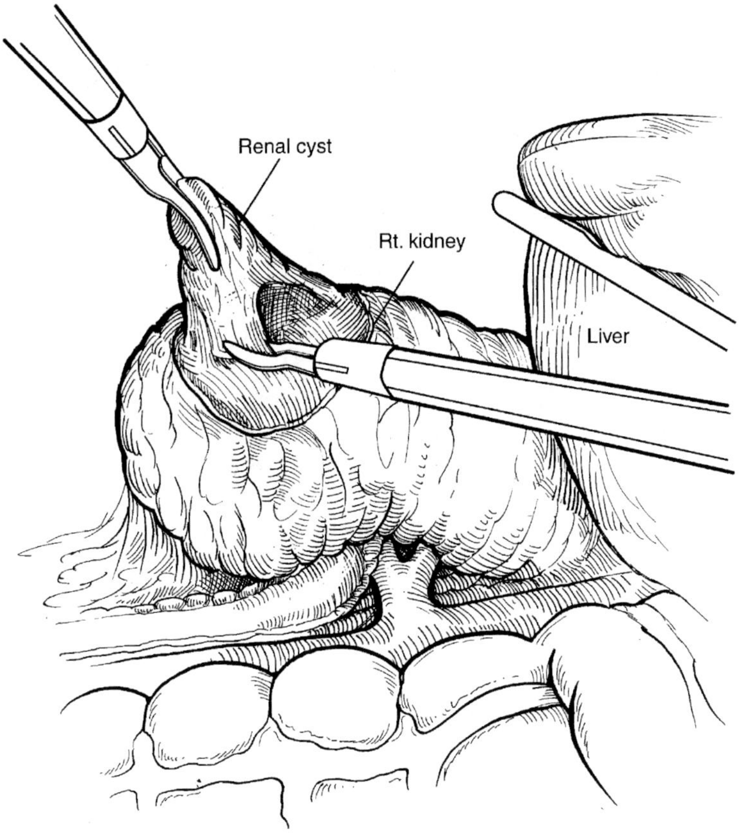

Fig. 6. On the right side, the colon is reflected medially and a Kocher maneuver may be necessary to fully expose the kidney. (Reprinted by permission from Fabrizio MD: Laparoscopic evaluation and treatment of symptomatic and indeterminate renal cysts. *In* Bishoff JT, Kavoussi LR, ed: Atlas of Laparoscopic Retroperitoneal Surgery. Philadelphia, W. B. Saunders, 2000.)

In the case of an intrarenal cyst, laparoscopic cyst decortication may be a challenge. The use of intraoperative ultrasound to locate the cyst or the preoperative placement of a percutaneous nephrostomy tube may facilitate localization of the cyst and help distinguish it from the collecting system; however, decortication involves transection of renal parenchyma and may result in significant hemorrhage. As such, internal renal cysts should be approached cautiously, if at all.

Peripelvic cysts are more difficult to approach laparoscopically than simple peripheral renal cysts. The location of the cysts near the hilum mandates that meticulous dissection be performed to avoid vascular injury or entry into the collecting system. A ureteral catheter may be placed prior to the procedure to enable injection of indigo carmine-stained saline to help distinguish the cyst from the collecting system. Use of electrocautery should be avoided during the dissection due to the close proximity to the renal vessels and collecting system. The use of laparoscopic ultrasound can help distinguish the cyst from the renal vein *(48)*.

For patients with ADPKD, direct laparoscopic vision facilitated by intraoperative ultrasound is critical in order to find, identify, and unroof as many cysts as possible (Figs. 11 and 12) Typically, hundreds of cysts will be unroofed or punctured in ADPDK (Figs. 13 and 14). If safe excision of a cyst wall is precluded by overlying parenchyma, aspiration of the cyst may be performed. It is important to limit spillage of cyst fluid in these cases, as many of the APKD cysts may be infected.

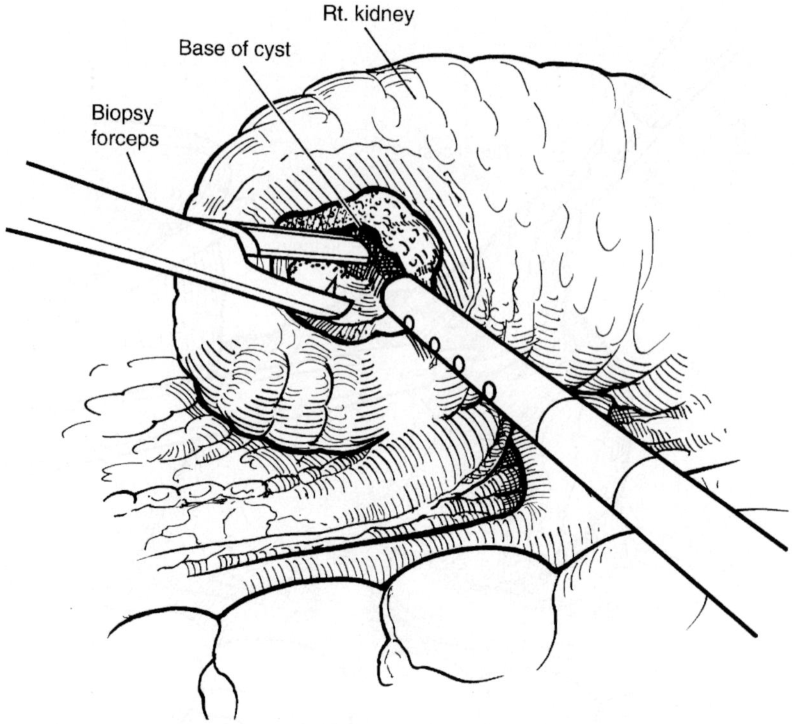

Fig. 7. The renal cyst can be identified through Gerota's fascia and the perinephric fat is mobilized until a rim of normal parenchyma is exposed. (Reprinted by permission from Fabrizio MD: Laparoscopic evaluation and treatment of symptomatic and indeterminate renal cysts. *In* Bishoff JT, Kavoussi LR, ed: Atlas of Laparoscopic Retroperitoneal Surgery. Philadelphia, W. B. Saunders, 2000.)

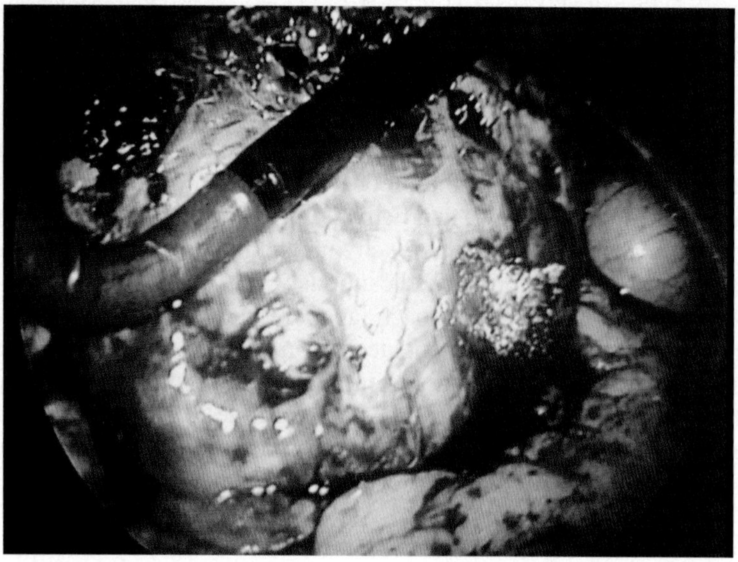

Fig. 8. For large cysts, dissection may be facilitated by partially decompressing the cyst using an 18 gauge spinal needle placed percutaneously and if necessary guided by laparoscopic vision. The cyst fluid is sent for cytopathologic evaluation.

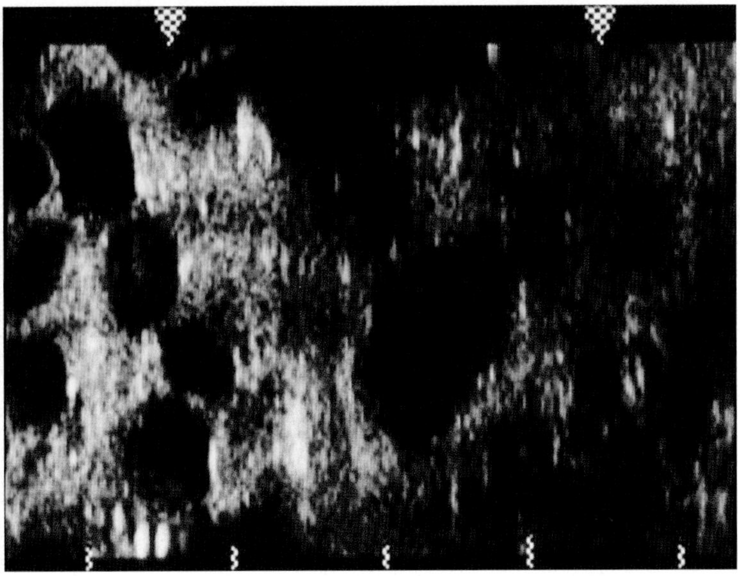

Fig. 9. The cyst wall is then grasped and electrocautery scissors used to excise the wall until it is flush with the renal capsule. (Reprinted by permission from Fabrizio MD: Laparoscopic Evaluation and treatment of symptomatic and indeterminate renal cysts. *In* Bishoff JT, Kavoussi LR, ed: Atlas of Laparoscopic Retroperitoneal Surgery. Philadelphia, W. B. Saunders, 2000.)

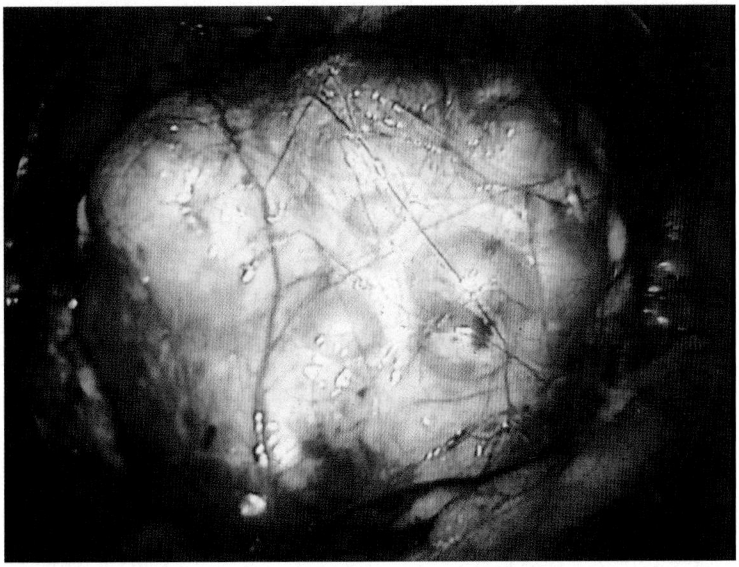

Fig. 10. The base of the cyst is inspected for suspicious nodules or irregularities that may be biopsied with cup biopsy forceps. (Reprinted by permission from Fabrizio MD: Laparoscopic evaluation and treatment of symptomatic and indeterminate renal cysts. *In* Bishoff JT, Kavoussi LR, ed: Atlas of Laparoscopic Retroperitoneal Surgery. Philadelphia, W. B. Saunders, 2000.)

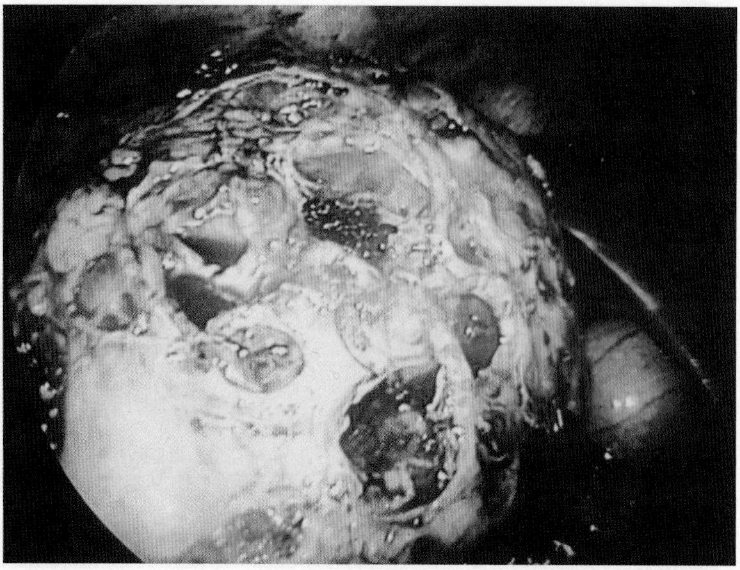

Fig. 11. The laparoscopic ultrasound facilitates detection of cysts and is particularly useful in ADPKD and for intra-parenchymal cysts.

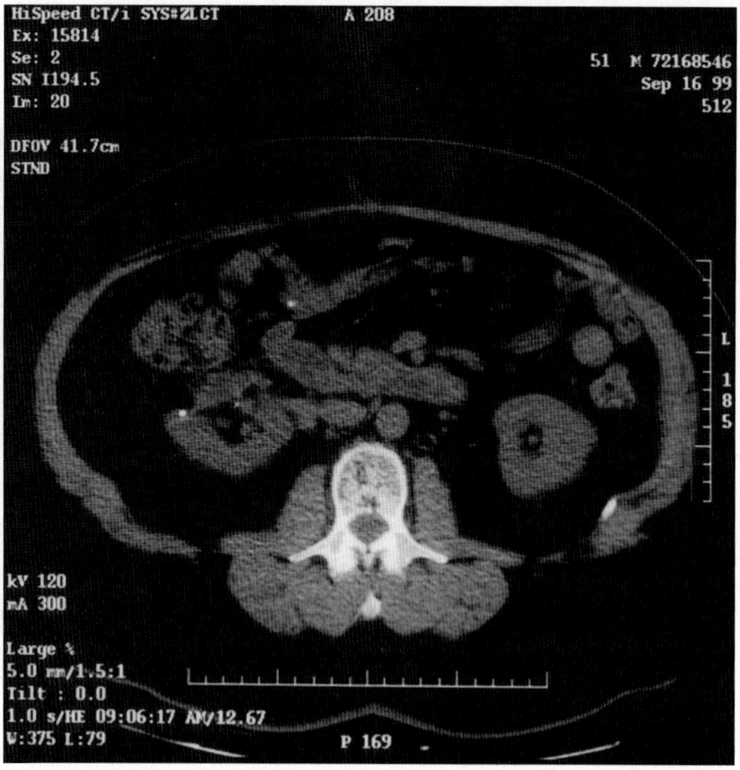

Fig. 12. Multiple subsurface cysts visualized using laparoscopic ultrasound.

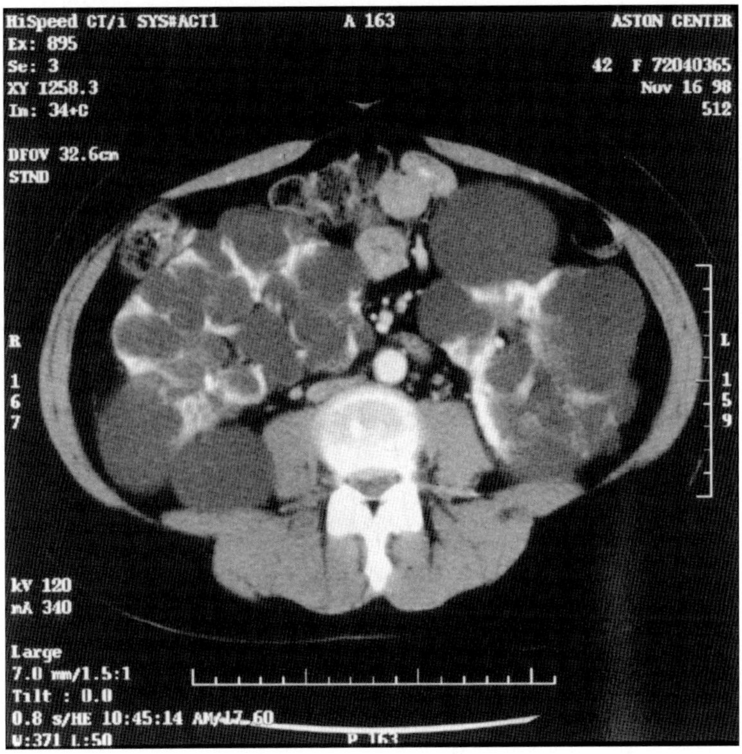

Fig. 13. Laparoscopic view of a kidney in a patient with ADPKD.

Retroperitoneal Approach

The retroperitoneal approach is used most commonly for posterior and lower pole cysts; however, some authors advocate this approach for any peripheral or peripelvic cyst *(49)*. After trocar placement, the peritoneum is swept medially and the psoas and quadratus lumborum muscles are identified, allowing Gerota's fascia to be opened. Perinephric fat may be used to elevate the kidney. Once the cyst is identified, it is managed similarly to the transperitoneal approach.

Postoperative Care

Most patients begin clear liquids on the night of surgery and the diet is advanced the next morning. The bladder catheter is removed the morning after surgery. Antimicrobial prophylaxis with a cephalosporin is continued for three additional doses postoperatively.

In the event of a persistent ileus, fever, or abdominal distention, an urinoma or retroperitoneal hematoma should be considered and is best diagnosed with a contrast-enhanced CT. If an injury to the collecting system is suspected intraoperatively, injection of indigo carmine-stained saline may confirm it and an indwelling ureteral stent should be placed at the conclusion of the case. For a previously unsuspected urinoma, a Foley catheter should be reinserted and a percutaneous nephrostomy tube or ureteral stent placed. For the rare retroperitoneal hematoma, conservative management with or without transfusion suffices in most cases; rarely, a renal arteriogram and transcatheter embolization is necessary to identify and treat the source of hemorrhage.

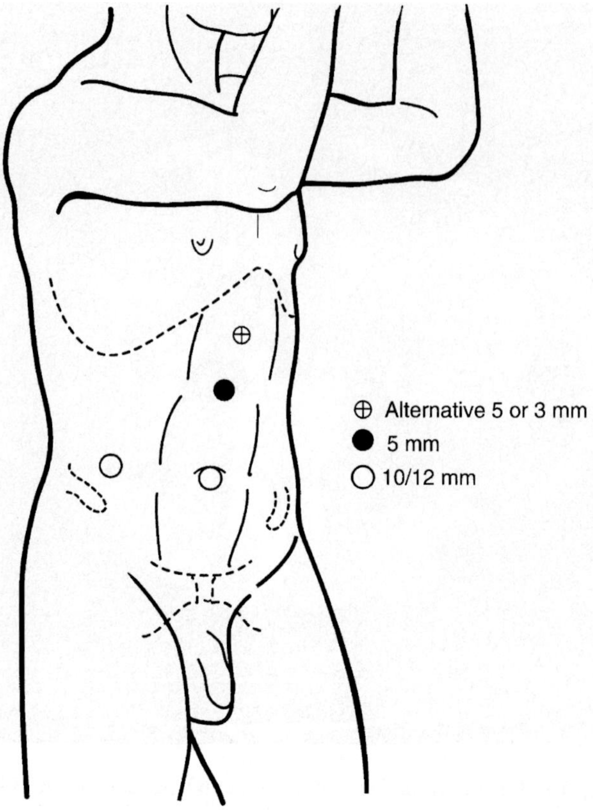

Fig. 14. Laparoscopic view of a kidney in a patient with ADPKD after decortication.

RESULTS

Simple Renal Cysts

Reports of laparoscopic cyst decortication for simple renal cysts using both the transperitoneal and retroperitoneal approaches abound in the literature *(42,44,50–56,60)*. Among series with at least ten patients, success rates of (77–100%) have been reported, although follow-up is short to intermediate in most series (Table 3). In most series, the indication for surgery was persistent pain requiring narcotic analgesics. Most investigators used cyst resolution as the primary outcome parameter and determinant of success; however, resolution of pain was reported in greater than 75% of patients in most series *(52,50,53,56,60)*.

Fahlenkamp reviewed 139 cases of laparoscopic cyst decortication at 4 centers and noted only 5 complications *(55)*. The need for transfusion was rare and most groups reported minimal blood loss, few complications and only rare cases required open conversion. Complications that have been reported include bleeding, open conversion, ileus, urinary fistula, and nerve paresthesia. The overall complication rate of 4.5% (Table 3) compares favorably with the 32% rate reported for open cyst decortication *(29)*.

Indeterminate Cysts

The laparoscopic management of complex cysts is controversial. While most Bosniak IV cysts require partial or radical nephrectomy, the incidence of malignancy in class II and III cysts is lower and

Table 3
Laparoscopic cyst decortication for symptomatic cysts

Author	*Pts*	*TP/RP*	*OR time (min)*	*Transf.*	*Conversion*	*Complic.*	*LOS (d)*	*Conval. (week)*	*F/U (mo)*	*Success (%)*
Rubenstein *(42)*	10	9/1	147	10%	10%	20%	2.2	1	10	100
Guazzoni *(50)*	20	TP	75	0%	0%	0%	2.2	1	3–6	100
Valdivia *(51)*	13	TP	–	–	0%	–	–	–	0–>12	–
Roberts *(56)*	21	13/8	164	0%	0%	14%	1.9	–	15.8	95
Atug *(17)*	45	TP	89	0%	1.8%	0%	1.1	–	58	91
Shiraishi *(60)*	36	29/7	–	0%	0%	0%	–	–	65	92
Wada *(52)*	13	TP	–	–	7.7%	7.7%	–	–	3	77
Ou *(53)*	14	RP	78	–	–	7	4.2	1	8	100
Denis *(54)*	10	8/2	92	–	10%	10%	5.4	–	8.3	100
Fahlenkamp *(55)*	139	–	–	–	–	3.5%	–	–	–	–
TOTAL	321	157/25	107	0.7% (1/132)	2.3% (4/168)	4.5% (14/308)	2.8	1	–	–

may warrant laparoscopic evaluation to rule out malignancy *(8,44,54,56–58)*. Santiago and colleagues reviewed their series of 35 patients with Bosniak II and III cysts who underwent laparoscopic cyst decortication. Among these patients, five (14.5%) were found to have renal cell carcinoma, of whom, four underwent immediate partial or radical nephrectomy and one patient underwent a delayed partial nephrectomy after a change in pathologic interpretation. No recurrences were detected in this group of patients at a mean follow-up of 20 months *(57)*.

Roberts and colleagues also performed laparoscopic cyst decortication in eight patients with Bosniak class II/III cysts. One patient with a finding of a 0.8-cm focus of papillary renal cell carcinoma on permanent histopathological examination subsequently underwent an open radical nephrectomy with excision of the trocar site that was used for specimen extraction. With 60 months follow-up, no recurrence has been detected *(56)*. Warren et al. reviewed the accuracy of the Bosniak classification and concluded that concordance between radiologic classification and malignancy is well established and accurate for class I and IV cysts, however, in the absence of large prospective studies, differentiating between class II and III cysts remains controversial *(58)*. Several groups reviewed by Warren utilized CT guided biopsy of class II–III renal cyst to aid in their decision making. Until longer follow-up and more patients are evaluated, laparoscopic cyst decortication for the intermediate cyst should be employed cautiously and selectively.

Peripelvic Cysts

Few reports are currently available regarding the outcome of laparoscopic decortication of peripelvic cysts *(33,42,48,56)*. The largest series to date was reported by Roberts and colleagues in which 11 patients with peripelvic cysts underwent laparoscopic decortication with no open conversions, no transfusions, and no recurrences. The only complication was a prolonged urine leak and associated ileus. Not surprisingly, operative time and mean blood loss were statistically greater for treatment of peripelvic cysts compared with simple cysts (164 vs. 233 min ($p = 0.003$), 98 vs. 182 ml ($p = 0.04$)) *(56)*.

Affonso recently described the University of California, San Francisco (UCSF) experience with laparoscopic renal cyst decortication on four men with peripelvic cysts. All patients underwent preoperative CT scan and retrograde pyelogram. Intraoperative ureteral catheters were placed to allow injection of methylene blue to ensure no communication between cyst and collecting system. At 6 months follow-up, all patients achieved both symptomatic and radiographic success *(33)*. Hoenig and associates also treated four patients with peripelvic cysts using both the transperitoneal ($n = 3$) and retroperitoneal ($n = 1$) approaches. The sole failure occurred in the only patient who underwent a retroperitoneal approach, and the authors concluded that this approach might offer less optimal visualization of the hilum *(48)*. From these small series it appears that with careful technique, laparoscopic decortication of peripelvic cysts is feasible and efficacious.

Autosomal Dominant Polycystic Kidney Disease

Laparoscopic cyst decortication for ADPKD has been reported in a few small series (Table 4) *(36,39,43–47,59)*. While the early series do not note the number of cysts decorticated, several recent studies emphasize the importance of extensive cyst decortication. Dunn and co-workers marsupialized on average 204 cysts/procedure with the hope that more aggressive cyst decortication may lead to more durable pain relief *(46,59)*. It should be noted that extensive cyst decortication is a time-consuming and tedious operation with an average published time of 226–300 min (Table 4). Lee and colleagues decorticated an average of 220 cysts per patient in 29 patients with ADPCKD with an average OR time of 5 h *(36)*.

Short and intermediate term pain relief is typical after laparoscopic cyst decortication. Lifson and colleagues reported complete pain resolution in 71 and 57% of 7 patients were pain-free at 6 months

Table 4
Laparoscopic cyst decortication for ADPKD

Author	*Pts*	*TP/RP*	*EBL (ml)*	*OR time (min)*	*Transf.*	*Convers.*	*Complic.*	*LOS (d)*	*Recur.*	*F/U (mo)*	*Pain relief*
Elzinga *(39)*	3	TP	–	–	–	–	–	–	–	–	–
Chehval *(45)*	3	TP	–	–	0	0	0	2.3	0	16.7	100% initial and at F/U
Brown *(47)*	8	TP	<150	164	0	0	0	<2	25%	12–28	85% initial, 50% at F/U
Elashry *(59)*	2 (5 proc)	TP	85	207	0	0	0	2.4	0	9	100% initial and 6–22 months
Lifson *(44)*	8 (11 proc)	10/1	116^	137^	9%	0	9%	2.2	28.6% (2/7)	11–65	71% at 6 mo, 57% at 2 years
Lee *(36)*	29	27/2	124	300	0	0	34%	3.2	–	32	81% with a 50% pain reduction
Dunn *(46)*	15 (21 proc)	TP	88	330	0	0	33%	3.2	13.30%	26.4	86.7% initial, 73% at 2 years
TOTAL	68 (80 proc)	77/3	112.6	228.6	2.5% (2/77)	0%	22% (17/77)	2.55	15.7% (6/38)	–	–

and 2 years, respectively *(44)*. Dunn and coworkers also noted a reduction in pain in 73% of 15 patients at 2 years, with an average pain reduction of 62% *(46)*. The impact, if any, of cyst decortication on the natural history of ADPDK-related hypertension and renal function is unclear. Dunn and colleagues found no change in blood pressure in 40%, improvement in 20%, resolution in 7% and worsening in 33% of 12 ADPDK patients undergoing extensive laparoscopic cyst decortication. Serum creatinine levels remained stable in 87% of patients *(46)*. In the review by Lee and colleagues, five patients were rendered normotensive, nine required a decrease dose of anti-hypertensive medication and six had worsening hypertension at 3 years of follow-up *(36)*.

CONCLUSIONS AND TAKE-HOME MESSAGES

Renal cysts diagnosed either as part of a workup in a symptomatic patient or as an incidental finding are common problems in urology. Percutaneous cyst aspiration and/or sclerotherapy, while associated with increased recurrence rates as compared to laparoscopic decortication, can be offered as first-line therapy for simple symptomatic renal cysts that fail conservative medical management. However, complex cysts, cysts associated with ADPKD, and peripelvic cysts may be best managed initially with laparoscopic or open exploration. Laparoscopic cyst decortication has been demonstrated to be a safe, efficacious and minimally invasive approach for treatment of renal cysts.

Take Home Messages:

1. A trial of conservative management or percutaneous sclerotherapy for simple cysts can precede laparoscopic cyst decortication.
2. The laparoscopic management of complex renal cysts is controversial and patient candidates for laparoscopic exploration and/or decortication require careful selection. For Bosniak II/III cysts, aspirated cyst fluid should be sent for cytology and samples of the cyst wall and base should be sent for histopathologic evaluation at the time of surgery.
3. Peripelvic cysts require careful dissection around the hilum and retrograde injection of methylene blue to rule out inadvertent injury to the collecting system.
4. Aggressive cyst decortication of as many surface and subsurface cysts as possible is advisable for ADPKD. Laparoscopic ultrasound will facilitate identification of accessible cysts.

REFERENCES

1. Tada S, Yamagishi J, Kobayashi H, Hata Y, Kobari T. The incidence of simple renal cyst by computed tomography. Clin Radiol 1983 Jul;34(4):437–439.
2. Laucks SP Jr, McLachlan MS. Aging and simple cysts of the kidney. Br J Radiol 1981 Jan;54(637):12–14.
3. Gabow PA. Autosomal dominant polycystic kidney disease. N Engl J Med 1993 Jul 29;329(5):332–342.
4. Bosniak MA. The current radiological approach to renal cysts. Radiology 1986 Jan;158(1):1–10.
5. Page IH. The production of persistant htn by cellophaneperinephritis. JAMA 1939;113:2046–2048.
6. Davies MC, Perry MJ. Urological management of 'page kidney'. BJU Int 2006 Nov;98(5):943–944.
7. Wolf JS Jr. Evaluation and management of solid and cystic renal masses. J Urol 1998 Apr;159(4):1120–1133.
8. Harisinghani MG, Maher MM, Gervais DA, McGovern F, Hahn P, Jhaveri K, Varghese J, Mueller PR. Incidence of malignancy in complex cystic renal masses (Bosniak category III): should imaging-guided biopsy precede surgery? AJR Am J Roentgenol 2003 Mar;180(3):755–758.
9. Israel GM, Bosniak MA. Follow-up CT of moderately complex cystic lesions of the kidney (Bosniak category IIF). AJR Am J Roentgenol 2003 Sep;181(3):627–633.
10. Gibbons RP, Bush WH Jr, Burnett LL. Needle tract seeding following aspiration of renal cell carcinoma. J Urol 1977 Nov;118(5):865–867.
11. Auvert J, Abbou CC, Lavarenne V. Needle tract seeding following puncture of renal oncocytoma. Prog Clin Biol Res 1982;100:597–598.
12. Kiser GC, Totonchy M, Barry JM. Needle tract seeding after percutaneous renal adenocarcinoma aspiration. J Urol 1986 Dec;136(6):1292–1293.

13. Wehle MJ, Grabstald H. Contraindications to needle aspiration of a solid renal mass: tumor dissemination by renal needle aspiration. J Urol 1986 Aug;136(2):446–448.
14. Shenoy PD, Lakhkar BN, Ghosh MK, Patil UD. Cutaneous seeding of renal carcinoma by Chiba needle aspiration biopsy. Case report. Acta Radiol 1991 Jan;32(1):50–52.
15. Abe M, Saitoh M. Selective renal tumour biopsy under ultrasonic guidance. Br J Urol 1992 Jul;70(1):7–11.
16. Slywotzky C, Maya M. Needle tract seeding of transitional cell carcinoma following fine-needle aspiration of a renal mass. Abdom Imaging 1994 Mar–1994 Apr 30;19(2):174–176.
17. Atug F, Burgess SV, Ruiz-Deya G, Mendes-Torres F, Castle EP, Thomas R. Long-term durability of laparoscopic decortication of symptomatic renal cysts. Urology 2006 Aug;68(2):272–275.
18. Ohkawa M, Tokunaga S, Orito M, Shimamura M, Hirano S, Okasho A, Kosaka S. Percutaneous injection sclerotherapy with minocycline hydrochloride for simple renal cysts. Int Urol Nephrol 1993;25(1):37–43.
19. Wahlqvist L, Grumstedt B. Therapeutic effect of percutaneous puncture of simple renal cyst. Follow-up investigation of 50 patients. Acta Chir Scand 1966 Oct;132(4):340–347.
20. Fontana D, Porpiglia F, Morra I, Destefanis P. Treatment of simple renal cysts by percutaneous drainage with three repeated alcohol injection. Urology 1999 May;53(5):904–907.
21. Hanna RM, Dahniya MH. Aspiration and sclerotherapy of symptomatic simple renal cysts: value of two injections of a sclerosing agent. AJR Am J Roentgenol 1996 Sep;167(3):781–783.
22. Ohta S, Fujishiro Y, Fuse H. Polidocanol sclerotherapy for simple renal cysts. Urol Int 1997;58(3):145–147.
23. Reiner I, Donnell S, Jones M, Carty HL, Richwood AM. Percutaneous sclerotherapy for simple renal cysts in children. Br J Radiol 1992 Mar;65(771):281–282.
24. Gelet A, Sanseverino R, Martin X, Leveque JM, Dubernard JM. Percutaneous treatment of benign renal cysts. Eur Urol 1990;18(4):248–252.
25. Okeke AA, Mitchelmore AE, Keeley FX, Timoney AG. A comparison of aspiration and sclerotherapy with laparoscopic de-roofing in the management of symptomatic simple renal cysts. BJU Int 2003 Oct;92(6):610–613.
26. Plas EG, Hubner WA. Percutaneous resection of renal cysts: a long-term followup. J Urol 1993 Apr;149(4):703–705.
27. Salas Sironvalle M, Gelet A, Viguier JL, Martin X, Sanseverino R, Marechal JM, Dubernard JM. [Percutaneous resection of benign renal cysts]. Actas Urol Esp 1990 Sep–1990 Oct 31;14(5):349–351.
28. Lopatkin NA, Martov AG. The percutaneous x-ray endoscopic surgery of simple kidney cysts. Urol Nefrol (Mosk) 1993 Mar–1993 Apr 30;2:2–5.
29. Kropp KA, Grayhack JT, Wendel RM, Dahl DS. Morbidity and mortality of renal exploration for cyst. Surg Gynecol Obstet 1967 Oct;125(4):803–806.
30. Morgan C Jr, Rader D. Laparoscopic unroofing of a renal cyst. J Urol 1992 Dec;148(6):1835–1836.
31. Jahnsen JU, Solhaug JH. Extirpation of benign renal cysts with laparoscopic technique. Tidsskr Nor Laegeforen 1992 Nov 20;112(28):3552–3554.
32. Hulbert JC. Laparoscopic management of renal cystic disease. Semin Urol 1992 Nov;10(4):239–241.
33. Camargo AH, Cooperberg MR, Ershoff BD, Rubenstein JN, Meng MV, Stoller ML. Laparoscopic management of peripelvic renal cysts: University of California, San Francisco, experience and review of literature. Urology 2005 May;65(5):882–887.
34. Grantham JJ. The etiology, pathogenesis, and treatment of autosomal dominant polycystic kidney disease: recent advances. Am J Kidney Dis 1996 Dec;28(6):788–803.
35. Murcia NS, Sweeney WE Jr, Avner ED. New insights into the molecular pathophysiology of polycystic kidney disease. Kidney Int 1999 Apr;55(4):1187–1197.
36. Lee DI, Andreoni CR, Rehman J, Landman J, Ragab M, Yan Y, Chen C, Shindel A, Middleton W, Shalhav A, et al. Laparoscopic cyst decortication in autosomal dominant polycystic kidney disease: impact on pain, hypertension, and renal function. J Endourol 2003 Aug;17(6):345–354.
37. Chapman AB, Gabow PA. Hypertension in autosomal dominant polycystic kidney disease. Kidney Int Suppl 1997 Oct;61:S71–S73.
38. Segura, J. W.; King, B. F.; Jowsey, S. G., et al. Chronic Pain and its medical and surgical management in renal cystic diseases. Polycystic Kidney Disease. New York: Oxford Medical Publications; p. 466.
39. Elzinga LW, Barry JM, Torres VE, Zincke H, Wahner HW, Swan S, Bennett WM. Cyst decompression surgery for autosomal dominant polycystic kidney disease. J Am Soc Nephrol 1992 Jan;2(7):1219–1226.
40. Ye M, Chen JH, Zhang L. Long-term results of cyst decapitating decompression (CDD) operation for autosomal dominant polycystic kidney disease (ADPKD). J Urol 157 (suppl):286.
41. Frang D, Czvalinga I, Polyak L. A new approach to the treatment of polycystic kidneys. Int Urol Nephrol 1988;20(1):13–21.
42. Rubenstein SC, Hulbert JC, Pharand D, Schuessler WW, Vancaillie TG, Kavoussi LR. Laparoscopic ablation of symptomatic renal cysts. J Urol 1993 Oct;150(4):1103–1106.
43. Teichman JM, Hulbert JC. Laparoscopic marsupialization of the painful polycystic kidney. J Urol 1995 Apr;153(4):1105–1107.
44. Lifson BJ, Teichman JM, Hulbert JC. Role and long-term results of laparoscopic decortication in solitary cystic and autosomal dominant polycystic kidney disease. J Urol 1998 Mar;159(3):702–705; discussion 705–706.

45. Chehval MJ, Neilsen C. Laparoscopic cyst decompression in polycystic kidney disease. J Endourol 1995 Jun;9(3):281–282.
46. Dunn MD, Portis AJ, Shalhav AL, McDougall EM, Clayman RV. Laparoscopic cyst marsupialization in patients with autosomal dominant polycystic kidney disease. J Urol 2001 Jun; 165(6 part 1): 1888–1892.
47. Brown JA, Torres VE, King BF, Segura JW. Laparoscopic marsupialization of symptomatic polycystic kidney disease. J Urol 1996 Jul;156(1):22–27.
48. Hoenig DM, McDougall EM, Shalhav AL, Elbahnasy AM, Clayman RV. Laparoscopic ablation of peripelvic renal cysts. J Urol 1997 Oct;158(4):1345–1348.
49. Gill IS, Rassweiler JJ. Retroperitoneoscopic renal surgery: our approach. Urology 1999 Oct;54(4):734–738.
50. Guazzoni G, Montorsi F, Bergamaschi F, Consonni P, Bellinzoni P, Centemero A, Rigatti P. Laparoscopic unroofing of simple renal cysts. Urology 1994 Feb;43(2):154–159.
51. Valdivia Uria JG, Baquero GA, Alebesque FM, Santamaria EL. Laparoscopic ablation of renal cysts. Arch Esp Urol 1994;47:246.
52. Wada T, Kamiryo Y, Tsuchida M, Kato M. Laparoscopic unroofing of a renal cyst. Hinyokika Kiyo 1995 Nov;41(11):861–865.
53. Ou YC, Yang CR, Chang YY, Kuo JH, Wu HC. The clinical experience of gaseous retroperitoneoscopic and gasless retroperitoneoscopy-assisted unroofing of renal cyst. Chung Hua I Hsueh Tsa Chih (Taipei) 1997 Apr;59(4):232–239.
54. Denis E, Nicolas F, Ben Rais N, Cloix P, Dawahra M, Marechal JM, Gelet A. Laparoscopic surgical treatment of simple cysts of the kidney. Prog Urol 1998 Apr;8(2):195–200.
55. Fahlenkamp D, Rassweiler J, Fornara P, Frede T, Loening SA. Complications of laparoscopic procedures in urology: experience with 2,407 procedures at 4 German centers. J Urol 1999 Sep;162(3 Pt 1):765–770; discussion 770–771.
56. Roberts WW, Bluebond-Langner R, Boyle KE, Jarrett TW, Kavoussi LR. Laparoscopic ablation of symptomatic parenchymal and peripelvic renal cysts. Urology 2001 Aug;58(2):165–169.
57. Santiago L, Yamaguchi R, Kaswick J, Bellman GC. Laparoscopic management of indeterminate renal cysts. Urology 1998 Sep;52(3):379–383.
58. Warren KS, McFarlane J. The Bosniak classification of renal cystic masses. BJU Int 2005 May;95(7):939–942.
59. Elashry OM, Nakada SY, Wolf JS Jr, McDougall EM, Clayman RV. Laparoscopy for adult polycystic kidney disease: a promising alternative. Am J Kidney Dis 1996 Feb;27(2):224–233.
60. Shiraishi K, Eguchi S, Mohri J, Kamiryo Y. Laparoscopic decortication of symptomatic simple renal cysts: 10-year experience from one institution. BJU Int 2006 Aug;98(2):405–408.

Laparoscopic Simple Nephrectomy

Transperitoneal and Retroperitoneal Approaches

Kevin C. Zorn and Arieh L. Shalhav

INTRODUCTION

Seventeen years after the first reported laparoscopic nephrectomy in 1990 by Clayman et al. *(1)* and over a decade since the first retroperitoneal approach using a dissecting balloon by Gaur et al. *(2)* minimally invasive approaches to renal pathology continue to prove as an effective alternative to traditional open nephrectomy. Wide dissemination of these surgical techniques and continued improvement in instrumentation has made laparoscopy the preferred approach for treating benign pathologic conditions of the kidney.

Today, laparoscopy has emerged as the standard of care for benign renal disease requiring surgical intervention. More than 1,600 cases have been reported in the literature *(3)*. The advantages of reduced blood loss, postoperative pain, a shorted hospital stay, earlier return to normal activities, and improved cosmesis compared to the open approach are well documented *(4–11)*.

Although the term "simple" has been associated with nephrectomies that are performed for benign indications, this description continues to be one of the great misnomers in the field of urologic surgery. Chronic inflammation with subsequent fibrosis and scarring often affect the surrounding tissues making the process of tissue plane identification much more difficult than that of the typical radical nephrectomy. When present, these factors make the laparoscopic approach to simple nephrectomy a challenge for even the most experienced laparoscopic surgeons.

This chapter provides a comprehensive overview of the laparoscopic simple nephrectomy, concentrating on critical dissection points when utilizing either the transperitoneal or retroperitoneal approach. In addition, technical considerations when dealing with specific pathologic entities will be discussed. It is hoped that this detailed review will facilitate the performance of the laparoscopic simple nephrectomy and assist in preventing the complications associated with this procedure.

Preoperative Assessment for Laparoscopic Simple Nephrectomy

The most common indication for laparoscopic renal surgery for benign disease is simple nephrectomy. Although laparoscopic removal of small atrophic kidneys are ideally suited for less experienced surgeons, simple nephrectomy in situations with dense inflammation and fibrosis could pose immense challenges toward surgical dissection. Patients with xanthogranulomatous pyelonephritis (XGP), tuberculosis (TB) nephritis and prior renal surgery should be reserved for the most experienced laparoscopic surgeons *(3)*. Such patients should be counseled regarding the increased likelihood of perioperative complications and open conversion.

From: *Current Clinical Urology: Essential Urologic Laparoscopy*
Edited by: S. Y. Nakada and S. P. Hedican, DOI 10.1007/978-1-60327-820-1_6

Most often, pain, hematuria, and/or chronic infections are the presenting symptoms. In addition, some benign processes, such as renal cysts and obstruction, cause massive enlargement leading to displacement of adjacent structures and symptoms such as dyspnea, early satiety, and gastroesophageal reflux. Indications for laparoscopic simple nephrectomy are summarized in Table 1.

Table 1
Benign indications for laparoscopic simple nephrectomy

1) Chronic pyelonephritis
2) Chronic renal obstruction (uretero-pelvic obstruction, ureteral obstruction)
3) Reflux nephropathy
4) Autosomal dominant polycystic kidney disease (ADPKD)
5) Multicystic dysplastic kidney
6) Renal dysplasia
7) Large stone burden with minimal residual renal function
8) Nephrosclerosis
9) Renovascular hypertension
10) Renal tuberculosis
11) Xanthogranulomatous pyelonephritis
12) Native nephrectomy before renal transplantation

Absolute contraindications are similar to those for open nephrectomy, which include uncorrected active peritonitis, coagulopathy, bowel obstruction, and severe cardiopulmonary disease. Renal anatomic anomalies, such as horseshoe *(12–14)* or ectopic kidney *(15)*, do not preclude the laparoscopic approach, provided adequate preoperative imaging is obtained to delineate renal vascular supply. Relative contraindications are directly related to the surgeon's experience and comfort level. Particularly related to a transperitoneal approach, a history of previous abdominal surgeries or a former ipsilateral kidney surgery may be considered a relative contraindication. If a significant number of intra-abdominal adhesions are suspected preoperatively, it is safest to proceed with an open Hasson trocar placement. A retroperitoneal technique may be preferred in such cases as the peritoneal contents are bypassed entirely.

In the past, obesity was considered to be a relative contraindication to laparoscopy *(16,17)* Initial access in obese patients (BMI>30 kg/m^2) can be difficult, resulting in a higher probability of abdominal wall vessel injury and subcutaneous dissection during pneumoperitoneal establishment. Longer trocars and Veress needle, as well as bariatric-size laparoscopic equipment should be requested during preoperative planning. Skin-to-peritoneal distance can easily be calculated from abdominal imaging. Furthermore, port placement location and distance to one-another, as well as entry angle to the subcutaneous tissue are essential to optimize instrument triangulation and freedom of movement. With increased experience, obese patients may be attempted.

Matin et al. previously published on the Cleveland Clinic experience in markedly and morbidly obese patients (BMI$\geq$30 kg/m^2) *(18)*. The authors concluded laparoscopic renal surgery is technically feasible in such patients when compared to the open surgery group, resulting in significantly decreased blood loss and analgesic requirement, quicker return of bowel function, shortened convalescence, and reduced hospital stay. Similar operative times and complications rates were observed. Doublet et al. examined the outcomes of retroperitoneal laparoscopic nephrectomies in nine obese patients, compared to those of 46 non-obese patients *(19)*. Again, postoperative complication rates were similar in the two groups, occurring in 11 and 8.5% of the obese and non-obese patients, respectively. No open conversions were required in the obese cohort when the retroperitoneal approach was utilized. Other authors have observed longer operative times and increased estimated blood loss, but similar complication and conversion rates and recovery period compared with the non-obese cohort *(20,21)*. In summary, in experienced hands, obese patients can have comparable outcomes to non-obese patients when undergoing laparoscopic nephrectomy. However, we recommend that experience should first be obtained in the non-obese population, in order to minimize complications. It is also prudent to emphasize the increased open conversion risk that is associated with the obese population, especially with the transperitoneal laparoscopic approach *(22)*.

The most difficult cases are related to the presence of severe scarring and fibrosis, which may completely obliterate normal anatomic planes for capsular and hilar dissection *(3)*. Examples include XGP, renal TB, and prior open abdominal/renal surgeries. Enlarged kidneys, such as autosomal dominant kidney disease (ADPKD) may also pose a challenge during mobilization. These situations are typically associated with higher complication and conversion rates *(23–25)* and should be reserved for the most experienced laparoscopic surgeons.

Preoperative Work-Up

As part of the preoperative work-up, all patients should have a complete history and physical examination, with particular attention to past surgical history. During the assessment, the patient's body habitus, location of previous surgical incisions, and the presence of skeletal deformities should be noted. Each of these factors can influence the choice of the laparoscopic approach, the surgical positioning of the patient as well as port placement.

Full informed consent must be obtained from the patient, with emphasis placed on the risks of the procedure, which include bleeding, injury to peritoneal contents, and the possibility for open conversion, which occurs in approximately 5% of laparoscopic nephrectomies *(23,26)*. For laparoscopic simple nephrectomies, however, the incidence of complications and open conversions is potentially higher (Table 2). In a series of 100 laparoscopic nephrectomies, Keeley et al. showed that the presence of an inflammatory process (XGP, pyonephrosis, staghorn calculus) increased the chances of conversion to 12% *(23)*. As a result, the patient must be made aware of the lower threshold for open conversion under these circumstances.

Preoperative laboratory studies include a complete blood count, serum chemistries, coagulation panel, urinalysis, and urine culture. Chest radiograph, electrocardiogram, and additional cardiac work-up (if warranted) are also obtained. A type and screen is obtained, and two units of packed red cells are cross-matched. Patients with active infection and obstruction require treatment with appropriate antibiotic coverage and percutaneous drainage before nephrectomy. All patients with renal TB should receive antituberculosis medication for at least 3–4 weeks before surgery.

All patients should have a preoperative imaging study to assist in choosing the appropriate laparoscopic approach. An abdominal/pelvic computed tomography (CT) scan, with and without intravenous contrast with a delay phase, is our imaging modality of choice. This study provides excellent representation of perirenal anatomy, including location and number of renal vessels and positioning of the ureter. CT scans are very helpful in delineating the presence of aberrant renal vessels, which are known to occur in 25–40% of kidneys *(27)*. If an accessory vessel is suspected but still not well-defined on CT, some groups recommend that an angiogram (CT, magnetic resonance, or traditional) should be performed to rule out the presence of vascular variants *(28)*. The surgeon can also assess the relationship of the kidney to adjacent structures and gain an accurate representation of the amount of perirenal and pararenal fat that is present. Finally, CT is very sensitive in detecting perirenal fat stranding, which is a hallmark of inflammation and fibrosis. In patients with a history of atherosclerosis, one should also carefully examine the non-contrast images of the CT scan to identify renal artery wall calcifications. If mural calcification is present, particularly at the ostium, the renal artery should be dissected and clipped at a point where the vessel is free of atherosclerotic disease. Vessel fracture during clip application can cause sudden, uncontrollable arterial hemorrhage.

Table 2
Outcomes of contemporary series ($n = 1{,}654$) of laparoscopic simple nephrectomy for benign disease

Study	*Year*	*Number of cases*	*Approach*	*Mean OR time (min)*	*Mean EBL (mL)*	*Open conversions (%)*	*Major complications (%)*	*Mean hospital stay (days)*	*Mean convalescence (days)*
Ono et al. *(100)*	1994	27	TP	265	455	6 (22%)	6 (22%)	10[a]	17α
Kerbl et al. *(7)*	1994	20	TP	355	200	1 (5%)	3 (15%)	3.7	28
Eraky et al. *(101)*	1994	60	TP	210	–	6 (10%)	4 (6.7%)	3.2	–
Parra et al. *(9)*	1995	12	TP	145	141	1 (8%)	2 (16.7%)	3.5	16
McDougal et al. *(102)*	1996	33	TP and RP	320	–	2	3 (9%)	2.9	14.7
Ono et al. *(103)*	1996	20	RP	198	135	0	1 (5%)	8	19
Doublet et al. *(104)*	1997	36	RP	95	–	0	1 (3%)	3.7	14
Rassweiler et al. *(76)*	1998	482[b]	TP and RP	188	–	46 (9.4%)	29 (6%)	5.4	–
Gill *(49)*	1998	36	RP	263	117	2 (5.6%)	0	2.9	16.1
Keely et al. *(23)*	1998	79	TP	147	–	5 (3.4%)	1 (1.3%)	4.8	–
Gaur*(31)*	2000	38	RP	132	84	6 (1.6%)	(45%)[c]	2.7	13.3
Hermal et al. *(105)*	2001	185[d]	RP	100	133	18 (9.7%)	7 (3.8%)	3	–
Sebe et al. *(106)*	2003	88	RP	114	98	3 (3.4%)	–	4.7	–
Gupta et al. *(6)*	2004	351	RP	98	65	4 (1%)	4 (1%)	3	–
Poulsen et al. *(107)*	2005	103[e]	TP and RP	190	150	7 (6.7%)	2 (1.9%)	4	–
Manohar et al. *(25)*	2007	84	TP	170	156	8 (9.5%)	4 (4.8%)	4.4	–

EBL – estimated blood loss; OR – operative room; RP – retroperitoneal; TP – transperitoneal.
[a]Cases completed laparoscopically.
[b]Series also included 38 radical nephrectomies for malignancy.
[c]Includes major and minor complications.
[d]Includes 31 nephroureterectomies performed for benign conditions.
[e]Series also included 39 radical nephrectomies and 23 nephroureterectomies for malignancy.

Gadolinium-enhanced MRI-imaging is also a suitable consideration for patients with renal impairment and contrast allergy. If there are concerns regarding the residual renal function, a MAG-3 nuclear scan with differential function is useful.

The need for preoperative bowel preparation depends on the anticipated difficulty of the case. At our institution, if the kidney is not involved with an inflammatory process (i.e., atrophic or hydronephrotic kidney), the patient is placed on a clear liquid diet the day before surgery and the bowel preparation omitted. Another option is a limited bowel preparation protocol consisting of a clear liquid diet and a bottle of magnesium citrate the day before surgery. If significant difficulty with dissection is expected, the patient should undergo a full mechanical bowel preparation along with antibiotics the day prior to surgery. If the kidney is suspected to be chronically infected (pyonephrosis, struvite calculi), appropriate antibiotics should be given for at least 1 week prior to surgery. All other patients should be given a parenteral antibiotic, usually a first-generation cephalosporin, in the preoperative holding area. Subcutaneous heparin and pneumatic compression stocking are administered prior to anesthesia induction. Oro-gastric decompression and Foley catheter placement are also performed prior to patient positioning.

SURGICAL TECHNIQUE

Laparoscopic simple nephrectomy can be performed either by transperitoneal ("pure" *(29)* or hand-assisted *(30)*) or retroperitoneal *(31)* approaches. The transperitoneal approach offers the advantage of more intuitive anatomic landmarks and greater working space. The retroperitoneal approach offers faster access to the renal hilum without the need to mobilize intra-abdominal structures and may be advantageous in patients with prior abdominal surgery. We describe the technical aspects of both approaches, with particular emphasis on the transperitoneal approach, our preferred choice. The hand-assisted approach is useful to bridge the steep learning curve needed to transition from open to pure laparoscopic surgery. Current hand-assisted ports are summarized in Table 3. Hand-assisted

Table 3
Characteristics of commercially available devices for hand-assisted laparoscopy *(108–111)*

Characteristic	*Gelport*	*Lap disc*	*Omniport*
Manufacturer	Applied Medical (Rancho Santa Margarita, CA)	Ethicon Endo-surgery (Cincinnati, OH)	Advanced Surgical Concepts (Ireland, distributed in US by Weck Closure, Raleigh, NC)
Device diameter (cm)	13	12	12
Number of components	Three pieces. -Flexible skirt, rigid base, gel cap	One piece.	Two pieces. Cuff with retention rings, insufflation device
Advantages	Gel cap maintains pneumoperitoneum with or without instruments and allows instrument to be placed directly through cap device	Small and simple to work. An iris configuration allows opening to be large enough for hand or tightly placed around a trocar	Able to maintain pneumoperitoneum even when incision too long
Disadvantages	Gas leak if incision too long	Gas leak if incision too long	Loss of pneumoperitoneum when hand is removed
Cost per device	$575	$490	$415

laparoscopic nephrectomy may also allow urologic surgeons with basic laparoscopic skills the capability to offer patients minimally invasive renal surgery and provide a platform on which to develop skill in advanced techniques. Furthermore, in situations where the surgeon failures to progress during a difficult case, conversion to a hand-assisted approach can help serve as a reasonable option prior to elective conversion. Hand-assisted laparoscopic surgery has the advantage of restoring tactile feedback and use of the hand to assist with dissection, retraction, extraction, and rapid control of bleeding if needed. Tan et al. have advocated its use upfront if severe fibrosis is anticipated *(32)* where manual, tactile sensation may assist with safe dissection. The technical aspect of the hand-assisted approach has been well-described elsewhere *(33)* and will not be further commented in this chapter.

Transperitoneal Nephrectomy

The transperitoneal route is considered the traditional laparoscopic approach to renal surgery. The greatest benefit of this approach includes good anatomic landmarks within the peritoneal cavity and a large working space that allows for optimal port placement. These advantages are important when treating enlarged kidneys or those involved with a generalized, massive inflammatory process. Disadvantages to this approach include the need to retract or dissect other intra-abdominal organs, such as the liver, spleen, and bowel, away from the kidney to provide adequate exposure. In addition, previous abdominal surgery can often make initial trocar placement difficult.

PROCEDURE

Essential equipment (Figs. 1 and 2) for laparoscopic transperitoneal simple nephrectomy includes:

- 15-Blade scalpel
- 14-Gauge Veress needle (both standard (12 mm) and bariatric length (15 mm))

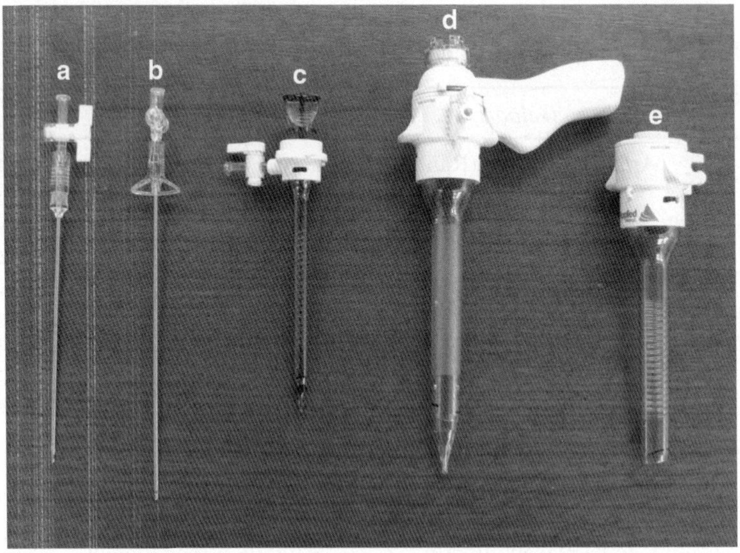

Fig. 1. Standard University of Chicago Medical Center pneumoperitoneal and trocar port access equipment. (From *left to right*): (**A**) 14 G × 12 mm Excel® (ConMed, Utica, NY); (**B**)14 G × 15 mm Surgineedle® (United States Surgical, Norwalk, CT) pneumoperitoneum insufflation needles; (**C**) 5 × 100 mm threaded cannula (Tyco Applied Medical, Rancho Santa Margarita, CA); Optical Separator System® with (**D**) non-threaded and (**E**) threaded 12 × 100 mm trocar ports (Tyco Applied Medical, Rancho Sanata Margarita, CA).

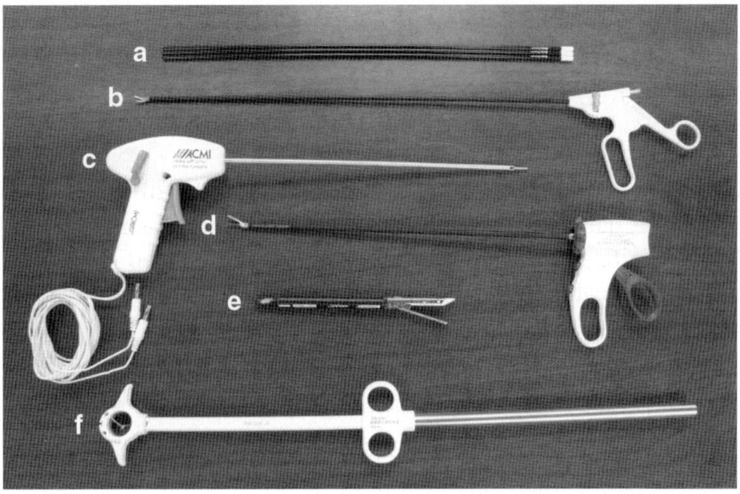

Fig. 2. Standard University of Chicago Medical Center dissection and hemostatic equipment. (From *top to bottom*): (**A**) Endopeanut® and (**B**) Endoshears® (Tyco Applied Medical, Rancho Sanata Margarita, CA); (**C**) Tripolar Ultra Cutting Forceps® (ACMI, Southborough, MA) which utilizes standard bipolar cautery coupled with a trigger-finger activated cutting blade; (**D**) Hand-activated 5 mm curved Harmonic Scalpel® (Ethicon Endosurgery, Cincinati, OH); (**E**) EndoGIA vascular stapler load (Tyco Applied Medical, Rancho Sanata Margarita, CA); (**F**) 15 mm Endocatch specimen retrieval bag (Tyco Applied Medical, Rancho Sanata Margarita, CA).

- **High-definition laparoscopes**
  - 5-mm (0° and 30°) Laparoscope
  - 10-mm (0° and 30°) Laparoscope
- **Blunt-ended trocar ports**
  - 12-mm Optical trocar
  - 12-mm Threaded trocars
  - 5-mm Trocars (3–4)
- **Dissecting instruments**
  - 5-mm Harmonic ultrasonic dissector
  - 5-mm Right-angle hook electrode
  - 5-mm Endoscopic scissors
  - 5-mm Maryland dissector
  - 5-mm Suction/irrigation probe
  - 5-mm Toothed, locking tissue graspers
  - 5-mm Kitner Endpeanuts
- **Hemostatic instruments**
  - 5-mm Bipolar grasper
  - 5- and 10-mm Weck Hemolock clips and applier
  - Endovascular GIA stapler (30 and 45 mm clips with reloads)
  - Argon-beam coagulator
  - Pre-loaded 6-in. 4–0 Vicryl suture end loaded with a Lapra-Ty Clip
  - Lapra-Ty clips with 10 mm applier
- **Specimen entrapment bag:**
  - 10- and 15-mm Endocatch bags (*U.S. Surgical Corporation, Norwalk, CT*)
- **Other equipment:**
  - Carter–Thomason® fascial closure device (*Inlet Medical Incorporated, Minneapolis,MN)*
  - Open laparotomy tray

- Vascular tray (clamps) and Prolene suture
- Hemostatic fibrin-based sealants (Tisseal (*Baxter, Deerfield, IL*), Evicel (*Johnson&Johnson, Somerville, NJ*))

Step 1: Initial Positioning

While in supine position, general anesthesia is established. A 16F Foley catheter is inserted for bladder drainage and urine output monitoring. In addition, an oro-gastric tube is placed for stomach decompression. When significant difficulty in dissection is anticipated due to existing inflammation (e.g., XGP or TB), a ureteral catheter can be placed to assist ureteral identification. We prefer to use a 6F open ended ureteral catheter. An occlusive ureteral balloon catheter with an inflatable balloon (2 cc of contrast maximum) can also be seated against the ureteropelvic junction, thus lessening the chance of dislodgement. If desired, additional catheter stiffness can be achieved by inserting a super-stiff guide wire through the balloon catheter *(34)*.

The patient's position is then adjusted on the bean-bag such that the break in the table on flexion is between the anterior superior iliac spine and the subcostal margin. The patient is then placed in a modified lateral decubitus position, with the thorax rotated back slightly at 30° (Fig. 3). The lower hand is padded and placed on an armrest. The lower leg is flexed at the knee 90°, while the upper leg is left extended. Pillows are placed between the legs for adequate support. Padding is placed under the lower ankle to relieve pressure in this area. An axillary roll is then placed 5 mm caudal to the axilla to protect the brachial plexus from a stretch injury. Additional padding is placed under the lower elbow to prevent ulnar nerve compression. The table is then flexed and placed in mild Trandelenburg such that exposure between the costal margin and iliac crest is optimized. At this point, the bean-bag is deflated

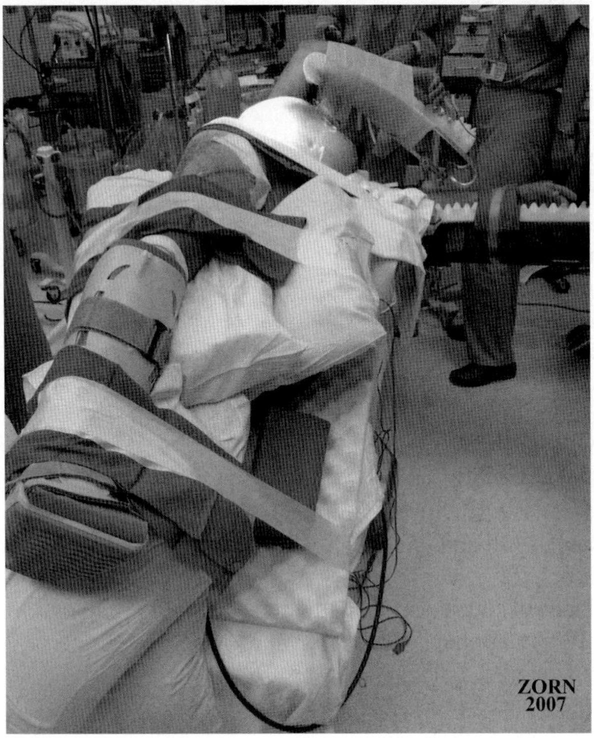

Fig. 3. Standard positioning for right-sided laparoscopic simple nephrectomy. Note the 30 rotational angle of the patient secured safely with the bean-bag support, pressure-point padding and silk tape wrapping.

to secure the final position. Care should be made to ensure visualization of the umbilicus and spine to ensure adequate exposure in the rare need for emergent open conversion. Surgical towels are placed over the skin at the hip, and knee levels, and 3-in. silk tape wrapped circumferentially at these levels to completely secure the patient to the table. Finally, an arm-rest (airplane) is then fastened to the table and secured to support the padded ipsilateral arm (Fig. 4). Careful attention to final position, pressure padding and security is essential, as bed rotation during surgery is often required to optimize exposure and assist with gravity bowel retraction.

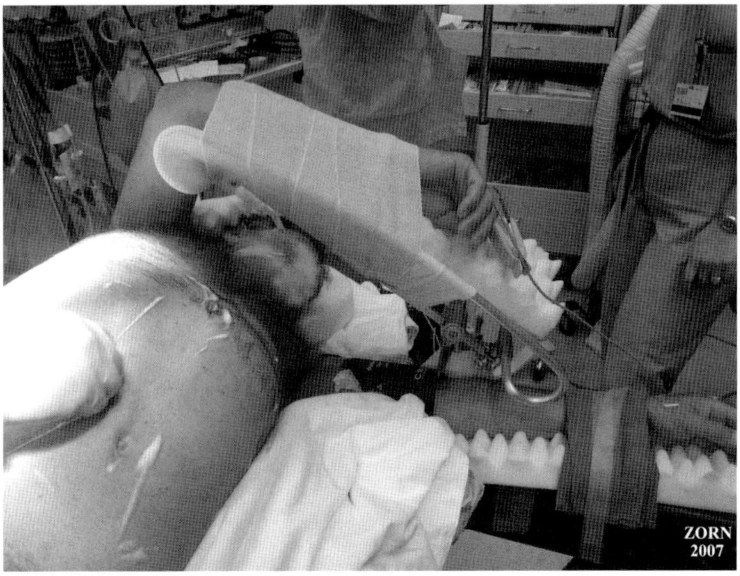

Fig. 4. Upper arm support with the air-plane table attachment. Note the natural bend in the elbow and appropriate padding. One must ensure the arm is supported as cephalad as possible to ensure maximal range of motion of laparoscopic equipment. The surgeon should simulate the expected port placement and instrument motions. If not considered appropriately before prepping the draping, lower pole dissection may be hampered by inference with the airplane device.

Without question, one should always ensure that an open laparotomy tray and vascular clamps are within the room and readily available before beginning the procedure. Skin preparation and site exposure should also take into account a possible open conversion. Finally, the patient's flank and abdomen are prepped and draped sterilely.

STEP 2: PNEUMOPERITONEAL ACCESS AND PORT PLACEMENT

Important anatomic landmarks for initial access are the subcostal margin, the umbilicus, and the rectus abdominus muscle. Standard port placement for right- and left-sided procedures is summarized in Figs. 5 and 6, respectively. Use of the skin marking pen and rule should be advocated prior to skin incisions. Furthermore, skin markings and port distances will significantly increase from 0 to 20 mmHg of peritoneal pressure. As such, one must reassess the port configuration after Veress access and pneumoperitoneal access. In patients with previous abdominal surgery, initial entry site should be well away from scars and prior surgical fields.

We favor the use of a 12 mm, 14-gauge Veress needle to insufflate the abdomen. Initial access is obtained at the level of the umbilicus, approximately 8–10 mm lateral to the midline. A further distance

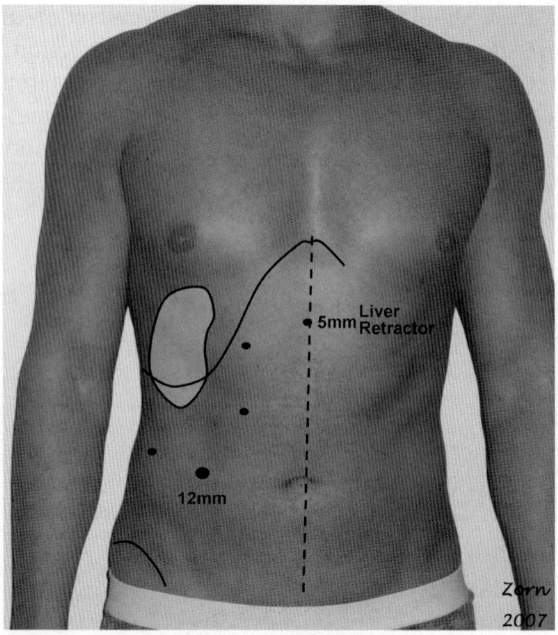

Fig. 5. Standard port placement for a laparoscopic right-sided nephrectomy. A total of five ports are routinely used (1–12 and 4–5 mm ports) in the above configuration.

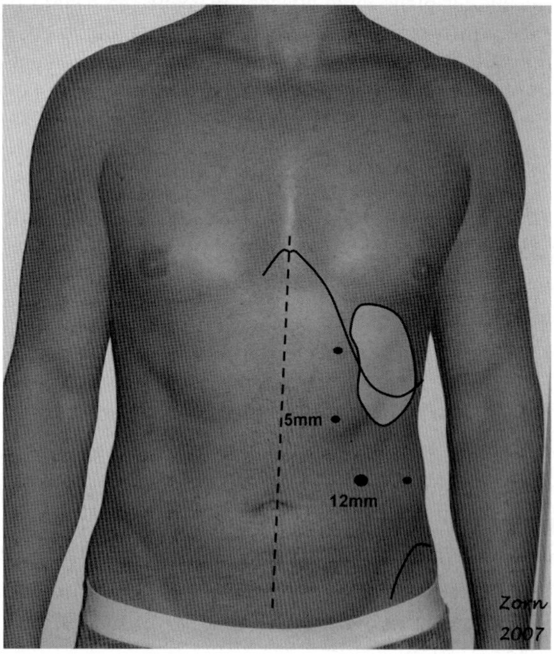

Fig. 6. Standard port placement for a laparoscopic left-sided nephrectomy. A total of four ports are routinely used (1–12 and 3–5 mm ports) in the above configuration.

should be used in obese patients, where the abdominal panus would fall with gravity. A 1.2 mm incision is made and a Hemostat instrument is used to spread the underlying subcutaneous tissues as well as permit the estimation of the skin-to-fascia distance. Counter-traction of the skin with two towel clamps elevating the skin will also help minimize the downward force of the needle, thereby decreasing the likelihood of vascular and visceral injury. The surgeon should feel two sequential points of resistance as the needle punctures the intervening fascial layers to enter the peritoneum. Until verification of proper position, absolutely no movement of the Veress needle tip should be made. At this point, the surgeon should confirm correct placement by first applying gentle suction through the needle using a 10-cc syringe, to insure that no bowel contents or blood is aspirated. Saline should then be injected, aspirated and upon release of the syringe, the fluid meniscus should drop secondary to the negative intra-abdominal pressure. It should be again stressed that at no point should the surgeon move the needle laterally in a back and forth motion or rotate the tip of the needle in an attempt to confirm position, as this can exacerbate potential inadvertent vascular or bowel injuries. If the needle is suspected to be in a suboptimal position, it should be removed and another placement attempt made. Failure to gain access should prompt an open approach with the Hasson technique.

Once the Veress needle is in proper position, insufflation is then initiated with CO_2 to raise the intra-abdominal pressure to 20 mmHg. The surgeon should examine and percuss the abdomen periodically during to confirm proper insufflation and that no significant subcutaneous emphysema is developing. When the intra-abdominal pressure is achieved, the needle is then removed.

The Optiview trocar (*Ethicon Endo-Surgical Corporation, Cincinnati, OH*) or the Optical Separator System® (*Tyco Applied Medical, Rancho Sanata Margarita, CA*) is then placed under camerascopic guidance. This instrument allows direct visualization of all layers of the abdominal wall during puncture. A standard progression of color-guided anatomy should be appreciated when placed (*yellow*– subcutaneous fat, *white*– pre-rectus fascia, *red*– muscle, *white*– transversalis fascia, *yellow*– pre-peritoneal fat, and *black*– pneumoperitoneum). We suggest ensuring all room-lights are off during this process to optimize tissue appreciation. A large enough incision should be ensured so that excessive downward port pressure is avoided. The Optiview trocar, along with a loaded, focused and white-balanced 10-mm 0° laparoscope, is then placed perpendicular to the fascia, using constant pressure and a continuous 180° twisting (supination and pronation) motion with the forearm. Steady pressure should be applied through the surgeon's shoulder, never with the elbow, as this has been shown to reduce the incidence of forceful trocar entry and the probability of vascular or bowel injury *(35)*. As the trocar passes through the abdominal wall, the blunt tip spreads apart intervening muscle and fascial layers until the peritoneum is penetrated. Intraperitoneal fat or bowel is easily visible once the peritoneal cavity is entered. At this point, the visual obturator is removed, and the 10-mm scope is quickly placed through the port. The intra-abdominal contents are examined, beginning with the area directly beneath the trocar entry point. The contents of the abdomen are then inspected carefully for signs of injury, beginning initially with the structures immediately beneath the point of trocar entry.

All remaining ports are then placed under visual guidance using the 5 mm 0° lens in a subcostal configuration (Figs. 5 and 6). We have developed a generalized approach for renal surgery in which near-identical trocar configurations are used for both extirpative and reconstructive procedures. Using this standard approach, we have successfully performed more than 1,200 laparoscopic renal surgery cases, including simple, donor, radical and partial nephrectomy, adrenalectomy, renal cyst decortication, and pyeloplasty. Adaptation of a standard approach simplifies surgical planning and facilitates transferring of laparoscopic techniques to the trainee.

We routinely place two 5 mm trocars through the para-rectus line so that all ports are distanced by at least 7–8 mm from one another. Only after the abdomen is insufflated, the final entry sites of the trocars are marked. A lateral trocar is then placed along the mid-axillary line, halfway between the anterior superior iliac spine and the costal margin. Particularly for right-sided procedures, another 5-mm port is placed in the midline 2–5 mm below the xiphoid process (subxiphoid port) to assist with liver retraction. Throughout the procedure, additional 5 mm ports can potentially be placed in the need for further tissue retraction.

Step 3: Initial Dissection

The camera is routinely placed through the lower, para-rectus 5 mm trocar allowing the working surgical instruments to be introduced through the 12 mm and upper para-rectus 5 mm ports. On the right and left sides, the ascending and descending colon, respectively, must be reflected off the anterior surface of the kidney as the initial step. This is accomplished by incising the line of Toldt along the axis of the colon, proceeding to the pelvic brim. We prefer using an ultrasonic dissector, as it allows the surgeon to grasp, incise, and dissect tissue securely with effective coagulation *(36)*. The hand-activated buttons also facilitate ergonomic positioning throughout the procedure. The blunt tip of the suction probe serves as an effective tool for downward traction against the mesenteric fat and bowel during initial dissection. When the plane between the lateral border of the colon and the abdominal wall is developed, the suction probe tip or a Kitner Endopeanut (*Tyco Applied Medical, Rancho Sanata Margarita, CA*) can then be used to bluntly reflect the colon medially while using the ultrasonic dissector to free any remaining flimsy attachments. Since there is likely an inflammatory response in the perinephric tissues, starting ones dissection at a lower point where tissue planes can be discriminated is a wise approach.

Once the kidney is exposed, dissection should be performed at the level of the renal capsule, if possible. In cases where significant inflammation and scarring is present, one must keep in mind that it will often be impossible to define planes within Gerota's fascia because of perirenal fibrosis. As such, dissection will likely be directed outside of this plane as would be done in a radical nephrectomy. It is essential to carefully dissect from points of known anatomy to points of unknown or difficult anatomy.

Step 4: Renal Dissection

Although tempting, one should avoid dissecting along the lateral border of the kidney initially, as early division of these attachments allows the kidney to drop medially, which can hinder hilar dissection. Use of the assistant's blunt-ended Kitner will facilitate tissue counter-traction while dissecting.

Right Kidney: In cases where the perinephric fat is easily dissected, it should be cleared away to expose the renal capsule. When significant inflammation is present, work should begin at the level of Gerota's fascia. Dissection proceeds medially, where the duodenum is located and lies anterior to the vena cava and hilar vessels. The surgeon should then define the duodenum, the lateral border of which must be carefully dissected and mobilized medially (*Kocher maneuver*). The duodenum is then reflected, exposing the underlying vena cava. As one progresses superiorly along the vena cava, the renal vein is located. Care should be made at identifying the gonadal vein for two important reasons. First, one can clip or bipolar coagulate followed by divide the vein early to prevent hemorrhage from this structure due to inadvertent tearing. In addition, this landmark can then be used to locate the ureter in close proximity.

If difficulty is encountered in initial dissection over the hilar region, one should commence with lower pole renal dissection and isolate the ureter (see Step 5). As will be discussed, a lower-pole-first dissection allows the surgeon to safely approach the hilum by progressing superiorly along the ureter or the gonadal vessel (known anatomy) after retracting the lower pole of the kidney off the psoas muscle, facilitating dissection.

Left Kidney: In patients with thin and uninflammed hilar tissues, dissection can begin medially over the hilar region. However, one must keep in mind that the long renal vein on this side travels over the aorta and will be the most anterior structure in this area. As such, care must be taken to avoid injuring this structure inadvertently. *Often because of significant fibrosis or inflammatory changes, safe dissection over the hilar region may be extremely difficult. As such, it is probably best to begin toward the lower pole of the kidney (see Step 5) to define the ureter and/or gonadal vein.* One can then proceed along these landmarks superiorly and define the hilar vessels. Once the renal vein is defined, the renal artery can then be isolated. Dissection of the periarterial tissue should begin bluntly, while looking for pulsations indicative of artery location.

Step 5: Isolation of the Lower Pole

The process of lower pole renal dissection is similar for both sides. Once the lower pole is defined, location and isolation of the ureter further medially is a key maneuver. This major anatomic landmark can be used not only as a traction point to assist in dissection toward the hilum, but also as a guide to other more medial structures such as the aorta on the left and the vena cava on the right. As a result, it is important not to clip and divide the ureter too early in the procedure. This should be only done once the hilar vessels are completely isolated and divided.

During ureteral dissection, the colon must be sufficiently retracted medially to improve exposure. Blunt dissection through the retroperitoneal fat using the closed tips of the Harmonic scalpel and the tip of the suction device allow visualization of the psoas muscle. The movements of the instruments should parallel the psoas muscle fibers. The ureter is then identified and isolated while the assistant's Kitner is used to retract all fatty tissue laterally. Thereafter, the Gerota's fat from the lateral border of the ureter to the body wall can safely be ligated, either using the bipolar, ultrasonic device or in difficult situations, the EndoGIA stapler, thus liberating the lower aspect of the renal specimen.

Dissection continues along the plane of the psoas muscle to the lower pole, posterior plane of the kidney. This avascular plane usually dissects very easily and creates a window superiorly to safely approach the hilar vessels. Consideration of lower pole accessory renal vessels must always be on the surgeon's mind during this dissection.

Step 6: Isolation of the Upper Pole

Left Kidney:On the left side, the splenorenal and phrenicocolic ligaments are located and divided, so as to allow mobilization of the splenic flexure of the colon and medial displacement of the spleen. One must incise the peritoneal reflection along the upper pole of the kidney in order to be able to define the plane between the adrenal and kidney. We advocate the use of bipolar energy along this plane to minimize troublesome venous bleeding.

During this aspect of the procedure, care must be made to avoid injury to the splenic capsule and diaphragm. In cases where splenic capsular bleeding is encountered, prompt increase of the pneumoperitoneal pressure to 20–25 mmHg coupled with compression using cellulose-based product should be initially performed. Coagulation with the argon-beam coagulator can then be attempted. Fibrin-based hemostatic agents, such as Tisseal (*Baxter, Deerfield, IL*) or Evicel (*Johnson&Johnson, Somerville, NJ*) can also be used.

Right Kidney:During a right-sided case, attachments to the inferior border of the right lobe of the liver are dissected in order to allow appropriate cephalad retraction of this structure. In certain instances, the right triangular ligament may also need to be partially divided to improve mobility of the right lobe. Use of a 5 mm locking-toothed grasper through the subxiphoid port, which should already be in position after port insertion, should be used to elevate the liver edge. The grasper shaft should be used to further retract the underside of the organ, and the lateral abdominal wall is engaged with the jaws of the grasper. The surgeon must take great care during positioning of the grasper to avoid traumatizing the liver with the instrument tip which can result in troublesome bleeding. The argon-beam coagulator can effectively manage hepatic bleeding. In addition, one must also avoid injuring the diaphragm with the graspers, as this may lead to a CO_2 pneumothorax should the pleura be inadvertently punctured, especially with thermal dissection of the lateral liver attachments. A diaphragmatic tear with pneumothorax should be suspected if the patient develops consistently high-end tidal CO_2 levels and end inspiratory pressures *(37)*. A floppy hemidiaphragm may also be appreciated during the procedure. Intra-operative repair of a diaphragmatic injury should involve intracorporeal suturing with needle drivers or the Endostitch device (*U.S. Surgical Corporation, Norwalk, CT*). Positive ventilatory pressure administered by the anesthesia team may help expel CO_2 prior to suture closure. Residual capnothorax may be treated either with a chest tube placement in symptomatic patients or conservatively in stable and asymptomatic patients. Due to the favorable absorptive properties of CO_2 gas, rapid resolution of a capnothorax can be expected within hours of the procedure (Fig. 7) *(38)*.

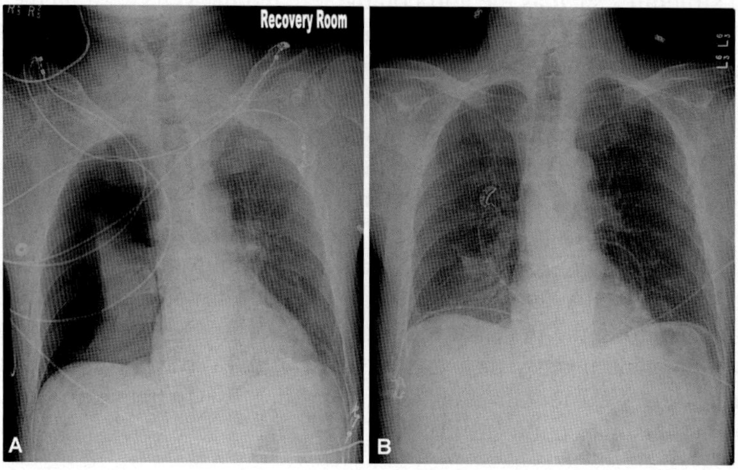

Fig. 7. Conservative management of a small diaphragmatic injuring during a right-sided laparoscopic renal procedure. **(A)** Postoperative chest X-ray taken while in recovery room demonstrating a large, right pneumothorax occupying 70% of the hemithorax. **(B)** Repeat chest X-ray taken 5 h later demonstrating complete right lung re-expansion.

The peritoneal reflection along the upper pole of the kidney should then be incised in order to commence dissection at the level of the renal capsule between the adrenal gland and the kidney. Once the peritoneal reflection along the upper pole of the kidney has been incised, dissection should proceed with the goal of finding the plane between the adrenal and the upper pole of the kidney. Use of the bipolar coagulator for dissection in this area is suggested, as the lower border of the adrenal should be well coagulated during dissection to minimize troublesome bleeding. Downward retraction of the kidney with the assistant's Kitner greatly assists with tissue tension and exposure. If significant bleeding or abundant, inflamed fatty tissue is encountered, another option is to use a GIA stapler to manage the plane between the adrenal and kidney. Ultimately, the dissection should ideally be taken down to the level of the psoas muscle, especially along the medial aspect. Creation of this window can provide the surgeon an option of rapid hilar control in the event of future trouble. Insertion along the psoas muscle of a vascular-loaded 45 mm EndoGIA stapler from the previously dissected lower pole with exposure of the device tip at the upper pole medial window can ensure safe, reliable clamping, and division of the hilar vessels *(39–40)*.

Step 7: Completion of Hilar Dissection

The surgeon should attempt to completely dissect the hilar vessels free from any surrounding tissue. By isolating the vessels from one another, precise and safe division of the vessels can be achieved. A helpful maneuver during hilar dissection is lateral traction of the kidney with the assistant's Kitner device.

Left Kidney:Numerous venous branches (adrenal, lumbar, gonadal) feed into the left renal vein which increases the complexity of its dissection. After careful dissection, we have previously controlled these branches with clips (two on the patient side, one on the specimen side), and divided before proceeding with dissection of the renal artery. We needed to be cognizant that the Hemolock clips can interfere with the engagement of an endovascular GIA staple load on the renal vein itself, leading to potentially catastrophic bleeding. Chan et al. found in a retrospective review that five of seven preventable causes of GIA stapler malfunction were caused by deployment of the stapler over unrecognized clips *(41)*. It is important to suspect stapler problems early, before disengaging the device, as one can place clips or another staple load further medially to ensure control of the vein. Due to such risk, we now favor the use of bipolar electrocautery using the ACMI Tripolar Ultra Cutting Forceps® (*ACMI, Southborough, MA*) to control the renal vein branches, which can then be divided without clips. Several authors have reported this technique during laparoscopic donor nephrectomies without complications *(42–43)*.

Right Kidney:Similar retraction and dissection maneuvers are employed during a right-sided procedure. The kidney needs to be retracted laterally to optimize exposure and tissue tension at the hilum. It is important, however, to first detach the adrenal gland from the upper pole of the kidney to prevent inadvertent injury to the right adrenal vein. The short renal vein can also make renal artery isolation a challenging task. If one is experiencing difficulty in renal artery dissection, the right ureter may need to be divided to allow cephalad and medial rotation of the lower pole. Once the renal artery and vein are circumferentially dissected, the artery must be clipped first. The artery can be controlled by placing two 10-mm Weck hemoclips (*Weck Closure Systems, Research Triangle Park, NC*) on the patient side and another clip on the specimen side prior to sharp division with endoscopic scissors. The additional security of a locking mechanism ensures the clip cannot be dislodged once engaged. The harmonic scalpel, however, is capable of burning through these clips. Prior to engaging a Hemolock clip, the vessel must be completely skeletonized, as any remaining periadvential tissue may become lodged within the locking mechanism and prevent clip engagement or worse, a delayed release. Ample space behind the artery should be ensured to allow proper placement of three clips. Once the artery is divided, flattening of the renal vein and renal discoloration should be observed. If the vein remains full, careful examination for an accessory renal artery should be performed. When the surgeon is satisfied that complete arterial control has been achieved, the renal vein is then ligated and cut. An endovascular GIA stapler or the use of hemolock clips can be used.

Should difficulty be encountered in isolating each of the renal vessels because of severe inflammatory changes, a renal pedicle isolation technique using a penrose drain can be implemented. Sufficient dissection anterior and posterior to the hilum, along the psoas muscle, must be performed in order to free the pedicle. At this point, the drain is placed around the pedicle such that lateral traction can be utilized to optimize exposure. An endovascular GIA staple load can then be used to cut and ligate the vessels en bloc. In this case, a wider staple load (3.5-mm) should be used. In their series examining the transperitoneal laparoscopic approach for inflammatory renal conditions, Shekarriz et al. managed five patients with this technique, with no subsequent development of an arteriovenous fistula after 2 years of follow-up *(24)*. More recently, White et al. reported on 94 patients who underwent en bloc renal hilar ligation during open ($n = 43$) and laparoscopic ($n = 51$) nephrectomy using a 45 mm titanium endovascular stapler *(40)*. With a mean follow-up of 35.2 months, no patient demonstrated any evidence of arteriovenous fistula formation. Furthermore, of the 40 patients who underwent CT arteriography, no fistulas were noted. As such, based on clinical follow-up and prospective radiographic evaluation, there appears to be a low risk of arteriovenous fistula formation after en bloc ligation of the renal hilum using a titanium endovascular stapler.

Step 8: Removal of Specimen

When the kidney is completely dissected, there are a number of options for specimen retrieval. The first is specimen morcellation to minimize skin incision length. This process is facilitated by incorporating the kidney within an Endocatch bag (*U.S. Surgical Corporation, Norwalk, CT*). To do this, the surgeon must maneuver the kidney over the liver after a right-sided nephrectomy or the spleen after a left-sided procedure to make room for the retrieval bag. Either the 10- or 15-mm Endocatch bag is used depending on the size of specimen. The 10 mm bag is placed through the 12-mm port, however, the 15-mm must be placed after removal of the 12-mm trocar and slight enlargement of the skin incision. The bag is then deployed inferior to the kidney with care not to rub the Endocatch over the ligated hilar vessels. The kidney is then grasped by the ureter and moved into the bag under direct vision. The drawstring is then pulled tight to cinch the edges of the bag closed, and the edges pulled out of the port.

If morcellation is desired, we prefer to manually morcellate the specimen using finger fragmentation and ring forceps. Morcellation with mechanical devices often takes longer in simple nephrectomy cases as inflammatory changes and renal calculi make the tissue very fibrous and scarred. If the specimen is large, as in cases of ADPKD, manual morcellation becomes less efficient. In these cases, a commercial morcellator, such as the Dyonics device (*Smith&Nephrew, Andover, MA*) described by Baughman et al. *(44)* can be used in concert with a Lapsac device (*Cook Urological, Incorporated, Spencer, IN*), which tends to be sturdier than the Endocatch bag. The process should be done under direct vision to ensure that the morcellator does not penetrate the sack and injure other intra-abdominal structures *(29)*.

A newer device, the WISAP morcellator (*WISAP America, Lenexa, KS*), allows efficient intracorporeal morcellation of specimens under direct vision, without the use of a laparoscopic bag. To utilize this approach, a 2-cm subumbilical incision is made and the 20-mm WISAP trocar placed with visual guidance. A serrated rotary sheath, along with grasping forceps, is placed within the trocar to perform morcellation. The specimen is grasped and pulled into the rotary sheath, which morcellates in a coring fashion. It is important to lift the specimen up and away from the bowel when engaging the kidney into the morcellator and to visualize the process carefully to prevent inadvertent injuries.

Varkarakis et al. have more recently described a novel prototype device that uses high-pressure (1,200–1,500 psi) water flow as a cutting/ablating tool (*HydroCision, Andover, MS*). *(45)* In all porcine cases, morcellation was performed inside a LapSac. By taking advantage of the Venturi effect, the vacuum created draws tissue into the space between the jet and the collector. The tissue captured in this space is completely macerated and consequently driven in a liquid form through the waste evacuation tubing to the connected waste container. Morcellation was significantly ($P< 0.0001$) faster in the water jet morcellator group than in the hand morcellation group (5.6 vs. 11.9 min). The macroscopic evaluation after filling the entrapment bags with normal saline revealed four (40%) and two (20%) pinhole perforations in the water jet and hand morcellation groups, respectively. The microscopic evaluation revealed an 80% perforation rate in the water jet group and a 20% rate in the hand morcellator group. Although promising, no clinic study has yet been published.

The second and ultimately the safest option for specimen extraction, which is used for unusually large specimens, is open extraction. This can be performed by lengthening the 12 mm port incision laterally, extending towards the lateral, mid-axillary 5 mm port. Finger elevation of the abdominal wall is required to avoid thermal injury to the specimen bag and abdominal viscera. The rectus fascia is then closed in a 2-layer fashion with 0-polydioxanone suture.

The use of a morcellator for specimen removal has not led to a significant reduction in operating or recovery time and remains as the surgeon's preference *(46)* Varkarakis et al. demonstrated in a series of 56 consecutive patients undergoing radical and simple nephrectomy, that despite a significantly longer extraction excision (7.1 vs. 1.2 mm, $p < 0.001$), no significant differences in pain or recovery between the intact extraction or morcellation groups were observed.

STEP 9: PORT CLOSURE AND PROCEDURE COMPLETION

Following specimen retrieval using the morcellation technique, a fingertip can be placed into the port through which the Endocatch device was removed. Pneumoperitoneum is reestablished and a final inspection of the abdominal contents is performed. We suggest decreasing the intra-abdominal pressure to 4 mmHg to confirm hemostasis prior to exiting the abdomen. The extraction site should then be closed using a 0-polydioxanone suture. The Carter–Thomason device (*Inlet Medical Incorporated, Minneapolis, MN*) also allows efficient suture placement with short-length or deep incisions. All 5-mm ports are then removed under direct vision, and the final para-rectus port withdrawn with the laparoscope left in the peritoneal compartment. The port should then be removed along side the scope followed by scope removal. This particular technique allows the surgeon to asses the wound edges for bleeding. If an additional 12 mm blunt tipped Optiview port was used throughout the procedure, we do not routinely close the fascial defect. When the port access tract is created by blunt dissection, the tissue planes tend to overlap upon removal of the trocar. At present, our experience of over 600 transperitoneal laparoscopic nephrectomies with unclosed12-mm trocar sites has yet to observe of clinical port herniation to date. All skin sites are typically closed with an absorbable 4-0 subcuticular suture and steri-stripped. Dermabond (*Ethicon, Piscataway, NJ*) can also be placed rather than the steri-strips to provide a water-tight seal.

Key Maneuvers

1. After incising the line of Toldt and providing medial colon reflecting, a lower pole first approach initial renal dissection with initial identification of the ureter should be performed. Although tempting, one should not begin at the postero-lateral aspect of the kidney. If this is done too early, the kidney will drop medially and make hilar dissection extremely difficult.
2. For right-sided nephrectomy, careful medial dissection to identify and mobilize the duodenum and vena cava allow safe identify of key vascular structures (gonadal, renal and adrenal veins).
3. In difficult situations, an endovascular GIA stapler can be used to divide the renal vessels en bloc. The surgeon must ensure that lower and upper pole dissection is well dissected down to the psoas muscle. A posterior plane along the psoas should also be ensured so that the lower blade of the stapler can safely be placed and visualized through the upper pole window. Once positioned, one must ensure that no clips are included within the staple jaws (e.g., clips on the stumps of the renal artery or left renal vein branches), as these can cause the stapler to misfire.

Retroperitoneal Nephrectomy

The retroperitoneal approach for laparoscopic nephrectomy was initially assessed by Clayman et al. *(47)*. However, multiple technical difficulties were encountered. The most significant of which was the lack of working space within the retroperitoneal space. Difficulty with orientation, visualization, and trocar spacing are other well-known challenges. As a result, most laparoscopic nephrectomies continued to be performed through the transperitoneal approach. It was not until Gaur described a technique of expanding the retroperitoneal space with a self-made balloon expander that this approach became more widely implemented *(48)*. Gaur went on to perform the first laparoscopic retroperitoneal nephrectomy in 1993 *(2)*. Since then, the advanced techniques of retroperitoneal nephrectomy have been well described *(31,49)*.

There are a number of advantages of the retroperitoneal route as compared to the more traditional transperitoneal approach. The lack of bowel mobilization with a resultant decrease in inadvertent bowel injury and ileus, rapid and direct kidney access, the avoidance of peritoneal cavity contamination and a lower risk of long-term complications (port site hernia and bowel obstruction) are noteworthy.

In addition, the renal artery can be identified much more readily as the kidney is approached from a posterior plane. The main disadvantages of the retroperitoneal approach include the lack of anatomic landmarks, a smaller working space (especially for a large kidney) with a significantly longer learning curve for the surgeon. With limited skin surface area in the lateral decubitus position, trocar placement is spaced closer together. Specimen entrapment after completion of dissection can also present a challenge.

In general, a retroperitoneal simple nephrectomy can be performed for any indication for which a transperitoneal approach is contemplated. However, larger kidneys will often cause problems in a retroperitoneal approach secondary to more limited hilar access and difficulty in specimen entrapment *(50)*. In addition, a known history of retroperitoneal inflammation (XGP, TB) can also limit this approach. As such, Gupta et al., with the largest reported series of retroperitoneoscopic nephrectomy for benign non-functioning kidney, considered a history of renal surgery, pyonephritis, XGP – a contraindication to retroperitoneal nephrectomy *(6)*. The majority of open conversions in their series of 351 consecutive cases were done in patients with XGP or a history of ipsilateral renal surgery. Prior placement of a percutaneous nephrostomy has also been considered a relative contraindication. Ultimately, surgeon preference and comfort coupled with patient characteristics should guide surgical approach.

PROCEDURE

Equipment list for laparoscopic retroperitoneal simple nephrectomy includes: **(Figs. 1 and 2)**

- 15-Blade scalpel
- Retroperitoneal (800 cc, kidney-shaped) balloon dilator
- **High-definition laparoscopes**
  - 5-mm (0 and 30°) Laparoscope
  - 10-mm (0 and 30°) Laparoscope
- **Blunt-ended trocar ports**
  - 12-mm Optical trocar
  - 12-mm Retroperitoneal blunt-tip trocar
  - 5-mm Trocars (3–4)
- **Dissecting instruments**
  - 5-mm Harmonic ultrasonic dissector
  - 5-mm Right-angle hook electrode
  - 5-mm Endoscopic scissors
  - 5-mm Maryland dissector
  - 5-mm Suction/irrigation probe
  - 5-mm Toothed, locking tissue graspers
  - 5-mm Kitner Endopeanuts
- **Hemostatic instruments**
  - 5-mm Bipolar grasper
  - 5- and 10-mm Weck Hemolock clips and applier
  - Endovascular GIA stapler (30 and 45 mm clips with reloads)
  - Argon-beam coagulator
  - Pre-loaded 6-in. 4-0 Vicryl suture end loaded with a Lapra-Ty Clip
  - Lapra-Ty clips with 10 mm applier
- **Specimen entrapment bag:**
  - 10- and 15-mm Endocatch bags (*U.S. Surgical Corporation, Norwalk, CT*)
- **Other equipment:**
  - Open laparotomy tray
  - Vascular tray (clamps) and Prolene suture

STEP 1: INITIAL POSITIONING

If one anticipates a difficult dissection secondary to perirenal inflammation, a ureteral catheter should be placed. The patient undergoes the same positioning steps as in the transperitoneal approach, along with placement of an axillary roll, Foley catheter and oro-gastric tube. A key difference, however, is the full lateral decubitus position (Fig. 8) to optimally mobilize the bowel and visceral structures with gravity.

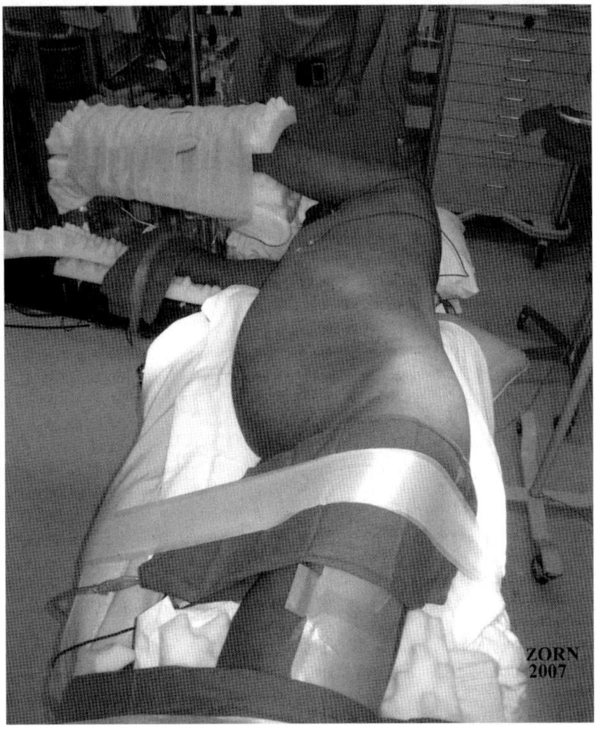

Fig. 8. Standard positioning for left-sided laparoscopic retroperitoneal nephrectomy. Note the full lateral decubitus patient position on the bean-bag support with pressure-point padding and silk tape wrapping.

Chiu et al. performed detailed CT studies of patients, looking specifically at differences in the antero-posterior distances between the quadratus lumborum and colon when patient positioning was changed. A significant increase in the distance between these structures was found with patients in lateral decubitus positions *(51)*. As a result, the patient should lie perpendicular to the table, with the table break between the anterior superior iliac spine and the costal margin prior to table flexion. Proper positioning is essential to maximize the abdominal working space to allow for optimal trocar placement. The spine, anterior superior iliac spine, costal margin, and umbilicus should be left exposed within the operative field to serve as anatomic landmarks. Leg positioning, padding of pressure points, and securing of the patient is then performed in the same fashion as described for the transperitoneal approach. The room and equipment setup differs in that during a retroperitoneal approach, the surgeon will stand facing the patient's back, with the video tower on the opposite side.

STEP 2: ESTABLISHMENT OF PNEUMOPERITONEUM

At our institution, we utilize the retroperitoneal approach described previously by Gill et al. from the Cleveland Clinic *(52,53)*. However, for initial access we prefer to use the blunt optical trocar with a 10-mm 0° laparoscope for direct visualization of the tissue layers, as opposed to the blunt separation

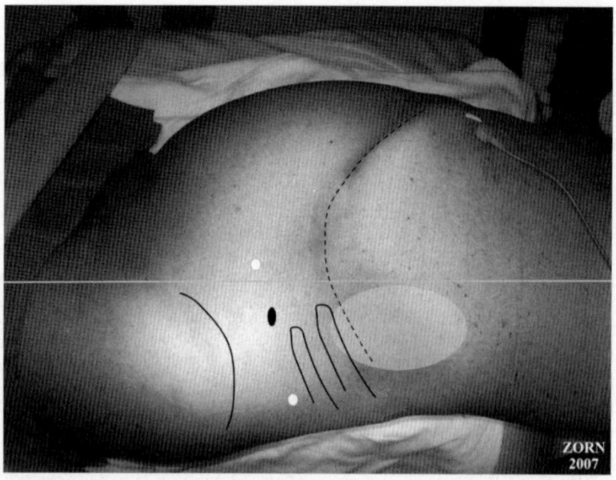

Fig. 9. Port configuration during left-sided laparoscopic retroperitoneal nephrectomy. Initial incision, retroperitoneal expansion and 12 mm port placement is performed 1 finger-breadth below and medial to the tip of the 12th rib. The two remaining 5 mm working trocars are placed at the junction of the 12th rib and paraspinous muscle as well as along the anterior axillary line.

technique using S retractors (open Hasson technique) *(54)*. The anatomic landmarks consist of the 12th rib and the angle between the 12th rib and paraspinous musculature (Fig. 9). Initial access is achieved approximately one fingerbreadth inferior to the tip of the 12th rib. A 15-blade is used to make a 1.5-cm transverse skin incision at this point. The optical trocar is then placed into the incision under direct vision, using the 10-mm 0° laparoscope. With the trocar pointed to the level of the umbilicus, 20° anteriorly, a twisting motion is applied until the retroperitoneum is entered through the intervening muscle layers and the lumbodorsal fascia. Visualization of the psoas muscle is helpful in identifying proper retroperitoneal access. Next, the surgeon's index finger is placed through the established tract to bluntly define the retroperitoneal space. It is important to begin the dissection by sweeping the finger under the tip of the 12th rib anteriorly, to ensure that the correct plane into the retroperitoneum has been entered. The goal is for the surgeon's finger to be between the internal surface of the transversalis fascia and the retroperitoneal fat at all times. As the space develops, blunt dissection continues posteriorly. The psoas and paraspinous muscles should be palpated with the tip of the index finger at this point, confirming that the correct plane outside of Gerota's fascia has been maintained. Lastly, the surgeon will sweep the finger further anteriorly to free any remaining attachments, with care taken to avoid inadvertent entry into the peritoneum.

Once the initial development of the retroperitoneal space is completed, the surgeon should be able to sweep the entire index finger in all directions without resistance. A 12 mm extraperitoneal space dissector (blunt-tipped trocar) is then placed into the tract and a 0° 10-mm laparoscope inserted into it, to allow direct visualization of the retroperitoneum during balloon expansion. We prefer the Spacemaker Plus Dissector System® *(Tyco Applied Medical, Rancho Sanata Margarita, CA)*, because the balloon is "kidney-shaped" and expands the retroperitoneum in an antero-posterior axis as well as a medio-lateral fashion (Fig. 10a). Approximately 800–1,000 cc (40 pumps) of air is required to fill the balloon in the adult patient (Fig. 10b) *(49,53)*. Correct placement anterior to the psoas muscle and posterior to the Gerota's fascia is required. Once the balloon has been fully expanded, the wrinkles along the midline seam of the balloon should no longer be visible. We advocate leaving the balloon expanded for 5 min to tamponade any small disrupted vessels. Time is spent during this period of identifying the ureter along the psoas muscle. The balloon is then deflated, and the bag removed. Unlike the former generation retroperitoneal space dissectors, where a separate device was required for the trocar, the Spacemaker Plus Dissector System® allows for an all-in-one device. After balloon removal, the

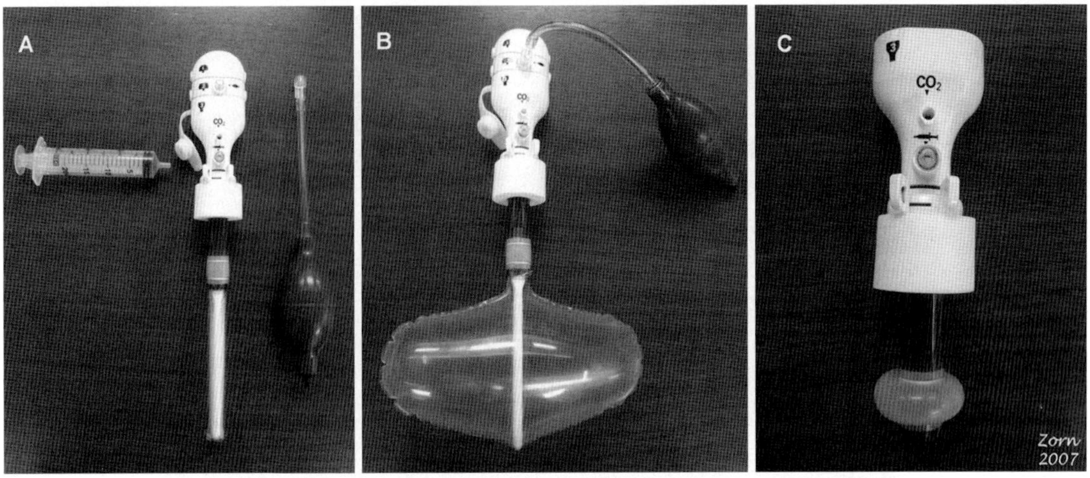

Fig. 10. Standard University of Chicago Medical Center retroperitoneal dissector and access trocar port (Spacemaker Plus Dissector System® (Tyco Applied Medical, Rancho Sanata Margarita, CA)). (**A**) Basic instrument components include an in-line, 12 mm blunt-tip obturator, balloon dissection mechanism and 12 mm trocar. (**B**) Insufflation of the balloon to 800 cc with the 10 mm obturator left in position. In the clinical setting, the 10 mm 0°scope would be in its position to visualize the retroperitoneum. (**C**) Final trocar setup with insufflation of the retaining cuff with 20 cc of air. The mid trocar foam can also be compressed downward toward the skin to optimize an air-tight seal.

remaining 12-mm trocar is left in situ and the retaining balloon inflated with 20 cc of air (Fig. 10c). The balloon rests against the transversalis fascia of the abdominal wall, and the adjustable foam cuff compressed at the skin level that prevents loss of pneumoperitoneum through the 1.5-cm skin incision. CO_2 extraperitoneal pressure is then established trocar at 14 mmHg.

A Veress needle can also be used to insufflate the retroperitoneum, creating an initial potential space before active balloon dilation is performed. The initial puncture point should be within Petit's triangle, which is formed by the medial border of the latissimus dorsi muscle, the lateral border of the external oblique muscle, and the superior border of the iliac crest *(47)*. Cadaveric and radiologic studies by Capelouto et al. further refined the access site within Petit's triangle *(55)*. Their report demonstrated that placement of the Veress needle approximately 1 mm above the iliac crest at the level of the posterior axillary line while angling the needle tip 10° anteriorly allows safe initial retroperitoneal entry. Once the retroperitoneum has been insufflated, an appropriately sized skin incision is made at the tip of the 12th rib to allow insertion of a balloon dilator, along with a 10-mm 0° laparoscope. After the retroperitoneal space is fully developed under direct vision, accessory ports are then placed as described in *Step 3*.

Step 3: Completion of Port Placement

With our method, two additional working trocars are placed with initial tactile guidance, using an index finger inserted into the initial port site. If possible, the trocars should be spaced at least 6–8 mm apart from one another in the subsequently described configuration (Fig. 9) *(53)*.

The first working port consists of a 5-mm trocar placed at the angle formed by the junction between the 12th rib and the paraspinous musculature. The surgeon, with the index finger placed in the initial port site to provide tactile guidance, places the trocar at the junction point approximately 1 mm below the 12th rib and 1 mm lateral to the paraspinous muscles (Fig. 11).

The second port, which is furthest anterior, should be placed approximately 3–5 mm above the iliac crest along the anterior axillary line. A linear configuration among the three ports is appreciated. The proposed insertion site is palpated from within the 1.5-cm port site to ensure that no intervening

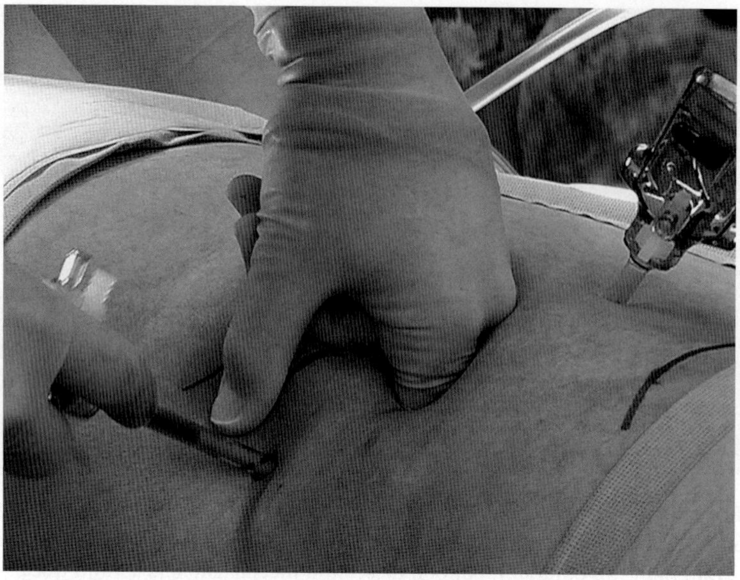

Fig. 11. Safe port placement with finger tip palpation at the junction of the 12th rib and paraspinous muscle.

structures are present. It is crucial to ensure that the border of the peritoneum has been swept as far medially as possible (both manually and by balloon dilation) to avoid puncture during insertion of this trocar. A defect in the peritoneum can cause CO_2 pressure equilibration with the peritoneal cavity, reducing an already limited working space. A 15-blade is used to make a 5-mm skin incision at this site, and a 5-mm trocar is then inserted under tactile guidance. Care must be made not to skive the port so that the internal port distance is reduced. If the surgeon anticipates that an endovascular GIA stapler will likely be required for renal vessel or en bloc division, a 12-mm trocar may be used at this site instead.

Step 4: Dissection of the Kidney

Dissection is begun by inserting the 0° 10-mm laparoscope into the Bluntip trocar, and the ultrasonic dissector and blunt-tipped suction/irrigation probe into the working ports. Initial orientation in the retroperitoneum can be difficult. The psoas muscle and ureter are often the only visible structures in the lower half of the visual field. Gerota's fascia (anteriorly and medially) comprises the remainder of the field. On the right side, the vena cava may be seen. With a left-sided approach, the aortic pulsations can usually be identified quite easily.

It is often simplest to begin dissecting toward the posterior surface of the kidney, which allows eventual access to the renal artery. Use of the suction/irrigation probe as a blunt dissector will allow the surgeon to define the plane between Gerota's fascia and the renal capsule. Any remaining perinephric fat can then be dissected away efficiently with the ultrasonic dissector. If significant inflammation is present, the goal of dissection should be to define Gerota's fascia around the kidney. Only if this fails should one attempt to define the renal capsule.

Proceeding inferiorly, the lower pole should be freed and the ureter identified. Once freed, the ureter should be grasped and torqued in an antero-lateral direction to provide traction for hilar exposure. Dissection should then proceed toward the hilum.

As hilar dissection progresses, the surgeon should work both superiorly and inferiorly to the hilum to disengage as much perinephric fat as possible. When sufficient investing fat is freed, the kidney can be also be elevated anteriorly with the suction/irrigation probe or a Kitner dissector to provide even further hilar exposure. Dissection should not progress to the anterior surface of the kidney until the artery and vein have been controlled. Doing so will drop the kidney posteriorly and block access to the hilum.

Vascular Control. *Right Side:*The renal artery should be the first major vascular structure encountered. It is important to watch for pulsations indicative of proximity to the artery. After the artery has been isolated, the renal vein is found anterior and likely inferior to the artery. One must remember that the structure immediately anterior and medial to the renal artery is likely the vena cava, not the duodenum, and avoid rough retraction, grasping, and dissection of this area. It is common for the vena cava to collapse under the pressure of the CO_2 pressure, making this structure difficult to distinguish from bowel, a gonadal vein, or a ureter.

Left Side: Branches of the left renal vein will complicate hilar dissection. The surgeon must be aware of the lumbar vein originating from the renal vein, which is often encountered prior to reaching the renal artery. This lumbar branch should be isolated, either bipolar coagulated or clipped (two on stay side, one on specimen side) and finally divided. The renal artery is isolated next. Once the renal artery is circumferentially exposed with no intervening neurolymphatic tissue present, the artery can be clipped. A total of two 10-mm clips should be placed on the patient side and one clip secured on the specimen side. The artery is then sharply divided with endoscopic scissors.

Finally, the renal vein is identified; care must be taken to dissect out, coagulate and divide the gonadal and adrenal branches, which are located inferior and superior to the renal vein, respectively. As an alternative to clipping the branches of the renal vein, Hemolock clips may be used to control the venous branches. If the renal vein is divided very close to the kidney, the gonadal and adrenal branches may be left intact. The vein is then engaged and cut with the articulated, endovascular GIA stapler (*U.S. Surgical Corporation*). This particular stapler has the advantage of adjustable angling of its jaws to optimize positioning.

If hilar dissection is difficult, the ureter can be isolated, clipped, and divided, as it can block mobilization of the lower pole from a retroperitoneal direction. Following this, the lower pole is dissected and freed, allowing retraction of this area superiorly to improve access to the hilum.

Step 5: Completion of Renal Dissection

The ureter is then divided between two 10-mm clips. Completion of the dissection involves careful division of the anterior and superior attachments of the kidney. This portion of the dissection poses the greatest risk of bowel injury, particularly when dense adhesions are present between the anterior aspect of the kidney and the peritoneal cavity. The superior dissection takes place in the plane between the kidney and adrenal, as the adrenal is left behind. Intermittent retraction of the kidney caudally, laterally, and medially will facilitate this process.

Step 6: Removal of Specimen

At this point, a 30° 5-mm laparoscope is placed through the posterior port. A 10-mm Endocatch bag is inserted through the 12-mm Bluntip port and deployed. Grasping forceps are then used through the anterior working port to maneuver the specimen into the bag. Unfortunately, the limited space within the retroperitoneum makes this step rather challenging. It is best to position the Endocatch bag directly inferior to the specimen and attempt to guide the kidney into the enclosure device using graspers. Once the bag has been drawn around the specimen, the edges are pulled out of the 12-mm Bluntip port. Morcellation or open extraction of the specimen is then performed.

Step 7: Port Closure and Completion of Procedure

When morcellation is complete and the Endocatch bag has been removed, a fingertip can be inserted into the 12-mm Bluntip port site and insufflation restarted to allow a final inspection of the retroperitoneum. The retroperitoneal pressure should be reduced to 4 mmHg to confirm hemostasis prior to case completion. The anterior trocar is first removed under direct vision. The posterior 5-mm trocar is then slipped out over the shaft of the laparoscope, leaving the 5-mm scope within the retroperitoneum. The laparoscope is then withdrawn slowly, allowing visualization of the access tract to confirm hemostasis.

If the peritoneum is intact, there is no need to close the fascia of the 12-mm port sites, as there is no retroperitoneal structure that is predisposed to herniation. All skin incisions are routinely closed with a subcuticular 4-0 absorbable suture and secured with either steri-strips or Dermabond.

Key Maneuvers

1. Ensure that initial finger dissection of the retroperitoneum (at initial port site at the tip of 12th rib) is done in the correct plane. Always begin by palpating under the 12th rib from within the retroperitoneum and continue with manual dissection along the psoas muscle.
2. Trocars should be spaced as far apart as possible to avoid instrument collision. The maximum distance between ports that will be achieved is likely only 6–8 mm.
3. Extreme care must be used when placing the anterior working trocar to avoid peritoneal entry or visceral injury. Insertion must be performed with tactile guidance.
4. Initial orientation within the retroperitoneum can be difficult. Key orienting structures are the ureter and psoas muscle posteriorly, the aorta on the left, and the vena cava on the right. During left-sided cases, try to look for arterial pulsations (renal artery or aorta) if structures are not immediately obvious.
5. When using the endovascular GIA stapler to divide the renal vein, the surgeon must ensure that no clips are in the staple path (e.g., clips on the stumps of the renal artery), as these can cause the stapler to misfire and cause renal vein bleeding.

SURGICAL CONSIDERATIONS FOR SPECIFIC PATHOLOGIC ENTITIES AFFECTING THE KIDNEY

Nephrectomy for XGP, TB, and ADPKD is a humbling experience even for the most experienced laparoscopic urologic surgeon, and it is crucial to have extensive laparoscopic experience before tackling such cases. Even with an open approach, a chronically infected kidney is a surgical challenge because of the loss of planes, the dense adhesions, and the severe fibrotic lymphadenopathy around the renal hilum. With ADPKD, the huge renal size, surrounding fibrosis, and proximity to several vital structures make for a technically difficult and prolonged operation.

The first step in the management of these cases is patient selection based on history, physical examination, and a spiral contrast-enhanced CT scan. One may attempt laparoscopy first for all comers and convert if needed. However, at our institution, the desire for laparoscopy declines as more of the following factors accumulate in the patient: previous open upper abdominal surgery, previous open surgery or percutaneous drainage of the kidney, a very large polycystic (to or across midline), a large (> 10 mm) inflammatory mass related to the kidney, extension of the inflammatory mass into adjacent organs (muscle, spleen, liver, bowel), presence of a frank nephric or perinephric abscess, and a large amount of perinephric and paranephric fat around the kidney, especially if massive stranding of this fat is present on CT imaging.

In general, when operating on these cases, one should do everything possible to make surgery easier. Bowel preparation is a good safety measure. The working space between the costal margin and anterior superior iliac spine should be maximized with breaking the table and elevating the kidney rest. We prefer a transperitoneal approach for all such cases. There is more working space and at least initially, there are known landmarks. The use of five trocars with an active assistant improves retraction and suction, and going from known to unknown following previously identified landmarks is helpful.

Herein, we describe the pathological process and technical aspects related to each pathologic entity.

Xanthogranulomatous Pyelonephritis

Xanthogranulomatous pyelonephritis (XGP) is a severe, chronic bacterial infection of the renal parenchyma that results in significant inflammatory changes within the kidney and surrounding tissues *(3)*. It is a process that occurs mainly in middle-aged females in the setting of chronic infection (most often with *Proteus mirabilis* or *Esherichia coli*) and obstruction *(56–60)*. Calculi are associated with 22–83% of involved kidneys in various XGP series in the literature *(57,58,61,62)*. XGP has been called the "great imitator" because it may mimic other inflammatory or neoplastic conditions of the kidney. The most common symptoms and signs that accompany the process are flank/abdominal pain, palpable mass, fever, anemia, leukocytosis, and weight loss *(59,62,63)*. The extensive inflammation that accompanies the process causes a severe reaction that involves contiguous structures such as the liver, spleen, colon, and psoas muscle. XGP is usually unilateral and often results in destruction of the kidney requiring nephrectomy. CT scan is the preferred diagnostic tool in the evaluation of XGP. Typical findings include a large staghorn calculus on the background of a large and non-excreting (non-functioning) kidney which appears as a "bear claw sign" on transverse view CT images (Fig. 12).

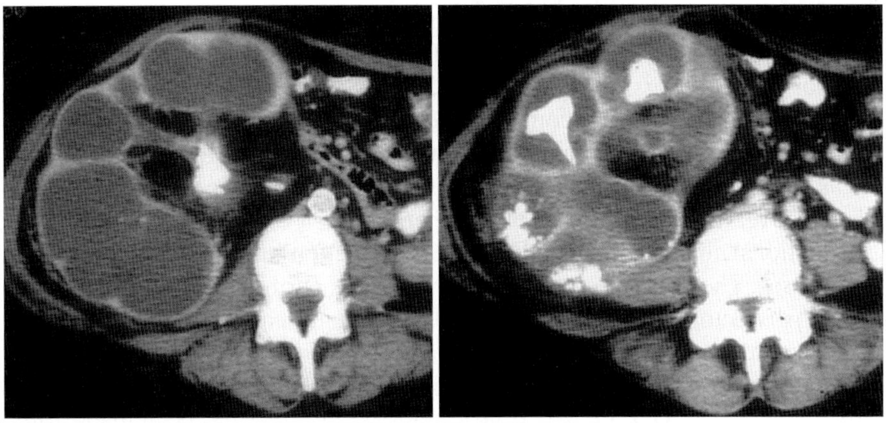

Fig. 12. Contrast CT-imaging of a 65-year-old white female with a history of recurrent urinary tract infections. Note the enlarged, poorly enhancing right renal unit with the presence of several calculi. XGP is an unusual, supurative granulomatous reaction to a chronic infection, frequently associated with a chronic obstruction due to a calculus, stricture or tumor. This process is more common in women.

Patients with XGP may also develop fistulous tracts to the skin or colon *(58)*. A Eastham et al. reviewed the results of 27 patients with a pathologic diagnosis of XGP *(59)*. In 23 of the patients, a CT scan had been performed. Overall, CT scan findings were sufficient to allow diagnosis of XGP in 20 of the 23 patients (87%). In addition, CT accurately revealed the presence of disease extension into the psoas and/or quadratus lumborum muscles in eight patients, into the descending colon in one patient, and involvement of the great vessels in five others. As such, an abdominal/pelvic CT scan should be a mandatory part of the preoperative work-up for a suspected case of XGP *(64)*. There is no question that the inflammatory nature of XGP predisposes the patient to a higher risk of complications.

Keeley et al. reviewed their first 100 laparoscopic nephrectomies and found that 87% of the patients without inflammatory conditions had no complications or open conversions, as compared to only 69% of patients with existing perirenal inflammation *(23)*. Notably, of the two patients undergoing laparoscopic nephrectomy for XGP, one had to undergo open conversion for lack of progression. In another series, Shekarriz et al. reported that one of three patients with XGP required open conversion for dense fibrosis *(24)*.

Bercowsky et al. performed a retrospective review comparing the results of a cohort of five patients undergoing laparoscopic nephrectomy for XGP (three transperitoneal approach, two retroperitoneal approaches) with four others treated with the traditional open approach *(65)*. Overall, when compared to the open group, mean operating time and blood loss was 360 vs. 154 min and 260 vs. 438 cc, respectively. Of note, complications occurred in 60% of the laparoscopic group, as compared to 0% of the open patients. One patient that underwent a retroperitoneal nephrectomy required conversion to a transperitoneal laparoscopic approach. The authors concluded that the benefits of minimally invasive surgery might not apply to this specific group of patients.

Khaira et al. have more recently reported on a small series of patients who underwent laparoscopic (n=3) vs. open (n=8) nephrectomy specifically for XGP *(66)*. Major complications rates were 33% for the laparoscopic group (vascular injury requiring open conversion) and 25% for the open group (unrecognized bowel injury, pneumothorax). The authors concluded that a laparoscopic approach, albeit challenging, does not necessarily pose a greater risk by an experienced laparoscopic surgeon.

It is noteworthy to point out that in recent report by Gupta et al., with the largest series of retroperitoneoscopic nephrectomy for benign non-functioning kidneys, the majority of conversions in an expert retroperitoneal surgeon's hand were done in patients with XGP *(6)*. The authors suggest that in such cases, open or transperitoneal laparoscopic surgery may be planned.

Preoperatively, all XGP patients should be counseled carefully about the increased complication rates associated with the laparoscopic treatment. In addition, there should be a clear understanding that the chance for open conversion may approach 50%. Once the laparoscopic approach has been chosen and the procedure initiated, it is common to encounter instances where dissection simply cannot proceed because of the inability to identify anatomic landmarks. It is important to attempt dissection in multiple areas, because freeing specific portions of the kidney can improve the overall exposure. Other helpful maneuvers include the use of a ureteral catheter with a super-stiff guide wire, intraoperative table rotational changes (i.e., medial or lateral rotation) and the addition of more 5-mm ports for retraction purposes. The hook electrode may be used as it permits very fine dissection, simulating a right-angled clamp dissector. It is prudent to get positive identification by additional dissection before cutting tubular structures or into new planes unless other previously identified landmarks indicate safe dissection. The surgeon should always have a conversion point in mind when undertaking an attempted laparoscopic dissection of an XGP kidney. If no significant progress has been made after 30 min, once the aforementioned maneuvers have been used, it is our policy to proceed with open conversion to safely complete the case.

Key Points

1. The laparoscopic approach to the XGP kidney can be fraught with difficulty and should be attempted only by very experienced laparoscopists.
2. The XGP patient should be made aware of the increased risks involved with the laparoscopic approach.
3. Preoperative CT scan is mandatory to assess the degree of inflammation present and involvement of any adjacent structures.
4. The transperitoneal approach should be used because it provides a large working space and helpful landmarks.
5. Finally, early conversion should always be considered, to facilitate completion of the nephrectomy.

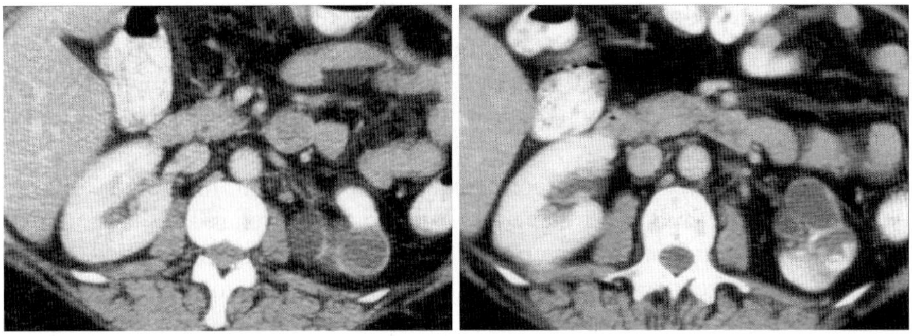

Fig. 13. Renal tuberculosis. Axial contrast-enhanced CT scan demonstrates left tuberculous pyonephrosis with minimal extension of the inflammatory process into the perinephric space. Significant parenchymal calcification is noted along with size reduction and loss of renal function with reduced contrast uptake. Transperitoneal laparoscopic nephrectomy was successfully completed in this patient.

Tuberculous Kidney

Until the mid-1980s, there was a steady decline in the prevalence of TB. Since that time, however, there has been a resurgence of TB due to the acquired immunodeficiency syndrome (AIDS) epidemic and increasing number of drug-resistant strains of *Mycobacterium tuberculosis (67)* In addition to immunocompromised individuals, other population groups who are at increased risk include minorities, the poor, alcoholics, immigrants from third-world countries, prisoners, the aged, nursing home residents, and the homeless *(68)*.

Although manifestations of TB are usually limited to the chest, the disease can affect any organ system and in patients infected with the HIV virus, it usually involves multiple extrapulmonary sites including the skeleton, genitourinary tract, and central nervous system *(68)*. TB demonstrates a variety of clinical and radiologic features depending on organ site involved and has a known propensity of dissemination from its primary site. Thurs, TB can mimic a number of other disease entities, and it is important to be familiar with the various radiologic features to ensure early, accurate diagnosis.

Genitourinary TB often results from secondary, hematogenous dissemination from the lungs. With regards to the kidneys, radiography may demonstrate calcifications within the renal parenchyma (Fig. 13). The calcifications may be amorphous, granular, curvilinear, or lobar *(69,70)*. Ulceration, wall thickening, and fibrosis characterize involvement of the collecting system. Intravenous urography and delayed-imaging CT demonstrate a variety of findings depending on the extent of renal involvement. The earliest urographic abnormality is a "moth-eaten" calyx due to erosion. Focal or global poor renal function, dilation of the collecting system, or irregular pools of contrast may also be seen *(68)*. Infundibular stenosis may lead to incomplete opacification of the calyx (phantom calyx) *(71)*. Advanced disease leads to cortical scarring with dilatation and distortion of adjoining calyces, and strictures of the pelvicaliceal system producing luminal narrowing either directly or by causing kinking of the renal pelvis (Kerr kink) *(72)*.

CT imaging is extremely helpful in identifying the manifestations of renal TB. Various patterns of hydronephrosis may be seen at CT depending on the site of the stricture and include focal caliectasis, caliectasis without pelvic dilation, and generalized hydronephrosis *(70)*. Other common findings include parenchymal scarring and low attenuation parenchymal lesions. CT is also useful in depicting the extension of disease into the extrarenal space as well as other genitourinary structures, such as the adrenal glands, ureter, bladder, and genitalia.

From a surgical perspective, tubercular pyelonephritis results in dense perinephric adhesions that complicate surgical dissection *(73)*. Surgical management of the involved kidney is necessary to eradicate a source of infection and prevent late complications such as hypertension and abscess formation *(74)*. Unfortunately, spillage of infectious caseous material is common during attempted laparoscopic dissection of the involved kidney *(73,75)*. Therefore, it is important to have initiated medical treatment well in advance of the surgery. Involvement of the infectious disease team is suggested during preoperative planning.

As with XGP kidneys, laparoscopic dissection can be very difficult. In a review of 482 laparoscopic nephrectomies, Rassweiler et al. found that four of five cases of renal TB that underwent attempted laparoscopic treatment required open conversion *(76)*. Hemal et al. reported a 22% conversion rate in their series *(77)*. A more recent study of 13 renal TB patients undergoing laparoscopic nephrectomy (9 transperitoneal, 4 retroperitoneal) showed that 12 were successfully completed, with only one open conversion. However, the authors noted that subcapsular dissection was required in some instances as a result of the intense adhesions to surrounding tissue *(75)*.

Lee et al. from Korea have published on their experience with laparoscopic nephrectomy for non-functional tuberculous kidneys *(78)*. Thirty (97%) of the 31 TB cases were successfully completed (10 transperitoneal and 21 retroperitoneal approaches). When compared to their control group of 45 laparoscopic nephrectomies for other benign etiologies (ureteral calculus and obstruction, hydronephrosis, reflux nephropathy, staghorn calculus, and polycystic kidney), the perioperative and postoperative parameters were comparable, except for the mean operative time, which at 244 min for the TB group was significantly greater than the 216 min for the control group. No significant intra-operative or postoperative complications were observed in either group. The authors conclude that laparoscopic nephrectomy be considered as an initial procedure for a tuberculous non-functioning kidney.

Theoretically, a retroperitoneal approach limits contamination resulting from spillage from the infected kidney and should be attempted if possible. A CT scan is very helpful in assessing the degree of inflammation that is present and can assist the surgeon in determining the appropriate laparoscopic approach. Again, there should be a low threshold for open conversion if lack of progression is experienced. If gross intra-operative spillage occurs, the patient should be placed on an antituberculosis regimen during the immediate postoperative period. These regimens should consist of multiple agents, most commonly isoniazid, rifampin, ethambutol, and pyrazinamide *(75)*.

Autosomal Dominant Polycystic Kidney Disease (ADPKD)

ADPKD is an autosomal dominant inherited disease, characterized by progressive enlarging renal cysts associated with hypertension, renal failure, pain, hematuria, and infection, with an incidence of 1:400 to 1:1,000 *(79)*. Genetic mutations in the PKD1 or PKD2 genes are responsible for the improper encoding of polycystin and other vital cellular membrane proteins *(80)*. Patients with the disease develop multiple, bilateral renal cysts, which progressively enlarge and eventually destroy remaining areas of renal parenchyma (Fig. 14) *(79)*. The cysts are thought to derive from an abnormal proliferation of renal tubular cells *(80)*.

Co-morbidities associated with ADPKD can be numerous. Up to 50% of patients with ADPKD develop end-stage renal disease that necessitates hemodialysis or renal transplantation by the age of 60 *(81)*. In addition, hypertension can develop in up to 50–70% of patients *(82,83)*. The pathogenesis of hypertension in ADPKD patients is complex, but is thought to be derived from progressive intrarenal ischemia through physical compression by enlarging cysts, thus activating the renin–angiotensin–aldosterone pathway *(80)*. Up to 60% of patients also have significant, chronic flank discomfort *(84)*. The etiology of the pain is thought to derive from progressively increased tension on the sensory nerves of the renal capsule as cysts enlarge over time *(85)*. Other potential causes of pain are cyst infection and hemorrhage, as well as nephrolithiasis *(86)*. Laparoscopic management of renal cysts not only has been shown to reduce pain in some patients, but also improves hypertension and stabilizes renal function, delaying renal replacement therapy *(87)*.

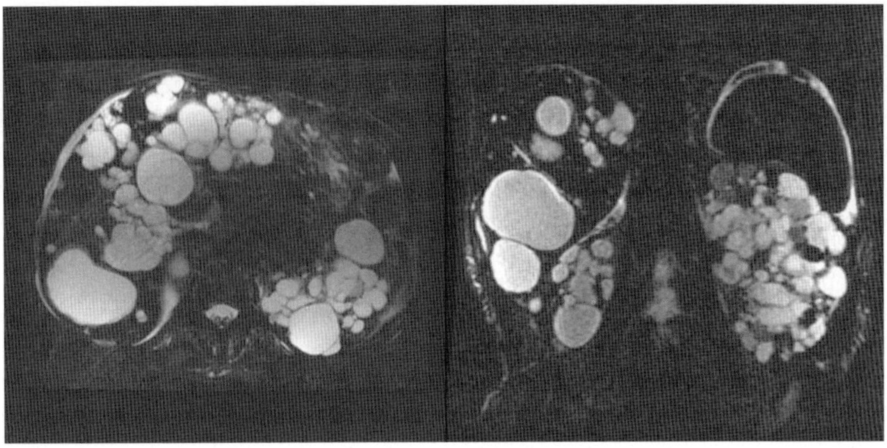

Fig. 14. Coronal MRI-imaging of a 54-year-old male with ADPKD. Both renal units are completely replaced by cyst formation. The liver is also involved with cyst formation.

In general, nephrectomy in a case of ADPKD is reserved for patients with end-stage renal disease and chronic pain that is refractory to medical therapy. Past studies have documented significant morbidity and mortality rates associated with conventional open nephrectomies for ADPKD *(88,89)*. However, the laparoscopic approach is well suited for the ADPKD kidney, because it results in much less morbidity for these patients *(90)*.

Early experiences with laparoscopic nephrectomy for ADPKD utilized the transperitoneal approach with intact specimen removal through the flank *(86)*. Because a large incision was required to remove the enlarged specimens, it was soon discovered that patients were prone to develop incisional hernias when a flank muscle cutting incision was used *(91)*. Current approaches for the laparoscopic treatment of ADPKD kidneys attempt to minimize the overall size of the specimen during dissection and limit the size of extraction incisions.

From a surgical perspective, extension of the kidney across the midline, obscuring underlying vital structures, the renal hilum and the ureter, and stretching of renal vessels in the grooves between cysts and embedded in fibrotic tissue make it difficult to identify the vessels. Helpful maneuvers for these situations include a complete bowel preparation and the placement of an occlusion balloon as described above to help identify the ureter. We prefer the transperitoneal route in these cases because of the optimal working space. When approaching an ADPKD kidney transperitoneally, initial port placement should be at an umbilical location (umbilical base), to avoid injury to the enlarged kidney, which may cross the midline *(90,92)*. Cyst decortication and drainage of fluid is a mandatory step prior to dissection of the kidney, in order to reduce its overall size so that mobilization and exposure of the hilum is facilitated. Sequential cyst puncture with the active blade of the ultrasonic dissector and removal of the cyst fluid using a suction probe is an efficient method of completing this task. One should expect the vessels to be collapsed and invested in fibrotic tissue and splayed between the cysts. Once the specimen is ready to be removed, aspiration of as many cysts as possible should be performed to decrease the kidney size. Morcellation should then be carried out to minimize the wound size as previously described.

CONCLUSIONS

The laparoscopic approach to simple nephrectomy is applicable to many forms of benign pathology, with significant patient benefits such as superior cosmesis, reduced analgesia requirements, shortened hospital stays, and decreased convalescent times over the open approach. Among the 1,654 reported laparoscopic nephrectomies for benign disease (Table 2), approximately equal have been done via the transperitoneal and retroperitoneal approaches. Review of the retrospective studies comparing the two approaches did not demonstrate significant differences in most outcomes measures *(11)*. Unfortunately, there in no randomized study comparing transperitoneal with retroperitoneal simple nephrectomy, as has been done for radical nephrectomy. In the recent review by Liao et al., no consistent advantages for either approach with respect to operative time, blood loss, conversion rate, and complications were observed across the past decade's published series *(3)*. Whereas there are theoretical advantages and disadvantages for either approach depending on patient characteristics and specific indication, surgeon experience and preference remains the primary driving force.

Prevention of complications requires careful attention to patient selection, positioning, access, intra-operative fluid balance, vascular injury, exiting the abdomen, and postoperative abdominal pain *(93)*. Several large series of laparoscopic renal surgery have addressed the issue of complication *(94–98)*. A recent meta-analysis compared complication rates related to different laparoscopic renal procedures and techniques *(99)*. Major complications include bleeding, vascular injury, injury to surrounding organs, embolism, open conversion, and death. Minor complications include ileus, wound cellulites, diaphragmatic irritation, urinary retention, and subcutaneous emphysema. The overall major and minor complication rates for all laparoscopic renal surgery were 9.5 and 1.9%, respectively. Of the 300 patients included in the analysis who underwent laparoscopic simple nephrectomy, the major and minor complication rates were 13.7 and 5.7%, respectively. Interestingly, the major and minor complication rates were higher for both laparoscopic radical nephrectomy (10.7, 3.3%) and donor nephrectomy (10.6, 0.5%), respectively, highlighting the challenging nature of "simple" nephrectomy *(3)*.

As with any surgical procedure, however, careful preoperative patient evaluation is necessary to plan the proper approach and maximize the chances for success. The surgeon should always keep in mind the limitations of laparoscopy and apply the approach judiciously when faced with a situation where significant inflammation may be involved.

Take Home Messages

1. If progression is hindered during a laparoscopic simple nephrectomy (transperitoneal or retroperitoneal), early open conversion is warranted.
2. When dealing with very large kidneys (e.g., ADPKD) or marked perirenal inflammation, the transperitoneal approach is preferred to maximize the available working space and improve orientation.
3. Always be aware of clips that may impede engagement of the GIA stapler when taking. the renal vein, causing it to misfire and forcing an open conversion.
4. The ultrasonic dissector can be used for almost all points of dissection during a laparoscopic nephrectomy. If difficulty is encountered or finer dissection is needed, switching to a right-angle hook electrode and grasping structures with a Maryland dissector can facilitate the process.

ACKNOWLEDGMENTS

The authors would like to thank Dr. Michael Vannier for his help with case study radiology materials for the specific pathologic entities.

REFERENCES

1. Clayman RV, Kavoussi LR, Soper NJ, Dierks SM, Meretyk S, Darcy MD, et al. Laparoscopic nephrectomy: Initial case report. J Urol 1991, 146: 278–282.
2. Gaur DD, Agarwal DK, Purohit KC. Retroperitoneal laparoscopic nephrectomy: Initial case report. J Urol 1993, 149:103–105.
3. Liao JC, Breda A, Schulam PG. Laparoscopic Renal surgery for benign disease. Curr Urol Rep 2007, 8:12–18.
4. Doehn C, Fornara P, Fricke L, Jocham D. Comparison of laparoscopic and open nephroureterectomy for benign disease. J Urol 1998, 159:732–734.
5. Doublet JD, Barreto HS, Degremont AC, et al. Retroperitoneal nephrectomy: Comparison of laparoscopy with open surgery. World J Surg 1996, 20:713–716.
6. Gupta NP, Goel R, Hemal AK et al. Should retroperitoneoscopic nephrectomy be the standard of care for benign nonfunctioning kidneys? An outcome analysis based on experience with 449 cases in a 5-year period. J Urol 2004, 172:1411–1413.
7. Kerbl K, Clayman RV, McDougall EM, et al. Transperitoneal nephrectomy for benign disease of the kidney: A comparison of laparoscopic and open surgical techniques. Urology 1994, 43:607–613.
8. McDougall EM, Clayman RV. Laparoscopic nephrectomy for benign disease: comparison of the transperitoneal and retroperitoneal approaches. J Endourol 1996, 10:45–49.
9. Parra RO, Perez MG, Boullier JA, Cummings JM. Comparison between standard flank versus laparoscopic nephrectomy for benign renal disease. J Urol 1995, 153:1171–1173.
10. Rassweiler J, Frede T, Henkel TO, et al. Nephrectomy: A comparative study between the transperitoneal and retroperitoneal laparoscopic versus the open approach. Eur Urol 1998, 33:489–496.
11. Traxer O, Pearle MS. Laparoscopic nephrectomy for benign disease. Semin Laparosc Surg 2000, 7:176–184.
12. Donovan JF, Cooper CS, Lund GO, Winfield HN. Laparoscopic nephrectomy of a horseshoe kidney. J Endourol 1997, 11:181–184.
13. Saggar VR, Singh K, Sarangi R. Retroperitoneoscopic heminephrectomy of a horseshoe kidney for calculus disease. Surg Laparosc Endosc Percutan Tech 2004, 14:172–174.
14. Yohannes P, Dinlenc C, Liatsikos E, et al. Laparoscopic heminephrectomy for benign disease of the horseshoe kidney. Jsls 2002, 6:381–384.
15. Gupta N, Mandhani A, Sharma D, et al. Is laparoscopic approach safe for ectopic pelvic kidneys? Urol Int 2006, 77:118–121.
16. Loffer FD Pent D. Laparoscopy in the obese patient. Am J Obstet Gynecol 1976, 125: 104–107.
17. Winfield HN, Donovan JF, See WA, Loening SA, Williams RD. Urological laparoscopic surgery. J Urol 1991, 146: 941–948.
18. Fazeli-Matin S, Gill IS, Hsu TH, et al. Laparoscopic renal and adrenal surgery in obese patients: Comparison to open surgery. J Urol 1999, 162:665–669.
19. Doublet J Belair G. Retroperitoneal laparoscopic nephrectomy is safe and effective in obese patients: A comparative study of 55 procedures. Urology 2000, 56: 63–66.
20. Anast JW, Stoller ML, Meng MV, et al.: Differences in complications and outcomes for obese patients undergoing laparoscopic radical, partial or simple nephrectomy. J Urol 2004, 172:2287–2291.
21. Klingler HC, Remzi M, Janetschek G, Marberger M: Benefits of laparoscopic renal surgery are more pronounced in patients with a high body mass index. Eur Urol 2003, 43:522–527.
22. Jacobs SC, Cho E, Dunkin BJ, Bartlett ST, Flowers JL, Jarrell B. Laparoscopic nephrectomy in the markedly obese living renal donor. Urology 2000: 56: 926–929.
23. Keeley FX, Tolley DA: A review of our first 100 cases of laparoscopic nephrectomy: Defining risk factors for complications. Br J Urol 1998, 82:615–618.
24. Shekarriz B, Meng MV, Lu HF, et al.: Laparoscopic nephrectomy for inflammatory renal conditions. J Urol 2001, 166:2091–2094.
25. Manohar T, Desai M, Desai M. Laparoscopic Nephrectomy for benign and inflammatory conditions. J Endourol 2007, 21:1323–1328.
26. Gill IS, Kavoussi LR, Clayman RV, Ehrlich R, Evans R, Fuchs G, et al. Complications of laparoscopic nephrectomy in 185 patients: A multi-institutional review. J Urol 1995, 154: 479–483.
27. Kabalin JN. Surgical anatomy of the retroperitoneum, kidneys, and ureters. In: Campbell's Urology vol. 1. (Wein AJ, ed.), W.B. Saunders, Philadelphia, 1998, pp 49–88.
28. Leder RA Nelson RC. Three-dimensional CT of the genitourinary tract. J Endourol 2001, 15: 37–46.
29. Kumar U, Albala DM. Simple nephrectomy: Transperitoneal approach. J Endourol 2000, 14: 779–785; discussion 785–786.
30. Stifelman M, Andrade A, Sosa RE, Shichman S. Simple nephrectomy: Hand-assisted technique. J Endourol 2000, 10:793–798.
31. Gaur DD. Simple nephrectomy: Retroperitoneal approach. J Endourol. 2000, 10:787–790.

32. Tan YH, Siddiqui K, Preminger GM, Albala DM. Hand-assisted laparoscopic nephrectomy for inflammatory renal conditions. J Endourol 2004, 18:770–774.
33. Kessler BD, Shichman SJ. Laparoscopic radical nephrectomy: Hand-assisted. In Essential urologic laparoscopy: The complete clinical guide. Edited by Nakada SY. Totowa: Humana Press; 2003:143–156.
34. Albala DM, Kavoussi LR Clayman RV. Laparoscopic nephrectomy. Semin Urol 1992, 10: 146–151.
35. Bhoyrul S, Vierra MA, Nezhat CR, Krummel TM, Way LW. Trocar injuries in laparoscopic surgery. J Am Coll Surg 2001, 192: 677–683
36. Helal M, Albertini J, Lockhart J, Albrink M. Laparoscopic nephrectomy using the harmonic scalpel. J Endourol 1997, 11: 267–268.
37. Potter SR, Kavoussi LR, Jackman SV. Management of diaphragmatic injury during laparoscopic nephrectomy. J Urol 2001, 165: 1203–1204.
38. Msezane LP, Zorn KC, Gofrit ON, Schade GR, Shalhav AL. Conservative Management of a Large Capnothorax following Laparoscopic Renal Surgery: A Case Report. J Endourol 2007, 21: 1445–1447.
39. Rapp DE, Orvieto MA, Gerber GS, Johnston WK 3rd, Wolf JS, Shalhav AL. En bloc stapling of renal hilum during laparoscopic nephrectomy and nephroureterectomy. Urology 2004, 64:655–659.
40. White WM, Klein FA, Gash J, Waters WB. Prospective radiographic follow-up after en bloc ligation of the renal hilum. J Urol 2007, 178:1888–1891.
41. Chan D, Bishoff JT, Ratner L, Kavoussi LR, Jarrett TW. Endovascular gastrointestinal stapler device malfunction during laparoscopic nephrectomy: Early recognition and management. J Urol 2000, 164: 319–321.
42. Schuster TG, Wolf JS, Jr. Use of bipolar electrocautery during laparoscopic donor nephrectomy. J Urol 2001, 165: 1968–1970.
43. Orvieto M, Chien GW, Harland R, Garfinkel MR, Galocy M, Shalhav AL. Bipolar electrocoagulation for clipless division of left renal vein branches during laparoscopic living donor nephrectomy. Transplant Proc. 2004, 36: 2625–2627.
44. Baughman SM, Bishoff JT. Novel direct-vision renal morcellation with orthopedic rotary shaver-blade instrumentation. J Endourol 2005, 19:86–89.
45. Varkarakis JM, McAllister M, Ong AM, Solomon SB, Allaf ME, Inagaki T, Bhayani SB, Trock B, Jarrett TW. Evaluation of water jet morcellation as an alternative to hand morcellation of renal tissue during laparoscopic nephrectomy: An in vitro study.
46. Varkarakis I, Rha K, Hernandez F, Kavoussi LR, Jarrett TW. Laparoscopic specimen extraction: Morcellation. BJU Int 2005, 95 Suppl 2:27–31.
47. Kerbl K, Figenshau RS, Clayman RV, Chandhoke PS, Kavoussi LR, Albala DM, Stone AM. Retroperitoneal laparoscopic nephrectomy: Laboratory and clinical experience. J Endourol 1993, 7: 23–26.
48. Gaur DD. Laparoscopic operative retroperitoneoscopy: Use of a new device. J Urol 1992, 148: 1137–1139.
49. Gill IS. Retroperitoneal laparoscopic nephrectomy. Urol Clin North Am 1998, 25: 343–360.
50. Pearle MS, Nakada SY. Laparoscopic nephrectomy: Retroperitoneal approach. Semin Laparosc Surg 1996, 3: 75–83.
51. Chiu AW, Chen KK, Wang JH, Huang WJ, Chang LS. Direct needle insuffl ation for pneumoretroperitoneum: Anatomic confirmation and clinical experience. Urology 1995, 46: 432–437.
52. Gill IS, Rassweiler JJ. Retroperitoneoscopic renal surgery: Our approach. Urology 1999, 54: 734–738.
53. Hsu TH, Sung GT, Gill IS. Retroperitoneoscopic approach to nephrectomy. J Endourol 1999, 13: 713–718; discussion 718–720.
54. Gill IS, Grune MT, Munch LC. Access technique for retroperitoneoscopy. J Urol 1996, 156:1120–1124.
55. Capelouto CC, Moore RG, Silverman SG, Kavoussi LR. Retro peritoneoscopy: Anatomical rationale for direct retroperitoneal access. J Urol 1994, 152: 2008–2010.
56. Anhalt MA, Cawood CD, Scott R, Jr. Xanthogranulomatous pyelonephritis: A comprehensive review with report of 4 additional cases. J Urol 1971, 105: 10–17.
57. Petronic V, Buturovic J, Isvaneski M. Xanthogranulomatous pyelonephritis. Br J Urol 1989, 64: 336–338.
58. Chuang CK, Lai MK, Chang PL, Huang MH, Chu SH, Wu CJ, Wu HR. Xanthogranulomatous pyelonephritis: Experience in 36 cases. J Urol 1992, 147: 333–336.
59. Eastham J, Ahlering T, Skinner E. Xanthogranulomatous pyelonephritis: Clinical fi ndings and surgical considerations. Urology 1994, 43: 295–299.
60. Tolia BM, Newman HR, Fruchtman B, Bekirov H, Freed SZ. Xanthogranulomatous pyelonephritis: Segmental or generalized disease. J Urol 1980, 124: 122–124.
61. Malek RS, Greene LF, DeWeerd JH, Farrow GM. Xanthogranulomatous pyelonephritis. Br J Urol 1972, 44: 296–308.
62. Tolia BM, Iloreta A, Freed SZ, Fruchtman B, Bennett B, Newman HR. Xanthogranulomatouspyelonephritis: Detailed analysis of 29 cases and a brief discussion of atypical presentations. J Urol 1981, 126: 437–442.
63. Nataluk EA, McCullough DL, Scharling EO. Xanthogranulomatous pyelonephritis, the gatekeeper'sdilemma: A contemporary look at an old problem. Urology 1995, 45: 377–380.

64. Anderson KR. Simple nephrectomy: Managing the difficult case: Xanthogranulomatous pyelonephritis and autosomal dominant polycystic kidney disease. J Endourol 2000,10:799–803.
65. Bercowsky E, Shalhav AL, Portis A, Elbahnasy AM, McDougall EM, Clayman RV. Is the laparoscopicapproach justified in patients with xanthogranulomatous pyelonephritis? Urology 1999, 54: 437–442; discussion 442–443.
66. Khaira HS, Shah RB, Wolf JS. Laparoscopic and open surgical nephrectomy for xanthogranulomatous pyelonephritis. J Endourol 2005,19:813–817.
67. Davis SD, Yankelevitz DF, Williams T, Henschke CI. Pulmonary tuberculosis in immunocomprimised hosts: Epidemiological, clinical, and radiological assessment. Semin Roentgenol 1993, 28:119–130.
68. Harisinghani MG, McLoud TC, Shepard JO, Ko JP, Shroff MM, Mueller PR. Tuberculosis from head to toe. Radiographics 2000, 20:449–470.
69. Premkumar A, Lattimer J, Newhouse JH. CT and sonography of advanced urinary tract tuberculosis. AJR Am J Roentgenol 1987, 148:65–69.
70. Wang LJ, Wong YC, Chen CJ. CT features of genitourinary tuberculosis. J Comput Assist Tomogr 1997, 21:254–258.
71. Brennan RE, Pollack HM. Nonvisualized ("phantom") renal calyx: Causes and radiological approach to diagnosis. Urol Radiol 1979, 21:163–170.
72. Skutil V, Gow JG. Urogenital tuberculosis: The present state in Europe-the report of round table discussion. Eur Urol 1977, 3:257.
73. Gupta NP, Agrawal AK, Sood S. Tubercular pyelonephritic nonfunctioning kidney – another relative contraindication for laparoscopic nephrectomy: A case report. J Laparoendosc Adv Surg Tech A 1997, 7: 131–134.
74. Flechner SM, Gow JG. Role of nephrectomy in the treatment of non-functioning or very poorly functioning unilateral tuberculous kidney. J Urol 1980, 123: 822–825.
75. Kim HH, Lee KS, Park K, Ahn H. Laparoscopic nephrectomy for nonfunctioning tuberculous kidney. J Endourol, 2000, 14: 433–437.
76. Rassweiler J, Fornara P, Weber M, Janetschek G, Fahlenkamp D, Henkel T, et al. Laparoscopic nephrectomy: The experience of the laparoscopy working group of the German Urologic Association. J Urol 1998, 160: 18–21.
77. Hemal AK, Gupta NP, Kumar R. Comparison of retroperitoneoscopic nephrectomy with open surgery for tuberculous nonfunctioning kidneys. J Urol 2000,164:32–35.
78. Lee KS, Kim HH, Byun SS, Kwak C, Park K, Ahn H. Laparoscopic nephrectomy for tuberculos nonfunctioning kidney: Comparison with laparoscopic simple nephrectomy for other diseases. Urology 2002, 60:411–414.
79. Arnaout MA. Molecular genetics and pathogenesis of autosomal dominant polycystic kidney disease. Annu Rev Med 2001, 52: 93–123.
80. Wang D, Strandgaard S. The pathogenesis of hypertension in autosomal dominant polycystic kidney disease. J Hypertens 1997, 15: 925–933.
81. Steinman TI. Pain management in polycystic kidney disease. Am J Kidney Dis 2000, 35: 770–772.
82. Bell PE, Hossack KF, Gabow PA, Durr JA, Johnson AM, Schrier RW. Hypertension in autosomal dominant polycystic kidney disease. Kidney Int 1988, 34: 683–690.
83. Milutinovic J, Fialkow PJ, Agodoa LY, Phillips LA, Rudd TG, Sutherland S. Clinical manifestations of autosomal dominant polycystic kidney disease in patients older than 50 years. Am J Kidney Dis 1990, 15: 237–243.
84. Gabow PA. Autosomal dominant polycystic kidney disease. N Engl J Med 1993, 329: 332–342.
85. McNally ML, Erturk E, Oleyourryk G, Schoeniger L. Laparoscopic cyst decortication using the harmonic scalpel for symptomatic autosomal dominant polycystic kidney disease. J Endourol 2001, 15: 597–599.
86. Elashry OM, Nakada SY, Wolf JS, Jr., McDougall EM, Clayman RV. Laparoscopy for adult polycystic kidney disease: A promising alternative. Am J Kidney Dis 1996, 27: 224–233.
87. Hemal AK. Laparoscopic management of renal cystic disease. Urol Clin North Am 2001, 28:115–126.
88. Bennett AH, Stewart W, Lazarus JM. Bilateral nephrectomy in patients with polycystic renal disease. Surg Gynecol Obstet 1973, 137: 819–820.
89. Rayner BL, Cassidy MJ, Jacobsen JE, Pascoe MD, Pontin AR, van Zyl Smit R. Is preliminary binephrectomy necessary in patients with autosomal dominant polycystic kidney disease undergoing renal transplantation? Clin Nephrol 1990. 34: 122–124.
90. Dunn MD, Portis AJ, Elbahnasy AM, Shalhav AL, Rothstein M, McDougall EM, Clayman RV. Laparoscopic nephrectomy in patients with end-stage renal disease and autosomal dominant polycystic kidney disease. Am J Kidney Dis 2000, 35: 720–725.
91. Elashry OM, Giusti G, Nadler RB, McDougall EM, Clayman RV. Incisional hernia after laparoscopic nephrectomy with intact specimen removal: Caveat emptor. J Urol 1997, 158: 363–369.
92. Seshadri PA, Poulin EC, Pace D, Schlachta CM, Cadeddu MO, Mamazza J. Transperitoneal laparoscopic nephrectomy for giant polycystic kidneys: A case control study. Urology 2001, 58: 23–27.
93. Gill IS, Kavoussi LR, Clayman RV, et al. Complications of laparoscopic nephrectomy in 185 patients: A multiinstitutional review. J Urol 1995, 154:479–483.

94. Matin SF, Abreu S, Ramani A, et al. Evaluation of age and comorbidity as risk factors after laparoscopic urological surgery. J Urol 2003, 170:1115–1120.
95. Parsons JK, Varkarakis I, Rha KH, et al. Complications of abdominal urologic laparoscopy: Longitudinal five-year analysis. Urology 2004, 63:27–32.
96. Soulie M, Salomon L, Seguin P, et al.: Multi-institutional study of complications in 1085 laparoscopic urologic procedures. Urology 2001, 58:899–903.
97. Soulie M, Seguin P, Richeux L, et al. Urological complications of laparoscopic surgery: Experience with 350 procedures at a single center. J Urol 2001, 165:1960–1963.
98. Vallancien G, Cathelineau X, Baumert H, et al. Complications of transperitoneal laparoscopic surgery in urology: Review of 1311 procedures at a single center. J Urol 2002, 168:23–26.
99. Pareek G, Hedican SP, Gee JR, et al. Meta-analysis of the complications of laparoscopic renal surgery: Comparison of procedures and techniques. J Urol 2006, 175:1208–1213.
100. Ono Y, Katoh N, Kinukawa T, Sahashi M, Ohshima S. Laparoscopic nephrectomy, radical nephrectomy and adrenalectomy: Nagoya experience. J Urol 1994, 152: 1962–1966.
101. Eraky I, el-Kappany H, Shamaa MA, Ghoneim MA. Laparoscopic nephrectomy: An established routine procedure. J Endourol 1994, 8: 275–278.
102. McDougall EM, Clayman RV. Laparoscopic nephrectomy for benign disease: Comparison of the transperitoneal and retroperitenel approaches. J Endourol 1996,10:45–49.
103. Ono Y, Katoh N, Kinukawa T, Matsuura O, Ohshima S. Laparoscopic nephrectomy via the retroperitoneal approach. J Urol 1996, 156: 1101–1104.
104. Doublet JD, Peraldi MN, Monsaint H, et al. Retroperitoneal laparoscopic nephrectomy of native kidneys in renal transplant recipients. Transplantation 1997, 64:89–91.
105. Hemal AK, Gupta NP, Wadhwa SN, Goel A, Kumar R. Retroperitoneoscopic nephrectomy and nephroureterectomy for benign nonfunctioning kidneys: A single-center experience. Urology 2001, 57: 644–649.
106. Sebe P, de la Taille A, Hoznek A, Chopin D, Abbou CC, Salomon L. Simple nephrectomy with retroperitoneal laparoscopy. Prog Urol 2003, 13:577–580.
107. Poulsen EU, Eddy B, Poulsen J. Laparoscopic nephrectomy. Scand J Urol Nephrol 2005, 39:138–142.
108. Wolf JS. Tips and tricks for hand-assisted surgery. AUA Update Series 2005,24:2
109. Rane A, Dasgupta P. Prospective experience with a second generation hand assisted laparoscopic device and comparison with first generation devices. J Endourol 2003,17:895–897.
110. Rupa P, Stifelman MD. Hand-assisted laparoscopic devices: The second generation. J Endourol 2004,18:649–653.
111. Bishoff JT, Kavoussi LR. Laparoscopic Surgery of the Kidney. (in Campbell-Walsh Urology, 9th ed, Saunders, Elsevier, 2007, p1761.

Laparoscopic Radical Nephrectomy

Retroperitoneal Approach

Andre Berger, Sidney Castro de Abreu, and Inderbir S. Gill

INTRODUCTION

At specialized centers worldwide, laparoscopic radical nephrectomy is now routine practice for management of indicated patients with localized renal cell carcinoma. Compared to open radical nephrectomy, the laparoscopic approach is associated with comparable operative time, decreased blood loss, superior recovery, improved cosmesis, and equivalent cancer control over a long-term follow-up *(1–3)*.

At the Cleveland Clinic, laparoscopic radical nephrectomy is preferentially performed by the retroperitoneal technique. Concerns about the smaller retroperitoneal working space not withstanding, our learning curve has allowed us to readily overcome this technical difficulty. Furthermore, retroperitoneoscopy offers several unique advantages, including expeditious access to renal artery and vein allowing early ligation, extra fascial mobilization of the kidney, and en bloc removal of the adrenal gland, recapitulating the principles of open surgery *(4)*. A prospective randomized study comparing retroperitoneal and transperitoneal approaches *(5)* showed shorter time to hilum control and shorter total operative time in the retroperitoneal group. In fact, it is the senior author's impression that graduating fellows from our institution are equally comfortable and adept at either the transperitoneal or the retroperitoneal laparoscopic approach to radical nephrectomy.

PREOPERATIVE ASSESSMENT

Attention to the patient's cardiorespiratory status, coagulation profile, history of prior operations, and bone or spinal abnormalities is imperative.

Our preoperative bowel preparation comprises two bottles of magnesium citrate administered the evening before the surgery. The patient reports to the hospital on the morning of surgery. Broad-spectrum antibiotics are administered intravenously 2 h preoperatively and intermittent compression stockings are placed bilaterally.

NECESSARY INSTRUMENTATION

- One 10-mm 30° laparoscope
- One 10-mm trocar-mounted balloon dissection device (U.S. Surgical, Norwalk, CT)
- One 10-mm Bluntip trocar (U.S. Surgical)

From: *Current Clinical Urology: Essential Urologic Laparoscopy*
Edited by: S. Y. Nakada and S. P. Hedican, DOI 10.1007/978-1-60327-820-1_7

- Two 10–12-mm trocars
- One 5-mm electrosurgical monopolar scissors
- One 5-mm electrosurgical hook
- One 5-mm atraumatic grasping forceps (small bowel clamp)
- One 10-mm right-angle dissector
- One 10-mm three-pronged reusable metal retractor (fan-type)
- One 11-mm Endoclip applier
- One 12-mm articulated endo-GIA vascular stapler (U.S. Surgical)
- One 5-mm irrigator/aspirator
- One 15-mm Endocatch II bag (U.S. Surgical)
- One Weck clip applicator with disposable clip cartridges (Weck Systems)

PATIENT POSITION

Following general anesthesia and Foley catheter placement, the patient is firmly secured to the operating table in a 90° full flank position. All bony prominences are meticulously padded and extremities carefully placed in neutral position to minimize postoperative neuromuscular sequelae. The kidney bridge is elevated moderately, and the operating table is flexed somewhat to increase the space between the lowermost rib and the iliac crest. To guard against the development of neuromuscular spinal problems, we make every attempt to minimize the time period for which the patient is placed in the lateral decubitus flexed position.

OPERATION ROOM SET-UP

The surgeon and the camera operator (assistant) stand facing the patient's back. The surgeon stands towards the patient's feet, while the assistant stands toward the patient's head. The cart holding the primary video monitor, CO_2 insufflator, light source, and recorder is placed on the side of the table contralateral to the surgeon. The scrub nurse is positioned toward the foot end of the operative table.

PORT PLACEMENT

During radical retroperitoneoscopic nephrectomy, three trocars are placed. The laparoscope is positioned in the primary port at the tip of the 12th rib. The surgeon works through the posterior and anterior secondary ports (Fig. 1).

Primary Port

The open (Hasson cannula) technique is ideal for obtaining initial access. A horizontal 1.5-cm skin incision is made just below the tip of the 12th rib. Using S-shaped retractors, the flank muscle fibers are bluntly separated. Entry is gained into the retroperitoneal space by gently piercing the anterior thoracolumbar fascia with the fingertip or hemostat. Limited finger dissection of the retroperitoneum is performed in a cephalad direction, remaining immediately anterior to the psoas muscle and fascia, and posterior to the Gerota's fascia to create a space for placement of the balloon dilator *(6)*. At this juncture, the tip of the lower pole of the kidney can often be palpated by the finger. We insert a trocar-mounted balloon dissection device (Origin Medsystems, Menlo Park, CA) for rapidly and atraumatically creating a working space in the retroperitoneum in a standardized manner (Fig. 2). The volume of air instilled into the balloon is typically 800–1,000 mL in adults (40 pumps of the sphygmomanometer bulb). The balloon dilatation outside Gerota's fascia (i.e., in the pararenal space between the psoas muscle posteriorly and Gerota's fascia anteriorly) effectively displaces the Gerota's

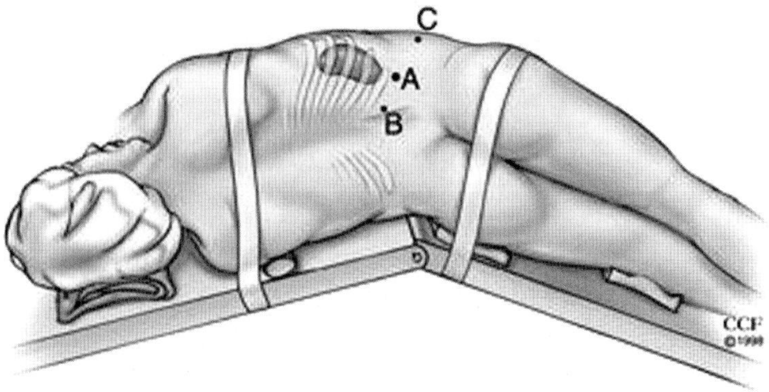

Fig. 1. Port placement during right retroperitoneoscopy radical nephrectomy. **A** primary 10-mm port is placed at the tip of 12th rib. **B** 10-/12-mm port is placed at the junction of lateral border of the erector spinae muscle with underside of 12th rib. **C** 10-/12-mm port is placed three finger-breadths cephalad to iliac crest, between mid and anterior axillary lines.

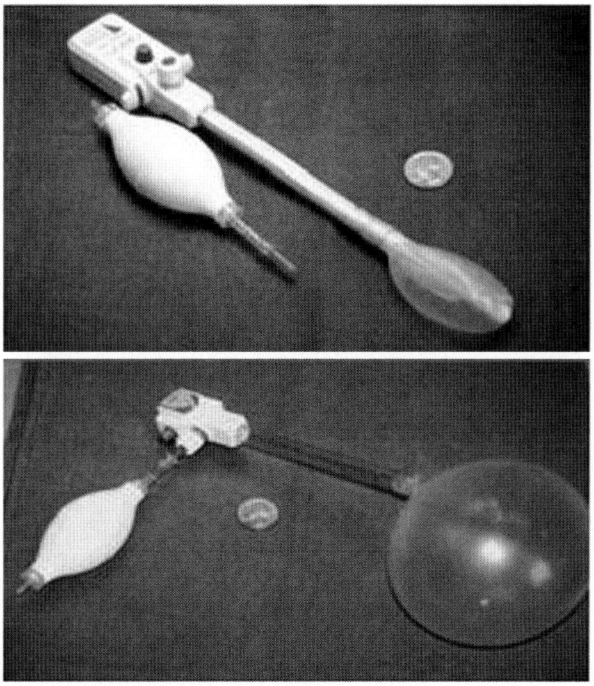

Fig. 2. Trocar-mounted preperitoneal dilator balloon (uninflated and inflated) device (Origin Medsystems).

fascia covered kidney anteromedially, allowing direct access to the posterior aspect of the renal hilum (Fig. 3). Laparoscopic examination from within the transparent balloon confirms adequate expansion of the retroperitoneum. Secondary cephalad or caudad balloon dilatation, as required by the clinical situation, further enlarges the retroperitoneal working space. For example, during a retroperitoneoscopic adrenalectomy the balloon is deflated and reinflated in a more cephalad location along the undersurface of the diaphragm to create a working space in the immediate vicinity of the adrenal gland. Similarly,

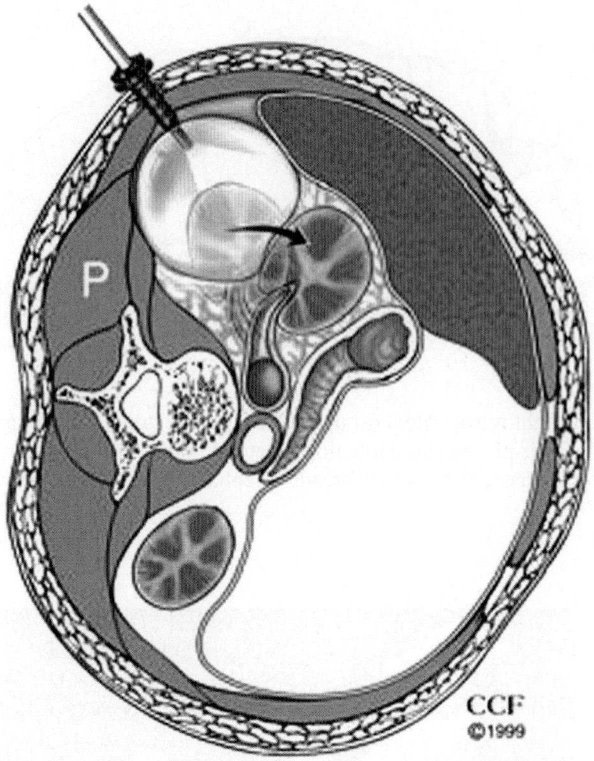

Fig. 3 Balloon dilator positioned between psoas fascia posteriorly and Gerota's fascia anteriorly. The distended balloon (800 cc) displaces Gerota's fascia/kidney anteromedially allowing access to renal vessels.

during a retroperitoneoscopic nephroureterectomy, secondary balloon dilation is performed caudally to expose the distal ureter.

Following balloon dilatation and removal, a 10-mm Bluntip trocar (Origin Medsystems) is placed as the primary port (Fig. 4). This trocar has an internal fixed fascial retention balloon and an external adjustable foam cuff, which combine to eliminate air leakage at the primary port site. The internal fascial retention balloon of the cannula is inflated with 30 cc of air, and the external adjustable foam cuff is cinched down to secure the primary port in an airtight manner *(7)*. In the author's experience, such

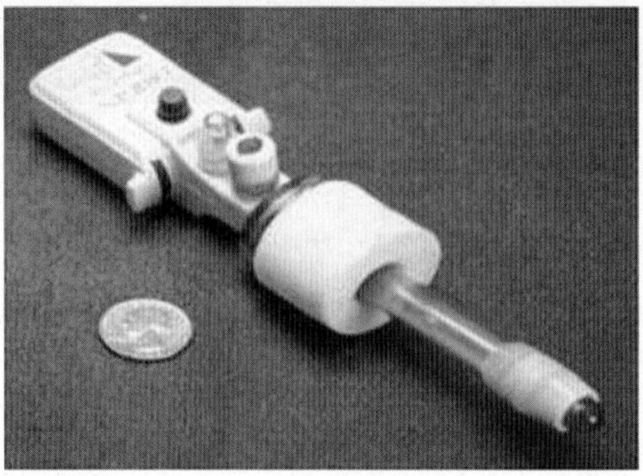

Fig. 4. A Bluntip trocar (Origin Medsystems) is employed to achieve an airtight seal for the primary port.

an airtight seal has been more difficult to achieve with a standard Hasson cannula. Pneumoretroperitoneum is established to 15 mmHg, and a 10-mm, 30° laparoscope is inserted. The psoas muscle and Gerota's fascia are identified immediately. In our experience *(8)*, one or more of these landmarks are identifiable in the following frequency: lateral peritoneal reflection (83%); ureter and/or gonadal vein (61%); pulsations of the fat-covered renal artery (56%); aortic pulsations of the left side (90%); and the compressed, ribbon-like inferior vena cava on the right side (25%).

Secondary Ports

Two secondary ports are placed under 30° laparoscopic visualization. The immediately adjacent undersurface of the flank abdominal wall is visualized endoscopically.

A 10-/12-mm port is placed three finger-breadths cephalad to the iliac crest, between the mid and anterior axillary lines. A second 10-/12-mm port is placed at the lateral border of the erector spinae muscle just below the 12th rib *(9)*. Frustrating "clashing of swords" occurs if the trocars, and therefore the laparoscopic instruments, are located in close proximity. Thus, the port placed between mid and anterior axillary lines can be positioned even more anteriorly to the anterior axillary line; however, the lateral peritoneal reflection must be clearly visualized laparoscopically and avoided before the port is inserted. If necessary, the lateral peritoneal reflection can be bluntly mobilized further anterior medially from the undersurface of the flank abdominal wall using the laparoscope's tip.

STEP-BY-STEP SURGICAL APPROACH

Renal Hilum Control

The kidney is retracted anterolaterally with a laparoscopic small bowel clamp or the fan retractor in the nondominant hand of the surgeon placing the renal hilum on traction. Gerota's fascia is incised longitudinally in the general area of the renal hilum, parallel and 1–2 cm anterior to the psoas muscle. Care must be taken to avoid dissection close by the psoas muscle, which may lead the surgeon to reach the retrocaval or the retroaortic space. The longitudinal incision of the Gerota's fascia opens the retroperitoneal space, thereby adding to the effect of the carbon dioxide insufflation, and exposing the renal hilum. Blunt and sharp dissection in this avascular area of loose areolar fatty tissue is performed to identify renal arterial pulsations. Visualization of the vertically oriented, distinct arterial pulsations indicates the location of the renal artery, which is circumferentially mobilized, clip-ligated (11-mm titanium clips: three on the "stay side" and two on the "go side") and divided. Subsequently, the renal vein, is stapled and divided with an Endo-GIA stapler (U.S. Surgical) (Fig. 5). Usually after division of the renal vein, some flimsy hilar attachments remain between the kidney and the great vessels. In order to avoid traction injury, which may lead to venous tear and bleeding, these remaining attachments should be precisely clipped and transected.

Intraoperative Trouble-Shooting

Problems with Orientation in the Retroperitoneum

To avoid problems with orientation in the retroperitoneum, the camera should be oriented such that the psoas muscle is always absolutely horizontal on the video monitor *(5)*. However, the retroperitoneal space is relatively small at this stage of the procedure, anteromedial retraction of the kidney serves to increase the retroperitoneal space, exposing the psoas muscle that can be identified most easily caudal to the kidney.

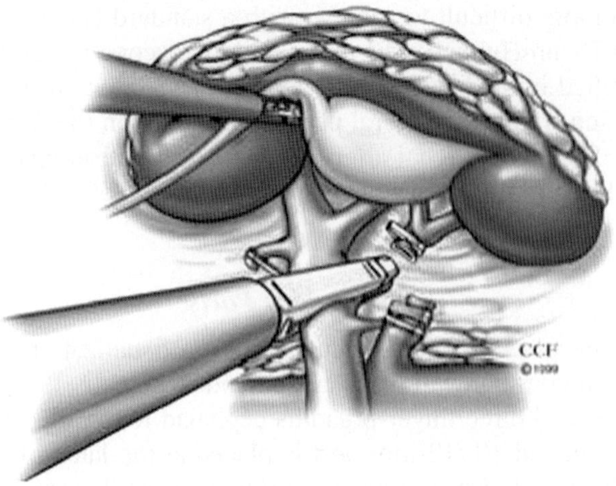

Fig. 5. Renal artery has been clip-ligated and divided. Renal vein is circumferentially mobilized and controlled with a gastrointestinal anastomosis stapler.

Difficulty in Finding the Renal Hilum

If the renal hilum cannot be located, the surgeon should reinsert the laparoscope slowly and identify the psoas muscle. The psoas muscle should then be crossed from lateral-to-medial in a cephalad direction and a search conducted for arterial pulsation near its medial border. Pulsations of the fat-covered renal artery or aorta are usually identifiable. Gentle dissection with the tip of the suction device or hook is performed directly toward the pulsations. The renal artery is identified and traced directly to the renal hilum. One must always be mindful of aberrant major vessels, such as the superior mesenteric artery, which arises from the aorta more medially and superiorly than the left renal artery. Alternatively, the ureter can be identified and followed cephalad to the hilum. Dissection through the perirenal fat may identify the surface of the kidney, which can then be dissected toward its hilum.

Persistent Renal Hilar Bleeding After Division of the Renal Artery and Vein

Persistent renal hilar bleeding generally indicates the presence of an overlooked, accessory renal artery. After flow is controlled from the main renal artery, the renal vein should appear flat and devoid of blood. A normally distended renal vein at this juncture indicates continued arterial inflow through an accessory renal artery. In this circumstance, division of the distended renal vein with an Endo-GIA stapler (U.S. Surgical) interrupts renal outflow, with a resultant increase in intrarenal venous back pressure. This causes persistent oozing during the remainder of the dissection. One should search for an accessory renal artery in this situation.

Endo GIA Malfunction

The GIA stapler is standard for control of renal hilar vessels. However, failure of the device can be associated with severe consequences, including emergency conversion to open procedure.

The most common cause of GIA failure is inadvertent placement of the device over a previously placed surgical clip *(10)*. In order to avoid this situation, extreme care must be taken when positioning and firing the Endo GIA stapler in the presence of surgical clips in the area of renal hilum.

CIRCUMFERENTIAL EXTRAFASCIAL MOBILIZATION OF THE EN BLOC SPECIMEN

Suprahilar dissection is performed along the medial aspect of the upper pole of the kidney and the adrenal vessels, including the main adrenal vein, are precisely controlled with clip-ligation. Dissection is next redirected towards the supralateral aspect of the specimen, including en bloc adrenal gland, which is readily mobilized from the underside of the diaphragm. In the avascular flimsy areolar tissue in this location, inferior phrenic vessels to the adrenal gland are often encountered and controlled. The anterior aspect of the specimen is mobilized from the underside of the peritoneum envelope. During this dissection, use of electrocautery must be avoided in order to avoid transmural thermal damage to the bowel located just beside the thin peritoneal membrane. The ureter, with or without the gonadal vein, is secured, and the specimen is completely freed by mobilization of the lower pole of the kidney. The entire dissection is performed outside Gerota's fascia, mirroring established oncologic principles of open surgery.

INTRAOPERATIVE TROUBLE-SHOOTING

Inadverted Peritoneotomy

A peritoneotomy does not necessarily mandate conversion to transperitoneal laparoscopy. Usually, a peritoneal rent does not cause significant problems, and the procedure can be completed retroperitoneoscopically. However, if operative exposure is compromised, a fourth port can be inserted to provide additional retraction of the billowing peritoneal membrane.

Also, intra-abdominal viscera must be thoroughly inspected by inserting the laparoscope trough the peritoneotomy to rule out iatrogenic injury.

SPECIMEN ENTRAPMENT

Organ entrapment is rapidly performed by using an Endocatch bag (U.S Surgical). This bag is an impermeable plastic and nylon sac designed to prevent tumor spillage during intact specimen removal. This bag should never be employed during tissue morcellation *(11)*. The specimen is tented up by the

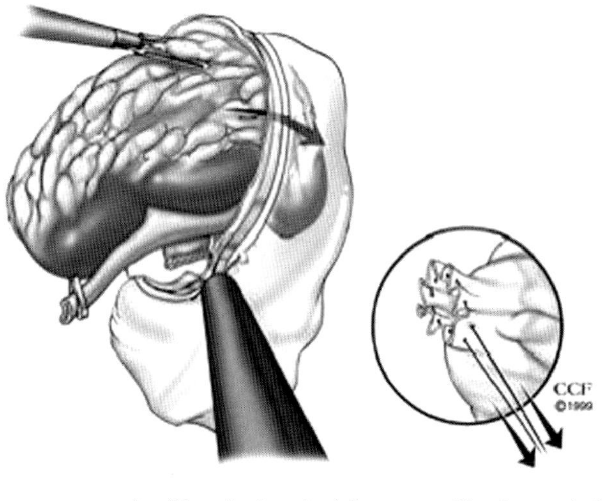

Fig. 6. After specimen entrapment, mouth of bag is detached from metallic ring and closed by pulling on built-in drawstring.

nondominant hand. The bag is introduced through the anterior port, the spring-loaded mouth of the sac is opened in the retroperitoneun, and the specimen placed within. After specimen entrapment, the mouth of the bag is detached from the metallic ring and closed (under laparoscopic visualization) by tightening the drawstring (Fig. 6).

Entrapment of Larger Specimens

An intentional peritoneotomy is occasionally created, strictly for entrapment of large specimens. The large specimen is inserted within the peritoneal cavity where it is entrapped within the 15-mm Endocatch II bag (U.S. Surgical).

SPECIMEN EXTRACTION

Currently, our routine practice for specimen extraction aims to achieve a superior cosmetic result while providing an intact specimen for precise pathologic staging. In this manner, we usually employ a low muscle-splitting Pfannenstiel incision *(12)*. For the appropriate female patient a vaginal extraction *(13)* of the specimen can be safely performed.

Pfannenstiel Incision

A Pfannenstiel skin incision (slightly lateralized towards the nephrectomy side) is made at or just below the level of the pubic hairline. Subsequently, the anterior rectus fascia is incised obliquely, rectus muscle fibers are retracted medially, posterior rectus fascia is incised, the peritoneal membrane is reflected cephalad using finger dissection, and extraperitoneal access is gained to the retroperitoneal space, to extracted the intact entrapped specimen (Fig. 7).

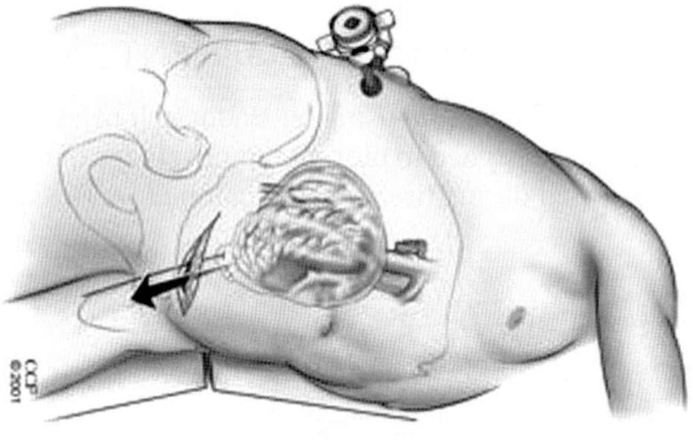

Fig. 7. A Pfannenstiel skin incision (at or just below the level of the pubic hairline) is used to retrieve the intact specimen entrapped in a bag.

Vaginal Extraction

After the specimen is entrapped in an Endocatch II bag, a generous longitudinal peritoneotomy is intentionally created along the undersurface of the anterior abdominal wall. The operating table is placed in a steep Trendelenburg position, and rotated such that the flank position is decreased to 60°. Bowel loops are retracted cephalad.

A sponge-stick is externally inserted into the sterilely prepared vagina and tautly positioned in the posterior fornix. Laparoscopically, a transverse posterior 3-cm colpotomy is created at the apex of the tented-up posterior fornix, and the drawstring of the entrapped specimen is delivered into the vagina

(Fig. 8). After laparoscopic exit is completed, the patient is placed in a supine lithotomy position. The specimen is extracted intact per vaginum, and the posterior colpotomy incision repaired transvaginally. This approach is contraindicated in patients with even a mild degree of pelvic or intraperitoneal adhesions from any etiology.

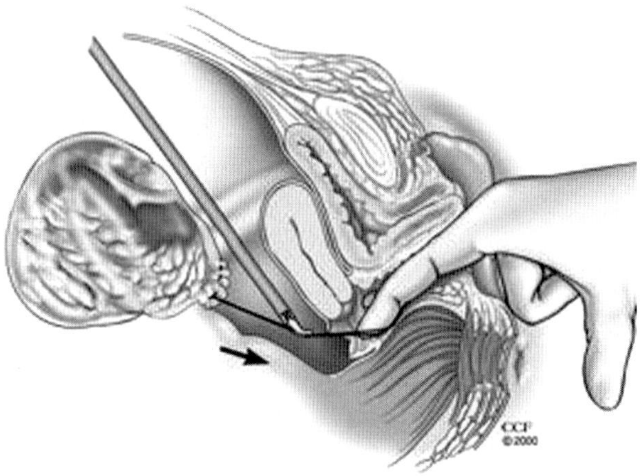

Fig. 8. The drawstring of the closed Endocach II bag, previously grasped by the laparoscopic clamp, is delivered into the vagina.

HEMOSTASIS

Hemostasis is confirmed under lowered retropneumoperitoneun (Fig. 9) and ports are removed under laparoscopic visualization. Fascial closure is performed for all 10-mm or larger port sites.

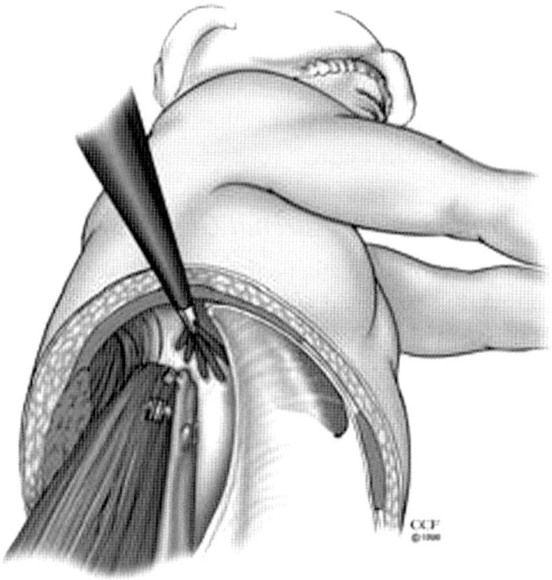

Fig. 9. Hemostasis of the renal bed is confirmed after 5–10 min without CO_2 pressure in the retroperitoneal space. Trocars are removed under laparoscopic visualization.

SPECIAL CONSIDERATIONS

Concerns About Tumor Size

As our initial approach is targeted towards the renal hilum, the size of the renal mass only becomes a significant issue at the time of specimen mobilization. In our series, 33% of the tumors were equal to or larger than 6 cm on CT scan (Fig. 10), including tumors up to 13–14 cm in size with overall specimen weight exceeding 1.5 kg.

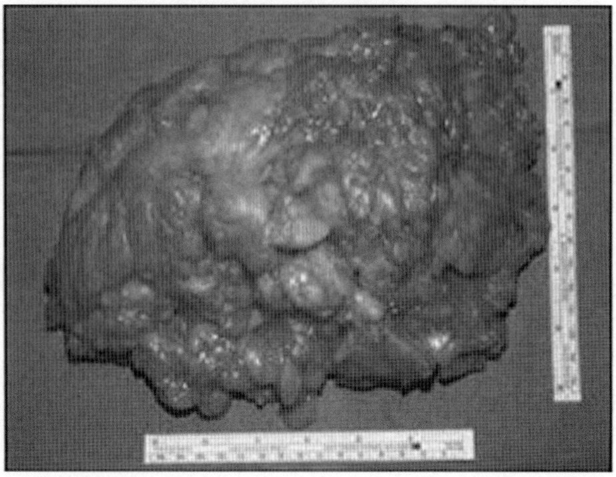

Fig. 10. Retroperitoneoscopic radical nephrectomy. Surgical specimen weighted 1,200 g.

Retroperitoneoscopy in Obese Patients

Although the excessive retroperitoneal fat increases the degree of technical difficulty, adherence to a standardized stepwise anatomical approach *(14)* allows retroperitoneoscopy to be performed effectively in markedly obese or morbidly obese patients. In fact, the retroperitoneal flank approach allows the gravitational pull to shift much of the weight of the pannus anteriorly, away from the ipsilateral flank (Fig. 11). In our series, 35% of the patients had body mass index (BMI) equal or greater than 30. However, the reader should be cautioned that these challenging procedures should be performed by surgeons facile with the laparoscopic technique.

Preservation of the Adrenal Gland (if Necessary)

To preserve the adrenal gland, Gerota's fascia is opened and a well-defined plane between the upper pole of the kidney and the adrenal is dissected using electrosurgical scissor (Fig. 12). In our series, en bloc adrenalectomy was not performed in 33 cases (30.5%). These included cases from bilateral radical nephrectomy, previous contralateral adrenalectomy, or elective preservation of the adrenal gland.

Oncologic Efficacy of Laparoscopic Radical Nephrectomy

Laparoscopic surgery for renal tumor does not result in an increased risk of port site seeding, local recurrences, or metastasis *(15)*. To achieve oncological safety, the classical rules of renal cancer surgery must be respected. Also the surgical specimen must be removed in a hermetic sac to avoid any contact with the abdominal wall. We prefer intact specimen extraction so as to allow precise pathologic staging. Laparoscopic lymph node dissection for RCC is feasible and safe and specially important in patients with advanced disease. The procedure can be useful for staging, decreasing recurrence rates

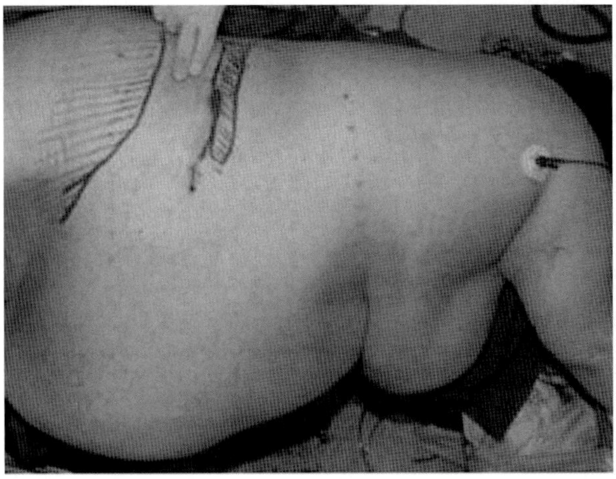

Fig. 11. With a patient in a full flank position a significant amount of abdominal pannus falls away from operative side. This patient had a BMI of 47.5.

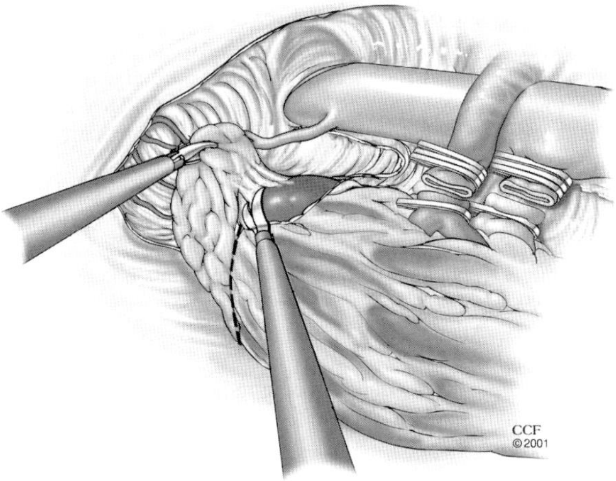

Fig. 12. If necessary the adrenal gland can be preserved Gerota's fascia is opened and adrenal is detached from renal upper pole using electrocautery scissors.

and even for improving survival *(16)*. Overall, cancer-specific and recurrence-free survival are similar in contemporary cohorts comparing laparoscopic and open approaches, even for T2 tumors *(2,3)*.

TAKE HOME MESSAGES

1. Compared with transperitoneal laparoscopy, retroperitoneoscopy may be associated with a somewhat sharper learning curve.
2. For efficacious performance of retroperitoneoscopic surgery, proper development of the retroperitoneal space and constant orientation with various anatomical landmarks is critical. It is abundantly clear that the retroperitoneal space can be readily developed and enlarged appropriately as the laparoscopic dissection proceeds.
3. Although out of sight, peritoneal organs must never be out of mind, because they are separated only by the peritoneal layer, and therefore are susceptible to injury.

4. Retroperitoneoscopy does offer straightforward and rapid exposure and control of the renal hilum, and nonviolation of the peritoneum, thus minimizing the chances of intraperitoneal organ injury. Prospective randomized study showed shorter time to control the hilum and shorter operative time when compared to transperitoneal approach *(4)*.

REFERENCES

1. Gill IS, Meraney AM, Schweizer DK, Savage SS, Hobart MG, Sung GT, et al. Laparoscopic radical nephrectomy in 100 patients: A single center experience from the United States. Cancer 2001; 92: 1843–1855.
2. Colombo JR Jr, Haber GP, Aron M, Cocuzza M, Colombo R, Kaouk J, Gill IS. Oncological outcomes of laparoscopic radical nephrectomy for renal cancer. Clinics 2007 Jun; 62(3):251–256.
3. Hemal AK, Kumar A, Kumar R, Wadhwa P, Seth A, Gupta NP. Laparoscopic versus open radical nephrectomy for large renal tumors: a long-term prospective comparison. J Urol 2007 Mar; 177(3):862–866.
4. Gill IS, Rassweiler JJ. Retroperitoneoscopic renal surgery: our approach. Urology 1999; 54, 734–738.
5. Desai MM, Strzempkowski B, Matin SF, Steinberg AP, Ng C, Meraney AM, Kaouk JH, Gill IS. Prospective randomized comparison of transperitoneal versus retroperitoneal laparoscopic radical nephrectomy. J Urol 2005 Jan;173(1):38–41.
6. Gaur DD. Laparoscopic operative retroperitoneoscopy: use of a new device. J Urol 1992; 148: 1137–1139.
7. Gill IS. Retroperitoneal laparoscopic nephrectomy. Urol Clin North Am 1998; 25: 343–360.
8. Sung GT, Gill IS. Anatomic landmarks and time management during retroperitoneoscopic radical nephrectomy. J Endourol 1998; 16: 165–169.
9. Gill IS, Schweizer D, Hobart MG, Sung GT, Klein EA, Novick AR. Retroperitoneal laparoscopic radical nephrectomy: the Cleveland Clinic experience. J Urol 2000; 163: 1665–1670.
10. Chan D, Bishoff L, Ratner L, Kavoussi LR, Jarrett TW. Endovascular gastrointestinal stapler device malfunction during laparoscopic nephrectomy: early recognition and management. J Urol 2000; 164, 319–321.
11. Urban DA, Kerbl K, McDougall EM. Organ entrapment and renal morcelation: permeability studies. J Urol 1993; 150: 1792–1794.
12. Kaouk JH, Gill IS. Laparoscopic nephrectomy: morcellate or leave intact. Rev Urol 2003.
13. Gill IS, Cherullo EE, Meraney AM, Borsuk F, Murphy DP, Falcone T. Vaginal extraction of the intact specimen following laparoscopic radical nephrectomy. J Urol 2002; 167: 238–241.
14. Matin SF, Gill IS, Hsu TH, Sung TK, Novick AC. Laparoscopic renal and adrenal surgery in obese patients: comparison to open surgery. J Urol 1999; 162: 665–669.
15. Cicco A, Salomon L, Hoznek H, Alame W, Saint F, Bralet MP, et al. Carcinological risks and retroperitoneal laparoscopy. Eur Urol 2000; 38: 606–612.
16. Simmons MN, Kaouk J, Gill IS, Fergany A. Laparoscopic radical nephrectomy with hilar lymph node dissection in patients with advanced renal cell carcinoma. Urology 2007 Jul; 70(1):43–46.

Laparoscopic Radical Nephrectomy: Transperitoneal Approach

Leslie A. Deane, David I. Lee, Jaime Landman, Chandru P. Sundaram, and Ralph V. Clayman

INTRODUCTION

Radical nephrectomy, as described by Robson et al. in 1963, is the traditional gold standard approach to the management of renal tumors *(1)*. This procedure has an established success rate but is associated with significant postoperative pain and prolonged convalescence, stemming from the flank, subcostal, Chevron or thoraco-abdominal incisions typically used. Laparoscopic radical nephrectomy, as introduced by Clayman and associates in 1991, has become a suitable alternative to open radical nephrectomy over the 16 years since this first reported case *(2)*. It is equally efficacious for small- to medium-sized tumors which are deemed not amenable to partial nephrectomy and also for larger tumors, in some cases as large as 25 cm (authors' experience) *(3,4)*. Cases with renal vein and limited subhepatic inferior vena caval thrombus can also be managed laparoscopically in high volume centers with extensive experience *(5–9)*. The advantages of minimally invasive surgery have been well demonstrated for laparoscopic radical nephrectomy. In a study comparing open and laparoscopic radical nephrectomy, McDougall and colleagues demonstrated significantly decreased postoperative analgesia requirement and a more rapid initiation of oral intake in favor of the laparoscopic approach. In addition, there was a shorter hospital stay, a shorter return to the pre-operative level of normal activity and full recovery *(10)*. Several other studies have corroborated these findings (Table 1) *(11–18)*. In addition, the long-term cancer free success rate of this approach is equivalent to open surgery at 5 and now 10 years' follow-up *(4)*. Furthermore, the laparoscopic approach is more cost effective than an open approach, by just over $1,000 *(19)*.

For all of these reasons, laparoscopic radical nephrectomy is now recognized worldwide as the standard of care and in many institutions, has almost completely replaced open radical nephrectomy.

Since the first edition of this book, as surgical experience has been accrued, greater expertise has been garnered and technology has advanced, numerous modifications to the original approach to transperitoneal radical nephrectomy have been attempted and some changes adopted, although the anatomically based templates have remained largely the same. Herein, we highlight the nuances of our technique as it exists in 2009.

From: *Current Clinical Urology: Essential Urologic Laparoscopy*
Edited by: S. Y. Nakada and S. P. Hedican, DOI 10.1007/978-1-60327-820-1_8

Table 1
Summary of major clinical series of laparoscopic transperitoneal radical nephrectomy

Technique	*Author*	*Number of patients*	*Tumor size (range) (cm)*	*Operative time (min)*	*Estimated blood loss (ml)*	*Mean analgesic requirement (mg morphine)*	*Mean length of hospital stay (days)*	*Mean time to resuming normal activity (weeks)*	*Mean length of follow up (months)*	*Recurrence rate (%)*	*Complication rate (%)*
Transperitoneal	Barrett et al., 1998 *(11)*	66	4.5 (1.0–9.0)	175	Two patients transfused	Not reported	4.4	Not reported	21.4	5	Minor 6.9
	Dunn et al., 2000 *(12)*	61	5.3	330	172	28	3.4	3.6	25	8	Major 3.3; minor 34.4
	Chan et al., 2001 *(13)*	67	5.1 (1–13)	256	289	Not reported	3.8	Not reported	35.6	3	Overall 15
	Ono et al., 2001 *(14)*	103	3.1 (1.1–4.8)	282	254	Not reported	Not reported	23	29 (Median)	3.9	Major 10.7; minor 1.9
	Wille et al., 2004 *(15)*	125	5.1 (2–14)	200	210	Not reported	6	Not reported	23.5 (Median)	3.7	Major 4; minor 3.2
	Jeschke et al., 2000 *(16)*	51	(2–9)	125			7.2		7.9	0	Major 4
	Cheung et al., 2005 *(17)*		4.6 (2–10)	120	100	Not reported	Not reported	Not reported	30 (Median)	2	Major 1; minor 6
	Permpongkosol et al., 2005 *(18)*	67	5.1	Not addressed	Not addressed	Not addressed	Not addressed	Not addressed	73	6	Not addressed

PRE-OPERATIVE EVALUATION, PATIENT PREPARATION AND POSITIONING

Patients are routinely evaluated with complete blood count, basic metabolic panel including serum creatinine and blood urea nitrogen, serum calcium, liver function tests, alkaline phosphatase, coagulation panel, type and screen, urinalysis, and urine culture. Radiographic investigations include a chest X-ray and computed tomography of the abdomen and pelvis before and after the administration of intravenous contrast showing non-contrast, arterial, venous and delayed excretion phases. Modern technology allows for 3-D reconstructed and volume rendered imaging and these are indispensable in the pre-operative planning, allowing the surgeon to "know" the exact hilar anatomy and tumor extent prior to entering the operating room. If there is a contrast allergy, magnetic resonance imaging with gadolinium is performed, provided the patient has normal renal function. In patients at risk for contrast-induced nephropathy (renal disease, diabetes mellitus, congestive cardiac failure, gout, proteinuria, and hypertension) low osmolality or iso-osmolar contrast agents can be used in addition to N-acetylcysteine, sodium bicarbonate and pre-procedure hydration *(20)*. An isotope renal scan may be performed to document adequate contra-lateral renal function. The images acquired are reviewed with the radiologist to rule out liver metastases, lymphadenopathy, renal vein and/or vena caval involvement, and to confirm a normal contra-lateral adrenal gland in the event that the ipsilateral gland has to be excised.

Bowel preparation is not routinely employed but a clear liquid diet and Dulcolax/bisacodyl suppository is administered the day prior to the scheduled surgery. Prophylactic antibiotics are given within 1 h of the skin incision and Cefazolin 1 g usually provides adequate coverage in the non-allergic patient. The recommended pharmacologic therapy for DVT prohylaxis for high risk patients is low molecular weight heparin 40 mg subcutaneously (SC) daily, low-dose unfractionated heparin 5000 units SC 2 times daily.

General anesthesia with endotracheal intubation followed by placement of an oro-gastric tube and Foley catheter precedes positioning. Then, the patient is secured to the operating table in the lateral decubitus position contra-lateral to the kidney being removed (Fig. 1). The table is half flexed and placed in Trendelenberg until the flank is parallel to the floor. An axillary roll is placed between the patient and the table just superior to the nipple and it is ensured that the axilla is empty. The lower leg is flexed and pillows are placed between the legs until there is no tension over the hip of the upper leg. The kidney rest is then raised and its elevation is timed for half of an hour at which time it is lowered. Two hip grips (SunMedica, Redding, CA) one at the buttock and the second at the shoulder, allow rotation of the table away from the surgeon without the fear of the patient slipping. Egg-crate or gel-pad padding is placed under the lateral malleolus and fibular head of the dependant leg. Next the patient is secured to the table using 3 in. cloth tape at the shoulder, hips, and legs and Velcro straps to reinforce this (Fig. 1). The table is no longer placed in full rotation but rather at 25°. During the case, we request that the urine output is maintained at a minimum of 100 cc/h, and use of intravenous fluids, furosemide, and mannitol can help in achieving this goal.

Access

Following appropriate positioning, sterile preparation and draping of the abdomen, the potential port insertion sites are marked. Each site is injected with 0.5% bupivacaine (Marcaine) prior to any incision *(21)*. We choose a point two finger-breadths medial and two finger-breadths superior to the anterior superior iliac spine for placement of the Veress needle. After infiltration with local anesthetic, a 12 mm skin incision is made followed by blunt dissection using a hemostat to expose the fascia of the external oblique muscle. This is then grasped using two Allis clamps and the Veress needle is passed between the clamps and into the peritoneum. A pneumoperitoneum of 25 mmHg is then established until the ports are placed and not exceeding 10 min at which time the pressure is lowered to 12 mmHg *(22)*.

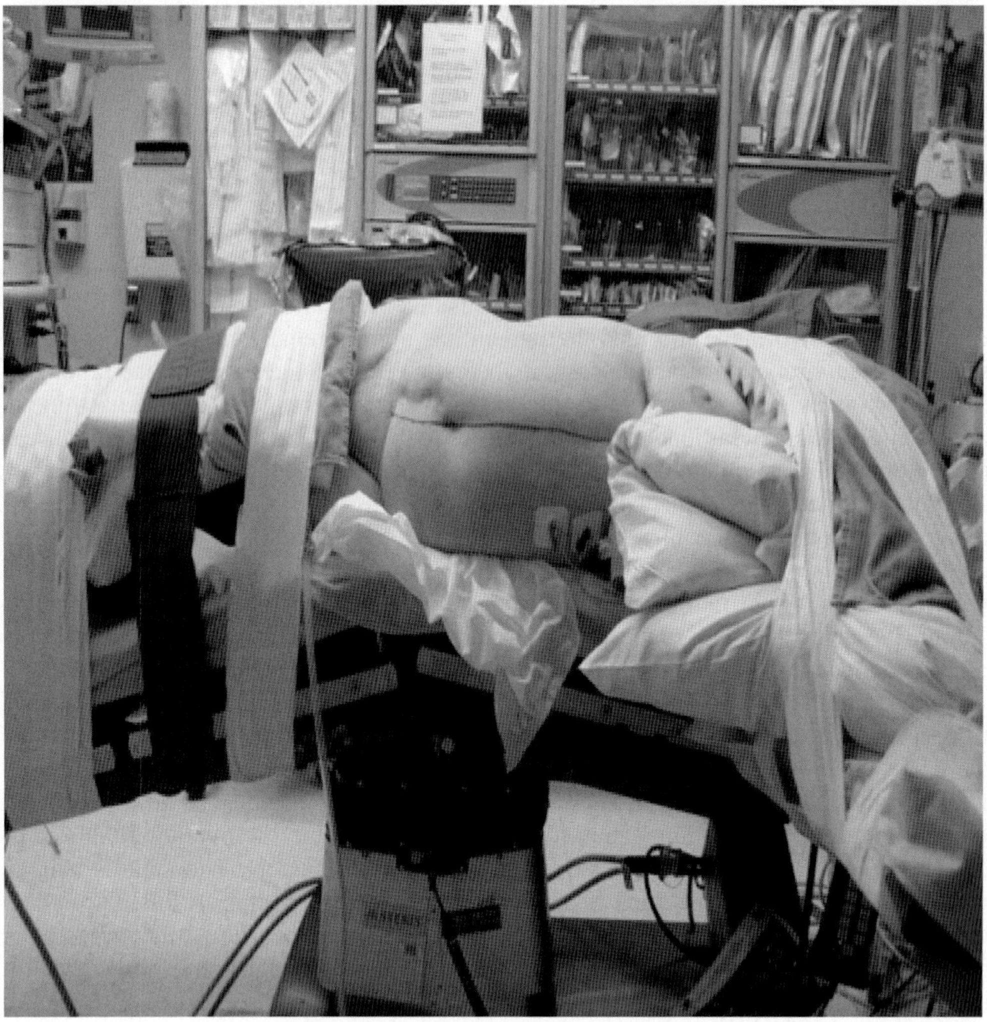

Fig. 1. Patient positioned for laparoscopic right radical nephrectomy.

The first 12 mm port to be placed is in the mid-clavicular line, approximately one finger-breadth below the costal margin using a 10 mm 0° lens through a visual non-bladed port such as an Endopath Xcel (Ethicon EndoSurgery, Cincinnati, OH). We believe that this is a safe approach to enter the peritoneal cavity as one can clearly identify each layer of muscle and intervening fascia followed by pre-peritoneal fat, prior to entry into the pneumoperitoneum. The 0° lens is immediately switched for a 30° lens and the site of Veress needle entry is carefully inspected to rule out inadvertent bowel injury. The needle is then removed and a second 12 mm port is placed the same site under direct vision. The third 12 mm port is then placed superior and lateral to the umbilicus (which is also lateral to the rectus muscle to avoid injury to the inferior epigastric vessels) in most patients as this will facilitate access to the renal hilum. In very thin patients, this port can be placed in the upper, outer quadrant of the umbilicus, making for a superior cosmetic result. On either side, a fourth port can be placed after the colon has been mobilized. Typically, this is a 5 mm port placed subcostally between the mid and posterior axillary lines. For right-sided nephrectomies a fifth port (5 mm) may be placed in a subxiphoid location and on the right side of, rather than through the falciform ligament. This port is used to provide retraction of the right lobe of the liver. The reader is referred to Figs. 2 and 3 for a schematic of the port placement.

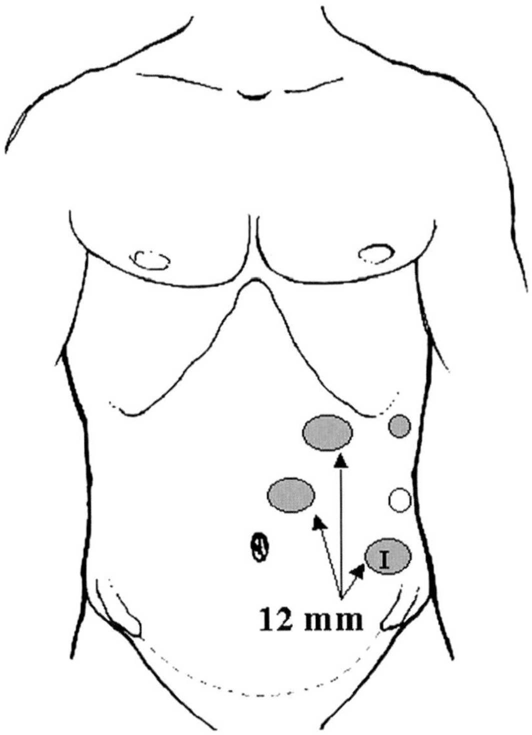

Fig. 2. Sites selected for placement of Veress needle (I) and subsequent 12 mm (*large grey circles*) and 5 mm (*small grey circle*) working ports for laparoscopic transperitoneal left radical nephrectomy. The fifth "clear circle" port site is "optional" and usually only placed if one is having difficulty entrapping a specimen. The "I" indicates the insufflation site.

There are some special circumstances in which we deviate from the aforementioned routine. In patients, who have had a prior appendectomy or right-sided colon resection, left colon resection or history of sigmoid and/or descending colonic diverticular disease, we opt to obtain Veress needle access in the mid-clavicular line one finger-breadth below the costal margin (Palmer's point) *(23)*. The needle is then removed and either a 12 mm non-bladed port is passed under endoscopic control, or, in the case when the quality of the pneumoperitoneum is not certain, then a 6 mm Ternamian Endo-TIP Cannula (Karl Storz Endoscopy America, Culver City, CA) with a 5 mm 0° laparoscope in its lumen, is rotated through the abdominal wall and into the pneumoperitoneum (Fig. 4) *(24)*.

This allows for more controlled and slow entry into the abdomen without the risk of slippage. Once the sites are selected for placement of the other ports, adhesions can be lysed safely and the Endo-TIP can be up-sized to a standard 12 mm port as needed. If one plans to keep the 5 mm Endo-TIP as a working port, then a 5 mm Kittner should never be used through this port since there is a risk of dislodging and losing the tip of the Kittner in the abdomen.

Instrumentation

Basic instrumentation for laparoscopic nephrectomy includes a standard laparoscopic tower (a carbon dioxide insufflator, light source, camera, monitor, and suction–irrigation setup) (Table 2). Ten millimeter 0 and 30° laparoscopes are used, the former for visual entry into the peritoneum and the latter to facilitate direct laparoscopic vision during challenging portions of the dissection such as the hilar dissection; with the 30° lens, the surgeon can see almost 270° around a particular structure.

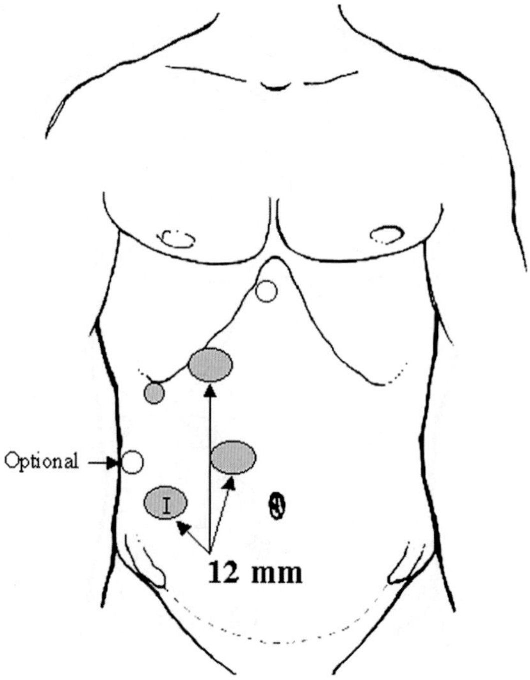

Fig. 3. Sites selected for placement of Veress needle (I) and subsequent working ports for laparoscopic transperitoneal right radical nephrectomy. The "clear circle" port site is "optional" and usually only placed if one is having difficulty entrapping a specimen. The "I" indicates the insufflation site. The unlabeled ports are 5 mm in size. Note the subxiphoid 5 mm port used for liver retraction.

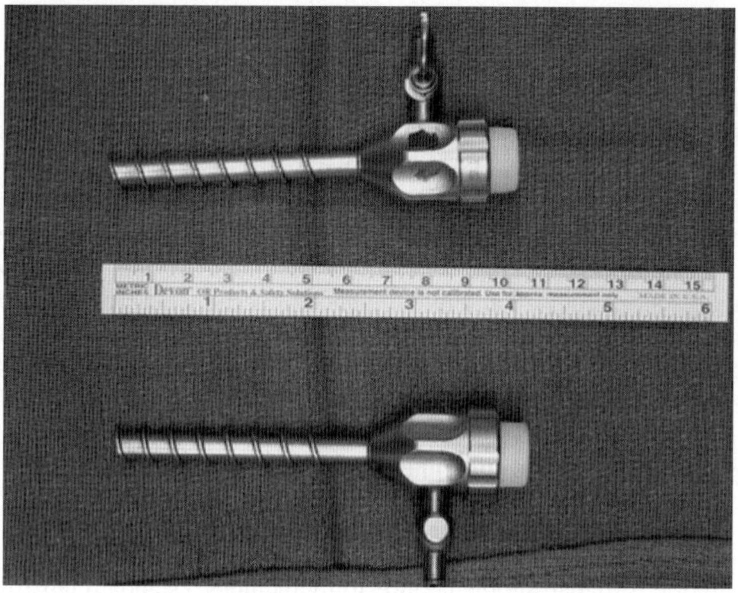

Fig. 4. Six millimeter Ternamian Endo TIP trocars.

Table 2
Laparoscopic instrumentation for standard transperitoneal radical nephrectomy (University of California, Irvine)

Disposable equipment:
- 45-mm Multifire Endovascular Stapler with reloads available. (Ethicon Endosurgery, Cincinnati, OH)
- Two 5-mm and three 12-mm Endopath XCEL (Ethicon EndoSurgery, Cincinnati, OH)
- 8 x 10 in. LapSac (Cook Urological, Spencer, IN)
- Veress needles (150 mm) (U.S. Surgical, Norwalk, CT)
- CO_2 insufflation tubing
- Ten sponges (Raytex)
- 5-mm Harmonic scalpel (curved jaws) (Ethicon EndoSurgery, Cincinnati, OH)
- 5-mm Ligasure Device (Valleylab, Boulder, CO)
- Argon beam coagulator (Conmed Corporation, Utica, NY)
- 5-mm Kittner Dissectors (Auto Suture, Norwalk, CT)
- 10-mm Kittner Dissectors (Ethicon EndoSurgery, Cincinnati, OH)

Nondisposable equipment:
- Two 6 mm Ternamian Endo TIP metal trocars (Karl Storz Endoscopy America, Culver City, CA)
- Endoholder (Codman, division of Johnson and Johnson) or CIVCO Laparostat – Laparoscope Holder (CIVCO Medical Solutions, Kalona, IA)
- Suction irrigator, extra long, 5-mm (Nezhat-Dorsey System, Davol Inc., Cranston, RI)
- Laparoscope: 10-mm (0 and 30°) lens and a 5-mm (0 and 30°) lens (Karl Storz Endoscopy America, Culver City, CA)
- Two atraumatic, non-locking 5-mm bowel forceps (Karl Storz Endoscopy America, Culver City, CA)
- Four traumatic (toothed), locking, 5-mm grasping forceps (Karl Storz Endoscopy America, Culver City, CA)
- LapSac two tine introducer (Cook Urological, Spencer, IN)
- 5-mm Hook electrode (Encision Inc., Boulder, CO)
- 5- and 10-mm PEER retractors (J. Jamner Surgical Instruments, Inc, Hawthorne, NY)
- 80-mm Snowden-Pencer Triangular Liver Retractor (Snowden-Pencer Brand, Cardinal Health, Dublin, OH) (also known as the “snake”)
- Two, 5-mm needleholders (Aesculap Inc., Center Valley, PA)
- 10-mm Soft curved angled forceps (Maryland dissector) (Karl Storz Endoscopy America, Culver City, CA)
- 10-mm Right angle dissector (Karl Storz Endoscopy America, Culver City, CA)
- 5-mm right angle dissector (Karl Storz Endoscopy America, Culver City, CA)
- Carter–Thomason needle suture grasper and closure cones (Inlet Medical, Eden Prairie, MN)
- 5 mm Hook dissector with active electrode monitoring (Encision, Boulder, CO)

Available but not opened equipment:
- Endostitch and all types of suture used (0,2-0,4-0, Polysorb, Polydac and Prolene) (U.S. Surgical, Norwalk, CT)
- Disposable Hasson trocar, 12-mm Blunt-Tip (U.S. Surgical, Norwalk, CT)
- 3-0 Cardiovascular silk (RB-1 needle) and 0-Vicryl sutures for fascial closure
- Lapra-Ty clips and 10-mm Laparo-Ty clip applier (Ethicon EndoSurgery, Cincinnati, OH)
- 10-mm Soft curved Satinsky clamp (49310 VC) (Karl Storz Endoscopy America, Culver City, CA)
- Two hip grips (SunMedica, Redding, CA)

For the majority of the pararenal dissection, we prefer ultrasound energy using a 5-mm curved ultrasonic shears (i.e., Harmonic Scalpel, Ethicon EndoSurgery, Cincinnati, OH). Thicker tissues that are likely to contain vessels are taken using the Ligasure device (Valleylab, Boulder, CO). This instrument combination allows for expedient dissection with excellent hemostasis. When the renal hilar neurolymphatic tissue is being dissected, the ultrasonic shears or Ligasure is preferred to minimize the risk of a lymphatic leak by adequately sealing these channels *(25)*. Additionally, monopolar electrosurgical energy with a right-angled hook electrode is used for delicate dissection on the surface of the artery and vein. This instrument allows the surgeon to perform safe and accurate dissection by engaging and retracting small strands of tissue around these vascular structures prior to the application of energy; the heel of this instrument is useful for gentle blunt dissection. In addition, we make ample use of the 10 and 5 mm Kittner dissectors from Ethicon EndoSurgery (Cincinnati, OH) and Auto Suture (Norwalk, CT), respectively. These provide excellent and safe blunt dissection around the hilum, often “dropping” into a fatty plane around the vessels with minimum effort. We have found a gentle forward, up and down plus twisting action to work well with this instrument.

For retraction, we have found the PEER Jarit retractor (J. Jamner Surgical Instruments, Inc, Hawthorne, NY) to be useful in a variety of locations (Fig. 5). The PEER retractor is secured in place using the Endoholder (Codman, Raynham, MA) or more recently the CIVCO Laparostat – Laparoscope Holder (CIVCO Medical Solutions, Kalona, IA) which allows maintenance of reliable, safe retraction. These instruments are invaluable because they both allow the surgeon complete control on the amount of retraction placed on vulnerable structures (i.e., liver, spleen, and renal hilum) and avoid the inevitable fatigue and instrument “drift” to which even the most diligent assistant is susceptible (Figs. 6 and 7).

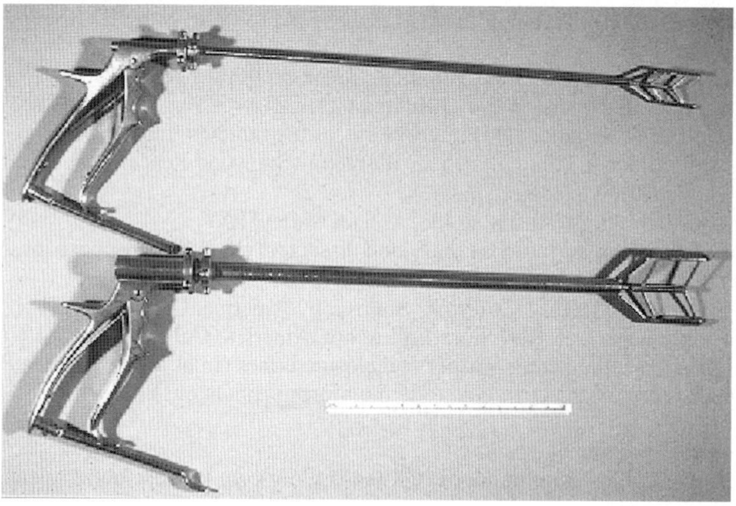

Fig. 5. The PEER retractors: 5-mm (*upper*) and 10-mm (*lower*) size. The 5-mm size opens to 2 × 3-cm surface area and the 10-mm size opens to a 4 × 3-cm surface area.

For veins ≤ 5 mm (i.e., gonadal, adrenal, and lumbar veins) the Ligasure device (Valleylab, Boulder, CO) allows efficient sealing and transection. If vessel length permits, we will apply one seal proximally without transection and a second seal distal to the first followed by transection. This gives the added security of three seals on the side of the vessel which will remain in situ and one seal on the specimen side. In addition, using this device avoids the potential problem of titanium clips interfering with subsequent deployment of the endoscopic stapling device.

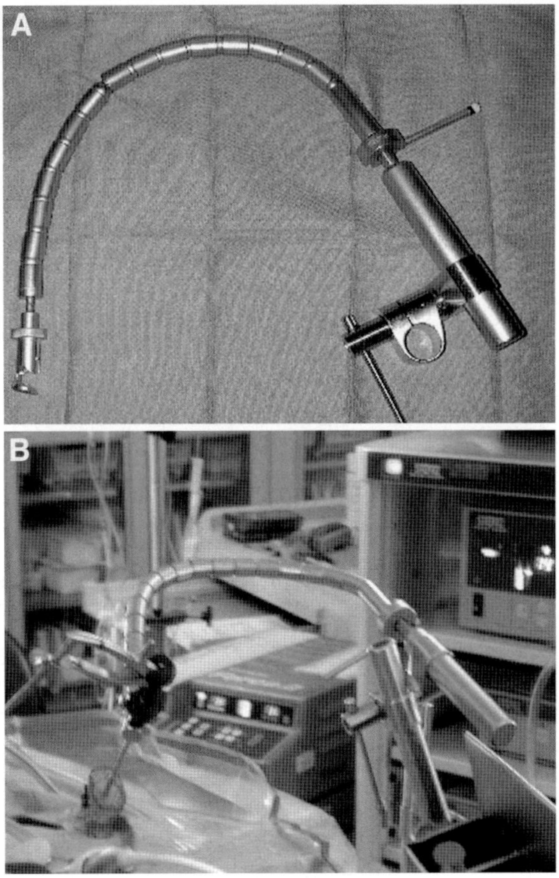

Fig. 6. The Endoholder by Codman. **A**The Endoholder before placement. **B** The Endoholder holding the PEER retractor during a laparoscopic procedure.

Control of major arteries and veins is achieved with the endovascular stapler. Typically, the 45 mm Endovascular stapler (Ethicon Endosurgery, Cincinnati, OH) is used for stapling the renal artery and then the renal vein. Prior to stapling, we routinely allow 10 s for compression of the tissue within the firmly closed jaws of the stapler.

Choosing a sack for specimen entrapment is dependent on the choice of extraction technique. If morcellation is to be performed, only the LapSac (Cook Urological, Spencer, IN) is used for organ entrapment, since no other entrapment sack has proven to be impermeable and resistant to tearing during intra-abdominal morcellation. Recently, due to the removal of the high-speed electrical tissue morcellator from the market, we have only been using ring forceps to perform morcellation. In this regard, the Sopher forceps, a gynecologic instrument, has been found to be a very efficient manual morcellator. Unlike a standard ring forceps (i.e., 12 × 22 mm), this re-enforced heavy duty ring forceps has a 14 × 45 mm jaw. The plastic sacks have not proven sufficiently durable for manual morcellation; to date, we have witnessed two bowel injuries associated with attempted morcellation in a plastic entrapment sack. However, if one elects to make a 3–4 cm incision on the abdominal wall, a broad expanse of the neck of the entrapment sack can be delivered through the triply draped wound and the specimen can be gently morcellated "above" the abdominal wall under direct vision *(26)*.

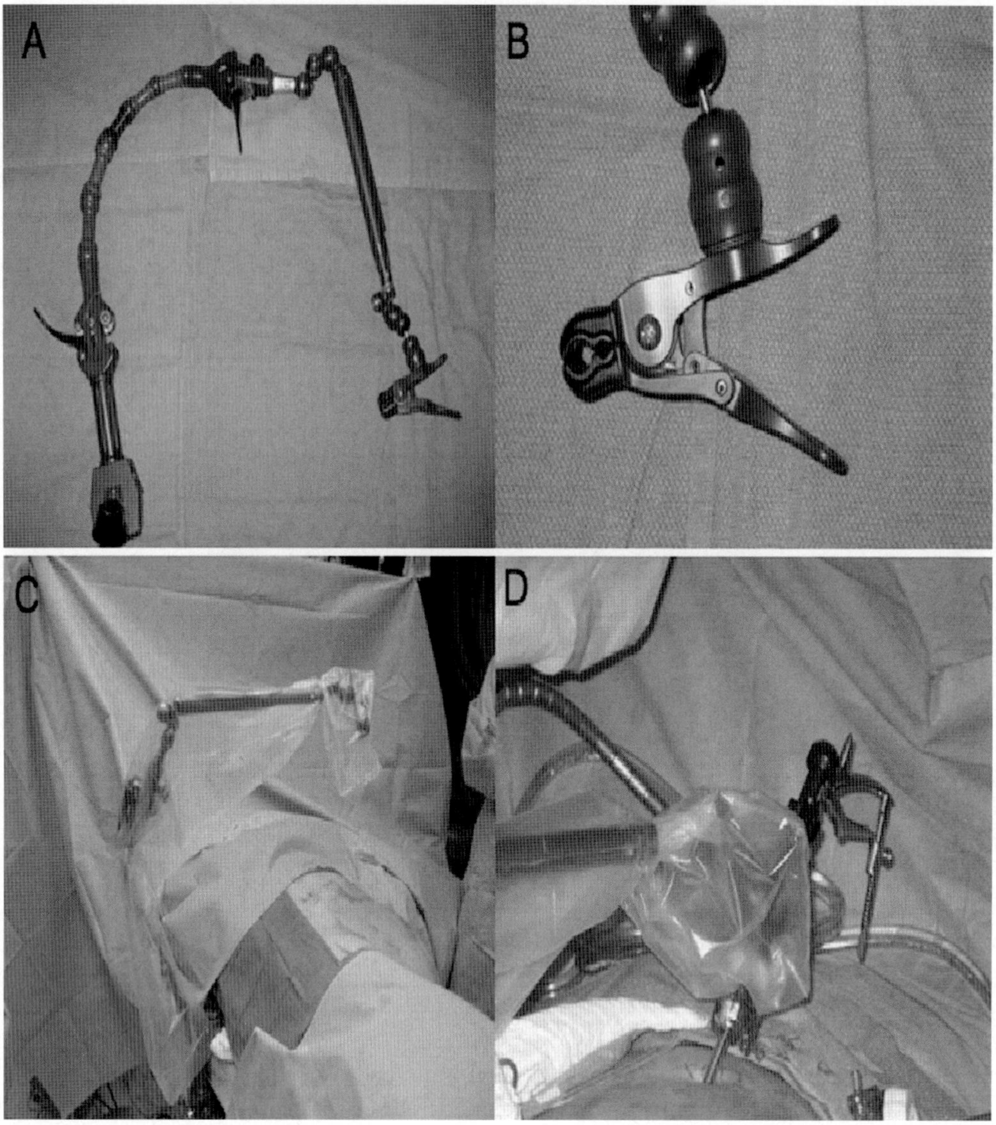

Fig. 7. The CIVCO Laparostat – Laparoscope Holder. **A** and **B** show device prior to placement. **C** and **D** show device attached to operating table (covered with sterile plastic drape) and holding a PEER retractor during a laparoscopic right radical nephrectomy, respectively. The arm of this device can be manually moved without having to unlock it, thereby facilitating its rapid repositioning.

If the specimen is to be extracted intact, use of an entrapment sack is still indicated because the sack prevents potential tumor seeding of the wound, which could occur when trying to extract a bare specimen through the incision. Under these circumstances, an appropriately sized bag is chosen (e.g. 15 mm Endocatch).

For closure of 12-mm ports, the Carter–Thomason® device is especially useful (Inlet Medical, Eden Prairie, MN). In adults, non-midline ports which are 12 mm or less, do not require closure provided that they were placed with a blunt trocar and there has not been excessive torque placed on the port during the dissection. As a rule, if the surgeon's index finger can be easily passed into the abdomen via the unoccupied port site, then the port should be closed. Table 1 provides a list of the instruments used at the University of California, Irvine for a laparoscopic transperitoneal radical nephrectomy.

Right Side

The peritoneal cavity is closely inspected. The liver is visualized for mass lesions. The protrusion of the kidney within Gerota's fascia is commonly visible behind the ascending colon and below the hepatic triangular ligament.

Step 1: Peritoneal Incisions and Pararenal Dissection

The key to en bloc resection of the kidney within Gerota's fascia lies in defining the borders of the dissection. On the right side, the dissection follows an anatomic template with a "wedge-shaped" configuration (Fig. 8). The sharp or thin edge of the wedge is the line of Toldt. The dissection is initiated using a 5-mm curved harmonic shears and atraumatic bowel grasping forceps for counter-traction. We also advocate liberal use of the both 5 mm (Auto Suture, Norwalk, CT) and especially 10 mm laparoscopic Kittner dissectors (Ethicon EndoSurgery, Cincinnati, OH) as they are not only useful atraumatic retractors but may also be used to help define natural tissue planes (Fig. 9). The harmonic shears is preferred for the majority of the dissection as it provides excellent hemostasis with minimal associated peripheral thermal injury to surrounding tissues. One must, however, be cognizant that the lower and active jaw of the ultrasonic shears becomes very hot and thus it must be kept a safe distance from structures such as the colon and duodenum. The line of Toldt is incised beginning at the pelvic brim; this incision is carried upward to the lower pole of the kidney at which point the incision is steered medially staying approximately 2–3 cm away from the ascending colon; in essence the latter half of this incision defines the lower side of the wedge as well as the upper medial border of the broad side of the "wedge." The colon is thus completely mobilized away from the kidney. As such, the lateral border of the kidney and its lateral retroperitoneal attachments are not disturbed; this results in the kidney remaining firmly attached to the abdominal sidewall, thereby facilitating the hilar dissection later in the procedure. The incision in the line of Toldt is continued cephalad from the upper pole of the kidney up to the level of the diaphragm to include the triangular ligament of the liver, thereby mobilizing the lateral aspect of the right lobe of the liver, and completing the "sharp" or thin edge of the wedge.

The broad or thick side of the wedge comprises three distinct levels of dissection along the medial aspect of the kidney (Figs. 8A and B): (*1*) the mobilized ascending colon; (*2*) Kocher maneuver of the duodenum to displace it medially (Fig. 10 A); and (*3*) dissection of the anterior and lateral surfaces of the inferior vena cava (IVC) (Fig. 10B). In performing this part of the dissection, it is important to realize that the duodenum may appear flattened against the medial aspect of the kidney; it is essential to move slowly during this part of the dissection in order to clearly identify the duodenum. Also, the surgeon should be cognizant that the duodenum MUST always be dissected away from the kidney before the anterior surface of the vena cava can be identified. To facilitate development of the third and deepest plane of dissection (i.e., the IVC dissection which defines the lower border of the "broad" edge of the wedge), it is helpful to first define the superior border of the wedge by incising the posterior coronary hepatic ligament from the line of Toldt, laterally, to the IVC, medially. This dissection is facilitated by the placement of the 5 mm subxiphoid port through which a 5 mm locking grasping forceps can be advanced under the inferior edge of the right lobe of the liver until the abdominal wall can be grasped along the upper edge of the incised line of Toldt. A second option for liver retraction is to use the 80 mm Snowden-Pencer Triangular Liver Retractor (Snowden-Pencer Brand, Cardinal Health, Dublin, OH); however, if this is passed via the subxiphoid port, then an Endoholder is needed on the surgeon's side of the table to hold it in place. If one uses the lateral 5 mm port for this retractor, then hilar retraction becomes more difficult as a Jarit PEER retractor can no longer be used via this port

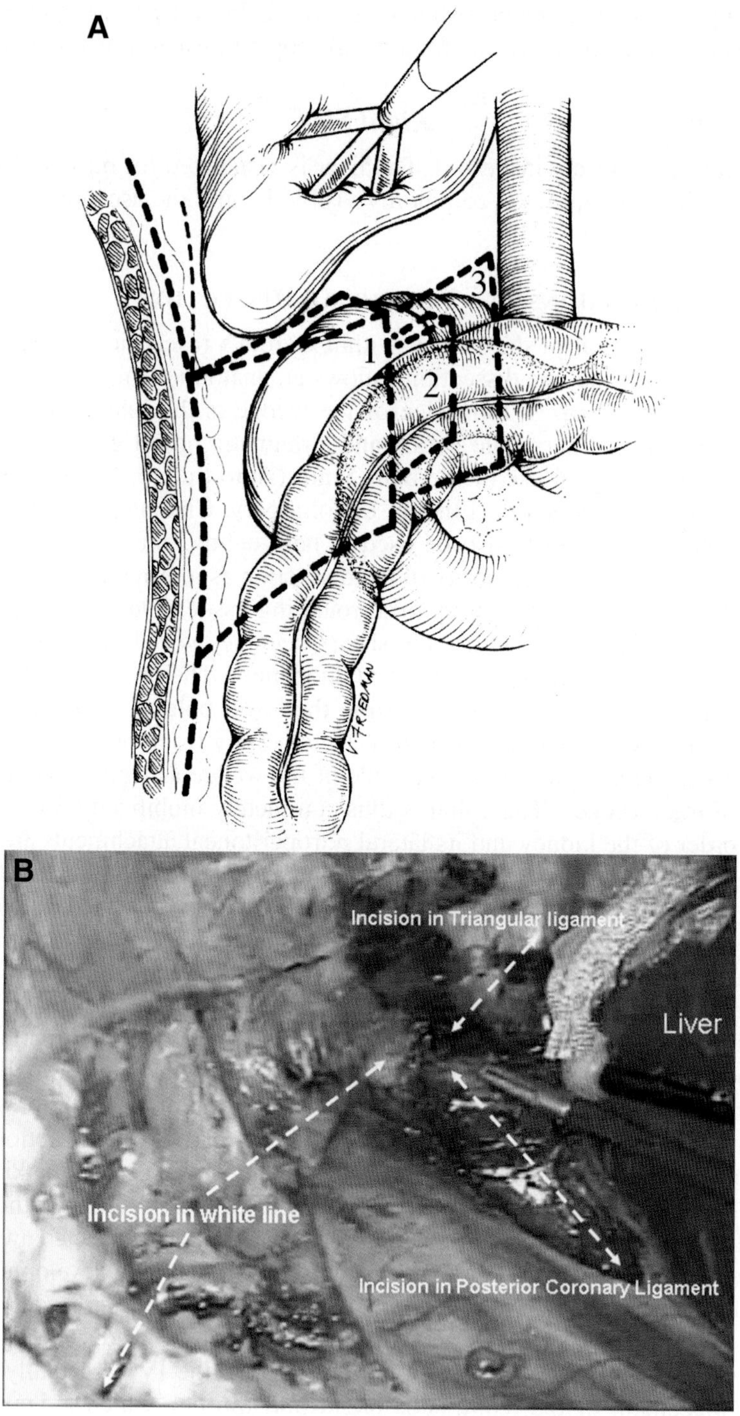

Fig. 8. Picture **A** and diagram **B** of the right-sided nephrectomy demonstrating the wedge-shaped configuration of the peritoneal incisions. The numbers in **B** refer to the three distinct levels of dissection along the medial aspect of the kidney: colon; duodenum; and inferior vena cava, which define the "broad" surface of the wedge. The lateral renal attachments are not dissected to prevent the kidney from falling medially and obscuring the renal hilum; however, the incision in the line of Toldt and its continuation up and through the triangular ligament of the liver, define the "sharp" edge of the wedge.

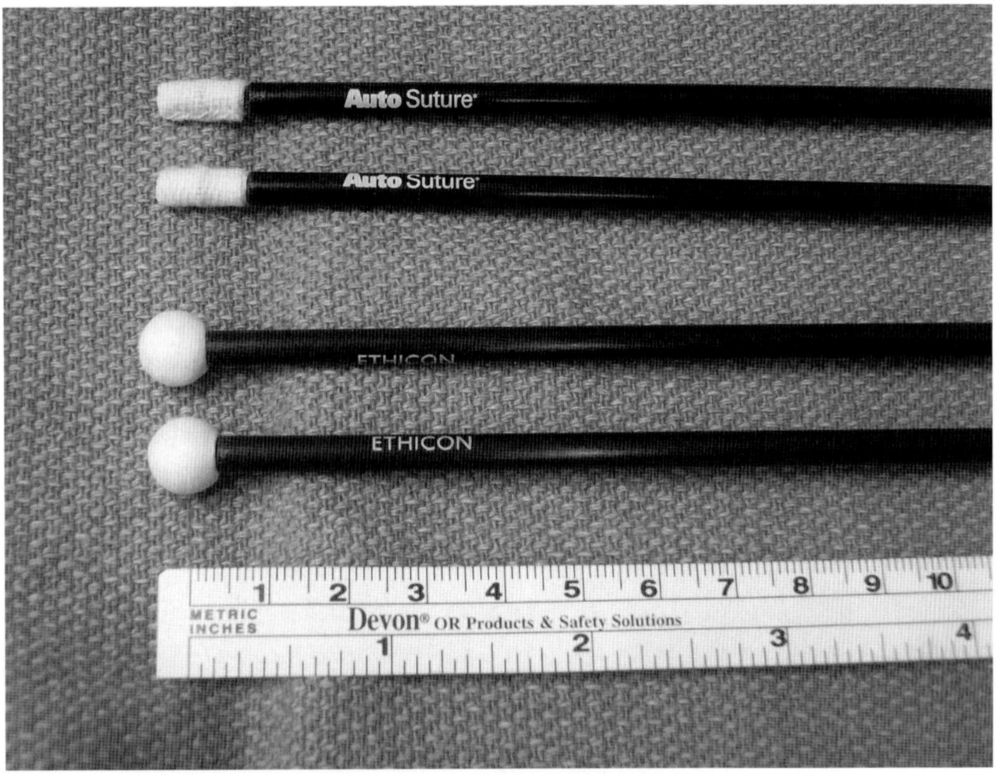

Fig. 9. Five and 10 mm laparoscopic Kittner dissectors.

to place traction on the hilum. Either of these maneuvers will atraumatically retract the liver allowing definition and visualization of the posterior coronary hepatic ligament. As the superior edge of the wedge is developed with further medial dissection of the posterior coronary hepatic ligament, the surgeon will come directly onto the lateral and anterior surface of the IVC well above the duodenum and the adrenal gland. At this point, the en bloc area of dissection of the specimen has been completely defined, ensuring removal of the kidney within Gerota's fascia, along with the pararenal and perirenal fat, the adrenal gland, and an anterior patch of peritoneum. Any minor bleeding which obscures view of the dissection can be controlled effectively by using the argon beam coagulator (Conmed Corporation, Utica, NY). One should always remember to have an assistant desufflate the abdomen while the argon beam coagulator is activated, to prevent sudden, significant elevation of intra-abdominal pressure. Alternatively, several small patches of Surgicel (2×3 cm) can be packed into any area of bleeding thereby providing hemostasis and a bit of additional blunt dissection; another alternative is to just place some Floseal (Baxter Inc., Irvine, CA) in the area to stop any small oozing and then revisit this point of dissection later.

Step 2: Securing the Gonadal Vein

The dissection on the IVC is continued caudally until the entry of the gonadal vein is identified. This vein is circumferentially dissected free from surrounding tissue with a combination of the hook electrode, blunt 5 and/or 10 mm Kittners and 5 or 10 mm right-angled forceps. We have moved away from clipping this vein and now routinely seal and transect it with the Ligasure device (Valleylab, Boulder, CO) as it is invariably <5 mm in diameter. During this portion of the dissection, if one encounters "caval" bleeding, it is more than likely due to inadvertent injury to the gonadal vein where it enters

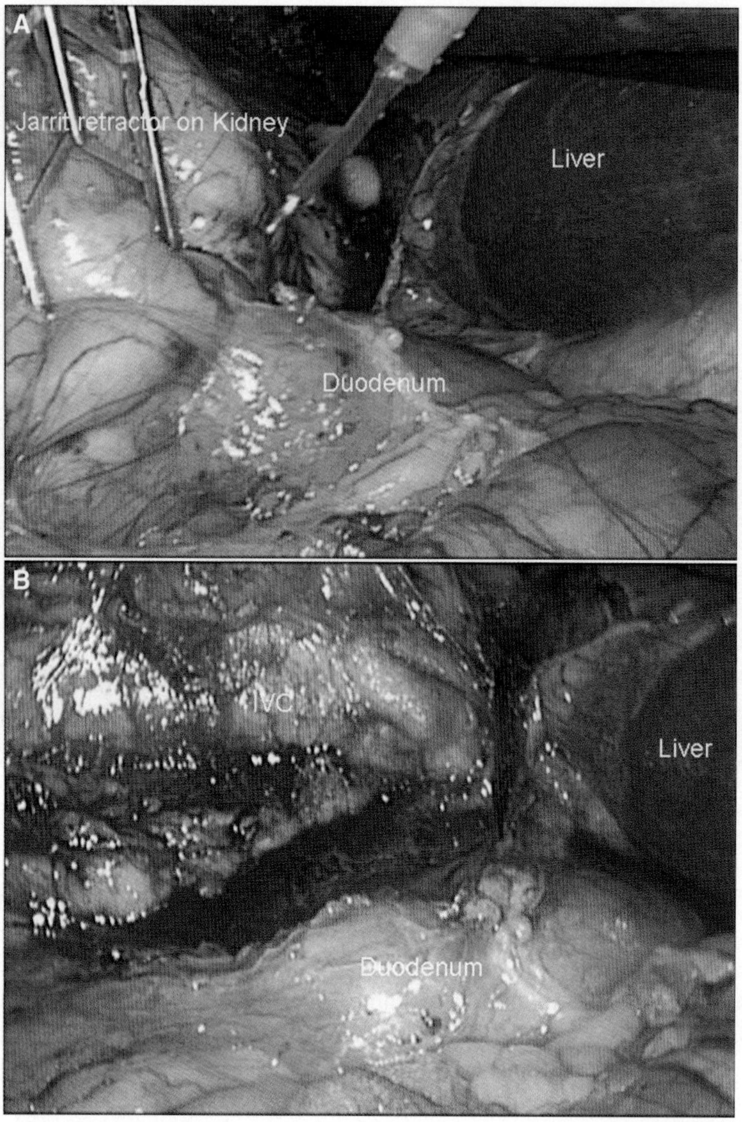

Fig. 10. Laparoscopic view of the duodenum being Kocherized. **A** Before; **B** After. The dissection of the IVC, which is in the *upper left* of the figure, is next. At this point the ascending colon and the colonic hepatic flexure, which were initially mobilized, lie inferior and medial to the duodenum.

the IVC. If this occurs, it is helpful to raise the pneumoperitoneum pressure to 25 mmHg (caveat: this pressure is never maintained for longer than 10 min by the clock – vide infra); this maneuver appears to effectively decrease any venous bleeding and facilitates identification of the venous injury. One can then more easily identify the gonadal vein lying lateral to the inferior vena cava and dissect it cephalad to define its termination. Clips or sutures can then be safely applied to control bleeding. When using a pneumoperitoneum pressure of 25 mmHg, it is helpful to have the circulating nurse inform the surgeon when 10 min at this pressure has elapsed so that the time at this pressure is limited thereby obviating the risks of hypercarbia and/or elevated airway pressures resulting in difficult ventilation. Also, in the event of a vena caval injury, aside from increasing the pressure to 25 mmHg, it is important to notify the anesthesiologist and request a liberal bolus of intravenous fluid, in accordance with studies by O'Sullivan and colleagues which have shown the importance of adequate hydration in prevention of carbon dioxide embolism *(27)*. Also, we believe that it is essential to have access to a laparoscopic Satinsky clamp which should always be available for immediate control of a major vascular injury; indeed, this particular laparoscopic clamp is present on the table during all of our renal surgery cases.

Step 3: Securing the Ureter

The gonadal vein can be traced distally from the vena cava. The right ureter usually lies just posterior and lateral to the right gonadal vein. It is carefully dissected from the retroperitoneal tissues. Another approach is to proceed to secure the ureter with four clips and divide it. However, we prefer to divide the ureter at the end of the procedure to provide a good length of ureter to which a grasping forceps can be affixed to facilitate subsequent specimen entrapment. However, if one is having any difficulty dissecting the hilum, earlier transection of the ureter can be helpful, as anterior traction on the ureter can help bring the renal artery and vein further anterior.

At this point, all of the caudal retroperitoneal attachments to Gerota's fascia can be dissected, thereby freeing the specimen inferiorly. This is also a helpful maneuver as by lifting upward on the dissected lower portion of Gerota's fascia with the kidney inside, the renal hilum is exposed inferiorly, such that the artery is seen lying parallel to the vein (vide infra).

Step 4: Securing the Adrenal Veins

Continued cephalad dissection of the IVC exposes the renal hilum and adrenal vein. The adrenal vein is dissected from the surrounding tissue and sealed proximally and distally. This is done by firing the Ligasure device once close to the IVC but not deploying the knife; the handles are then released and the Ligasure device is moved towards the adrenal and closed again on the vein. A second firing is completed, and now the Ligasure knife is pushed forward and the vein is then transected thereby leaving three seals on the caval stump of the vein and one seal on the specimen side. Alternatively, if the supra-adrenal area just medial to the IVC has been cleanly dissected down to the diaphragm and the lateral border of the supra-adrenal IVC has been identified in this area, then once the inferior border of the adrenal has been cleared of tissue, an Endo-GIA vascular load can be used to secure all of the tissue medial to the adrenal and lateral to the IVC, thereby "taking" the adrenal vein in the 4.5 cm line of vascular staples.

If one wishes to spare the adrenal gland, then the upper medial border of the kidney needs to be identified. As such, Gerota's fascia in this area is incised. Once the renal parenchyma of the medial and anterior part of the upper pole of the kidney is seen, an Endo-GIA stapler or Ligasure can be used to further define the horizontal margin of dissection from medial (i.e., IVC side) to lateral below the adrenal gland, thereby preserving the adrenal gland and adrenal vein.

Step 5: Securing the Renal Hilum

Attention is then turned to the dissection of the right renal vein from the surrounding tissue. If the IVC has been cleanly dissected, the origin of the renal vein is usually quite evident. The 5 mm PEER retractor is a useful instrument to retract the kidney laterally and place the renal hilum on gentle stretch, facilitating the dissection of the renal artery and vein. The PEER retractor is secured with either an Endoholder or CIVCO unit to maintain its position and tension. The right renal artery is subsequently identified behind the renal vein and dissected circumferentially. Mobilization of the renal artery must be adequate for comfortable placement of a 45 mm Endo-GIA stapler (vascular load). The renal vein is then dissected circumferentially and secured with an Endo-GIA vascular stapler (45 mm load) (Fig. 11).

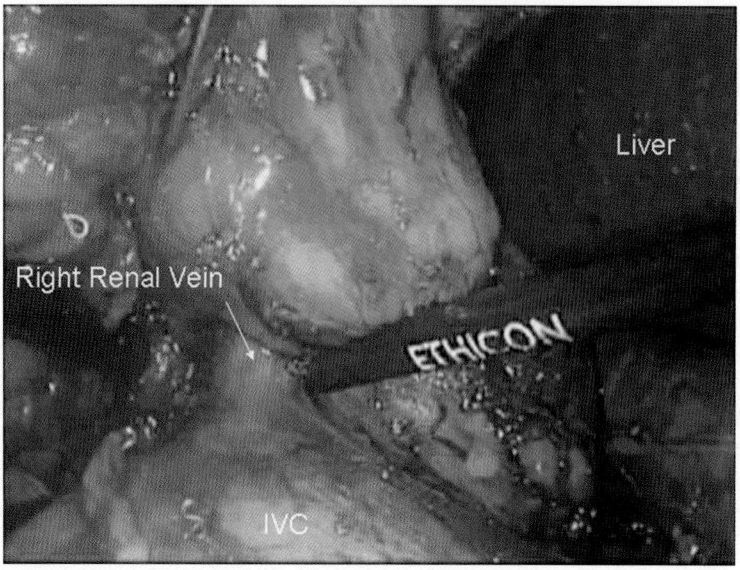

Fig. 11. The right renal vein is dissected and isolated prior to stapling and transection with an Endo-GIA stapler containing a vascular load.

One modification described by Chan and colleagues is to just free the posterior, inferior, and superior borders of the renal artery and then secure it with an laparoscopic stapler vascular load; however, when doing this it is important for the surgeon to develop the plane of dissection deeply along the upper and lower borders of the renal artery until the muscles of the retroperitoneum and posterior body wall can be clearly seen. The thin jaw of the Endo-GIA should then be placed anteriorly between the artery and vein with the larger jaw along the posterior body wall *(28)*.

Occasionally, an adequate length of the renal artery cannot be exposed in the presence of the overlying renal vein. In this situation, one or two clips can be applied across the artery to occlude the artery without transection. Now that the main renal artery is occluded, the renal vein is divided with the Endo-GIA stapler. One must be careful to avoid these clips while applying the Endo-GIA stapler. The artery is then further dissected and now allows easy placement of the Endo-GIA.

Rarely, the artery cannot be accessed from the anterior approach. It is then necessary to dissect the kidney laterally, rotate the entire specimen medially, and approach the artery from posterior. In this case, the artery is often dissected further medially, where it crosses the posterior surface of the IVC. Great care must be used in dissecting the anterior surface of the renal artery in this location in order not to inadvertently injure the IVC.

A third, and possibly the simplest approach to the renal hilar dissection, involves lifting the ureter and tracing it up to the hilum to identify the artery posterior to the vein. With this inferior approach, the artery and vein are seen to lie parallel to each other, allowing for easier dissection, as opposed to the anterior approach where the vein invariably covers the artery.

A fourth, and rarely used, approach to the right renal artery is to identify its origin from the aorta in the inter-aorto-caval space. This requires extensive mobilization of the duodenum such that the medial wall of the vena cava is seen. Much of this inter-aorto-caval dissection can be facilitated by using the laparoscopic Kittners for blunt dissection and the hook electrode in this region. The left renal vein is identified and retracted upward to reveal the right renal artery. A single 11 mm titanium clip can be applied to the artery in its inter-aorto-caval location; this is followed by stapling and transaction of the right renal vein. The artery can then be identified again once the vein is transected, and secured with an laparoscopic stapler load *(29)*.

STEP 6: FREEING THE SPECIMEN AND SECURING THE URETER

The specimen, within Gerota's fascia, is then freed from the retroperitoneum using electrocautery, the harmonic dissector, and blunt dissection. At this time, the lateral attachments of the kidney to the abdominal sidewall, which were kept intact at the beginning of the procedure, are incised. At the inferior border of the dissection, the ureter is secured with the Ligasure device; a locking grasping forceps, passed via the 5-mm subcostal posterior axillary line port, is placed on the ureter. Using the locking grasping forceps on the ureter, the entire specimen is moved cephalad until it rests on the anterior surface of the liver. Once in this position, the shaft of the grasping forceps is fixed in place by attaching it to the Endoholder or CIVCO Laparostat – Laparoscope Holder.

STEP 7: ENTRAPMENT FOR MORCELLATION

If specimen morcellation is planned, a LapSac is used. The 8 × 10 in. LapSac is appropriately sized for the majority of renal specimens (i.e., = 1,500 g). On the back table, a nitinol glidewire is passed through each of the holes in the edge of the LapSac such that the two free ends exit the edge of the sack at the same point that the blue nylon drawstring exits the edge of the sack (Fig. 12); this method was initially described to the authors by Yoshinari Ono from Nagoya University *(30)*. The nitinol glidewire passed around the holes in the neck of the sack greatly facilitates initiation and maintenance of a wide-open entrance to the sack. If one wishes, the nitinol glidewire can be passed twice around the neck of the sack via every other hole; this may provide improved opening of the sack. The LapSac is tightly wrapped onto the two tine introducer. For the right kidney, the sack is rolled clockwise from the bottom of the sack upward, onto the tines. The uppermost 12 mm port is removed and the entrapment sack on its introducer is passed into the abdomen. The sack is directed toward the lower quadrant of the abdomen under endoscopic control. The two tine introducer is then rotated counterclockwise thereby loosening the sack from the introducer; the sack can then be slid off of the introducer until it clears the port site and lies totally within the abdominal cavity. The introducer is removed and the 12 mm port is replaced. The two ends of the glidewire, and the nylon drawstring should all be parallel to one another and on the same side of the sack. Alternatively, once the glidewire is positioned properly through the holes in the neck of the sack, the nylon drawstring can be cut and removed.

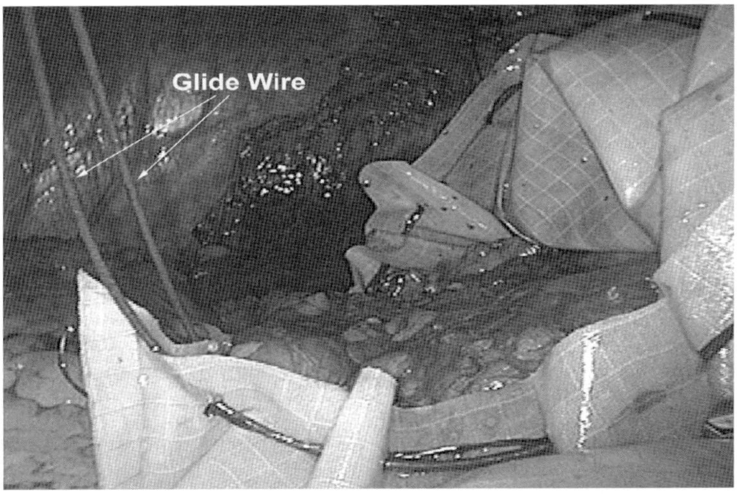

Fig. 12. Appearance of LapSac with nitinol guidewire (i.e., Glide Wire) passed through the holes along the neck of the sack.

The 5 mm traumatic grasping forceps that was passed via the subxiphoid port to support the liver is now removed allowing the liver to return to its natural position. The laparoscope is passed via the uppermost 12 mm port, while two 5 mm atraumatic bowel forceps are passed via the para-rectus and lowermost abdominal ports. These graspers are used to unfurl the LapSac.

Next two traumatic, 5 mm locking grasping forceps are introduced, one via the subxiphoid 5 mm port and one via the lowermost 12 mm port; the two lower tabs on the mouth of the LapSac are grasped. The LapSac is opened broadly such that its inferior edge is pulled just beneath the edge of the liver via the para-rectus 12 mm port, a 5 mm traumatic grasper is passed and the apex of the sack is pulled anterior. The laparoscope can be passed into the triangulated LapSac, and with circular motions the entrapment sack is further opened. The specimen is then rolled off of the liver into the mouth of the sack; the forceps on the ureter is directed at the locking grasping forceps holding the apex of the sack. As the specimen enters the sack, the two forceps creating the inferior edge of the sack's mouth are moved slightly cephalad and anterior to trap and push the specimen deeper into the sack. The LapSac is essential if one is planning to manually morcellate the specimen.

If LapSac entrapment using this approach is difficult, then a sixth right trocar (5-mm) is placed just above or at Petit's triangle. Now the LapSac is opened again using three points of fixation; however, the middle grasper (i.e., lowermost 12 mm port) pulls the lip of the sac upward against the underside of the abdominal wall, forming the apex of a tent-like opening in the sac; the medial (i.e., para-rectus 12 mm port) and lateral (i.e., port above Petit's triangle) 5-mm graspers are used to pull the bottom of the sac in either direction, respectively, while displacing the sack posteriorly, thereby creating the base of the tent. As such, this triangular opening of the sack results in the base of the triangle running parallel with the edge of the liver while the apex of the triangle lies at the anterior portion of the underside of the abdominal wall. The base of the sack is then positioned further posterior and cephalad until it lies just under the lower edge of the liver. The surgeon now moves the ureteral grasper towards the grasper on the apex of the sack. In doing this, the specimen rolls off of the liver and into the sack; as this occurs, the assistant holding the medial and lateral graspers on the sack moves the base of the sack anterior, thereby pushing the specimen deeper into the sack. Specimen entrapment in this manner requires three people: the surgeon, who controls the ureteral grasper and thus guides the specimen into the sack; the camera operator to hold the laparoscope and the middle grasper on the sack (apex of the triangle); and an assistant to hold the medial and lateral graspers (base of the triangle) on the sack (Fig. 13).

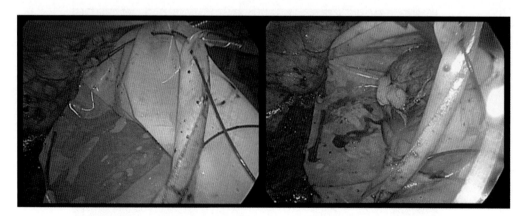

Fig. 13. Technique of grasping mouth of LapSac such that the opening is held in a triangular configuration; the lowermost medial grasper can not be seen in this view. The grasper on the left is pulling the sack upwards toward the abdominal wall creating the "apex" of a triangle, while the two other graspers, lateral and medial (unseen) are deployed deep in the abdomen to form the base of the triangle, which is moved upward until it lies under the lip of the inferior edge of the liver or spleen. The specimen is then easily advance into the sack.

STEP 8: ENTRAPMENT FOR INTACT REMOVAL

If intact removal is planned, then a 15-mm Endocatch II (U.S. Surgical) is introduced and opened just beneath the liver; the self-opening design of this entrapment sack facilitates the entrapment process. The Endocatch II entrapment sac cannot be passed through a 12-mm trocar. As such, the trocar is removed and the barrel of the 15-mm entrapment sack deployment mechanism is gently passed through the trocar incision site under direct endoscopic vision. This is usually done via the 12 mm para-rectus port site. Endocatch sac insertion is facilitated by 2-3 mm extension of the skin incision, and a minimal partial deployment of the Endocatch II sack prior to insertion to give the device a "point."

STEP 9: MORCELLATION VS INTACT REMOVAL

If morcellation of the specimen is planned, then the neck of the LapSac is delivered through the lowermost port which has been enlarged to 2 cm. The surgical field around the port site is further isolated by the sequential placement over the neck of the sac of a sterile adhesive "10 × 10" drape, a fenestrated absorbent towel, and a nephrostomy drape; the neck of the sac is passed through a hole in each of these drapes. These precautions are taken to help prevent possible wound contamination with any "spilled" tumor cells.

If at any time during the morcellation process, there is loss of the pneumoperitoneum, the morcellation should be immediately terminated, as it is likely that the sack has been perforated. *Failure to heed this early warning sign may well lead to catastrophic damage to bowel and any other organs lying outside of the sack as well as tumor spillage into the peritoneal cavity.*

If the LapSac is perforated, then the port site incision is immediately enlarged so the remainder of the specimen within the LapSac can be delivered immediately and intact. In the senior author's experience spanning 16 years, this has occurred in only two cases; in both cases the perforation was identified immediately and the leakage from the sack was scant; to date, neither patient has developed a port site or intraperitoneal metastasis.

After completion of morcellation, the surgeon and all other members of the surgical team who participated during morcellation, re-gown, and re-glove. Using this technique over the past decade, the authors have not experienced a wound seed or peritoneal contamination in any of their renal cell cancer patients, nor have there been any complications associated with morcellation in the LapSac.

Manual intra-abdominal morcellation should not be used with the currently available plastic sacks (vide infra) as these sacks can be easily punctured with resultant injury to bowel or other intra-abdominal organs, and tumor spillage. If one wishes to morcellate in a plastic entrapment sack, then the incision through which the neck of the sack is delivered, after entraping the specimen, should be widened to 3–4 cm; the neck of the sack is then triply draped and the specimen is morcellated under direct vision. The ring forceps are used to only grasp and fragment tissue that is literally lying *above* the abdominal wall in direct view of the surgeon *(26)*.

For intact removal, it is recommended to make a lower midline abdominal or a Pfannenstiel incision. The specimen is then extracted intact within the entrapment sack. One should resist the temptation to connect the medial and lateral upper or lower port sites for extraction purposes. The former will result in a more cephalad and possibly more painful incision, whereas the latter is a "weaker" incision and may result in a delayed hernia postoperatively.

Left Side

After laparoscopic abdominal inspection, the outline of the left kidney within Gerota's fascia can commonly be identified posterior to the descending colon.

Step 1: Peritoneal Incisions and Pararenal Dissection

The template for anatomic dissection of the left kidney assumes the configuration of an inverted cone (i.e., a water scooper) (Fig. 14). The lateral side of the cone is formed by the white line of Toldt which is incised from the pelvic brim, cephalad to the level of the diaphragm; this incision includes any spleno-phrenic attachments too. On the left side, the colon covers more of the surface area of the anterior portion of the kidney than on the right side; hence this incision in the white line of Toldt is made throughout the length of the retroperitoneum at the outset of the procedure. There are often adhesions from the descending colon at the splenic flexure to the anterior abdominal wall; these attachments need to be sharply released in order to carry the incision in the white line cephalad alongside the spleen and up to the diaphragm. This cephalad incision serves to release the spleno-

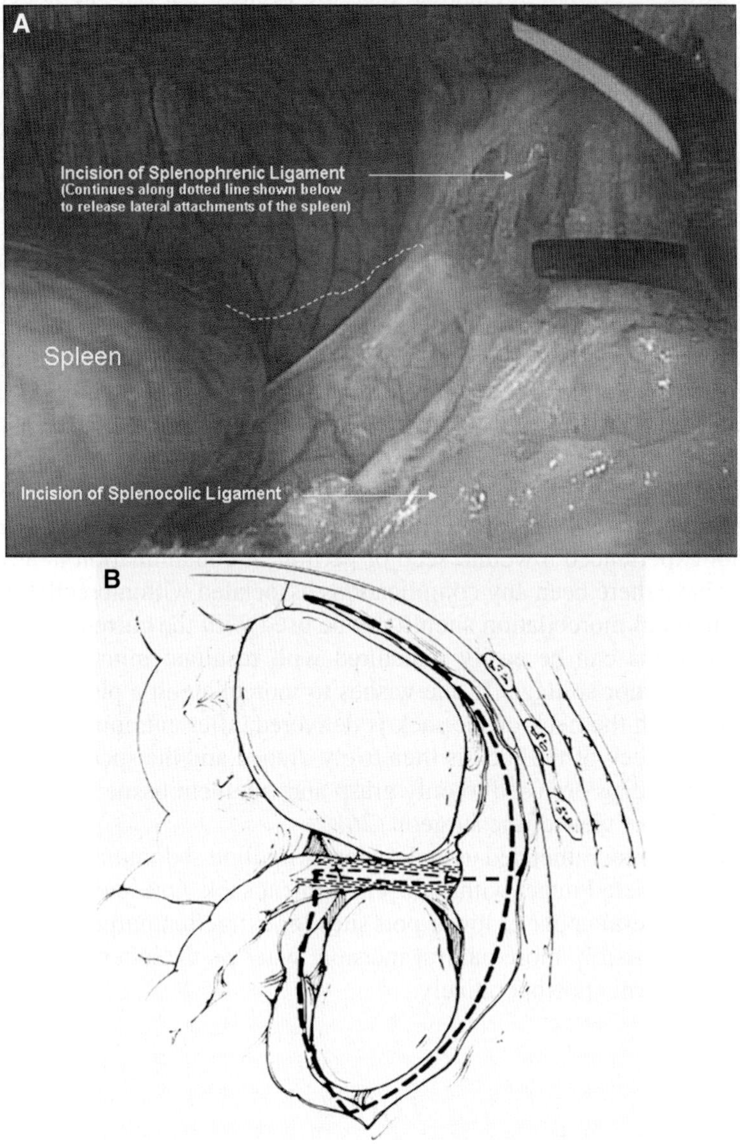

Fig. 14. Picture **A** and diagram **B** showing the template for left renal dissection.

phrenic attachments, thereby mobilizing the spleen from the abdominal sidewall (Fig. 14). As the upper most extent of the incision in the spleno-phrenic attachments is defined, the surgeon should exercise caution as the stomach can be nearby.

The medial aspect of the cone is then formed by retracting the peritoneal reflection of the descending colon medially and developing the plane between Gerota's fascia and the colonic mesentery. This natural plane between the mesentery of the descending colon and Gerota's fascia is most easily identified and entered along the lower pole of the kidney or just inferior to the kidney. The colon is then mobilized medially and cephalad up to the spleen.

The anterior upper curve of the cone is formed by the spleno-colic ligament, which is incised in order to fully mobilize the descending colon medially. The posterior upper curve of the cone is formed by the spleno-renal ligament that is incised to further release the spleen and thus precludes any inadvertent tearing of the splenic capsule. Incision of the spleno-renal ligament may be difficult at outset of the procedure and, is thus usually performed later in the procedure after the renal vessels have been secured. This part of the dissection clearly separates the spleen from the superior portion of Gerota's fascia. The dissection thus incorporates all of Gerota's fascia, the pararenal and perirenal fat, and the adrenal gland.

Step 2: The Gonadal Vein

The left gonadal vein is an important structure to identify during a left nephrectomy because it reliably leads the surgeon to the renal vein. The gonadal vein can most easily be exposed inferiorly from where it is traced up to its insertion into the renal vein (Fig. 15). If necessary, the surgeon can carry the dissection down to the level of the inguinal ring in order to reliably identify the gonadal vein and trace it cephalad; this maneuver is particularly helpful in the morbidly obese patient with a large amount of retroperitoneal fat. Anteriorly along the gonadal vein, there are rarely if ever, any tributaries, thereby providing the surgeon with a safe plane of dissection all the way up to the insertion of the gonadal vein into the main renal vein.

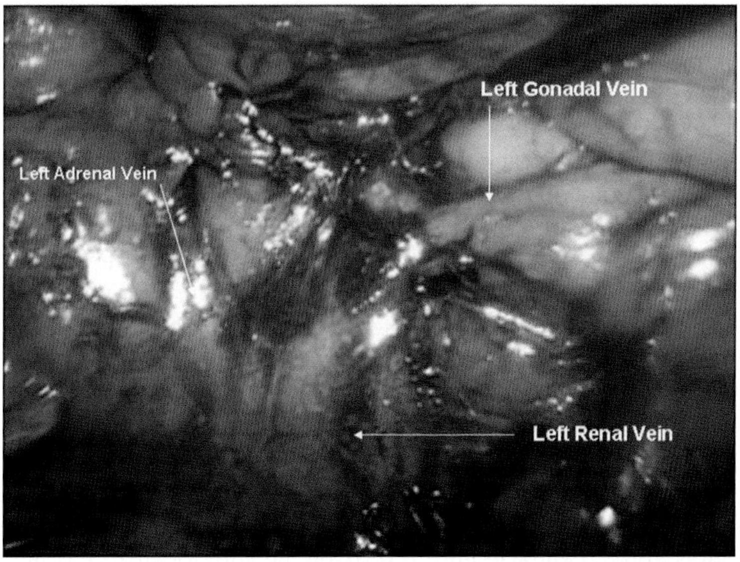

Fig. 15. Appearance after the left gonadal vein is identified and followed cephalad to its insertion into the left renal vein. The adrenal vein is almost directly opposite or slightly medial to the insertion of the gonadal vein. The renal artery will be identified posterior to the renal vein after the adrenal and gonadal veins are secured and transected.

Step 3: Securing the Ureter

The left ureter usually lies just posterior and lateral to the gonadal vein. It is carefully dissected from the retroperitoneal tissues and treated in the same manner as the right ureter was for a right nephrectomy.

Step 4: Securing the Renal Hilum

After tracing the gonadal vein to its junction with the main renal vein, it is secured with the Ligasure and divided (Fig. 15). Care should be taken to identify the ascending lumbar vein that may enter the renal vein posteriorly in the area of the gonadal vein or may even join the gonadal vein near its insertion into the renal vein. This vein is likewise secured with the Ligasure and transected. The superior border of the renal vein is then freed by dissection of the adrenal vein; this vein usually lies parallel with or just medial to the insertion of the gonadal vein; the adrenal vein is sealed with the Ligasure and divided. Using the Ligasure, precludes the need to use clips to secure these vessels.

All too often, when the surgeon tries to identify the left renal hilum by dissecting the area, where it "should be", the dissection drifts medially. This can become quite problematic and indeed, one may even risk injury to the duodenum, which often lies at the bottom of this "medial dissection." Also, the superior mesenteric artery may be encountered during inadvertent medial dissection. One should never proceed to staple and transect what is presumed to be a renal artery unless it is clearly located posterior to the renal vein and the gonadal, lumbar and adrenal veins have been identified, isolated and transected. Again, the surest way to the renal vein is to trace the left gonadal vein cephalad.

Inferior retraction of the superior border of the renal vein will usually expose the renal artery posterior. The renal artery is dissected free and stapled with a 45 mm vascular Endo-GIA. The renal vein is then also secured with the 45 mm laparoscopic vascular stapler.

However, if clips are used and the surgeon, in securing the renal vein, subsequently inadvertently deploys the stapler across a clip, the device may malfunction, precluding its release and removal. This problem is usually heralded by a "feeling" or sound that the stapler has not fired properly. If this should occur, the stapler should not be opened until adequate measures are in place either to convert to an open procedure or to proceed with more medial dissection of the vein. The decision of how best to manage this situation is dependent on the surgeon's experience. However, often it is possible to dissect the renal vein more medial, to where it crosses the aorta. A second stapler can then be used in this "clip free" area. Once the hilum is thus secured, the "frozen" stapler can be cut free of the stump of the renal vein and removed.

Alternatives to this anterior approach to the hilum, such as the posterior or inferior approach, are discussed in the previous section on right nephrectomy (vide supra: Step 5: Securing the Renal Hilum). Also, if the surgeon so desires, early ligation of the left renal artery can be achieved prior to mobilization of the colon and the formal dissection of the kidney. This requires elevation and retraction of the transverse colon followed by identification of the inferior mesenteric vein and the ligament of Treitz. An incision is made medial to the inferior mesenteric vein and extended to the ligament of Treitz. This exposes the anterior surface of the aorta which can be traced to the crossing of the left renal vein. The origin of the left renal artery is posterior to the vein and the artery can then be isolated and clipped. As a result, during the ensuing formal renal dissection, the surgeon can staple and transect the renal vein as soon as it is identified *(31)*.

Specimen dissection, entrapment, and removal of the left kidney are all identical to the description for the right side, except that the LapSac is rolled onto the tines in a counterclockwise direction and the left kidney specimen is moved cephalad until it rests on the anterior surface of the spleen just prior to entrapment. Also, a fifth port is routinely placed above Petit's triangle to facilitate LapSac entrapment.

Once the specimen has been removed, the extraction incision is closed in layers using multiple 0 – Vicryl figure-of-eight interrupted sutures, or in more obese patients the Carter–Thomason device can be used. The final check for hemostasis mandates close inspection of the vascular staple lines, the spleen, liver, and the inferior surface of the adrenal gland (if a total nephrectomy has been performed) at a pneumoperitoneum of 5 mmHg. We irrigate the renal bed with saline and carefully observe for "rivulets", a sure sign of bleeding that requires attention; the rivulet is a small stream of red seen coming upward into the clearer irrigation fluid. This area of red should be traced to its origin; usually a "missed" bleeding vessel. Liberal use of Floseal (Baxter Inc., Deerfield, IL) along the vessels and in the resection bed is useful for controlling minor oozing and providing the senior surgeon with an additional "peace of mind" factor. More significant bleeding can usually be controlled with the argon beam coagulator (Conmed Corporation, Utica, NY). During the hemostatic search, the pneumoperitoneum must be lowered to 5 mmHg to ensure that the tamponade effect is relieved and that any potential bleeding sites are unmasked and controlled. Using this approach, in the past 5 years, there has not been a single instance in which a patient has had to be re-explored for bleeding following any laparoscopic renal procedure.

Postoperative Care

Patients without contraindications receive 15–30 mg of ketorlac (Toradol) intravenous, every 6 h. This should be given around the clock for 36 h, in addition to an oral narcotic if necessary. Diet is resumed immediately postoperatively with clear fluids and advanced as tolerated. The patient is ambulated on the first postoperative day and once there is adequate mobility, the Foley catheter is removed. Discharge is routinely planned for the evening of postoperative day 1 or the morning of postoperative day 2 provided the patient has active bowel sounds and flatus. Parenteral antibiotics are stopped on postoperative day 1. The patient is discharged on oral narcotics as needed. Of note, it is not uncommon for these patients to develop some constipation postoperatively; as such, use of a Dulcolax suppository as needed as well as a stool softener (e.g., Colace one tablet twice a day) is recommended. Indeed, most patients do not have their first bowel movement until postoperative day 3 or 4, when they are already at home.

CONCLUSIONS

For small- and medium-sized renal tumors without main renal vein or vena caval involvement, the laparoscopic radical nephrectomy has become an accepted alternative to open radical nephrectomy. Using the anatomic templates and techniques herein described and illustrated, the laparoscopic urologic surgeon can successfully extract the affected kidney and the ipsilateral adrenal gland within Gerota's fascia while adhering to traditional oncologic principles. The laparoscopic approach meets all oncologic technical criteria while providing the patient with a more comfortable and expedient recovery. Also, its long-term effectiveness has now been corroborated by several investigators providing 5–10 year follow-up. Lastly, recent reports have shown that the laparoscopic approach is more cost effective than its open counterpart.

REFERENCES

1. Robson CJ, Churchill BM, Anderson W. Results of radical nephrectomy for renal cell carcinoma. J Urol. 1969; 101: 297–301.
2. Clayman RV, Kavoussi LR, Soper NJ, Dierks SM, Meretyk S, Darcey MD, et al. Laparoscopic nephrectomy: initial case report. J Urol. 1991; 146: 278–282.
3. Portis AJ, Yan Y, Landman J, et al. Long-term followup after laparoscopic radical nephrectomy. J Urol. 2002 Mar;167(3):1257–62.
4. Permpongkosol S, Chan DY, Link RE, et al. Long-term survival analysis after laparoscopic radical nephrectomy. J Urol. 2005 Oct;174(4 Pt 1):1222–5.

5. Varkarakis IM, Bhayani SB, Allaf ME, et al. Laparoscopic-assisted nephrectomy with inferior vena cava tumor thrombectomy: preliminary results. Urology 2004 Nov;64(5):925–9.
6. Hammond L, Powell TM, Schwartz BF. Pure laparoscopic radical nephrectomy for stage t(3b) renal-cell carcinoma: more than 2-year follow-up. J Endourol. 2007 Apr;21(4):4.
7. Romero FR, Muntener M, Bagga HS, et al. Pure laparoscopic radical nephrectomy with level II vena caval thrombectomy. Urology 2006 Nov;68(5):1112-4.08-10.
8. Hsu TH, Jeffrey RB Jr, Chon C, et al. Laparoscopic radical nephrectomy incorporating intraoperative ultrasonography for renal cell carcinoma with renal vein tumor thrombus. Urology 2003 Jun;61(6):1246–8.
9. Desai MM, Gill IS, Ramani AP, et al. Laparoscopic radical nephrectomy for cancer with level I renal vein involvement. J Urol. 2003 Feb;169(2):487–91.
10. McDougall E, Clayman RV, Elashry OM. Laparoscopic radical nephrectomy for renal tumor: the Washington University experience. J Urol. 1996; 155: 1180–5.
11. Barrett PH, Fentie DD, Taranger LA. Laparoscopic radical nephrectomy with morcellation for renal cell carcinoma: the Saskatoon experience. Urology. 1998 Jul;52(1):23–8.
12. Dunn MT, Portis AJ, Shalhav AL, et al. Laparoscopic versus open radical nephrectomy: a 9-year experience. J Urol. 2000 Oct;164(4):1153–9.
13. Chan DY, Caddedu JA, Jarrett TW, et al. Laparoscopic radical nephrectomy: cancer control for renal cell carcinoma. J Urol. 2001 Dec;166(6):2095–9.
14. Ono Y, Kinukawa T, Hattori R, et al. The long-term outcome of laparoscopic radical nephrectomy for small renal cell carcinoma. J Urol. 2001 Jun;165(6 Pt 1):1867–70.
15. Wille AH, Roigas J, Deger S, et al. Laparoscopic radical nephrectomy: techniques, results and oncological outcome in 125 consecutive cases. Eur Urol. 2004 Apr;45(4):483–8.
16. Jeschke K, Wakonig J, Pitzler C, et al. Laparoscopic radical nephrectomy: a single-center experience of 51 cases. Tech Urol. 2000 Mar;6(1):9–11.
17. Cheung M-C, Lee Y-M, Rindani R, et al. Oncological outcome of 100 laparoscopic radical nephrectomies for clinically localized renal cell carcinoma. ANZ J Surg. 2005 Jul;75(7):593–6.
18. Permpongkosol S, Chan DY, Link RE, et al. Laparoscopic radical nephrectomy: long-term outcomes. J Endourol. 2005 Jul–Aug;19(6):628–33.
19. Lotan Y, Gettman MT, Roehrborn CG, et al. Cost comparison for laparoscopic nephrectomy and open nephrectomy: analysis of individual parameters. Urology. 2002 Jun;59(6):821–5.
20. Pannu N, Wiebe N, Tonelli M. Prophylaxis strategies for contrast-induced nephropathy. JAMA. 2006 Jun 21;295(23):2765–79.
21. Khaira HS, Wolf JS. Intraoperative local anesthesia decreases postoperative parenteral opioid requirements for transperitoneal laparoscopic renal and adrenal surgery: a randomized, double-blind, placebo controlled investigation. J Urol. 2004 Oct;172(4 Pt 1):1422–6.
22. Mertens zur Borg IR, Lim A, Verbrugge SJ, et al. Effect of intraabdominal pressure elevation and positioning on hemodynamic responses during carbon dioxide pneumoperitoneum for laparoscopic donor nephrectomy: a prospective controlled clinical study. Surg Endosc. 2004 Jun;18(6):919–23.
23. Chang FH, Lee CL, Soong YK. Use of Palmer's Point for Insertion of the Operative Laparoscope in Patients with Severe Pelvic Adhesions: Experience of Seventeen Cases J Am Assoc Gynecol Laparosc. 1994 Aug;1(4, Part 2):S7.
24. Vilos GA. The ABCs of a safer laparoscopic entry. J Minim Invasive Gynecol. 2006 May–Jun;13(3):249–51.
25. Box GN, Lee HJ, Abraham JBA, et al. Comparative Study of In-Vivo Lymphatic Sealing Capability of the Porcine Thoracic Using Ligasure V, Gyrus Trissector, Harmonic Ace Scalpel, EnSeal and Monopolar Scissors. J Urol. 2007 April;177(4)Supplement:317; Abstract 960.
26. Landman J, Venkatesh R, Kibel A, et al. Modified renal morcellation for renal cell carcinoma: laboratory experience and early clinical application. Urology. 2003 Oct;62(4):632–4.
27. O'Sullivan DC, Micali S, Averch TD, Buffer S, Reyerson T, Schulam P, et al. Factors involved in gas embolism after laparoscopic injury to inferior vena cava. J Endourol 1998; 12: 149–154.
28. Chan, D. Y., Su, L. M. and Kavoussi, L. R.: Rapid ligation of renal hilum during transperitoneal laparoscopic nephrectomy. Urology 2001; 57: 360–362.
29. Porpiglia F, Terrone C, Cracco C, et al. Early ligature of renal artery during radical laparoscopic transperitoneal nephrectomy: description of standard technique and direct access. J Endourol. 2005 Jul–Aug;19(6):623–6.
30. Sundaram CP, Ono Y, Landman J, et al. Hydrophilic guide wire technique to facilitate organ entrapment using a laparoscopic sack during laparoscopy. J Urol. 2002 Mar;167(3):1376–7.
31. Porpiglia F, Terrone C, Cracco C, et al. Direct access to the renal artery at the level of Treitz ligament during left radical laparoscopic transperitoneal nephrectomy. Eur Urol. 2005 Aug;48(2):291–5.

Laparoscopic Radical Nephrectomy

Hand-Assisted

Tricia D. Greene, Edward G. Myer, and Steven J. Shichman

INTRODUCTION

The first hand-assisted laparoscopic nephrectomy (HALN) *(1,2)* and nephroureterectomy *(3)* in a human were reported in 1997. Many prior attempts to perform laparoscopic abdominal surgery while enabling the surgeon to retain tactile sensation had already been made, including finger dissection via a laparoscopic port site, insertion of a gloved hand into the abdomen *(4)*, hand-assistance using an "extra-corporeal pneumoperitoneum access bubble" *(5)*, intra-abdominal manipulation as an adjunct to laparoscopic nephrectomy *(6)*, and HALN performed in a porcine model.

Hand-assisted laparoscopy uses all the principles of standard laparoscopy, while maintaining the ability to use the most versatile instrument of all, the surgeon's hand. The surgeon's non-dominant hand is inserted through a small incision and used for retraction, counter-traction, palpation, dissection, and hemostasis. With tactile feedback, the surgeon is better able to palpate vessels and adjacent organs, minimizing the chance of injury to vital structures, particularly during difficult laparoscopic dissections. If bleeding occurs, the hand helps to quickly locate the source and apply definitive hemostasis. The hand may assist in more advanced laparoscopic techniques such as intracorporeal suturing and knot tying. The incision for the hand also permits rapid and intact specimen removal. In essence, HALN combines the advantages of both laparoscopic and open techniques.

The argument is no longer whether straight laparoscopic or hand-assisted techniques are comparable to or better than open surgery. The debate has now turned to the proper role of hand-assisted techniques in contemporary urologic surgery, and what benefit, if any, they hold over straight laparoscopic procedures *(7)*. Advocates argue that hand-assisted techniques allow better control by the surgeon. The hand is beneficial for tactile feedback and retraction, which facilitate dissection, thereby leading to shorter operative times and decreased hospital costs. Shortening of operative times is beneficial for patients with multiple medical comorbidities, where it is important to minimize anesthesia time. There is also (at least early in the learning curve) better vascular control by the surgeon, so a decreased rate of conversion to open surgery. Advocates maintain that a hand-assisted technique is particularly useful when intact specimen retrieval is necessary or when the size of the pathologic process could make the standard laparoscopic case difficult or prolonged. It is also beneficial in donor nephrectomy to have an incision for specimen extraction already made to minimize ischemia time. HALN has also been thought of as a "bridge" technique for surgeons who are making the transition from open to straight laparoscopic nephrectomy. This is true to a degree, as pure laparoscopy has a steep learning curve, can be quite demanding, and the quantity of cases necessary to become proficient is routinely performed

From: *Current Clinical Urology: Essential Urologic Laparoscopy*
Edited by: S. Y. Nakada and S. P. Hedican, DOI 10.1007/978-1-60327-820-1_9

at only large centers. When compared to open procedures, HALN allows for a faster procedure that is at least as safe, while affording the benefit of minimally invasive surgery with faster recovery times, shorter hospital stays, quicker return to full activity, and decreased need for narcotic pain relievers. Additionally, despite the added cost of the hand port, HALN actually cost less because of shorter anesthesia times and less overall equipment *(8)*.

Laparoscopic purists, on the other hand, argue that the hand incision contributes to a longer hospital stay and more postoperative pain than straight laparoscopic nephrectomy. Additionally, with increasing experience of an individual surgeon, the time benefit of hand-assisted techniques decreases even to the point where straight laparoscopic procedures are faster *(9)*. It may also be argued that the hand port has significant disadvantages, namely device malfunction, air leak, and time to set up (although in the setting of the newer generation access devices, these arguments hold less weight). Other criticisms of HAL techniques are that the hand port can interfere with optimal trocar placement, it is not in a cosmetic location, and neuromuscular strain and ischemic hand pain may become problematic in prolonged cases *(10)*.

A few words should be said about intact specimen retrieval in a cancer operation. When operating on bulky tumors, it may be difficult to adhere to principles of oncologic surgery using standard laparoscopy. Additionally, removal of an intact specimen requires an incision usually at least as large as that for the hand, made either by extending a port site for extraction, or making a Pfannenstiel or transvaginal incision. Is removal of an intact specimen necessary? We consider the jury is still out about the propriety of morcellation in a cancer operation *(11–14)*. It is our argument that if an incision is going to be made to remove an intact kidney, there is a clear benefit in making this incision early on in the operative procedure and using the hand to facilitate the entire procedure.

INDICATIONS, CONTRAINDICATIONS, AND PREOPERATIVE ASSESSMENT

The indications for HALN can include any situation where a radical nephrectomy is warranted. The most common indications include nephrectomy for renal masses, non-functioning kidneys, and renovascular hypertension. Hand-assisted techniques can also be applied to live donor renal transplants, nephroureterectomy for upper-tract transitional cell carcinoma, or partial nephrectomy, and during the early learning phase of reconstructive procedures, such as pyeloplasty, where intracorporeal suturing is required.

Care must be taken to evaluate whether a patient is an appropriate candidate for HALN. The most favorable patients are thin, lack a muscular abdominal wall, have virgin abdomens, and have small tumors located away from the renal hilum. Relative and absolute contraindications are listed in Table 1. What were considered relative contraindications in the previous edition of this chapter, it should be noted, have been shown to be feasible with experience, such as nephrectomy in morbidly obese patients *(15)*, presence of a renal vein or small caval thrombus *(16)*, patients with larger tumors *(17)*, and patients in whom dissection would be difficult due to location of tumor, prior surgeries with accompanying adhesions, and inflammatory or infectious conditions *(7)*. Obesity may even be considered an indication for HALN; at this point, it has been shown not only to be feasible, but actually safer in experienced hands when compared to open surgery for renal or adrenal lesions *(15)*. It should be emphasized, however, that minor modifications are in order in obese patients, such as shifting instruments and the hand-port cephalad and towards the side of the lesion.

Absolute contraindications include IVC thrombus above the level of the hepatic veins or direct extension of the tumor into the body wall or adjacent viscera. Contraindications to transperitoneal HALN include prior extensive abdominal procedures, presence of prior intra-abdominal abscesses, abdominal wall hernias repaired with mesh, although HALN may be accomplished retroperitoneally.

Table 1
Favorable aspects, relative contraindications, and absolute contraindications to performing hand-assisted laparoscopic nephrectomy

Favorable aspects	*Relative contraindications*	*Absolute contraindications*
Thin body habitus	Morbid obesity	Caval thrombus extending above hepatic veins
Small tumors	Severe intraperitoneal adhesions	Direct extension of tumor into
Left-sided tumors	Severe perirenal and perihilar adhesions	Body wall or adjacent viscera
Lower pole tumors	Muscular abdominal wall	Uncorrectable bleeding disorder
Tumors located away from the renal hilum	Extremely large tumors (>15 cm)	
Minimal or no previous abdominal surgery	Renal vein or IVC thrombus	
	Ipsilateral abdominal wall stoma	
	Pregnancy	

Though any of the above may increase the risk of the procedure, all factors must be taken into account when weighing the risks and benefits of different techniques. Ultimately, only the surgeons themselves can determine what they are comfortable doing and what they consider their own contraindications to HALN.

The preoperative assessment of a patient for HALN is the same as for an open nephrectomy. Abdominal and pelvic CT scan with IV contrast defines the anatomic details necessary for hand-assisted techniques. If a renal vein or caval thrombus is suspected, or renal insufficiency precludes CT scan with IV contrast, magnetic resonance imaging (MRI) or venogram will further assist in preoperative planning. For malignancies, the routine metastatic evaluation is mandated. Additionally, GFR should be estimated, either by the Modification of Diet in Renal Disease Study (MDRD) Equation or Cockcroft-Gault equation or by 24-h urine collection for creatinine clearance. In the event of an abnormal contralateral kidney on imaging or a poor creatinine clearance, a nephron sparing procedure should be considered. Preoperative discussion and informed consent should always include the possibility of conversion to an open nephrectomy.

A blood specimen should be sent for type and screen. Patients should be off any anti-platelet, anticoagulant, or anti-inflammatory agents for the appropriate amount of time. They are instructed to take a clear liquid diet starting the day prior to surgery and to have nothing to eat or drink after midnight. They may take a sip of water with medications the morning of surgery. Because an empty bowel helps maximize working space, we routinely use a mechanical bowel prep of an 8-ounce bottle of magnesium citrate the afternoon before surgery followed by a Fleets enema in the evening.

PREPARATION AND POSITIONING

Prior to induction of general anesthesia and endotracheal intubation, pneumatic anti-embolic stockings are applied. An orogastric tube and a Foley catheter are placed to keep the stomach and bladder decompressed. Prophylactic antibiotics are administered and 5,000 units of subcutaneous heparin are injected. For a transperitoneal procedure, the patient is placed into a modified lateral decubitus position

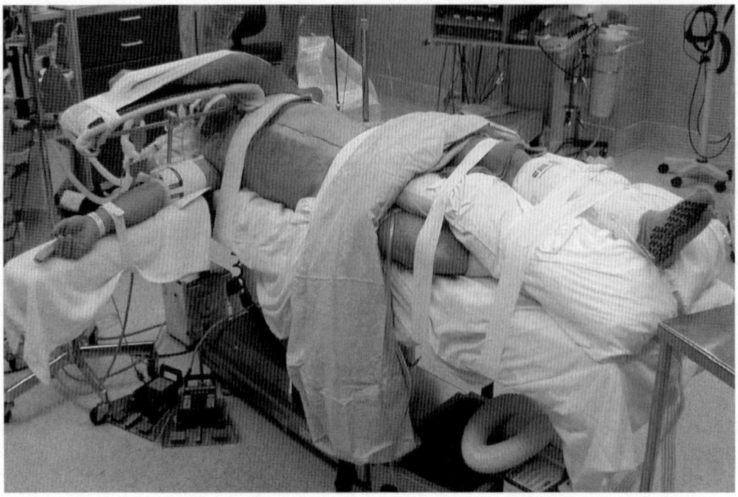

Fig. 1. Patient positioning for a hand-assisted left radical nephrectomy.

at a 45° angle and supported with gel pads (Fig. 1). The table is not flexed. The patient is positioned with the umbilicus over the kidney rest, but the kidney rest is not elevated. If conversion to an open procedure is needed, this position allows elevation of the kidney rest and flexion of the table to facilitate exposure. A padded neuro armrest is used to support the upper arm. An axillary role is not needed with the patient in a semilateral decubitus position. The lower leg is flexed and the upper leg extended with a slight bend to the knee with pillows placed in between.

In order to allow the patient to be rolled intraoperatively from a near supine position to the full flank position, 3 in. silk or cloth tape is wrapped over the patient and passed under the operating room (OR) table several times to secure the patient's shoulders, chest, hips, and legs. Upper and lower body warming blankets are used to maintain core body temperature. The patient should be shaved and prepped using a wide field to allow for placement of the hand-access device and trocars.

EQUIPMENT AND HAND-ASSIST DEVICES

The operating room is assembled in a manner similar to that for any laparoscopic procedure (Fig. 2A, B). Table 2 outlines the most important equipment used in hand-assisted surgery. Two important instruments exclusive to hand-assisted surgery include a ringless laparotomy pad and the hand-assist device.

A clean, rolled up laparotomy pad with the ring removed is placed into the abdomen through the hand incision. This is used to retract and to dry tissues, as drier tissue is easier to grasp and dissect, and tissue planes are easier to identify. It also saves time by avoiding frequent insertion of the suction/irrigation device. If the laparotomy pad becomes excessively bloody, it can absorb a significant amount of light, which can darken the video image. Replacing a blood-soaked laparotomy pad with a clean one can dramatically brighten the video image.

Hand-assist devices allow the hand to be introduced into an insufflated abdominal cavity while maintaining pneumoperitoneum. Technology evolves quickly and new devices and modifications are introduced frequently. Some devices have a mechanism to protect the abdominal incision, often called a wound retractor or protractor. Devices vary in the way in which they are affixed to the abdomen and in how the pneumoperitoneum is maintained. Early devices used an adhesive applied directly to the patient's abdomen to secure the device. As technology evolved, adhesive was replaced with

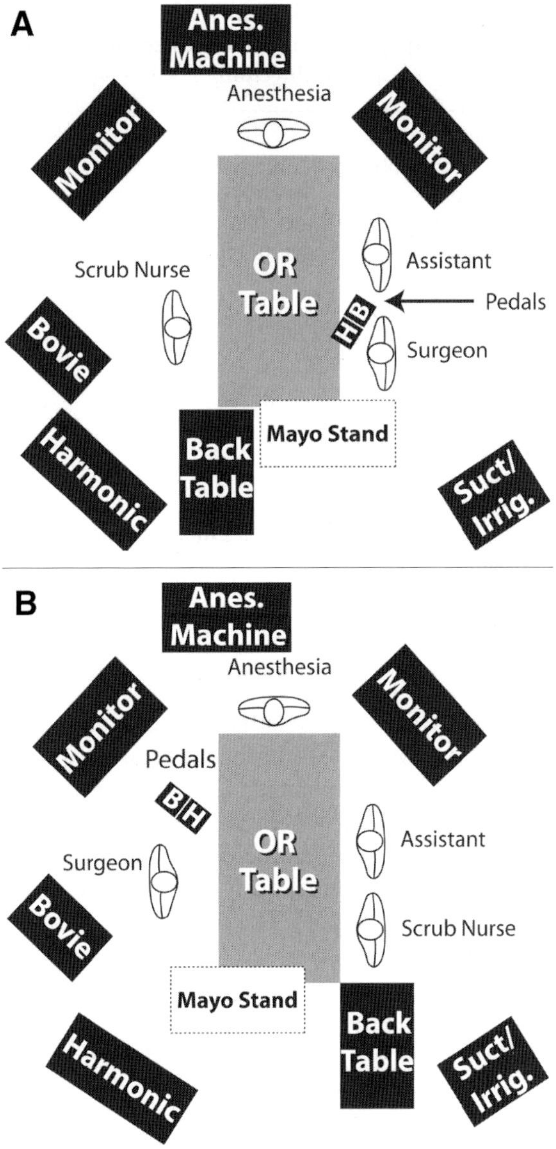

Fig. 2. Schematic drawing of the OR set-up for a hand-assisted (**A**) right and (**B**) left laparoscopic nephrectomy. *H*, harmonic scalpel foot pedal; *B*, electrocautery foot pedal.

self-retaining devices that both secure the device to the abdomen and protect the incision. The first device, introduced in 1997, was the PneumoSleeve® (Dexterity, Atlanta, GA). Other first generation devices include the HandPort® (Smith and Nephew, Laguna, CA), and the Intromit (Applied Medical, Rancho Santa Margarita, CA). Second generation devices include the GelPort™ (Applied Medical, Rancho Santa Margarita, CA), the Omniport™ (Advanced Surgical Concepts, County Wicklow, Ireland), and the Lap Disc (Ethicon Endo-Surgery, Cincinnati, OH). The Lap Disc has recently been replaced with the Dextrus™ (Ethicon Endo-Surgery, Cincinnati, OH) minimally invasive access system. All of the hand-assist devices are effective, and selection depends on surgeon preference, location of hand incision, body habitus, and patient's history of prior abdominal surgery. Each has its

Table 2
Essential equipment for hand-assisted laparoscopic nephrectomy

Pillows and gel pads
Pneumatic anti-embolic stockings
Neuro armrest
3-in. Silk or cloth tape (three rolls)
Upper and lower body warming blankets
Hand-assist device
Trocars (5-, 12-mm)
Ringless laparotomy pad
30° Camera
Liver retractor
Harmonic scalpel
Right-angle dissector
Maryland dissector
Laparoscopic scissors
Endoscopic linear stapler with vascular cartridges
Laparoscopic needledriver
Electrocautery

advantages and disadvantages *(18–20)*. The three latter devices have the additional advantage of being able to accommodate a laparoscopic port instead of the surgeon's hand. The Gelport and Dextrus can maintain pneumoperitoneum during hand exchange. The Gelport, additionally, has received statistically significant superior ratings to the first generation devices and the Omniport in all parameters evaluated and to the LapDisc in five of ten parameters, including ability to maintain pneumoperitoneum and overall satisfaction *(20)*. The original design of the Gelport had a larger footprint (16 cm), making it a bit more cumbersome in thin patients. The current design has an equivalent footprint when compared to other devices (13 cm).

TRANSPERITONEAL PROCEDURE: TROCAR AND HAND-PORT CONFIGURATION

Numerous factors must be considered when determining the optimal position of the hand port and trocars, including the patient's renal anatomy and body habitus, the surgeon's experience, the surgeon's hand and forearm size, and the side of the surgeon's dominant hand. Careful preoperative review of imaging studies is imperative in planning trocar placement. The midline should always be marked. This not only aids in trocar placement, but, if necessary, provides a guide for emergent laparotomy. Placement of the hand incision and trocars is made with the patient rolled into a near supine position because it allows for easier access to the peritoneal cavity and ensures better cosmetic results.

The hand incision should be at a distance from the operative target to allow insertion of the entire hand and wrist into the peritoneal cavity. The surgeon's wrist should have free range of motion. The fingers should comfortably reach the hilum. The hilum is typically 8–12 cm superior to the umbilicus, but this distance can vary widely based on patient size and vascular anatomy. If the distance on CT scan between the superior aspect of the renal vein and the umbilicus is greater than 12 cm, the surgeon has short arms, the patient is obese, or if the girth of the abdominal cavity is larger than normal, the hand incision should be moved cephalad. If the hand incision is placed too close to the kidney, however, the hand cannot be completely inserted into the abdomen and the surgeon will lose optimal maneuverability of the wrist and fingers. A low-hand incision decreases postoperative discomfort and respiratory compromise. Additionally, a midline or muscle splitting incision avoids cutting muscle fibers thereby reducing postoperative morbidity and incisional hernias.

The length of the hand incision in centimeters is usually equal to the surgeon's glove size. In other words, a surgeon who wears size 7½ gloves will generally need a 7.5-cm incision. If the incision is too small, paresthesia and cramping of the surgeon's hand can result. If it is too large, on the other hand, loss of pneumoperitoneum or dislodgement of the hand device may result. Once the hand incision is made and the peritoneal cavity is entered, the size and length of the incision is tested for comfort. A ringless, rolled laparotomy pad is placed into the abdomen. The hand device is inserted. The insufflation tubing is temporarily inserted through the hand port and a pneumoperitoneum is established to a pressure of 12–15 mmHg.

We use a midline hand incision at the level of the umbilicus for a left nephrectomy and a muscle splitting incision in the right lower quadrant, lateral to the rectus and just below the level of the umbilicus for a right nephrectomy (Fig. 3). This configuration allows the surgeon to approach both right and left kidneys in a similar fashion. The trocar configuration is essentially rotated depending on the side of the abdomen. A mirror image configuration, in which a midline incision is used for both sides, may also be used. We find the right nephrectomy somewhat more cumbersome, however, through a midline hand port, because either the dominant hand is inserted into the abdomen and the non-dominant hand controls the instruments (for the right-handed surgeon) or the non-dominant hand is inserted into the abdomen and the working and camera trocars are shifted cephalad. Other positions for the hand port include subcostal and transverse suprapubic *(21)*.

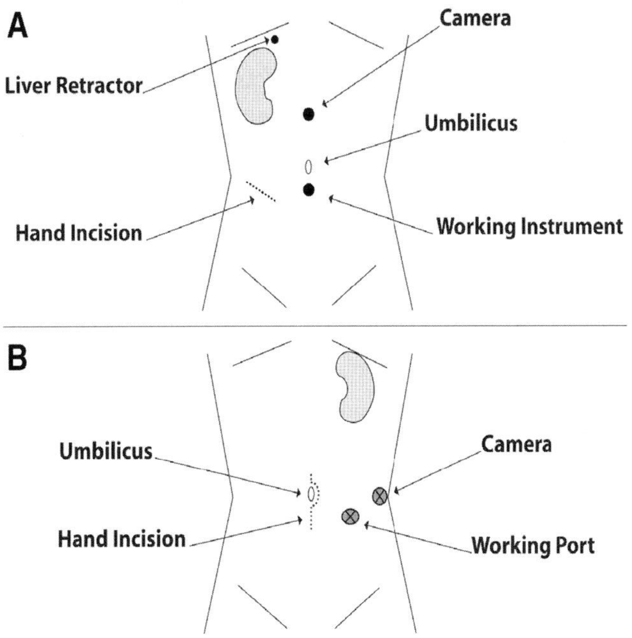

Fig. 3. Schematic drawing depicting placement of the hand incision and trocars for a right-handed surgeon for hand-assisted (**A**)right and (**B**) left laparoscopic nephrectomy.

Trocars are then placed. The intra-abdominal hand palpates the anterior abdominal wall and protects the intraperitoneal contents while guiding them in. The use of 12-mm trocars in all port sites enables the camera and endoscopic stapler to be placed through any trocar to allow maximal flexibility. For a right-sided nephrectomy, a 5-mm trocar is used in the right upper quadrant for placement of a liver retractor, since a camera or stapler would never be used at this site. For a right nephrectomy, the working instrument port is placed in the midline just superior to the umbilicus and the camera port is placed in the midline approximately 10 cm cephalad to the working trocar. The camera and working instruments may be switched at any time to facilitate the dissection. A third (5 mm) port is placed in the right midclavicular line, two fingerbreadths below the costal margin, to allow placement of a liver retractor (see Fig. 3A).

For a left nephrectomy (see Fig. 3B), the camera port is placed in the anterior axillary line at the level of the umbilicus, while the working instrument port is placed in the midclavicular line, just below the level of the umbilicus, lateral to the rectus muscle belly. For very large upper pole tumors, an additional superior midclavicular working port may be used for the most cephalad part of the dissection.

As in other laparoscopic surgery, trocars must not be placed too close to the hand-assist device or to one another because they may impede maneuverability of the hand and other instruments ("chop sticking"). In the case of an obese patient, the entire template is shifted laterally and cephalad to assure that instruments will reach the operative bed.

If adhesions are palpated, we carefully place the first trocar, then the camera to allow for direct visualization when placing the other accessory trocar(s). Inspection of the abdominal cavity is performed and surgical lysis of adhesions is performed. Taking down extensive intra-abdominal adhesions through the hand incision can save a significant amount of time as compared to using a purely laparoscopic technique.

TRANSPERITONEAL PROCEDURE: LEFT RADICAL NEPHRECTOMY

The majority of the dissection is carried out with the surgeon's non-dominant hand in the patient's abdomen and a harmonic scalpel in the surgeon's dominant hand. The colon is first released from the lateral sidewall by incising along the white line of Toldt from the splenic flexure to the iliac vessels. The colon is retracted medially using the back of the hand, while the fingertips and harmonic are used to establish the plane between the mesocolon and the anterior aspect of Gerota's fascia. The splenorenal ligaments and lateral splenic attachments are divided to the level of the gastric fundus, which allows the entire spleen and splenic colonic flexure to fall medially. The plane between the tail of the pancreas and the anterior aspect of Gerota's fascia is then developed, which allows the tail of the pancreas to rotate medially with the spleen. Care is taken to leave the entire anterior aspect of Gerota's fascia intact throughout the dissection.

Further mobilization of the mesocolon exposes the aorta and anterior aspect of the renal hilum. The investing tissue overlying the hilar vessels is grasped with the fingertips, held anteriorly, and divided, thereby exposing the anterior wall of the renal vein. The gonadal and left adrenal veins may be identified entering the renal vein at this point and clipped and divided. Care must be taken not to place the clips, where they may interfere with the subsequent firing of the linear stapling device across the hilar vessels later in the case.

The lateral attachments of the kidney to the body wall have been left intact to this point for traction during the medial dissection of the renal hilum. Dissection is now continued bluntly with the fingertips under Gerota's fascia inferolateral to the lower pole of the kidney, identifying the body sidewall and psoas muscle. The fingertips and the Harmonic scalpel are used to reflect the perinephric fat in a medial and anterior direction off the psoas muscle. The surgeon works from a lateral to medial direction. If a radical nephrectomy is performed, the ureter is identified, clipped, and transected at this point. Obviously, during a nephroureterectomy the ureter is left intact. If a donor nephrectomy is being performed, the periureteral tissue is left intact adjacent to the ureter and dissection of the ureter with all of its surrounding tissue is continued into the true pelvis below the iliac vessels. The gonadal vein is then encountered, doubly clipped proximally and distally, and divided. If the hilum has not already been identified, following the gonadal vein cranially will direct the surgeon to the renal vein.

The surgeon continues reflecting the inferior pole of the kidney, with the adjacent perinephric fat, and overlying Gerota's fascia, anteriorly and medially with the back of the hand while continuing to release the posterior and lateral attachments to the body sidewall. All lateral attachments are taken up to the level of the adrenal gland.

If the main renal artery is easily accessible anteriorly, it should be ligated and divided at this point in the procedure. The key to success of the HALN, however, is obtaining vascular control from a posterior approach. The tips of the second and third finger are placed just above the exposed anterior aspect of the renal vein. Using the thumb and dissecting instrument, the kidney may now be rolled anteriorly and medially and the thumb is placed on the posterior aspect of the renal vessels (Fig. 4). This maneuver helps identify the renal artery by direct palpation and allows for presentation of the artery to the dissecting instruments. Additionally, if bleeding is encountered, the fingers can compress the pedicle achieving rapid hemostasis. The lymphatic tissue surrounding the renal artery is divided with curved electrocautery shears, a Maryland dissector, or a Harmonic scalpel. Often, a lumbar vein draining into the renal vein is encountered coursing across the posterior aspect of the artery. This is clipped and divided. Once the artery has been freed circumferentially, it is divided with a vascular endoscopic linear stapling device.

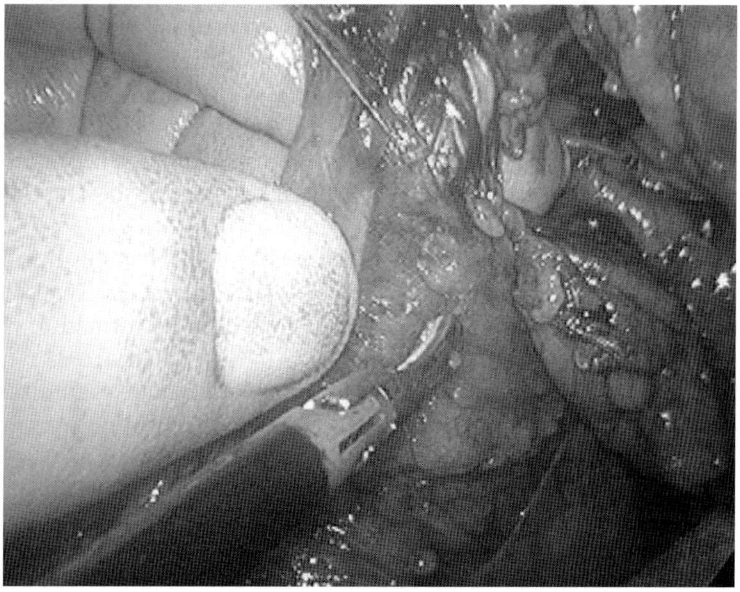

Fig. 4. The posterior approach to the left renal hilum.

The renal vein is then freed of all surrounding tissue and likewise controlled with an endoscopic linear stapling device. When the endoscopic stapler is used, great care must be taken not to engage any previously placed clips in between the jaws of the stapler. This will result in malfunction of the stapler and significant bleeding.

At this point, the adrenal gland is identified and the decision made to preserve the gland or to remove it with the specimen. If the adrenal gland is to be removed with the kidney, the most superior phrenic attachments and vessels feeding the adrenal gland should now be controlled and ligated with clips or the Harmonic scalpel. The superolateral attachments should be left intact and dissection should continue medially. The remaining posterior and lateral attachments can easily be transected using the Harmonic scalpel. On the left side, care is taken to avoid the tail of the pancreas and splenic vein during the medial dissection. On the right side, the medial plane of dissection is along the IVC, and the adrenal vein should be identified draining into it and ligated. The liver may need to be aggressively mobilized superiorly and medially for adequate exposure.

If the adrenal gland does not need to be removed, the groove separating the adrenal gland from the kidney can be located with visual inspection and palpation. The attachments are divided using the Harmonic scalpel.

The kidney is removed through the hand incision. We typically do not bag the kidney, however, if there is any concern about the integrity of the specimen, it should be placed into a retrieval bag prior to removal. Adequate hemostasis should be ensured at lower insufflation pressures (5–8 mmHg) and by Valsalva. All hilar stumps are re-examined and any bleeding staple lines can be controlled with suture ligation.

TRANSPERITONEAL PROCEDURE: RIGHT RADICAL NEPHRECTOMY

The procedure is modified on the right side to account for the presence of the liver and duodenum, the short stump of the renal vein, and the fact that the gonadal, adrenal, and lumbar veins drain directly into the vena cava. After insertion of the hand device and trocars as previously described, the liver retractor is inserted and the liver is retracted superiorly and medially. The right lobe of the liver is released from the body sidewall by incising the triangular ligament and, if necessary, the anterior and posterior divisions of the coronary ligaments with a harmonic scalpel. There may also be significant attachments between the undersurface of the right lobe of the liver to the anterior/superior aspect of Gerota's fascia that must be released.

Once the liver is adequately mobilized, the attachments of the hepatic flexure to the overlying Gerota's fascia are released and the colon reflected medially and caudally as described above. At this point, the duodenum is identified and a Kocher maneuver is performed to mobilize it medially exposing the underlying renal hilum and vena cava.

The inferior, lateral, and posterior attachments of Gerota's fascia are then dissected free. We start this part of the dissection by directing our attention to the perinephric fat inferior to the lower pole of the kidney. Using fingertip dissection, the psoas muscle is identified and the fingers are passed lateral to medial, raising the most caudal attachments of the kidney off the psoas muscle. This large pedicle of tissue may include the right gonadal vein and ureter. The entire pedicle can be divided using an endoscopic linear stapling device. Alternatively, individual pedicles of fat can be divided using the Harmonic scalpel while the gonadal vein and ureter are individually clipped and sharply divided. The gonadal vein may be identified draining into the IVC, dissected out along its lateral aspect, and reflected medially toward the vena cava.

With the hand placed posterior to the kidney, the kidney is elevated. Any remaining inferior medial attachments to the vena cava or lower pole accessory veins are identified and divided. For a right-handed surgeon, the second and third fingers are curled behind the renal pedicle and the thumb is placed anterior to it (Fig. 5). This is in distinction to the left nephrectomy, where the thumb is posterior to the hilum at this point. The renal artery can be palpated, and, using gentle traction with the index finger, can be moved out from beneath the renal vein and dissected free of surrounding lymphatic tissue. The artery and vein are ligated individually with an endoscopic stapler. The specimen is removed as described above.

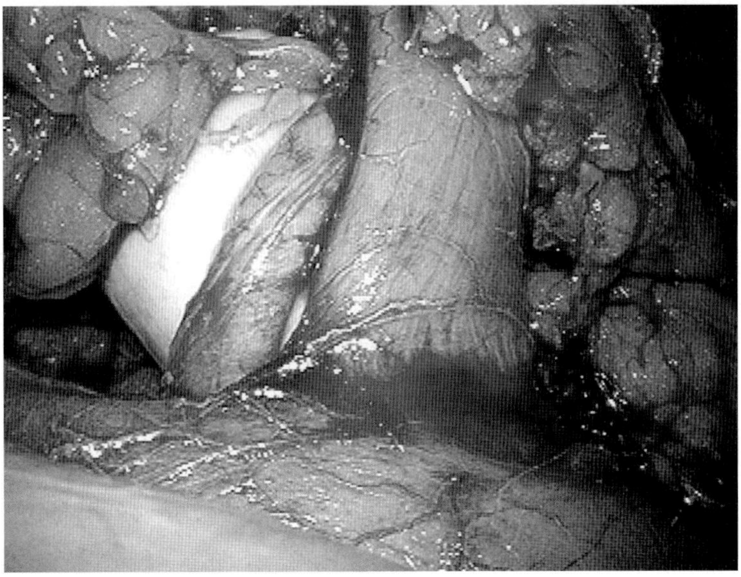

Fig. 5. The approach to the right renal hilum.

RETROPERITONEAL PROCEDURE

Hand-assisted laparoscopic retroperitoneal techniques are not commonly used, but have also been described for radical nephrectomy, nephroureterectomy, and living donor nephrectomy *(22)*. Retroperitoneoscopic HALN may be used in patients with ostomies, intraperitoneal shunts or an extensive surgical history. Advantages of retroperitoneoscopic surgery include more rapid access into the retroperitoneum, a lower risk of bowel injury, and potentially an earlier return of bowel function and hospital discharge. Disadvantages to this approach are the limited working space of the retroperitoneum, the lack of familiar intra-abdominal landmarks, and, in comparison with the transperitoneal approach, a longer operative time and a steeper learning curve *(23)*.

The patient is placed in a full flank position with the umbilicus over the break in the table. The table is flexed and the kidney rest is elevated, opening the space between the superior iliac crest and costal margin. The retroperitoneal space is then created, either manually through the hand incision or with balloon dissection through a smaller incision. If the space is made with the hand, a paramedial incision is made at the level of the umbilicus high enough for the surgeon to reach the upper pole of the kidney. Midline abdominal incisions or Pfannenstiel incisions have also been described. The peritoneum is then displaced with the hand to just above the upper pole of kidney and over to midline.

If the space is created with a balloon, a 2-cm incision is made at the tip of the 12th rib in the anterior axillary line. This site provides the most direct access to the retroperitoneum. A finger is inserted to initially create the retroperitoneal space by sweeping peritoneal contents anteromedially, followed by open trocar insertion for the balloon dilator or for insertion of the laparoscope. Pneumoretroperitoneum is created at 10–12 mmHg. A paramedial incision is subsequently made for the hand after the space has been created. A second 12-mm port in placed in the posterior axillary line for the camera. Usually the trocar template assumes a diamond configuration (Fig. 6).

A dissecting instrument and laparoscope are inserted. The plane between Gerota's and the psoas fascia is then developed with the harmonic scalpel. In doing so, the surgeon can march upwards from the inferior pole. The ureter and gonadal vein can be dissected together or separately and divided.

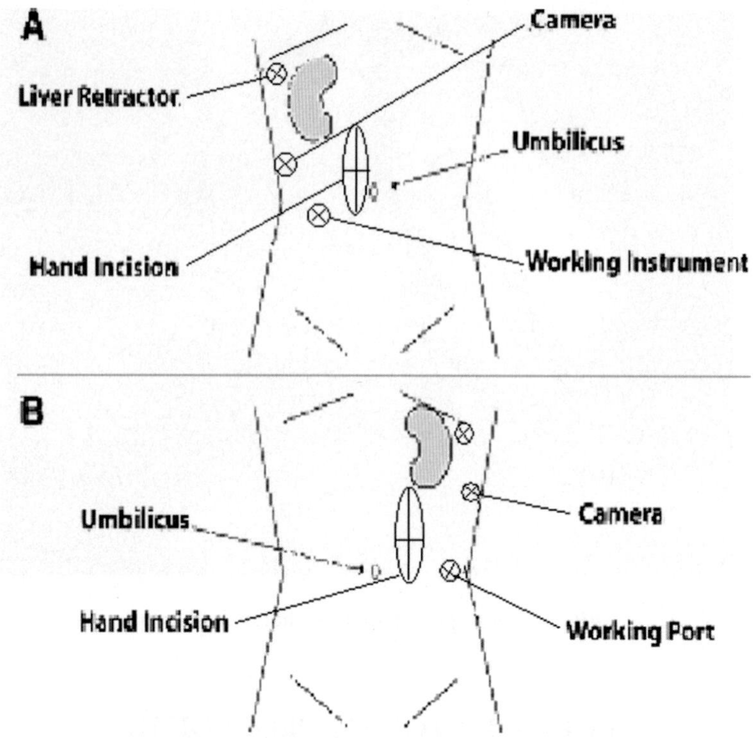

Fig. 6. Schematic drawing depicting placement of the hand incision and trocars for retroperitoneal hand-assisted **A**right and **B** left laparoscopic nephrectomy.

Palpation should be used to identify the hilar region. Similarly to the transperitoneal approach, the renal artery and vein should be exposed and isolated posteriorly. Once these vessels are controlled and divided, the kidney and adrenal are further mobilized, using the hand to sweep the peritoneum off Gerota's fascia and free the specimen superomedially. It is then removed intact through the hand port.

OUTCOMES: PERIOPERATIVE RESULTS

From March 1998 to January 2002, we performed 305 hand-assisted laparoscopic renal procedures including 174 radical nephrectomies. Operative times averaged 167 min, while estimated blood loss was 182 cc. Only two cases required conversion to an open approach. On average oral intake was started on postoperative day 1, average parenteral narcotic requirements were 41 mg equivalents of morphine sulfate, while length of stay averaged 3.6 days. Minor and major complication rates were 11 and 4%, respectively.

Early in our experience, we compared our HALN outcomes to a contemporary group of patients who underwent open nephrectomy (Table 3). Estimated blood loss, parenteral narcotic requirements, oral narcotic requirements, length of stay, and time of convalescence were all significantly less in the HALN group ($p < 0.05$). No statistical difference was shown between operative time and complication rate. These results have been confirmed in a number of other studies *(24,25)*. HALN, moreover, has been shown to be not only comparable to open nephrectomy for larger tumors, but also have significantly less blood loss, OR time, time to oral intake and time to discharge, with no increase in complication rates *(17)*.

Table 3
HALN vs open renal surgery

	Operative time (min)	*Estimated blood loss (cc)*	*Parenteral narcotics (mg MSO4)*	*Oral narcotics (tablets)*	*Length of stay (day)*	*Comp*	*Convalescence (week)*
HALN ($n = 74$)	198 ± 77	131 ± 66[a]	32.8 ± 24.6	4.6 ± 3.3	3.7 ± 1.3	6 (8%)	< 4
Open ($n = 20$)	196 ± 37	372 ± 68	208.5 ± 73[a, b]	8.8 ± 4.5[a]	5.2 ± 1.4[a]	2 (10%)	NR

NR, not reported.
[a] $p < 0.05$.
[b] Patients in the open group required an epidural for an average of 2.7 days; no patient in the HALN group received an epidural.

Several studies have compared HALN to standard laparoscopic nephrectomy. In the first published study, HALN was demonstrated to have a significantly shorter operative time than standard lap. Complication rates, hospital stay, and abdominal pain were not significantly different *(26)*. Shorter operative times have been consistently demonstrated in subsequent comparisons *(27–29)*, even for more challenging cases *(30)*.

ONCOLOGIC OUTCOMES

Although there are few long term studies comparing the oncologic outcomes of HAL with open nephrectomy, they appear equivalent in the short term. A retrospective study of 108 patients with a mean follow up of 10.8 months showed two recurrences, amounting to a 92.9% overall 3 year disease-free survival. No port-site, extraction site, or local recurrences were noted *(31)*. A subsequent study of 48 patients with a mean follow up of 25.1 months showed no cancer-specific deaths *(32)*. A recent study comparing the oncologic outcomes of retroperitoneal HAL against open nephrectomy with a median follow up of 41 months for the HALN group revealed no difference in 5-year disease-free (92 vs 91%) and cancer-specific (92 vs 94%) survival rates *(33)*.These results are similar to those reported for in comparisons of straight lap vs open nephrectomy.

COMPLICATIONS

Complications of HALN include (a) standard surgical complications such as urinary retention, prolonged ileus, small bowel obstruction, incisional hernia, reintubation, deep venous thrombosis, and pulmonary embolus, (b) complications of nephrectomy such as splenic capsular injury and diaphragmatic injury, and (c) complications of laparoscopy such as open conversion, subcutaneous emphysema, port-site hernias, hypercapnea, and diaphragmatic injury *(34)*. The incision site complication rate is reported at 9.3−10.4% *(35,36)*, and include infections (6.8%), hernias (3.5%), and wound dehiscences (0.5%). These complications have been shown to have a statistically significant correlation to omission of perioperative antibiotics, obesity, increased operative time, and smoking *(36)*. Other rare wound complications include enterocutaneous fistula *(35)* and hand-port metastases [Chen].

TAKE HOME MESSAGES

1. With the proper training, hand-assisted laparoscopic radical nephrectomy is a safe, reproducible, minimally invasive technique for performing extirpative renal surgery.

2. When performing extirpative laparoscopic renal surgery, making the hand incision at the beginning of the procedure will enable the surgeon to use the hand to operate quickly and safely, minimize blood loss, and allow intact specimen removal.
3. Hand-assisted laparoscopy is easier to learn and is applicable to larger tumors and more complex cases as compared to standard laparoscopy.
4. Vascular control of the renal hilum should be achieved from the posterior approach.
5. Data have shown decreased blood loss, narcotic use, length of hospital stay, and time to convalescence as compared to open techniques.

REFERENCES

1. Wolf JS, Moon TD, Nakada SY. Hand-assisted laparoscopic nephrectomy: comparison to standard laparoscopic nephrectomy. J Urol 1998; 160:22–27.
2. Nakada SY, Moon TD, Gist M, Mahvi D. Use of the pneumo sleeve as an adjunct in laparoscopic nephrectomy. Urology 1997; 49 (4): 612–613.
3. Keeley FX, Sharma NK, Tolley DA. Hand-assisted laparoscopic nephroureterectomy. J Urol 1997; 157 (Suppl): 339.
4. Tschada RK, Rassweller JJ, Schmeller N, Theodorakis J. Laparoscopic tumor nephrectomy-the German experiences (abstract). J Urol 1995; 153 (suppl): 479A.
5. Cuschieri A, Shapiro S. Extracorporeal pneumoperitoneum access bubble for endoscopic surgery. Am J Surg 1995; 170 (4): 391–394.
6. Tierney JP, Oliver SR, Kusminsky RE Tiley E, Boland J. Laparoscopic radical nephrectomy with intra-abdominal manipulation. Minimal Invas Ther 1994; 3:303–305.
7. Wolf JS. Selection of patients for hand-assisted laparoscopic surgery. J Endourol 2004: 18(4): 327–332.
8. Lindstrom P, Haggman M, Wadstrom J. Hand-assisted laparoscopic surgery for live donor nephrectomy is more time and cost effective than standard laparoscopic nephrectomy. Surg Endosc 2002; 16:422–425.
9. Gill IS. Hand-assisted laparoscopy: Con. Urology 2001; 58:313–317.
10. Johnston WK, Hollenbeck BK, Wolf JS. Comparison of neuromuscular injuries to the surgeon during hand-assisted and standard laparoscopic urologic surgery. J Urol 2005; 19(3): 377–381.
11. Shalhav AL, Leibovitch I, Lev R, Hoenig DM, Ramon J. Is laparoscopic radical nephrectomy with specimen morcellation acceptable cancer surgery? J Endourol 1998; 12(3): 255–257.
12. Cohen DD, Matin SF, Steinberg JR, Zagone R, Wood C. Evaluation of the intact specimen after laparoscopic radical nephrectomy for clinically localized renal cell carcinoma identifies a subset of patients at increased risk for recurrence. J Urol 2005; 173:1487–1491.
13. Landman J, Lento P, Hassen W, Unger P, Waterhouse R. Feasibility of pathologic evaluation of morcellated kidneys after radical nephrectomy. J Urol 2000; 164:2086–2089.
14. Varkarakis I, Rha K, Hernandez F, Kavoussi LR, Jarrett TW. Laparoscopic specimen extraction: morcellation. BJU Int 2005; 95 (Suppl 2): 27–31.
15. Hedican SP, Moon TD, Lowry PS, Nakada SY. Hand-assisted laparoscopic renal surgery in the morbidly and profoundly obese. J Endourol 2004; 18 (3): 241–244.
16. Phelan M, Hrebinko R. Hand-assisted laparoscopic nephrectomy in two cases of renal cell carcinoma with renal vein thrombus. J Endourol 2002; 16 (Suppl 1): 10–13.
17. Malaeb BS, Sherwood JB, Taylor GD, Duchene D, Broder K, Koeneman K. Hand-assisted laparoscopic nephrectomy for renal masses > 9.5 cm: Series comparison with open nephrectomy. Urol Oncol 2005; 23:323–327.
18. McGinnis De, Gomella LG, Strup SE. Comparison and clinical evaluation of hand-assisted devices for hand-assisted laparoscopy. Tech Urol 2001; 7(1): 57–61.
19. Stifelman M, Nieder AM. Prospective comparison of hand-assisted laparoscopic devices. Urology 2002; 59(5): 668–672.
20. Patel R, Stifelman MD. Hand-assisted laparoscopic devices. The second generation. J Endourol 2004; 18(7): 649–653.
21. Lopez-Pujals A, Leveillee RJ. Trocar arrangement for HALS. J Endourol 2004; 18:319.
22. Wadsrom J, Lindstrom P. Hand-assisted retroperitoneoscopic living donor nephrectomy: Initial 10 cases. Transplantation 2002; 73:1839.
23. Shiraishi K, Eguchi S, Mohri J, Kamiryo Y. Hand-assisted laparoscopic radical nephrectomy: Comparison of the transperitoneal and retroperitoneal approaches. J Laparosc Endosc Percutan Tech 2005; 15 (4): 216–219.
24. Nakada SY, Fadden P, Jarrard DF, Moon TD. Hand-assisted laparoscopic radical nephrectomy: comparison to open radical nephrectomy. Urology 2001; 58:517–520.
25. Lee SE, Ku JH, Kwak C, Kim HH, Paick SH. Hand-assisted laparoscopic radical nephrectomy: comparison with open radical nephrectomy. J Urol 2003; 170:756–759.

26. Wolf JS, Moond TD, Nakada SY. Hand-assisted laparoscopic nephrectomy: comparison to standard laparoscopic nephrectomy. J Urol 1998; 160:22–27.
27. Ruis-Deja G, Cheng S, Palmer E, Thomas R, Slakey D. Open donor, laparoscopic donor, and hand-assisted laparoscopic donor nephrectomy: a comparison of outcomes. J Urol 2001; 166:1270–1274.
28. Landman J, Lev R, Bhayani S, et al. Comparison of hand-assisted and standard laparoscopicradical nephroureterectomy for the management of localized transitional cell carcinoma. J Urol 2002; 167:2387–2391.
29. Nadler RB, Loeb S, Clemens JQ, Batler RA, Gonzalez CM, Vardi IY. A prospective study of laparoscopic radical nephrectomy for T1 tumors-Is transperitoneal, retroperitoneal, or hand-assisted the best approach? J Urol 2006; 175:1230–1234.
30. Nelson CP, Wolf JS. Comparison of hand-assisted versus standard laparoscopic radical nephrectomy for suspected renal cell carcinoma. J Urol 2002; 167:1989–1994.
31. Stifelman MD, Cohen MS, Taneja S, et al. A retrospective multi-institutional study evaluating the oncological efficacy of hand-assisted laparoscopic nephrectomy. J Endourol 2002; 16 (Suppl 1): 10–11.
32. Lowry PS, Nakada SY. Hand-assisted laparoscopic radical nephrectomy. J Endourol 2004; 18(4): 337–343.
33. Kawauchi A, Yoneda K, Fujito A, et al. Oncologic outcome of hand-assisted laparoscopic radical nephrectomy. Urology 2007; 69(1):53–56.
34. Hedican, SP, Wolf JS, Moon TD, et al. Complications of hand-assisted laparoscopy in urologic surgery. J Urol 2002; 167(Suppl):22.
35. Terranova SA, Siddiqui KM, Preminger GM, Albala DM. Hand-assisted laparoscopic renal surgery: hand-port incisional complications. J Endourol 2004: 18.
36. Montgomery JS, Johnston WK, Wolf JS. Wound complications after hand-assisted laparoscopic surgery. J Urol 2005; 174:2226–2230.

Laparoscopic Partial Nephrectomy

J. Stuart Wolf, Jr.

INTRODUCTION

Historically, renal cell carcinoma has been managed with open surgical radical nephrectomy *(1)*. Over the past decade partial nephrectomy, initially applied in settings of solitary kidney or bilateral disease *(2)*, has come to play a more prominent role, even on an elective basis in the setting of a normal contralateral kidney *(3, 4)*. Cancer cure appears to be equivalent to that achieved with radical nephrectomy *(5, 6)*, and the patient benefits from preservation of renal function *(7–9)*. Despite the rising incidence of renal tumors, especially small localized ones *(10)*, and the expansion of criteria for elective partial nephrectomy to include some masses up to 7 cm in size *(11, 12)*, evidence suggests that partial nephrectomy is underutilized *(13)*.

Laparoscopy in urology has been steadily expanding over the past decade. It was only 2 years following publication of the report of the first laparoscopic radical nephrectomy in 1991 *(14)* that the first successful laparoscopic partial nephrectomies were reported in a child *(15)* and an adult *(16)*. The success of open surgical partial nephrectomy for small renal masses and increasing confidence in laparoscopic techniques led to laparoscopic partial nephrectomy for renal cell carcinoma, first reported only a year later, in 1994 *(17)*. Although laparoscopic radical nephrectomy is now accepted as a standard of care, with cancer cure rates equivalent to that of open surgical radical nephrectomy *(18–20)*, acceptance of laparoscopic partial nephrectomy has lagged behind. This is predominantly owing to the technical challenges of obtaining parenchymal hemostasis and closing the collecting system laparoscopically. Even so, experience with laparoscopic partial nephrectomies is growing rapidly, and appears to be justified by reports of 5-year cancer control that is similar to that of open surgical partial nephrectomy *(21, 22)*.

INDICATIONS

Although the imperative (solitary kidney, bilateral tumors, renal insufficiency), relative (presence of medical disease that threatens renal function), and elective (mass less than 4 cm, with some supporting increasing the limit to 7 cm) indications for partial nephrectomy for suspected malignancy are the same for the open surgical and laparoscopic approaches, the technical limitations of laparoscopy are such that some tumors still are approached best with open surgery. At the author's institution, of the 65 partial nephrectomies performed for suspected malignancy in adults in 2006, 47 were laparoscopic and 18 were open surgical.

From: *Current Clinical Urology: Essential Urologic Laparoscopy*
Edited by: S. Y. Nakada and S. P. Hedican, DOI 10.1007/978-1-60327-820-1_10

Early in a surgeon's experience, it is best to restrict laparoscopic partial nephrectomy to superficial, exophytic masses, less than 4 cm in diameter and without penetration near the renal sinus, collecting system, or hilar vessels, that are located at the lower pole, anterior, or lateral surface of the kidney. Such tumors can be identified and accessed well with a transperitoneal approach and are technically straightforward in terms of resection and closure. As experience is gained larger, less exophytic and deeper masses, located posteriorly, medially, or at the upper pole, can be considered. For such lesions, renal ischemia, challenging access and resection, management of large open vessels, and closure of collecting system may be required.

Laparoscopic partial nephrectomy can be used for benign diseases as well. Indications include duplicated collecting systems with poorly functioning segments, benign masses such as angiomyolipoma, and calculi associated with cortical atrophy.

INSTRUMENTATION

The instruments needed for laparoscopic partial nephrectomy include general instruments and those needed for the particular technique being employed. General instruments should include, in addition to a standard laparoscopic instrument set, an argon beam coagulator, and a laparoscopic ultrasound probe. For most of the surgery preparing the operative site for resection, we prefer sharp dissection with a bipolar hook electrode (Gyrus-ACMI, Maple Grove, MN) in one hand of the surgeon and either a long-tipped "bowel grasper" or an irrigator–aspirator in the other. The utility of skilled use of the latter cannot be over-emphasized.

Depending on the technique of tumor excision and defect closure, various other supplies are needed. The availability of a hand-assistance device may be useful, even if use is not planned, as conversion from standard transperitoneal laparoscopy to hand-assistance facilitates the procedure if the perinephric fat is extremely adherent to the kidney. For procedures without renal ischemia, a coagulating/cutting device such as bipolar forceps or ultrasonic shears might be useful for tumor resection. To obtain renal ischemia, the hilum can be occluded with a handheld "bulldog" clamp, a laparoscopic "bulldog" clamp, or a laparoscopic Satinsky clamp. There are a variety of materials that can be used for hemostasis and sealing the collecting system, including: thrombin/collagen granules (Costasis, Orthovita, Malvern, PA), polyethylene glycol hydrogel (Coseal, Baxter, Deerfield, Illinois), bovine albumin/glutaraldehyde (BioGlue, CryoLife BioGlue Surgical Adhesive, Kennesaw, GA), fibrin glue (Tisseel, Baxter), thrombin/gelatin granules (Floseal, Baxter), gelatin sponge (Gelfoam, Pfizer, New York, NY), oxidized cellulose fabric (Surgicel Nu-Knit, Johnson & Johnson, New Brunswick, NJ), and sutures. For laparoscopic suturing, high-quality laparoscopic needle holders are needed. Clips, either plastic (Hem-o-lok clips, Weck, Raleigh, NC) or resorbable (Lapra-Ty II clips, Ethicon, Somerville, NJ) can be used as alternatives to knot-tying.

PREOPERATIVE PREPARATION

Review the imaging studies of the renal lesion carefully, or obtain new ones if adequate detail is not provided. Direct particular attention to the location and shape of the lesion, the mass of tumor extending above the renal surface (i.e., exophytic or not), the depth of penetration into the renal parenchyma, and the proximity to renal sinus, collecting system, and hilar vessels. Select the laparoscopic approach, intended handling of the renal hilum, and the intended technique of tumor bed management (see Choice of Technique and Approach below). The day prior to the scheduled date of surgery, the patient scheduled for a transperitoneal laparoscopic procedure should drink only clear liquids and receive a mild bowel preparation (i.e., magnesium citrate). The goal is to reduce the volume of the intestines and to minimize contamination if a bowel injury does occur. Bowel preparation is not needed for retroperitoneoscopy. After adequate anesthesia, place a urethral catheter to decompress the bladder and to monitor urine output. Insert an orogastric tube to decompress the stomach for transperitoneal cases. Avoid nitrous oxide inhalational anesthetic, which can distend the bowels.

CHOICE OF TECHNIQUE AND APPROACH

Based on the experience at the author's institution with our initial 100 partial nephrectomies *(23)*, we have developed a tailored system to laparoscopic partial nephrectomy, modifying the laparoscopic approach, handling of the renal hilum, and the technique of tumor bed management based upon tumor characteristics. Figure 1 illustrates the decision algorithm applied at the author's institution *(24)*. Make the decision of whether or not to clamp the renal hilum, how to manage the tumor bed, and what laparoscopic route to take based upon tumor depth, proximity to renal sinus, and tumor location, respectively. For tumors with < 5 mm of penetration into the renal parenchyma, do not clamp the hilum and manage the tumor bed with argon beam coagulation and hemostatic agents. For tumors with > 5 mm of penetration but still > 5 mm from the sinus/collecting system, visualization of the resection bed is poor and hemorrhage is excessive if the hilum is not clamped. In these cases, clamp the renal hilum to achieve temporary renal ischemia. If the resection does not enter the renal sinus/collecting system (which is usually the case when the deepest aspect of the lesion is > 5 mm from the sinus/collecting system), then still manage the tumor bed management with argon beam coagulation and hemostatic agents. For tumors within 5 mm of the renal sinus or collecting system, clamp the hilum and, because

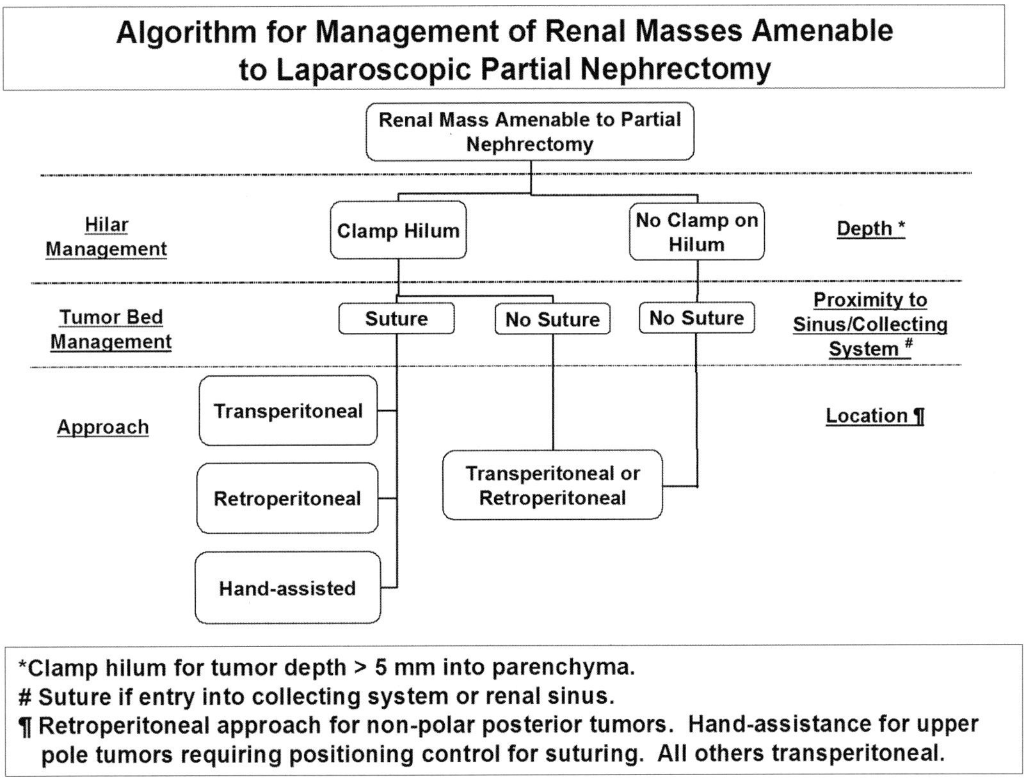

Fig. 1. Algorithm demonstrating selective use of hilar clamping, tumor bed management, and approach for laparoscopic partial nephrectomy based upon tumor depth, proximity to renal sinus, and tumor location, respectively.

the resection of such a mass with a negative margin often requires entry into the renal sinus/collecting system, suture into place a bolster for tumor bed management. Data from our institution suggest that resections that enter the renal sinus/collecting system are associated with a 41% rate of hemorrhage or urinary leak if only argon beam coagulation and hemostatic agents are used to manage the tumor bed *(23)*, compared to an incidence of 9% if a sutured bolster is applied *(24)*.

In terms of laparoscopic approach to the procedure, the default is a standard (not hand-assisted) transperitoneal one. This provides the benefit of a familiar anatomic orientation, a larger working space, and the ability to convert to hand-assistance. Disadvantages occur in the previously operated abdomen with the potential for bowel injury and the time-consuming task of dividing adhesions. Furthermore, the colon and other structures need to be mobilized to expose the kidney and renal hilum. The hand-assisted transperitoneal approach is useful in two situations. An upper pole tumor can be difficult to orient to the laparoscope and working instruments, and the intra-abdominal hand can facilitate positioning of the kidney for resection and tumor bed management (we typically use this approach only when sutured bolster placement is required). Secondly, as noted earlier, conversion from standard transperitoneal laparoscopy to hand-assistance is useful if the perinephric fat is extremely adherent to the kidney. Finally, a retroperitoneoscopic approach offers easier access to the renal hilum, and is the most direct approach for posterior tumors *(25)*. It requires less dissection than the transperitoneal approach and less visceral manipulation. An additional advantage is that any extravasated urine or blood spreads into only a limited area. The main disadvantages of the retroperitoneoscopic approach are that the orientation of the anatomy is unfamiliar and that the working space is less than with a transperitoneal approach. As indicated in Fig. 1, we recommend a retroperitoneal approach for non-polar posterior tumors, a hand-assisted transperitoneal approach for upper pole masses that would benefit from positioning control for resection and suturing, and the standard transperitoneal for all others.

A final approach to partial nephrectomy that has only recently been introduced is robot-assisted laparoscopic partial nephrectomy *(26, 27)*. Reported advantages of the technique include greater surgeon comfort and improved facility with intra-corporeal suturing. Further experience is required before the optimal use of this technique can be ascertained.

TRANSPERITONEAL STANDARD APPROACH

Place the patient in the lateral decubitus position, allowing the torso to fall back to a 45° angle from the horizontal. Do not flex the table, or do so only minimally. Full-flank positioning and table flexion are associated with increased incidence of neuro-muscular injuries and do not improve transperitoneal exposure *(28)*. Obtain transperitoneal access with a Veress needle or other similar method and insufflate the abdomen with carbon dioxide. The port positions for transperitoneal partial nephrectomy at the author's institution are illustrated in Fig. 2 (other port placements have been described). Insert the primary video-laparoscope port (12 mm) at the lateral border of the rectus muscle, approximately at the level of the umbilicus. Place three working ports along a line extending from the xiphoid process to the anterior superior iliac spine. For cases when suturing the tumor bed is not anticipated, use as working ports two 5-mm ports and one 12-mm port (as in Fig. 2). When suturing is planned, switch the 5- and 12-mm working ports, such that there is a 12-mm port cephalad, a 5-mm port in the middle, and a 12-mm port lowest down, to provide better angles and more ports for needle passage.

Incise the line of Toldt and reflect the colon medially to expose Gerota's fascia. If vascular clamping is planned, mobilize the descending colon to the aorta or the ascending colon to the duodenum and then incise Gerota's fascia medially and below the level of the hilum. Once the renal hilum is isolated (see below), incise Gerota's fascia over the kidney and reflect perinephric fat to generously expose the renal mass, with as much mobilization of the kidney as needed to turn the mass toward the video-laparoscope and working instruments. Evaluate the tumor with laparoscopic ultrasonography for shape, depth of

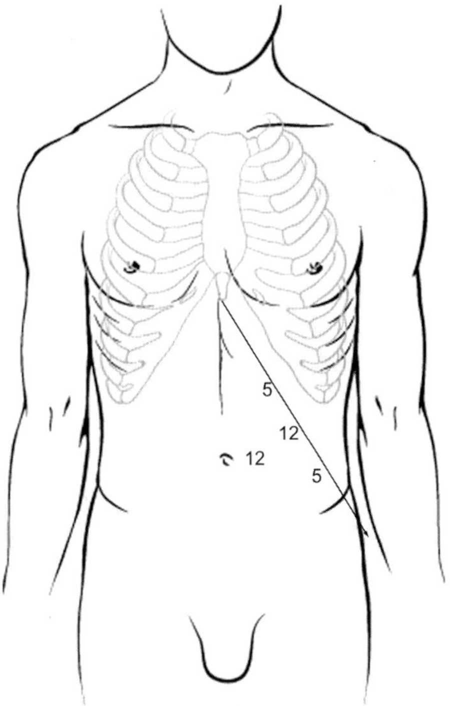

Fig. 2. Port placement for standard transperitoneal partial nephrectomy. The primary video-laparoscope port is at the lateral border of the rectus muscle, approximately at the level of the umbilicus. The three working ports are along a line extending from the xiphoid process to the anterior superior iliac spine (see text for sizes). Other port placements have been described.

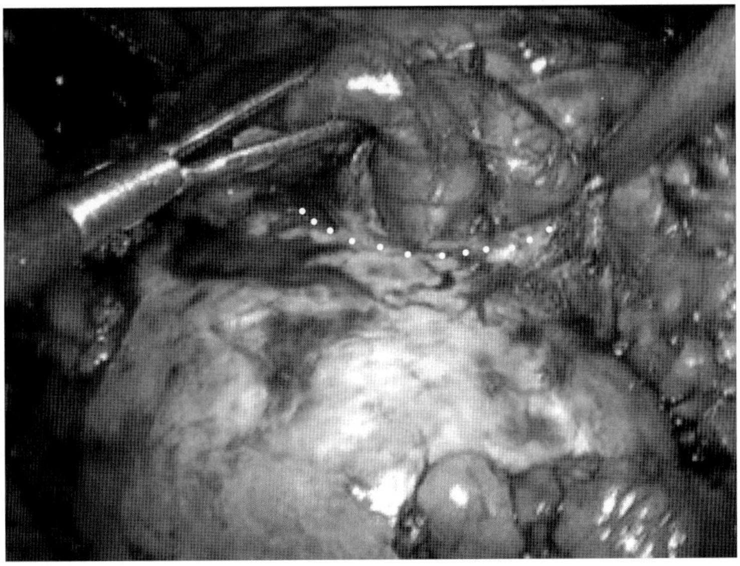

Fig. 3. Renal mass exposed, with a patch of perinephric tissue attached (*dotted white line* indicates tumor margin).

penetration, and proximity to renal sinus, collecting system, and large blood vessels. When exposing the mass, leave a patch of perinephric tissue attached if possible (Fig. 3). In cases where the fat is very mobile, it sometimes is best to remove the perinephric patch and send it as a separate specimen.

TRANSPERITONEAL HAND-ASSISTED APPROACH

Mark the midline of the patient prior to moving the patient from the supine position into the same partial flank position as described above for the standard transperitoneal laparoscopic approach. The typical hand-assistance device position in a non-obese patient is peri-umbilical in the midline. In obese patients use a paramedian incision. We prefer that right- and left-sided hand-assistance incisions are mirror images of each other (using the left hand intra-abdominal for left-sided surgery, and the right hand intra-abdominal for right-sided surgery), but some right-handed surgeons prefer to place the hand-assistance device in the right lower quadrant for right renal surgery, in order to use the left hand in the abdomen. Most commonly the incision for the hand-assistance device is made first, although some surgeons prefer entry as for a standard transperitoneal approach (as above) so that the peritoneal cavity can be inspected and port placements altered as need be. Insert the hand-assistance device and the laparoscopic ports. Figure 4 illustrates port placements for hand-assisted laparoscopic partial nephrectomy in a non-obese patient at the author's institution (other port placements have been described). Place the hand-assistance device peri-umbilical in the midline, the 12-mm port for the video-laparoscope 2 cm lateral to the device, and the working 12-mm port on a line from the primary port to the ipsilateral shoulder, 2 cm below the costal margin. Insert a 5-mm assisting port laterally in the ipsilateral lower quadrant. Use a 12-mm port at this site if suturing is anticipated.

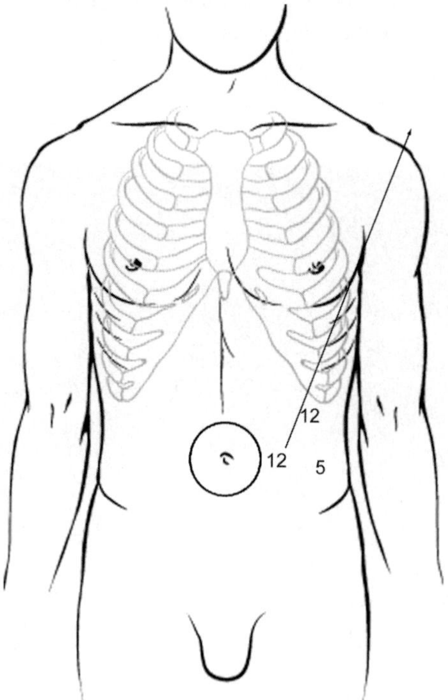

Fig. 4. Port placement for hand-assisted transperitoneal partial nephrectomy. The hand-assistance device is peri-umbilical in the midline, the video-laparoscope port is 2 cm lateral to the device, the primary working port is on a line from the primary port to the ipsilateral shoulder (2 cm below the costal margin) and an assisting port is lateral in the ipsilateral lower quadrant (see text for sizes). Other port placements have been described.

The steps of renal and hilar mobilization are the same as described above for the standard transperitoneal laparoscopic approach. The intra-abdominal hand facilitates many of these steps, particularly mobilizing the kidney to orient the renal mass toward the video-laparoscope and working instruments.

RETROPERITONEAL APPROACH

Position the patient in the full lateral decubitus position with the table flexed and the kidney rest elevated. As opposed to the transperitoneal approach, where such extreme positioning offers no advantage, for the retroperitoneal approach this position provides a larger working area between the ribs and the hip through which to access the retroperitoneum. Make the first incision (2-cm) just in front of or caudal to the tip of the 12th rib. Using a hemostat, spread tissue until the lumbodorsal fascia is exposed. Penetrate this fascia with the hemostat and spread to open this (usually dense) layer. Insert an index finger to penetrate the psoas fascia and then explore the retroperitoneal space. Palpate the psoas muscle, underside of the 12th rib, and the lower pole of the kidney to define the anatomy. Insert a dilating balloon (Spacemaker, Autosuture, Norwalk, CT) behind the kidney and expand the retroperitoneum with approximately 800 cc of air. Place a self-retaining balloon port or Hasson-type cannula (12-mm) at this site for the video-laparoscope, and inflate the retroperitoneum with carbon dioxide.

There is considerable variation in reported port placement for retroperitoneal renal surgery. We usually place a 12-mm working port just anterior to the palpable paraspinous muscles, entering the working space just anterior to the psoas muscle, 1 or 2 cm below the 12th rib. Use caution to avoid traumatizing the ilio-hypogastric nerve, which is often visible on the postero-lateral abdominal wall at this location. Insert a third 5-mm working port in the anterior axillary line in the same line as the first two ports. Place this port well above the iliac crest to ensure that it can be used optimally. If needed to retract the kidney anteriorly, or for other assistance, insert a fourth port (5-mm) in front of the tip of the 10th or 11th rib. Either of the 5-mm ports can be increased to a larger one for suturing as needed.

Keeping the psoas muscle horizontal on the monitor, to maintain orientation, mobilize and rotate the kidney anteriorly. If hilar clamping is needed, identify the renal artery. It is usually located straight in from the posterior-most port. After elevating the kidney and incising Gerota's fascia, the renal artery is often recognized by its pulsations. Then, incise Gerota's fascia and dissect perinephric fat off of the kidney to expose the mass. The same principles of management of peri-tumor fat and renal mobilization as described for the transperitoneal approach apply here.

RESECTION WITHOUT HILAR CLAMPING

For tumors that penetrate less than 5 mm into the renal parenchyma, hilar clamping is not necessary (Fig. 5). The minor bleeding that occurs at this depth usually can be controlled with a cutting/coagulation device such as monopolar electrocautery scissors, contact tip neodymium:yttrium–aluminum–garnet (Nd:YAG) laser, ultrasonic shears, or bipolar cautery forceps with and without impedance control, with additional use of an argon beam coagulator and/or hemostatic agents as needed. First, use an electrocautery instrument to incise the renal capsule 2-mm around the edge of the tumor to demarcate the resection line (Fig. 6). Then, slowly use the cutting/coagulation device to carve out the tumor with a 2-mm margin. Gently use the irrigator–aspirator to assist in both visualization and counter-traction on the mass. An alternative to a cutting/coagulation device is to coagulate the mass with radiofrequency ablation *(29)* or microwave tissue coagulation *(30)* and then resect the coagulated mass. This technique maximizes hemostasis. A disadvantage of any coagulation technique is that the margin of resection cannot be monitored easily. Recently, for small, shallow, and perfectly spherical

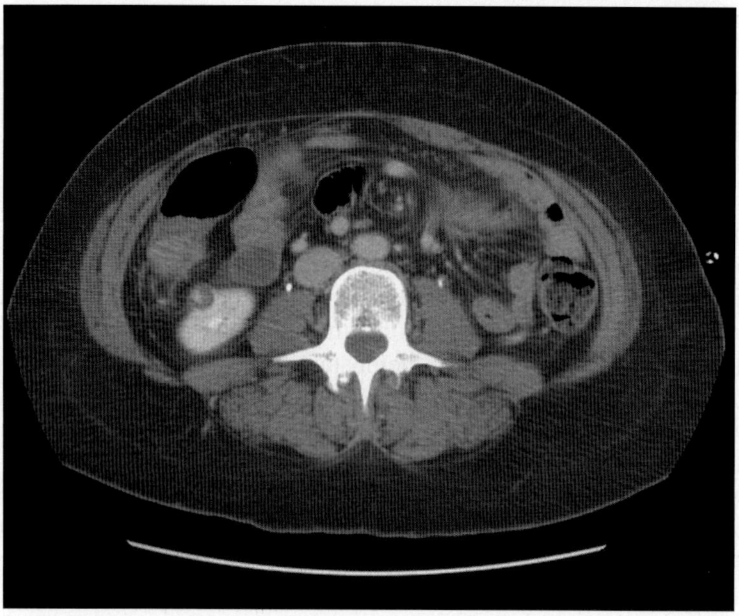

Fig. 5. Anterior right renal tumor penetrating less than 5 mm into the renal parenchyma.

tumors that appear to have a defined pseudocapsule, we have started enucleating the mass with the backside of laparoscopic scissors. If the mass rolls out easily, then our experience is that the margin is uniformly negative. Bleeding is minimal and can be controlled with an argon beam coagulator and application of hemostatic products such as thrombin/gelatin granules (Fig. 7).

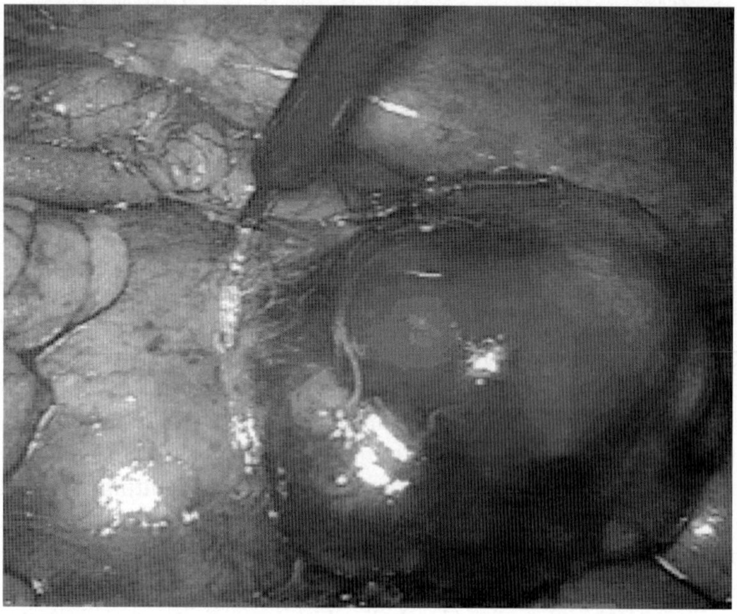

Fig. 6. Electrocautery is used to score the renal capsule 2-mm around the edge of the tumor.

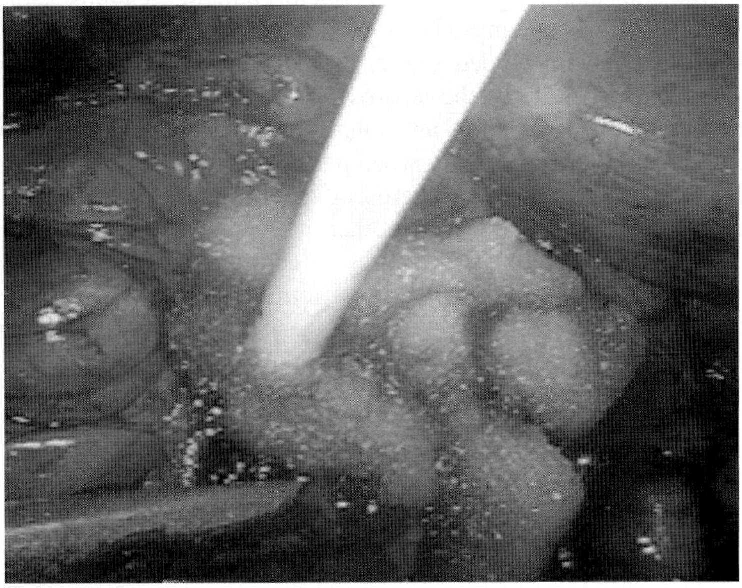

Fig. 7. After application of the argon beam coagulator, thrombin/gelatin granules are used to fill the renal defect for hemostasis.

RESECTION WITH HILAR CLAMPING BUT NO SUTURING

For tumors that penetrate more than 5 mm into the renal parenchyma, hemostasis is often not adequate without hilar clamping to occlude renal blood flow (Fig. 8). Preoperative imaging assessment is important in this regard, but ultimately it is the laparoscopic ultrasonographic evaluation of the mass that is most important. If the tumor's depth of penetration into the parenchyma exceeds 5 mm, then the renal hilum should be exposed. If there is any uncertainty in this regard, then dissect out the renal hilum.

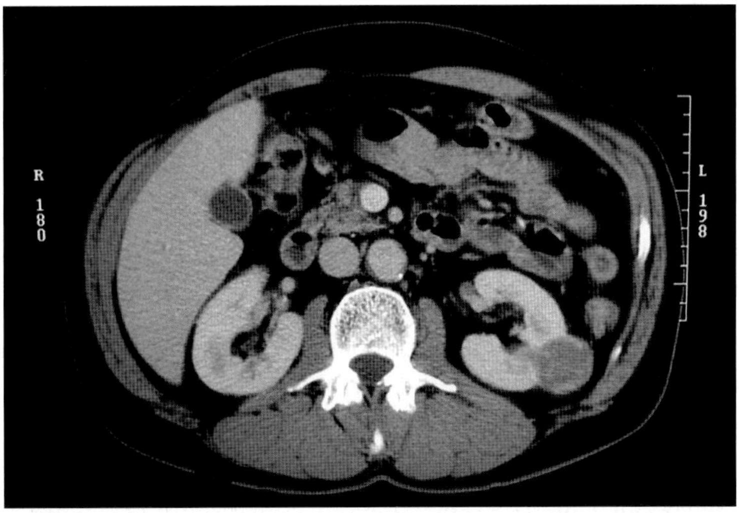

Fig. 8. Lateral left renal tumor penetrating more than 5 mm into the renal parenchyma, but located > 5 mm from the renal sinus.

The instruments for hilar clamping include handheld "bulldog" clamps, laparoscopic "bulldog" clamps, and laparoscopic Satinsky clamps. The former are used for hand-assisted transperitoneal procedures. A single "bulldog" clamp is adequate for the renal artery alone, but if the hilum is clamped en bloc then use two clamps. Similarly, the laparoscopic "bulldog" clamp is best applied to a single vessel. The laparoscopic "bulldog" clamps are often difficult to remove quickly, so many urologists prefer a laparoscopic Satinsky clamp (Fig. 9) when performing standard laparoscopy. For a transperitoneal approach the port through which the laparoscopic Satinsky clamp is placed can be positioned in such a manner that it does not interfere with the other instruments, and as such the only disadvantage of a laparoscopic Satinsky clamp is that it requires an additional port. Position this port below and just lateral to the umbilicus in most cases. During a retroperitoneal approach, however, the laparoscopic Satinsky clamp can be unwieldy in the small working space and, although it can be used in some cases, for many retroperitoneoscopic procedures the laparoscopic "bulldog" clamp applied to the isolated renal artery is best.

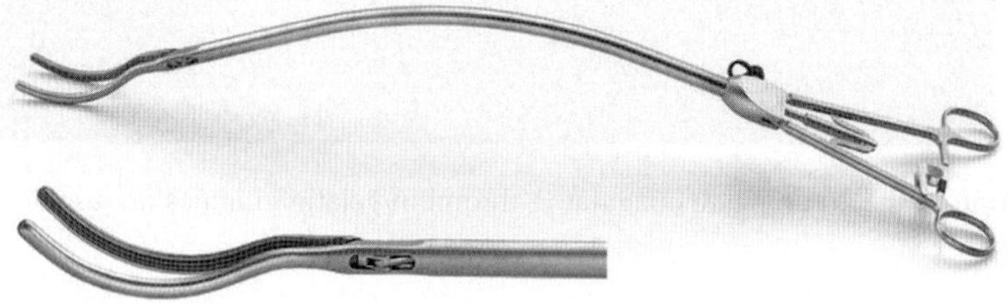

Fig. 9. Laparoscopic Satinsky clamp. This one is curved and requires a flexible port. Straight clamps can be inserted through a rigid port.

There is no consensus as to whether to clamp the renal artery alone, the renal artery and vein en bloc, or the renal artery and renal vein separately. We have not noted any consistent difference in intra-operative hemostasis among the techniques, and we decide on how to clamp the hilum based upon the accessibility of the vessels. One important point, however, is that the hilum must be adequately thinned out for en bloc clamping. If too much tissue remains around the renal vessels, then the clamp manages to occlude the vein but not the artery, resulting in more rather than less hemorrhage.

Renal hilar exposure is straightforward with the retroperitoneal approach, as the renal artery is usually located directly medially from the posterior-most port. After elevating the kidney and incising Gerota's fascia, identify the renal artery aided by its pulsations. For the retroperitoneal approach, we dissect out the artery individually for clamping, without manipulating the renal vein. For the transperitoneal approach, dissect sharply and bluntly to expose the psoas muscle immediately below the renal hilum. Then work upwards to and then around the renal hilum. We decide whether to clamp the renal artery alone or the artery and vein en bloc based upon the renal hilar anatomy. If the artery is easily accessible, then isolate it for individual clamping. Otherwise, thin out the renal artery and vein as a single structure for en bloc clamping (Fig. 10). In some cases of a polar tumor, there may be an arterial branch that can be isolated for clamping.

The options for cooling the kidney during laparoscopic partial nephrectomy are not standardized, and their use is not routine. Several techniques have been described, including: intra-corporeal ice slush around the kidney held within an endoscopic entrapment sac *(31)*; retrograde instillation of iced saline irrigation through a ureteral catheter into the renal pelvis *(32)*; intra-arterial cannula with infusion of cold lactated Ringer's solution *(33)*; and irrigation of the clamped kidney with either a

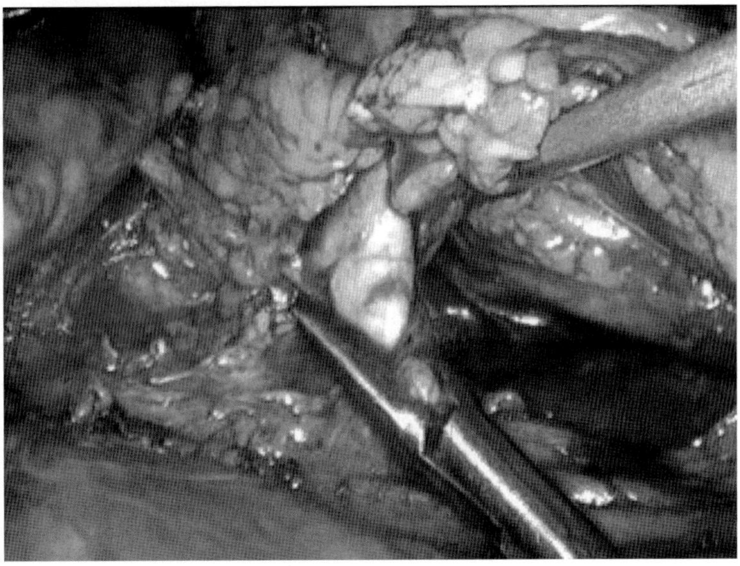

Fig. 10. The left renal artery and vein are clamped en bloc with a laparoscopic Satinsky clamp placed through a port below and just lateral to the umbilicus.

fine slurry of iced saline *(34)* or simply very cold saline *(35)*. None of these methods, however, have been widely accepted. Moreover, the benefit of cold ischemia over warm ischemia is not yet clear. The study of Jablonski and associates *(36)*, on renal damage in a rat model with variable warm ischemia times, is often referenced when considering the effect of warm ischemia time on renal function. In this study, immediate recovery of renal function after 30 min of warm ischemia was consistent, but 60 min of warm ischemia produced renal impairment (as measured by creatinine clearances) that lasted for 30 days, and 90 min of warm ischemia was associated with 83% mortality from uremia. Shekarriz and associates *(37)* used renal scans 3 months after laparoscopic partial nephrectomy to demonstrate that, with a mean hilar clamping time of 22.5 min (range 10–40), renal function was preserved in the operated kidneys. Kane and associates *(38)* found, in their experience with 15 laparoscopic partial nephrectomies which included temporary arterial occlusion for a mean time of 43 min, that renal function was not altered. A very useful report from Bhayani and associates *(39)*, comparing the change in serum creatinine 6 months after laparoscopic partial nephrectomy without warm ischemia, with warm ischemia less than 30 min, and with warm ischemia greater than 30 min (up to 55 min) revealed no significant differences between the groups (mean creatinine increases of 0.05, 0.06, and 0.08 mg/dl, respectively). Although the general goal is to maintain warm ischemia less than 30 min, slightly longer times do not appear to have a substantial effect.

As the hilum is being prepared for clamping, administer 12.5 g of mannitol intravenously (and give an additional 12.5 g after the hilum is unclamped). Once the hilum is ready for clamping, score the capsule with electrocautery for a 2–5 mm margin around the tumor. Ischemia is not necessary for this step, and performing it before hilar clamping reduces ischemia time and gives the surgeon a feel of the instrument angles that will be needed during subsequent resection. Clamp the renal hilum and then begin resection with laparoscopic scissors (no cautery) on the nearest edge of the tumor. A wide margin is not necessary, but there is a tendency to direct the scissors across rather than down into the parenchyma, depending on the angles available to the laparoscopic instrument. As such, start widely enough (usually not more than 5 mm is needed) to avoid this. If laparoscopic suturing is to be avoided, then the resection must be kept close to the tumor to avoid entry into the renal sinus or collecting system. Assuming the renal sinus/collecting system is not entered, manage the tumor bed with argon beam coagulation and application of hemostatic material such as thrombin/gelatin granules.

Resection of large or irregular tumors, or those within 5 mm of the renal sinus/collecting system, calls instead for a resection line that maintains a more generous margin, often entering the renal sinus, to prevent cutting into the tumor; in such cases a laparoscopic bolster should be used to manage the tumor bed (see below). Additionally, our "cut-off" of 5 mm from the renal sinus/collecting system before those structures are likely entered is only an approximation. The choice for management of the tumor bed is made after tumor resection, and in some "borderline" cases a lesion which was thought to be resectable without entry into the renal sinus/collecting system does require incision to this level. If a surgeon is not prepared to suture, such cases should be avoided. We have found that lesions between 5 and 10 mm from the renal sinus on imaging occasionally are associated with resection into the renal sinus/collecting system, but that lesions > 10 mm from the renal sinus on imaging can reliably be managed without laparoscopic suturing.

RESECTION WITH HILAR CLAMPING AND SUTURING

For tumors within 5 mm of the renal sinus or collecting system (Fig. 11), not only clamp the hilum but prepare to manage the tumor bed with a sutured bolster, since adequate resection of such tumors often requires entry into the renal sinus/collecting system (Fig. 12). Prepare the material for suturing before resection, including: 8-in. length of 2-0 polyglycolic acid suture on a SH needle; a rolled piece of oxidized cellulose fabric (the bolster) secured with 0-polyglycolic acid suture and with two 2-in. lengths of 0-polyglycolic acid suture on a CT-1 needle attached on one side of the mid-portion of the bolster (Fig. 13); and two 3-in. lengths of 0-polyglycolic acid suture on a CT-1 needle with a plastic or resorbable clip on the free end. Additionally, have ready one unit of thrombin/gelatin granules and one additional piece of oxidized cellulose fabric.

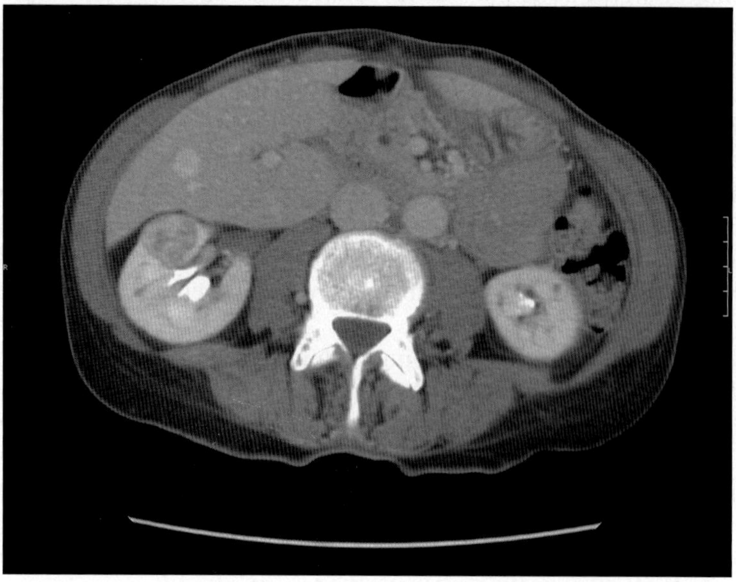

Fig. 11. Anterior right renal tumor abutting the renal sinus and collecting system.

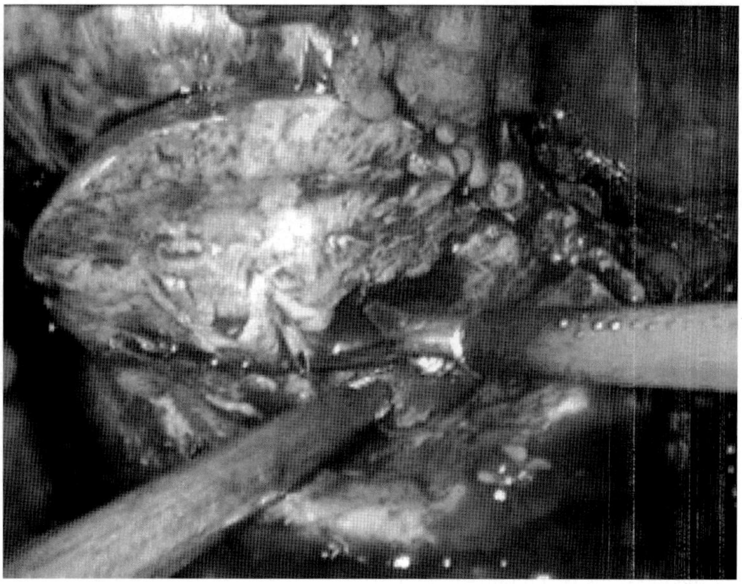

Fig. 12. Resection of a deep renal mass requiring wide entry into renal sinus.

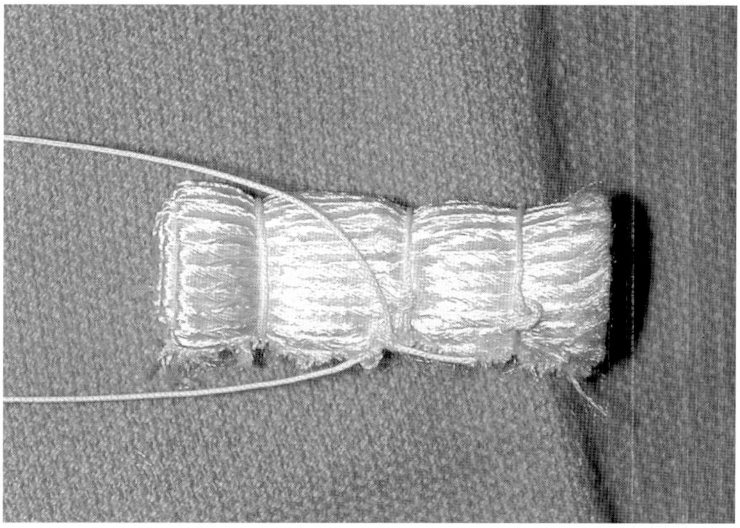

Fig. 13. The bolster is a rolled piece of oxidized cellulose fabric secured with 0-polyglycolic acid suture and with two 2-in. lengths of 0-polyglycolic acid suture on a CT-1 needle attached on one side of the mid-portion of the bolster.

After resection using laparoscopic scissors without cautery, fulgurate the outer rim of parenchyma with an argon beam coagulator. If the renal sinus is widely entered, such that the base of the section site exposes more than a cm or two of renal sinus, then loosely approximate the parenchymal edges around the sinus defect with a running suture of 2-0 polyglycolic acid on a SH needle (Fig. 14). Additionally, close any large entry into the collecting system with a figure-of-eight stitch of the same suture. Place the bolster with the two pre-loaded sutures into the renal defect, taking care that the "top" side of the bolster, the one to which the two sutures are attached, is most superficial. Pass each needle through the middle of one side of the parenchymal defect, "inside-out." Place a small amount

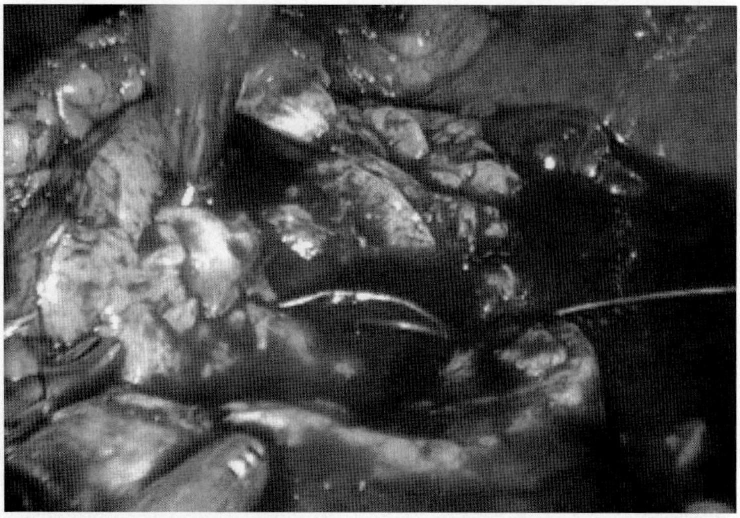

Fig. 14. One bite with a 2-0 polyglycolic acid suture on a SH needle has been placed (*right side of figure*) and the second bite (*left side of the figure*) is being pulled through.

of thrombin/gelatin granules underneath the bolster, and then secure the bolster – dimpling the renal surface but not pulling so hard as to tear the tissue – by placing a plastic or resorbable clip snugly on the parenchymal side of the suture. Complete the bolster placement by inserting one of the 3-in. segments of 0-polyglycolic acid suture on a CT-1 needle "outside-in" on the parenchyma at one apex of the resection defect, over or through the end of the bolster, and then "inside-out" on the parenchyma on the other side of the bolster (Fig. 15). Secure this stitch with a clip (Fig. 16), and then repeat with the

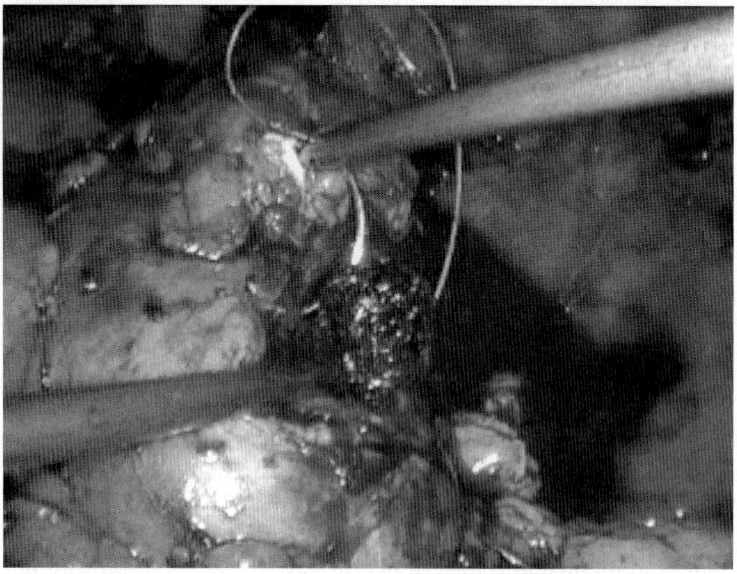

Fig. 15. A 0-polyglycolic acid suture on a CT-1 needle has been passed "outside-in" on one edge of the parenchyma (*right side of figure*) at the near apex of the resection defect, and is now being passed "inside-out" out on the opposite edge (*left side of the figure*).

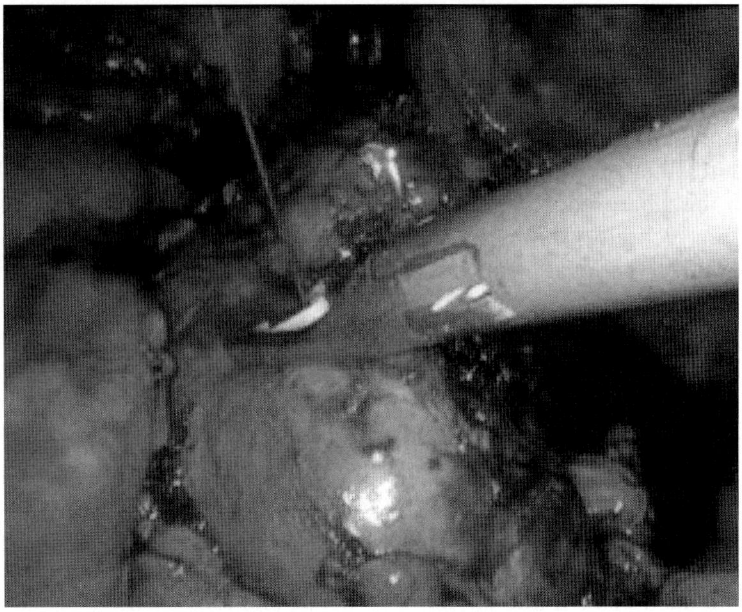

Fig. 16. A plastic clip is used to secure the suture.

other suture at the other apex. Only occasionally, for large defects, are more than these three fixation points (counting the first two pre-attached sutures as one fixation point) needed. Place the remaining aliquot of thrombin/gelatin granules on top of the bolter, cover the entire site with the remaining sheet of oxidized cellulose fabric (which allows gentle pressure to be placed on the entire resection site without disturbing the thrombin/gelatin granules), and remove the renal hilar clamp (Fig. 17).

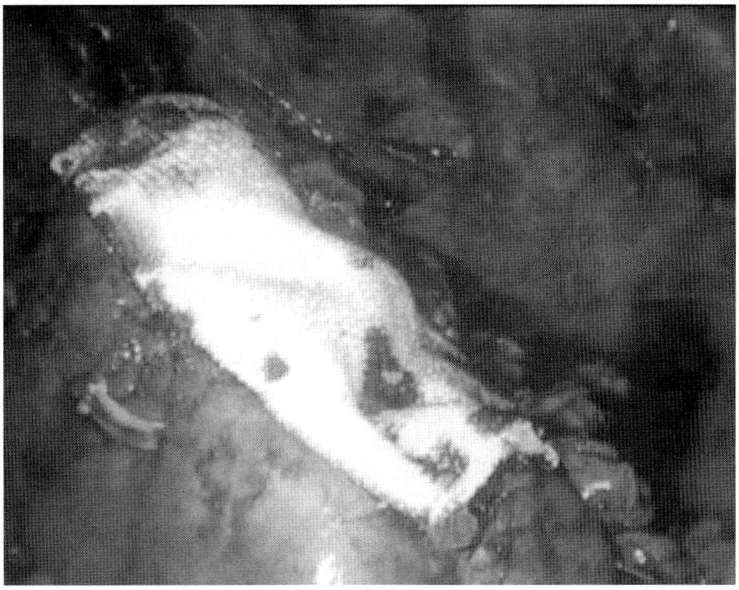

Fig. 17. Completed repair.

TUMOR EXTRACTION AND EXITING

Handling of the specimen depends on its appearance and the approach to the procedure. Hand-assistance allows rapid removal of the specimen and the ability to inspect it directly and get frozen sections or at least inking of the margin and gross examination. To extract all but the smallest specimens during standard laparoscopy, however, requires enlarging a port site. Rather than do this, inspect the specimen with the laparoscope, which provides an acceptable estimate of margin status in most cases. Routine frozen sections of biopsies of the tumor bed after partial nephrectomy do not appear to be useful *(40)*. Moreover, the focal positive margins that can occur when the resection appears grossly acceptable are not necessarily indicative of tumor remaining in the kidney. In a combined series of 511 laparoscopic partial nephrectomy patients with confirmed renal cell carcinoma from Johns Hopkins and Cleveland Clinic, there were nine (1.8%) positive margins *(41)*. Of these patients, two underwent radical nephrectomy (residual tumor was found in neither), one had von-Hippel-Lindau disease and died of metastatic renal cancer, and the other six are disease-free with a median follow-up of 32 months. In the author's series, two patients with positive margins of the laparoscopic partial nephrectomy specimen underwent completion radical nephrectomy and neither had residual tumor. Thus, if the resection appears adequate – with no exposure of the tumor on gross inspection – then complete the procedure without additional resection or biopsy. Set the tumor off to the side, and once tumor bed management is completed place it into an entrapment sac and remove it.

As in any laparoscopic procedure, reduce the intra-abdominal pressure to 5 mmHg in order to assess completely for hemostasis. This is especially important after partial nephrectomy. Since renal blood flow is reduced even at the typical operative pnemoperitoneum pressure of 15 mmHg, reduction of pressure might uncover hemorrhage from the operative site. Additionally, ask the anesthesiologist to lighten anesthesia to allow the systolic blood pressure to exceed 120 mmHg. It has been demonstrated experimentally that some partial nephrectomy operative sites that appear to have adequate hemostasis at low-blood pressure will bleed at higher pressures *(42)*. If the renal sinus/collecting system has been entered, place a closed suction drain placed through a lateral 5-mm port site.

SPECIFIC COMPLICATIONS

Hemorrhage

Management of parenchymal bleeding is perhaps the greatest challenge of laparoscopic partial nephrectomy. Novel instruments and techniques have been developed to achieve hemostasis more readily. These techniques fall into three categories based on the timing of their use: before resecting the tumor, while resecting the tumor, and after resecting the tumor.

The most obvious way to maximize hemostasis prior to resecting the renal mass is to clamp the renal hilum as described above. If renal hilar clamping is to be avoided, then the mass can be coagulated prior to resection with radiofrequency ablation *(29)* or microwave tissue coagulation *(30)*. Many laparoscopic instruments have been developed to provide hemostasis during resection of the renal tumor. Options include the argon beam coagulator, monopolar cautery devices, ultrasonic shears, the Nd:YAG laser, and bipolar electrocautery. These devices can be used singly or in combination. Coagulation during resection, however, obscures the surgical margin, and thus should be used only with small, spherical lesions where the margin can be anticipated. The most important methods of hemostasis are those that are applied after tumor resection, including the argon beam coagulator, hemostatic agents, and sutured bolster.

The majority of cases of early post-operative hemorrhage after partial nephrectomy can be managed with red blood cell transfusions and expectant management *(43)*. Delayed hemorrhage, however, should raise the suspicion of an arterio-venous fistula (renal artery pseudoaneursym). This is best treated with selective percutaneous angioembolization *(44)*.

Urinary Fistula

To most assuredly avoid a urinary fistula, do not enter the collecting system with the resection. For tumors more than 5 mm from the renal sinus, if small violations of the collecting system do occur urinary leakage usually is prevented by routine management of the tumor bed with hemostatic agents as described above. The more difficult situation is when the renal sinus and collecting system are entered widely in the process of achieving adequate resection of a deep renal mass. In the author's series, urinary fistula (defined as urine from the drainage tube beyond post-operative day 2) occurred in 1.6% of cases when the renal sinus/collecting system is not entered, compared to 4% when there is such entry *(24)*. Application of tumor bed management techniques as described above should keep the rate of urinary fistula to this level. Although some authors advocate insertion of a ureteral access catheter so that saline stained with methylene blue or indigo carmine can be instilled into the collecting system to assess for entry *(45)*, our group and others *(46)* have not found this to be necessary.

In our experience, most urinary fistulae occurring in association with laparoscopic partial nephrectomy resolve spontaneously within a week or two. Occasionally, ureteral stent placement (if one is not already in place) and urethral catheter drainage are required, and only rarely are additional maneuvers necessary.

Acute Tubular Necrosis

Prolonged renal ischemia can result in post-operative acute tubular necrosis and acute renal failure. This is especially problematic if the partial nephrectomy is being performed for absolute indications (solitary kidney, poor renal function). Because suturing is required for deeper resections, the likelihood of prolonged ischemia times during laparoscopic partial nephrectomy is greater in the setting of deep tumors. In expert hands, even solitary kidneys can be addressed in this manner with a low incidence of acute renal failure *(47)*. Nonetheless, given the long learning curve of sutured bolster application, it is recommended that early in a surgeon's experience the procedure should be limited to small, superficial tumors to minimize ischemia time.

RESULTS

Laparoscopic partial nephrectomy provides the same reduction in the intensity and duration of convalescence (compared to open surgery) that laparoscopic radical nephrectomy does *(48, 49)*. For the procedure to be acceptable, though, there are at least two additional issues to be addressed. First, is the operation routinely feasible, as measured by complications rates and technically successful resections? Second, how does it compare to the "gold standard" open surgical partial nephrectomy in terms of cancer control and other parameters?

Several groups have reported series that attest to the routine feasibility of laparoscopic partial nephrectomy. A common theme is that the procedure is straightforward for small superficial tumors, and difficult when larger and deeper tumors are addressed, but that with experience the latter lesions can be addressed equally as well. Nadu and associates *(50)* recently reported results in 140 laparoscopic partial nephrectomy patients, with an analysis that revealed lower rates of complications, conversions to open surgery, and positive margins in their last 110 patients compared to their first 30 patients, despite tumors being 50% larger on average. The experienced Cleveland Clinic group has noted a significant decrease in overall, urologic, and hemorrhagic complications in their most recent 200 patients compared to their first 200 patients, despite increased tumor complexity in the more recent patients *(51)*. The University of Chicago group compared their laparoscopic partial nephrectomies that did and did not require sutured collecting system repair (52 and 32 patients, respectively) *(52)*. Warm ischemia and operative times were longer in the group that required suturing, but complications and conversions to open surgery were similar in the two groups. The experience is the same at the author's institution; comparing 61 partial nephrectomies that did not require a sutured bolster (mean 1.9 cm tumor size and 7 mm depth of penetration into the parenchyma) with 113 patients that did require sutured bolster (mean 2.6 cm tumor size and 16 mm depth of penetration into the parenchyma), the warm ischemia and operative time were longer in the latter group but complications and conversions to open surgery were similar *(24)*.

A multi-institutional group has reported a comparison of 771 laparoscopic partial nephrectomies with 1,028 open surgical partial nephrectomies *(53)*. Despite being performed for smaller tumors (mean, 2.7 vs. 3.5 cm) that were less frequently "central" (34 vs. 53%), the laparoscopic approach was associated with longer ischemia time (31 vs. 20 min) and more post-operative complications, both urologic (9.2 vs. 5.0%) and non-urologic (16 vs. 14%). Laparoscopic patients, however, benefited from a shorter operative time (mean, 201 vs. 266 min) and duration of hospitalization (mean, 3.3 vs. 5.8 days). The frequency of loss of ipsilateral renal function (2.1 vs. 0.4%) and 3-year cancer death rate (0.7 vs. 0.8%) was low in both the laparoscopic and open surgical groups, respectively. Similarly, a report from Johns Hopkins found no difference in 5-year disease-free and patient survival between 85 laparoscopic and 58 open surgical partial nephrectomies *(21)*. These reports, and others, suggest that laparoscopic partial nephrectomy – in experienced hands – has technical success and oncologic efficacy similar to that of open surgical partial nephrectomy, but that the complication rate is greater than that of open surgical partial nephrectomy.

SUMMARY

Laparoscopic partial nephrectomy is an excellent management option for small, superficial renal masses. With experience, larger and deeper tumors can be addressed as well. Intermediate-term follow-up (3 and 5-year) suggests cancer control similar to that of open surgery. The benefit of laparoscopy over open surgery is a briefer and less intense convalescence. The disadvantage of laparoscopic partial nephrectomy, at least with current techniques, is a complication rate that is somewhat greater than for open surgery. Careful preoperative assessment and planning is of utmost importance. A successful procedure can be performed through a variety of approaches (transperitoneal, retroperitoneal, and hand-assisted), with or without renal hilar clamping, and using any of a number of methods for tumor bed management (coagulation instruments, hemostatic products, and suturing), with the optimal selection of technique determined by the tumor characteristics.

TAKE HOME MESSAGES

1. Assess the preoperative imaging carefully, considering tumor depth, proximity to renal sinus, and tumor location, to determine optimal plan for hilar clamping, tumor bed management, and approach.
2. Intra-operatively, study the mass with laparoscopic ultrasound to determine the relationship of the mass to the renal sinus, collecting system and vasculature.
3. Know the various instruments/techniques that may be useful for hemostasis, including energy-based devices, hemostatic agents, and – the most important technique for management of deep renal tumors – the use of hilar clamping and placement of a sutured bolster.
4. Appreciate that current data suggest that laparoscopic partial nephrectomy, compared to open surgical partial nephrectomy, is associated with superior convalescence, equivalent cancer control, and a greater complication rate.

REFERENCES

1. Robson CJ. Radical nephrectomy for renal cell carcinoma. J Urol 1963;89:37–42.
2. Buttarazzi PJ, Devine PC, Devine CJ, Jr., Poutasse EF. The indications, complications and results of partial nephrectomy. J Urol 1968;99:376–378.

3. Filipas D, Fichtner J, Spix C, et al. Nephron-sparing surgery of renal cell carcinoma with a normal opposite kidney: long-term outcome in 180 patients. Urology 2000;56:387–392.
4. Uzzo RG, Novick AC. Nephron sparing surgery for renal tumors: indications, techniques and outcomes. J Urol 2001;166:6–18.
5. Herr HW. Partial nephrectomy for unilateral renal carcinoma and a normal contralateral kidney: 10-year follow-up. J Urol 1999;161:33–34.
6. Fergany AF, Hafez KS, Novick AC. Long-term results of nephron sparing surgery for localized renal cell carcinoma: 10-year follow-up. J Urol 2000;163:442–445.
7. Clark PE, Schover LR, Uzzo RG, Hafez KS, Rybicki LA, Novick AC. Quality of life and psychological adaptation after surgical treatment for localized renal cell carcinoma: impact of the amount of remaining renal tissue. Urology 2001;57:252–256.
8. McKiernan J, Simmons R, Katz J, Russo P. Natural history of chronic renal insufficiency after partial and radical nephrectomy. Urology 2002;59:816–820.
9. Huang WC, Levey AS, Serio AM, et al. Chronic kidney disease after nephrectomy in patients with renal cortical tumours: a retrospective cohort study. Lancet Oncol 2006;7:735–740.
10. Hollingsworth JM, Miller DC, Daignault S, Hollenbeck BK. Rising incidence of small renal masses: a need to reassess treatment effect. J Natl Canc Inst 2006;98:1331–1334.
11. Russo P, Goetzl M, Simmons R, Katz J, Motzer R, Reuter V. Partial nephrectomy: the rationale for expanding the indications. Ann Surg Onc 2002;9:680–687.
12. Patard JJ, Shvarts O, Lam JS, et al. Safety and efficacy of partial nephrectomy for all T1 tumors based on an international multicenter experience. J Urol 2004;171:2181–2185.
13. Hollenbeck BK, Taub DA, Miller DC, Dunn RL, Wei JT. National utilization trends of partial nephrectomy for renal cell carcinoma: a case of underutilization. J Urol 2006;67:254–259.
14. Clayman RV, Kavoussi LR, Soper NJ, et al. Laparoscopic nephrectomy: Initial case report. J Urol 1991;146:278–282.
15. Jordan GH, Winslow BH. Laparoendoscopic upper pole partial nephrectomy with ureterectomy. J Urol 1993;150: 940–943.
16. Winfield HN, Donovan JF, Godet AS, Clayman RV. Laparoscopic partial nephrectomy: initial case report for benign disease. J Endourol 1993;7:521–526.
17. Luciani RC, Greiner M, Clement JC, Houot A, Didierlaurent JF. Laparoscopic enucleation of a renal cell carcinoma. Surg Endosc 1994;8:1329–1331.
18. Portis AJ, Yan Y, Landman J, et al. Long-term followup after laparoscopic radical nephrectomy. J Urol 2002;167: 1257–1262.
19. Saika T, Ono Y, Hattori R, et al. Long-term outcome of laparoscopic radical nephrectomy for pathologic T1 renal cell carcinoma. Urology 2003;62:1018–1023.
20. Permpongkosol S, Chan DY, Link RE, et al. Long-term survival analysis after laparoscopic radical nephrectomy. J Urol 2005;174:1222–1225.
21. Permpongkosol S, Bagga HS, Romero FR, Sroka M, Jarrett TW, Kavoussi LR. Laparoscopic versus open partial nephrectomy for the treatment of pathological T1N0M0 renal cell carcinoma: a 5-year survival rate. J Urol 2006;176: 1984–1988.
22. Lane BR, Gill IS. 5-year outcomes of laparoscopic partial nephrectomy. J Urol 2007;177:70–74.
23. Johnston WK, III, Montgomery JS, Seifman BD, Hollenbeck BK, Wolf JS, Jr. Fibrin glue v sutured bolster: lessons learned during 100 laparoscopic partial nephrectomies. J Urol 2005;174:47–52.
24. Weizer AZ, Gilbert SM, Roberts WW, Hollenbeck BK, Wolf JS, Jr. Tailoring technique of laparoscopic partial nephrectomy to tumor characteristics. J Urol 2008;180:1273–1278.
25. Kieran K, Montgomery JS, Daignault S, Roberts WW, Wolf JS, Jr. Comparison of intraoperative parameters and perioperative complications in retroperitoneal and transperitoneal approaches to laparoscopic partial nephrectomy: support for a retroperitoneal approach in selected patients. J Endourol 2007;21:754–759.
26. Caruso RP, Phillips CK, Kau E, Taneja SS, Stifelman MD. Robot assisted laparoscopic partial nephrectomy: initial experience. J Urol 2006;176:36–39.
27. Kaul S, Laungani R, Sarle R, et al. da Vinci-assisted robotic partial nephrectomy: technique and results at a mean of 15 months of follow-up. Eur Urol 2007;51:186–191.
28. Wolf JS, Jr., Marcovich R, Gill IS, et al. Survey of neuromuscular injuries to the patient and surgeon during urologic laparoscopic surgery. Urology 2000;55:831–836.
29. Gettman MT, Bishoff JT, Su LM, et al. Hemostatic laparoscopic partial nephrectomy: initial experience with the radiofrequency coagulation-assisted technique. Urology 2001;58:8–11.
30. Yoshimura K, Okubo K, Ichioka K, Terada N, Matsuta Y, Arai Y. Laparoscopic partial nephrectomy with a microwave tissue coagulator for small renal tumor. J Urol 2001;165:1893–1896.
31. Gill IS, Abreu SC, Desai MM, et al. Laparoscopic ice slush renal hypothermia for partial nephrectomy: the initial experience. J Urol 2003;170:52–56.
32. Landman J, Venkatesh R, Lee D, et al. Renal hypothermia achieved by retrograde endoscopic cold saline perfusion: technique and initial clinical application. Urology 2003;61:1023–1025.

33. Janetschek G, Abdelmaksoud A, Bagheri F, Al-Zahrani H, Leeb K, Gschwendtner M. Laparoscopic partial nephrectomy in cold ischemia: renal artery perfusion. J Urol 2004;171:68–71.
34. Webster TM, Moeckel GW, Herrell SD. Simple method for achieving renal parenchymal hypothermia for pure laparoscopic partial nephrectomy. J Endourol 2005;19:1075–1081.
35. Weld KJ, Koziol S, Montiglio C, Sorenson P, Cespedes RD, Bishoff JT. Feasibility of laparoscopic renal cooling with near-freezing saline irrigation delivered with a standard irrigator aspirator. Urology 2007;69:465–468.
36. Jablonski P, Howden BO, Rae DA, Birrell CS, Marshall VC, Tange J. An experimental model for assessment of renal recovery from warm ischemia. Transplantation 1983;35:198–204.
37. Shekarriz B, Shah G, Upadhyay J. Impact of temporary hilar clamping during laparoscopic partial nephrectomy on postoperative renal function: a prospective study. J Urol 2004;72:54–57.
38. Kane CJ, Mitchell JA, Meng MV, Anast J, Carroll PR, Stoller ML. Laparoscopic partial nephrectomy with temporary arterial occlusion: description of technique and renal functional outcomes. Urology 2004;63:241–246.
39. Bhayani SB, Rha KH, Pinto PA, et al. Laparoscopic partial nephrectomy: effect of warm ischemia on serum creatinine. J Urol 2004;172:1264–1266.
40. Kubinski DJ, Clark PE, Assimos DG, Hall MC. Utility of frozen section analysis of resection margins during partial nephrectomy. Urology 2004;64:31–34.
41. Permpongkosol S, Columbo JR, Jr., Gill IS, Kavoussi LR. Positive surgical parenchymal margin after laparoscopic partial nephrectomy for renal cell carcinoma: oncological outcomes. J Urol 2006;176:2401–2404.
42. Johnston WK, III, Kelel KM, Hollenbeck BK, Daignault S, Wolf JS, Jr. Acute integrity of closure for partial nephrectomy: comparison of 7 agents in a hypertensive porcine model. J Urol 2006;175:2307–2311.
43. Rosevear HM, Montgomery JS, Roberts WW, Wolf JS, Jr. Characterization and management of post-operative hemorrhage following upper retroperitoneal laparoscopic surgery. J Urol 2006;176:1458–1462.
44. Wright JL, Porter JR. Renal artery pseudoaneurysm after laparoscopic partial nephrectomy. Urology 2005;66:1109.
45. Gill IS, DeSai MM, Kaouk JH, et al. Laparoscopic partial nephrectomy for renal tumor: duplicating open surgical techniques. J Urol 2002;167:469–475.
46. Bove P, Bhayani SB, Rha KH, Allaf ME, Jarrett TW, Kavoussi LR. Necessity of ureteral catheter during laparoscopic partial nephrectomy. J Urol 2004;172:458–460.
47. Gill IS, Columbo JR, Jr., Moinzadeh A, et al. Laparoscopic partial nephrectomy in solitary kidney. J Urol 2006;175: 454–458.
48. Wolf JS, Jr., Seifman BD, Montie JE. Nephron-sparing surgery for suspected malignancy: open surgery compared to laparoscopy with selective use of hand-assistance. J Urol 2000;163:1659–1664.
49. Schiff JD, Palese M, Vaughan ED, Jr., Sosa RE, Coll D, Del Pizzo JJ. Laparoscopic vs open partial nephrectomy in consecutive patients: the Cornell experience. BJU International 2005;96:811–814.
50. Nadu A, Mor Y, Laufer M, et al. Laparoscopic partial nephrectomy: single center experience with 140 patients – evolution of the surgical technique and its impact on patient outcomes. J Urol 2007;178:435–439.
51. Simmons MN, Gill IS. Decreased complications of contemporary laparoscopic partial nephrectomy: use of a standardized reporting system. J Urol 2007;177:2067–2073.
52. Zorn KC, Gong EM, Orvieto MA, Gofrit ON, Mikhail AA, Shalhav AL. Impact of collecting-system repair during laparoscopic partial nephrectomy. J Endourol 2007;21:315–20.
53. Gill IS, Kavoussi LR, Lane BR, et al. Comparison of 1,800 laparoscopic and open partial nephrectomies for single renal tumors. J Urol 2007;178:41–46.

Laparoscopic Nephroureterectomy

Jaime Landman

SUMMARY

The gold standard for management of patients with upper ureteral or renal transitional cell carcinoma (TCC), who have two kidneys and normal renal function, is radical nephroureterectomy with excision of an ipsilateral periureteral cuff of bladder. While highly efficacious for disease control, the open nephroureterectomy, which involves a long muscle splitting incision, results in significant pain and an extended convalescence. Laparoscopic radical nephroureterectomy was introduced by Clayman et al. *(1)*. Compared to open nephroureterectomy, the laparoscopic approach results in decreased post-operative analgesic requirements, a shorter hospital stay, and improved convalescence *(2–5)*. Despite these advantages to the patient, there are two drawbacks to the laparoscopic approach: lengthy operative time, and the need for significant laparoscopic experience on the part of the surgeon. These disadvantages may be partially offset by the application of hand-assisted technique for nephroureterectomy. Indeed, hand-assisted nephroureterectomy is the most commonly reported technique for performing minimally invasive nephroureterectomy. Herein are described the techniques for transperitoneal laparoscopic nephroureterectomy and hand-assisted nephroureterectomy. Management options for the distal ureter and ipsilateral bladder cuff are reviewed.

INTRODUCTION

Transitional cell carcinoma (TCC) of the renal pelvis is responsible for 4.5–9% of all renal tumors and accounts for 5–6% of all urothelial tumors *(6–10)*. Traditionally, the management of upper tract TCC has involved open nephroureterectomy including an ipsilateral bladder cuff which is performed either with two separate incisions (a flank or upper abdominal incision and a lower abdominal incision) or via one extended muscle splitting incision. Advances in minimally invasive technologies have provided viable alternative management strategies. Antegrade and retrograde endoscopic excision and ablation of TCC have been described, and are accepted conservative management strategies in highly selected cases, including patients with a solitary kidney, renal insufficiency, or patients who are a poor surgical risk *(11–14)*. Along with technological advances in ureteroscopy, the indications for upper tract TCC ablation have expanded to include small, less than 1.5 cm, low grade Ta lesions *(15,16)*. However, the majority of patients will ultimately require nephroureterectomy.

In 1990, the introduction of laparoscopic renal surgery by Clayman, Kavoussi and colleagues enabled traditional management strategies (i.e., radical ablative surgery) to be performed in a less invasive manner *(17)*. This same innovative group subsequently described application of laparoscopy

From: *Current Clinical Urology: Essential Urologic Laparoscopy*
Edited by: S. Y. Nakada and S. P. Hedican, DOI 10.1007/978-1-60327-820-1_11

for nephroureterectomy *(1)*. The laparoscopic approach for control of upper tract TCC has afforded the urologic surgeon the opportunity to perform a highly effective form of surgical cancer control, yet minimize post-operative pain and convalescence. With the addition of the hand-assisted devices, which facilitates tactile sensation, surgeons less experienced with laparoscopic technique have been able to offer laparoscopic nephroureterectomy to their patients *(18)*.

The major series describing the results of laparoscopic nephroureterectomy are listed in Tables 1 and 2. Table 1 reviews the experience of seven trials incorporating 241 patients undergoing laparoscopic or hand-assisted laparoscopic nephroureterectomy. These trials demonstrate that the procedure can be safely performed with limited blood loss and with a relatively expeditious convalescence.

Table 1
Non-comparative laparoscopic nephroureterectomy trials

Series	*Operative approach*	*n*	*OR time (h)*	*EBL (mL)*	*Analgesic (mg MSO$_4$)*	*Hospital stay (days)*	*Complete convalescence (weeks)*	*Follow-up (years)*	*Major complications (%)*
1. Stifelman et al. *(35)*	Hand-assist	22	4.5	180	55	4.1	2.7	1.1	5
2. Jarrett et al. *(36)*	Laparoscopic	25	5.5	440	NA	4.0	NA	>1	12
3. Lee et al.	Laparoscopic	18	3.0	351	NA	2.5	NA	1.66	5
4. Wolf et al. *(37)*	Hand-assist	54	4.6	330	NA	4.1	4.4	2.3	6
5. Cannon et al. *(38)*	Hand-assist	34	5.28	252	33	5	NA	1.16	6.8
6. Kurzer et al. *(39)*	Hand-assist	49	NA	200	NA	3	NA	0.8	9
7. Muntener *(40)*	Laparoscopic	39	5.2	300	NA	4	NA	6.0	10.2

NA – Data not available.

Table 2 reviews results of six comparative trials contrasting open nephroureterectomy and laparoscopic or hand-assisted nephroureterectomy. Overall, 161 open nephroureterectomies were compared to 195 laparoscopic or hand-assisted laparoscopic procedures. While operative time favored the open approach by a mean of 42 min, hospital stay and post-operative analgesic requirements were significantly decreased in the cohort undergoing laparoscopic nephroureterectomy. Most striking, however, full convalescence was expedited by more than 4 weeks with laparoscopic or hand-assisted laparoscopic nephroureterectomy.

Application of hand-assisted laparoscopy to nephroureterectomy may offer the urologic surgeon advantages. First, the technique provides the novice laparoscopist a logical segue into minimally invasive surgery by allowing one hand to remain in the realm of open surgery while the other hand and the surgeon's field of view are in a laparoscopic milieu. Second, the hand-assisted laparoscopic technique affords the laparoscopist the use of tactile sensation, blunt manual dissection, and broad retraction. Thus, hand-assist technique decreases operative time and may allow experienced laparoscopic surgeons to expand the scope of cases performed laparoscopically (i.e., larger and more extensive tumors). Furthermore, the aggressive nature of TCC precludes morcellation, thus intact removal of the kidney, ureter, and bladder cuff are mandatory. Given the mandatory incision for extraction, and the potential advantages of hand-assisted technique, hand-assisted laparoscopic nephroureterectomy is appealing.

A multi-center retrospective comparison of 11 patients undergoing standard laparoscopic and 17 patients undergoing hand-assisted laparoscopic nephroureterectomy for localized TCC was completed at Washington University *(19)*. In this series, the hand-assisted technique decreased operative time by 1 h without significantly affecting blood loss (Tables 3 and 4). Patients in both cohorts manifested

Table 2
Comparative nephroureterectomy trials (laparoscopic and hand-assisted laparoscopic versus open trials)

Series	*Operative approach*	*n*	*OR time (h)*	*EBL (mL)*	*Analgesic (mg MSO_4)*	*Hospital stay (days)*	*Complete convalescence (weeks)*	*Follow-up (years)*	*Major complications (%)*
1. Shalhav et al. *(41)*	Laparoscopic	25	7.7	199	37	3.6	2.8	2.0	8
	Open	17	3.9	441	144	9.6	10	3.6	29
2. Seifman, et al. *(42)*	Hand-assist	16	5.3	557	48	3.9	2.5	1.5	19
	Open	11	3.3	345	81	5.2	7.5	1.2	27
3. Keeley and Tolley *(43)*	Laparoscopic	22	2.4	NA	NA	5.5	NA	NA	NA
	Open	26	2.3	NA	NA	10.8	NA	NA	NA
4. Hattori et al. *(44)*	Hand-assist	36	5.1	580	NA	NA	5	5	2
	Pure laparoscopic	53	4.3	354	NA	NA	4	5	1
	Open	60	5.4	665	NA	NA	8	5	3
5. Rassweiller et al. *(45)*	Retroperitoneal laparoscopy	23	3.3	450	18	10	NA	5	9
	Open retro	21	3.1	600	33	13	NA	5	10
6. Roupert et al. *(46)*	LNU	20	2.7	274	NA	3.7	NA	5.75	15
	Open	26	2.6	338	NA	9.2	NA	6.5	15
Total	Laparoscopic	195	4.5	389	29.3	5.5	3.9	4.4	6.6
Total	Open	161	3.8	538	82	10.1	8.4	4.8	10.4

NA – Data not available.

Table 3
Comparison of hand-assisted and laparoscopic nephroureterectomy: operative parameters ***(19)***

Parameter	*Hand-assisted laparoscopy*	*Laparoscopy*	*P-value*
Laparoscopy time (h)	4.4	5.3	0.09
Cystoscopy time (min)	29	46	0.15
Total operative time (h)	4.9	6.1	0.055
Estimated blood loss (mL)	201	190	0.78
Specimen weight (g)	576	335	0.36

Table 4
Comparison of hand-assisted and laparoscopic nephroureterectomy: convalescence parameters ***(19)***

Parameter	*Hand-assisted laparoscopy*	*Laparoscopy*	*P-value*
Time to oral intake (h)	20	13	0.45
Analgesics (Mg MSO_4)	33.0	29.3	0.83
Hosptial stay (days)	4.5	3.3	0.59
Partial recovery (weeks)	3.5	2.4	0.29
Complete recovery (weeks)	8.0	5.2	0.27

similar short-term convalescence. While not achieving statistical significance in this small cohort, the time to return to full activity was expedited by 3 weeks in the standard laparoscopic group.

The advantages of laparoscopic and hand-assisted laparoscopic nephroureterectomy over open nephroureterectomy are clear. This chapter will describe a practical guide to performing these procedures including equipment suggestions, surgical technique, and alternative surgical management strategies for the distal ureter and bladder cuff.

SURGICAL TECHNIQUE

Patient Preparation and Positioning

Prior to performing laparoscopic or hand-assisted nephroureterectomy, informed consent must be obtained. Patients should be made aware of the risks and benefits of the laparoscopic approach. The discussion should include review of possible complications, including conversion to an open surgical approach due to reasons such as failure to progress, vascular injury, or bowel injury, post-operative paresthesias (i.e., brachial plexus of downside arm, sciatic stretch injury of upside leg), bowel injury with possible need for diversion, and other potential problems associated with laparoscopy (i.e., CO_2 embolism). Two units of packed red blood cells should be available in the operating room.

Preoperative staging of upper tact TCC includes a chest radiograph and a CAT scan as part of a metastatic evaluation. The CAT scan should be carefully evaluated for the following: liver metastases; lymphadenopathy; extension into surrounding organs; and to assess the adrenal glands. A bone scan, chest CT, or head CT are indicated if there is an increased suspicion for metastatic disease. Depending on the surgeon's level of experience, direct extension of the tumor into surrounding structures may preclude the laparoscopic approach. As TCC is a field defect of the urothelium, cystoscopy should be performed to evaluate the lower urinary tract for TCC. Lower tract lesions need to be addressed prior to performing a nephroureterectomy. This is especially true if the bladder is to be opened to handle the distal ureter, as this is a risk for tumor seeding. Preoperative blood work includes a serum creatinine, liver function studies, alkaline phosphatase, and calcium levels. If the last two values are elevated or the patient complains of site-specific bone pain, a bone scan is obtained.

With the routine availability of small caliber flexible ureteroscopes and improvements in biopsy devices such as the Bigopsy (Cook, Spencer, IN) and Piranha (Boston Scientific, Marlbourough, MA), tumor visualization and possible biopsy is recommended to preclude the possibility of alternative benign pathology (i.e., fibroepithelial polyp, sloughed papilla, etc.). Special care must be taken to avoid ureteral injury and potential tumor extravasation. The use of a ureteral access sheath for evaluation and biopsy of renal pelvic tumors is highly recommended, as the sheath will protect the ureter from injury during the procedure, and has been shown to decrease renal pelvic pressures during ureteroscopy *(20)*. Tissue biopsy can be facilitated by the application of a nitinol basket to entrap and "avulse" an adequate specimen for histopathologic evaluation. Frequently, a characteristic appearance by endoscopic tumor inspection is adequate for diagnosis if other clinical evidence of malignancy is available (i.e., positive urinary cytology). As such, when there is a high degree of preoperative suspicion for upper tract TCC, it is possible to perform the ureteroscopic evaluation and the laparoscopic nephroureterectomy under a single anesthetic.

Bowel preparation with a bottle of magnesium citrate and a clear liquid diet for 24 h prior to surgery is advised, and a Dulcolax suppository is administered on the day prior to surgery. If the patient has a previous history of abdominal surgery or radiation, a full antibiotic and mechanical bowel preparation may be indicated. One gram of cefazolin is administered preoperatively. All patients should have pneumatic compression boots placed and activated prior to induction of anesthesia.

General endotracheal anesthesia is induced and the patient's stomach and bladder are decompressed with an orogastric tube and a Foley catheter, respectively. Due to the prolonged length of the procedure early in the learning curve, proper patient positioning and padding are of utmost importance. The patient is carefully positioned in a 70-degree flank position with the affected kidney on the upside. If hand-assisted laparoscopy is planned, the prepared surgical area must be extended to accommodate the external component of the hand-assist device (i.e., extended past the midline to the patient's right side for left-sided nephroureterectomy). The operating table is fully flexed and the kidney rest is fully raised beneath the iliac crest. The downside leg is flexed at the knee and separated from the extended up-side leg by pillows; the upside leg is placed on a sufficient number of pillows until it is level with the flank, thereby precluding any strain on the upside leg when the table is flexed and the kidney rest raised. The downside heel, hip, and knee are cushioned. The downside arm is padded and an axillary roll is carefully positioned. The upside arm is placed on a well-padded arm-board; the arm-board is positioned such that there is no tension on the brachial plexus. Once the patient has been properly positioned, he/she is secured to the operating table by padded safety straps that are passed over the chest, hip, and knee. As patient rotation is sometimes very helpful during laparoscopic procedures, securing the patient to the table is of great importance. After the patient has been secured, the table should be rotated steeply in both directions to assure the patient remains completely immobilized.

Access: Laparoscopic and Hand-Assisted Laparoscopic Nephroureterectomy

Laparoscopic Nephroureterectomy

Laparoscopic access can be obtained via a direct vision (Hasson) or Veress needle technique. Templates for trocar positioning for both right and left renal access are presented in Figs. 1 and 2. However, each patient's individual body habitus must be considered for thoughtful trocar deployment. In the virgin abdomen, a site medial and superior to the anterior superior iliac spine is typically used for primary access. Alternatively, if there has been prior surgery in the lower abdomen, the subcostal trocar site is suitable for primary access. A 12-mm incision is made approximately two fingerbreadths medial and

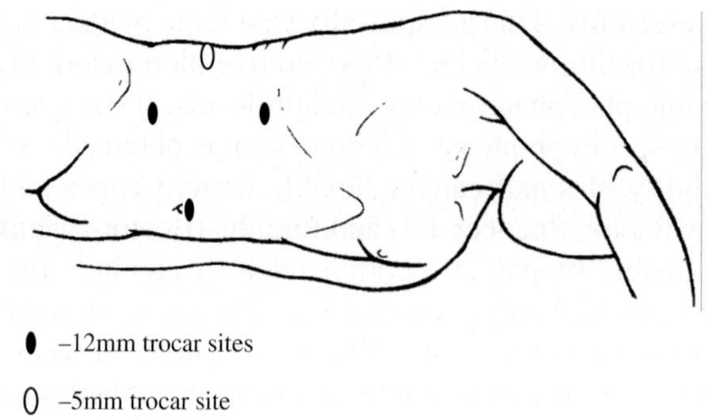

Fig. 1. Template for trocar sites used for right transperitoneal laparoscopic nephroureterectomy.

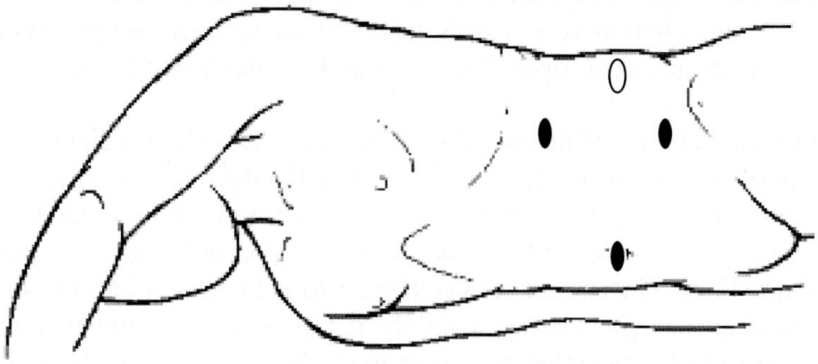

Fig. 2. Template for trocar sites used for left transperitoneal laparoscopic nephroureterectomy.

cranial to the anterior superior iliac spine. The subcutaneous tissue is spread with a Kelly clamp and a Veress needle pneumoperitoneum of 25 mm Hg is obtained. A 12-mm trocar is placed at this same site, and after access to the abdominal cavity has been obtained, the abdominal pressure is immediately reduced to 12 mmHg. A dilating trocar (blunt tip for penetrating the fascia) is preferred to a cutting trocar. A number of dilating trocars are commercially available, however, a visual dilating trocar affords the surgeon the additional advantage of direct vision dilation when desired. Occasionally, in the non-virgin or morbidly obese abdomen, visual dilation can be useful for obtaining access. Dilating trocars may reduce the probability of injury to the abdominal wall vasculature, and usually do not require closure as they result in smaller fascial defects (the defect is one-half the size of the diameter of the trocar).

A 10-mm 30° laparoscope is inserted and the underlying bowel is closely inspected for any injury that may have occurred during Veress needle or trocar placement. Subsequently, two additional 12-mm trocars are placed under direct endoscopic vision. A second trocar is placed 2 cm below the costal margin in the midclavicular line. The third trocar is placed either at the umbilicus or immediately lateral to the margin of the rectus abdominus muscle approximately 3–5 fingerbreadths above the umbilicus. This medial trocar site is used during the majority of the case for the laparoscope as it is midway between the two "working" trocar sites and thus it provides the surgeon with the most intuitive perspective on the operative field. Lastly, after mobilization of the colon from the abdominal sidewall, a fourth trocar (5 mm) is placed subcostally in the posterior axillary line. When all trocars have been placed, the primary access site is inspected laparoscopically as this is the only site of "blind" access.

Although trocar placement templates are helpful, the laparoscopic surgeon must tailor trocar placement to the individual patient. Patients with previous surgery should have primary access established

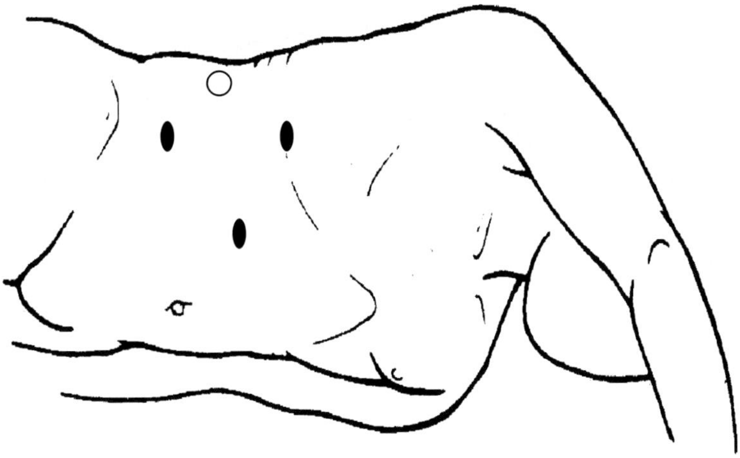

Fig. 3. Modified template for trocar sites for right transperitoneal laparoscopic nephroureterectomy in patient with alternative body habitus.

away from scar sites to avoid adhesions that may increase the probability of injury to underlying structures. Similarly, patient body habitus may alter trocar positioning. Figure 3 demonstrates movement of the optical trocar site medially which helps avoid the pannus in the obese patent. In this situation, care should be taken to remain lateral to the rectus abdominus muscle to avoid injury to the inferior epigastric vessels.

If a complete laparoscopic approach to the distal cuff with scissor excision and intracorporeal suture reconstruction is planned, the trocar configurations can be adjusted slightly. In these cases, the authors move the entire template 2 cm caudad. Additionally, the 5-mm lateral trocar site that is used for lateral retraction during the renal component of the nephroureterectomy is placed slightly more lateral and inferior to its standard position (near the anterior superior iliac spine) so that it can be used for suturing during the bladder reconstruction.

HAND-ASSISTED NEPHROURETERECTOMY

Primary access for hand-assisted procedures is gained by creating the hand-assist incision. Figures 4 and 5 demonstrate templates for hand-assist device and trocar placement sites for right- and left-sided nephroureterectomy. Prior to positioning for the procedure, the hand-assist incision site is marked, as the location of the skin incision may be difficult to discern with the patient in the lateral decubitus position (Fig. 6). The length of the hand-assist incision is equal to the surgeon's glove size

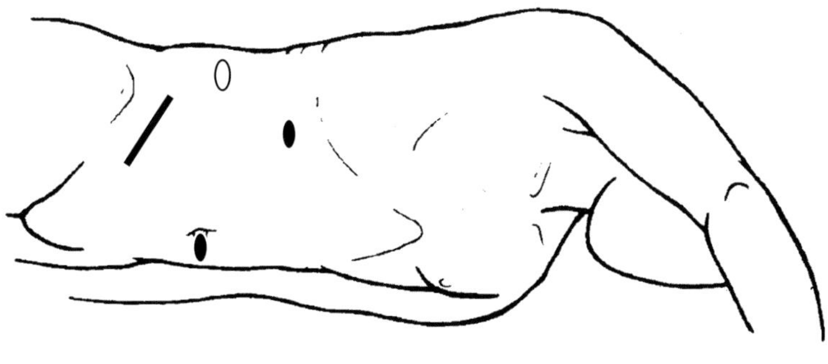

Fig. 4. Template for trocar sites used for right hand-assisted laparoscopic nephroureterectomy.

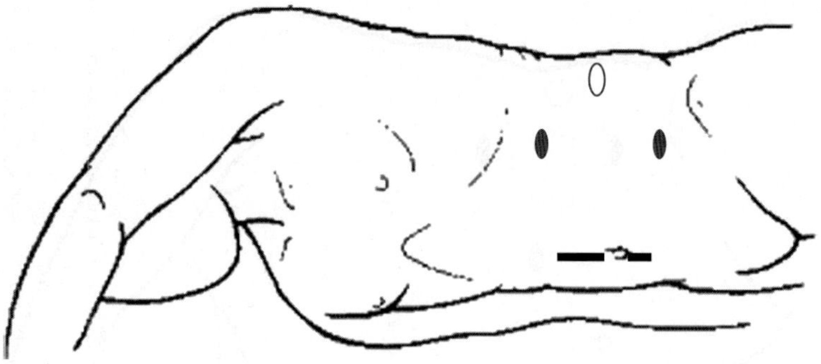

Fig. 5. Template for trocar sites used for left hand-assisted laparoscopic nephroureterectomy.

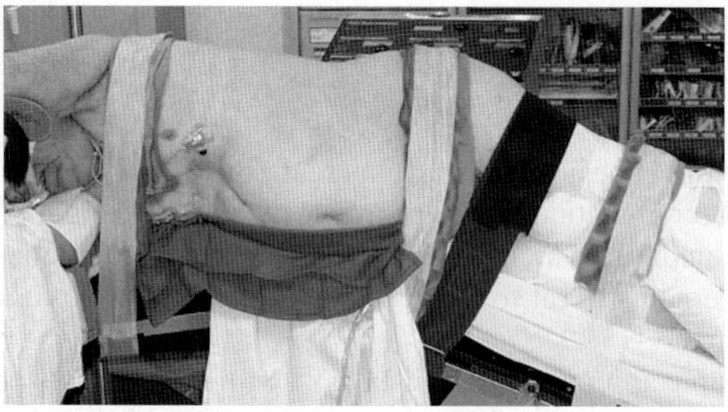

Fig. 6. Photograph of patient in the modified lateral decubitus position in preparation for left laparoscopic or hand-assisted nephroureterectomy.

in centimeters. Alternatively, some devices come supplied with a measuring template. Presently, there are a number of hand-assist devices available from different manufacturers. If there has been previous surgery at the anticipated site of hand-assist device placement, the surgeon may insufflate the abdomen at a virgin site (i.e., anterior superior iliac spine or subcostal trocar sites). After a primary trocar site has been established, the abdomen may be inspected for adhesions at the planned hand-assist device site. If present, adhesions may be lysed at the proposed hand-assist device location and prior to device placement.

Instrumentation

Basic instrumentation for laparoscopic nephrectomy includes a standard laparoscopic tower (a carbon dioxide insufflator, light source, camera, monitor, and suction–irrigation setup). A complete list of useful disposable and non-disposable equipment is presented in Table 5. A 10-mm laparoscope with a 30-degree lens can be exclusively used as the angled lens facilitates direct laparoscopic vision during challenging portions of the dissection such as the renal hilum.

The majority of dissection during the case can be performed expeditiously and safely with the use of ultrasound and bipolar energy. While there are many excellent energy devices available, the authors prefer to use ultrasound energy using a 5-mm curved end-effector (Harmonic ACE, Ethicon Endo-Surgery, Cincinnati, OH) in the dominant hand. This instrument allows for expeditious dissection with acceptable hemostasis. In the non-dominant hand, a 5-mm bipolar grasper (Aesculap, Center Valley,

Table 5
Laparoscopic instrumentation for laparoscopic nephroureterectomy

Disposable equipment:
End-effectors
Laparoscopic stapler (U.S. Surgical or Ethicon)
Clip appliers (11-mm titanium clips) (U.S. Surgical or Ethicon)
Harmonic ACE (5 mm curved jaws) (Ethicon)[a]
Endocatch II (15 mm) entrapment sack (Ethicon)
Others
Trocars (three 12- and 1 5-mm)
Veress needles (150 mm)
Hand-assisted device (Applied Medical Resources or Ethicon Endosurgery)
Non-disposable equipment:
End-effectors
Bipolar grasping forceps (Aesculap)[a]
Suction irrigator, extra long, 5 mm (Nezhat system: Storz)
Maryland grasping forceps 5 mm (2)
5-mm Endoshears
5-mm PEER retractor (Jarit)[a]
10-mm right angle dissector (Storz or Jarit)
Others
Laparoscope: 10 mm 30° lens
Endoholder (Codman)[a]
Open surgical tray (not open, but available for emergent conversion)

[a]Speciality instruments that greatly facilitate laparoscopic nephroureterectomy.

PA) (Fig. 7) serves well for both tissue manipulation (simple grasping) and for control of small to medium sized vessels that the harmonic scalpel does not easily control. The Aesculap bipolar grasper (Macrobipolar) is particularly useful as it is an excellent grasping device, has a well-engineered reticulating mechanism, and is ergonomically designed for the surgeon's hand. The simultaneous application of two energy end-effectors facilitates expeditious and safe dissection. Ultrasound and bipolar energy sources are preferred to monopolar energy as the peripheral thermal damage from the harmonic scalpel (0–1 mm) and bipolar end-effectors (2–6 mm) are known to be limited in comparison with monopolar energy (up to 10 mm) *(21)*. Monopolar electrosurgical energy with a right-angled hook end-effector is, however, occasionally useful for delicate dissection of hilar structures. This instrument allows the surgeon to perform safe, fine dissection by engaging and retracting small strands of tissue around vascular structures prior to the application of energy.

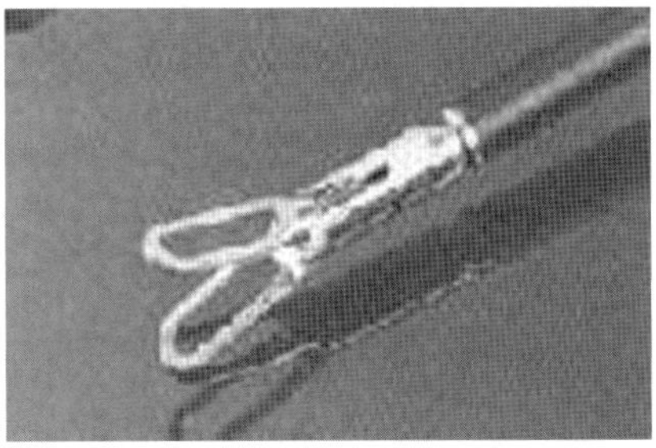

Fig. 7. Bipolar grasping forceps (Aesculap).

The 5-mm lateral trocar site is particularly important as it facilitates retraction of the specimen or surrounding structures. For retraction, the PEER retractor (J. Jamner Surgical Instruments) is useful and reliable (Fig. 8). The PEER retractor can be used in conjuction with the Endoholder (Codman) (Fig. 9) that allows consistent safe retraction. These instruments are invaluable as they both allow the surgeon complete control on the amount of retraction on vulnerable structures (i.e., liver and spleen) and avoid the inevitable fatigue of even the most diligent assistant. Application of these instruments for retraction allows the surgeon the use of both hands for dissection and tissue manipulation.

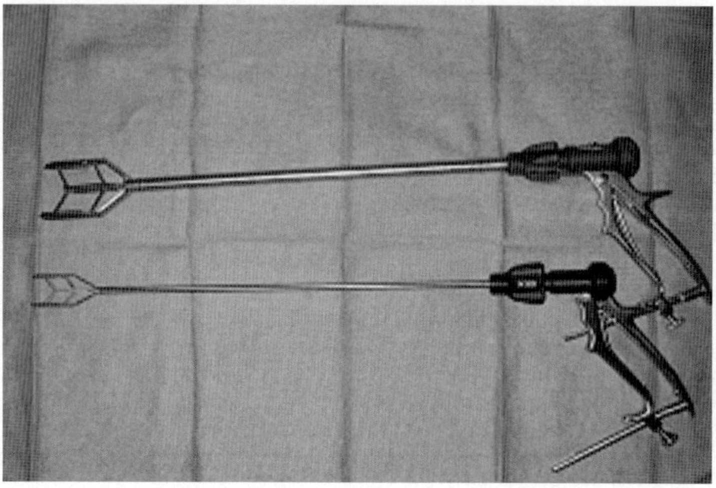

Fig. 8. The PEER retractors: 5- and 10-mm size. The 5-mm size opens to 2×3 cm surface area and the 10-mm size opens to a 4×3 cm surface area.

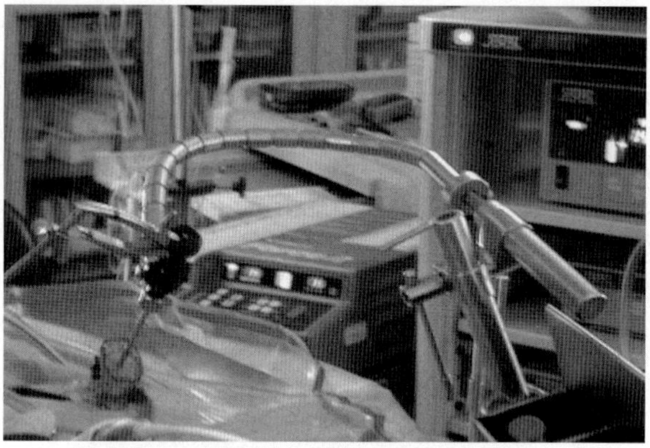

Fig. 9. The Endoholder by Codman holding the PEER retractor during a laparoscopic procedure.

Control of major arteries and veins is achieved with titanium clips or staples. Typically, an 11-mm titanium clip applier is used for clipping the renal artery and a stapler with a vascular load is used for division of the renal vein. Alternatively, a vascular stapler can be used for both the artery and the vein. The majority of smaller vessels (i.e., the gonadal vein, adrenal vein, and distal lumbar veins) may be controlled with the harmonic scalpel on the variable setting.

As *morcellation of the specimen is contraindicated* due to the biologically aggressive nature of TCC, entrapment of the specimen after mobilization is safely and easily performed with the Endocatch II (15 mm) sack (Ethicon Endosurgery) or with a LapSac (Cook, Spencer, Indiana). These sacks are large enough for the majority of specimens (up to 1,000 g) and the Endocatch device includes a simple deployment mechanism for the bag that allows the surgeon to "scoop-up" the specimen. The sack's deployment mechanism does, however, have a 15-mm diameter requiring trocar extraction and minimal dilation of the fascia. While easy to use, special care must be taken, as the sack may prematurely eject from the deployment mechanism. Additionally, the sack is made of plastic and is easily perforated by excessive tension, sharp edges, or electrosurgery (heating of peripheral structures may melt the plastic). Even with hand-assisted nephroureterectomy the use of an entrapment sack is recommended as application of the sack avoids contact between the specimen and the incision site. Additionally, the slick surface of the sack may facilitate the extraction and thus help minimize the size of the extraction incision.

Surgical Technique: Laparoscopic and Hand-Assisted Laparoscopic Nephroureterectomy – Right Side

After gaining access, the peritoneal cavity is closely inspected, and the liver is visualized for mass lesions. With hand-assisted nephroureterectomy, palpation of abdominal structures is possible. The outline of the kidney within Gerota's fascia is commonly visible behind the ascending colon.

Step 1: Peritoneal Incisions and Pararenal Dissection

The key to en bloc resection of the kidney within Gerota's fascia lies in defining the borders of the dissection. On the right side, the dissection follows an anatomic template with a "wedge-shaped" configuration (Fig. 10). While traditional teaching describes mobilization of the line of Toldt, this line is located quite laterally. Attention should be turned to the thin mesentery extending from the line of Toldt, draped over Gerota's fascia, and attaching medially to the lateral edge of the ascending colon. Gentle traction with a laparoscopic grasper will allow the surgeon to laparoscopically visualize this thin mesentery sliding over Gerota's fascia. Meticulous adherence to the plane between this filmy mesentery and Gerota's allows this portion of the procedure to proceed expeditiously and almost bloodlessly. There is a tendency to "wander" medially into the fatty mesenteric tissue that will result in increased bleeding. If the dissection appears to have more "oozing" than usual, it is likely that the proper plane has been abandoned. Re-evaluation of the surgical planes or attempting to enter this plane in a virgin area will usually allow the colonic mobilization to proceed in a bloodless fashion.

The dissection is initiated using a 5-mm curved harmonic scalpel and the bipolar grasping forceps for counter-traction. With the hand-assisted technique, placing a gauze pad in the abdominal cavity will provide superior tissue traction as well as assistance with hemostasis. The harmonic ACE is preferred for the majority of the dissection. The colon is mobilized medially beginning over the lower pole area of Gerota's fascia, where the plane between the colon and specimen is usually most distinct. Care must be taken to stay at least 1 cm from the edge of the colon to prevent thermal or mechanical injury. The colon should be mobilized from the pelvic brim with the incision is extending upward above the specimen through the triangular ligament to the diaphragm. This incision defines the medial upper border of the broad side of the "wedge". The colon is thus completely mobilized away from the kidney. The time spent in complete mobilization of the colon is particularly well invested, as it later defines a broad field for hilar dissection and prevents the surgeon from working "in a hole." The lateral border of the kidney and its lateral retroperitoneal attachments are not disturbed; this results in the kidney remaining firmly attached to the abdominal sidewall thereby facilitating the hilar dissection later in the procedure.

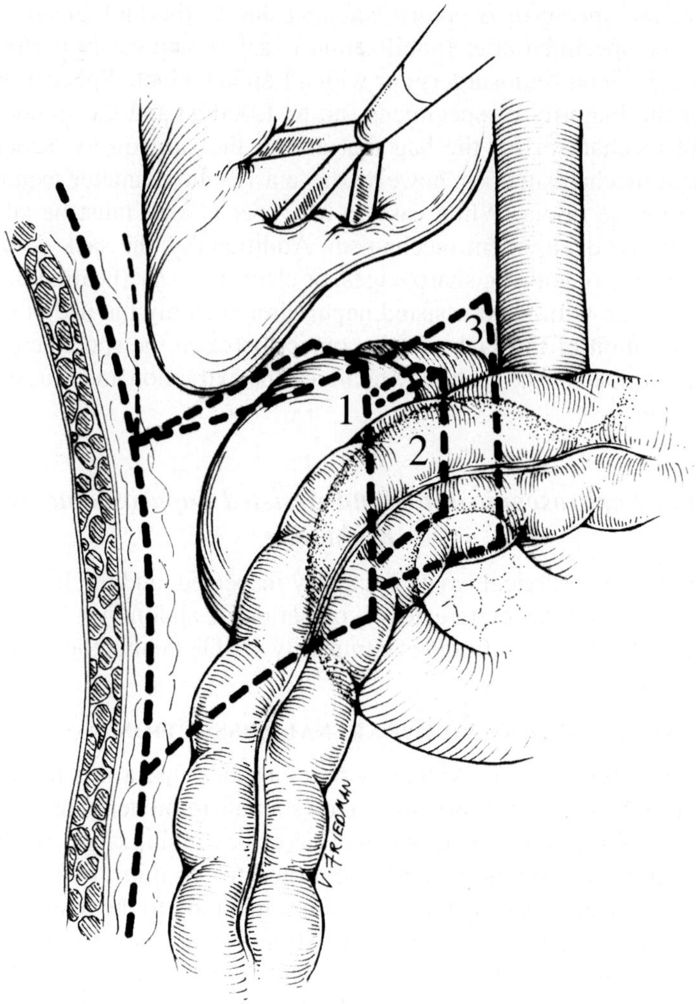

Fig. 10. Diagram of the right-sided nephrectomy demonstrating the wedge-shaped configuration. The numbers refer to the three distinct levels of dissection along the medial aspect of the kidney: colon; duodenum; and inferior vena cava.

The broad side of the wedge comprises three distinct levels of dissection along the medial aspect of the kidney: (1) the mobilized ascending colon; (2) Kocher maneuver on the duodenum to move it medially; and (3) dissection of the anterior and lateral surfaces of the inferior vena cava (IVC) (Fig. 11). As the colon is mobilized, special attention should be directed at identification of the duodenum. The duodenum may appear flattened against the medial aspect of the kidney; it is very important to move slowly during this part of the dissection in order to clearly identify the duodenum. The duodenum will always be identified before the anterior surface of the vena cava can be isolated. To facilitate development of the deepest plane of dissection (i.e., the IVC dissection), it is helpful to first define the superior side of the wedge by incising the posterior coronary hepatic ligament from the line of Toldt, laterally; to the level of the inferior vena cava, medially; at this cephalad level, the surgeon will come directly onto the lateral and anterior surface of the inferior vena cava well above the duodenum and the adrenal gland. This incision in the posterior coronary hepatic ligament provides access to the inferior vena cava well above the adrenal gland. This portion of the dissection is facilitated by inferior

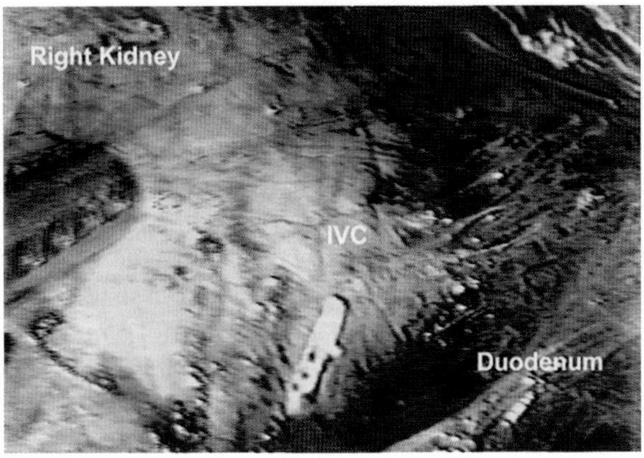

Fig. 11. Laparoscopic view of the duodenum Kocherized. The dissection of the IVC which is identified in the center of the figure is next. At this point, the ascending colon and hepatic flexure, which were initially mobilized, lie medial to the duodenum.

and lateral traction on the renal specimen with the PEER retractor. If hand-assisted technique is used, the surgeon's non-dominant hand can be used to retract the liver superiorly and medially providing excellent exposure. At this point, the en bloc area of dissection of the specimen has been completely defined, ensuring removal of the kidney within Gerota's fascia, along with the pararenal and perirenal fat, the adrenal gland, and an anterior patch of peritoneum.

Step 2: Identifying the Proximal Ureter

The dissection on the inferior vena cava (IVC) is continued caudally until the entry of the gonadal vein is identified. The gonadal vein can be traced distally from the vena cava; the right ureter usually lies just posterior and lateral to the right gonadal vein. It is carefully dissected from the retroperitoneal tissues. After the ureter has been dissected, the lower pole of the kidney can be easily mobilized below the renal hilum. By mobilizing the lower pole early in the procedure, the hilar dissection can be performed with both the inferior and lateral aspects of the hilum being exposed simultaneously. The combined inferior and lateral approach assures that the hilar dissection is in a wide and open surgical field, thus minimizing the risk and making small bleeding sites easier to identify and control.

Step 3: Securing the Adrenal Vein

Continued cephalad dissection of the IVC exposes the renal hilum and adrenal vein. The adrenal vein is dissected from the surrounding tissue and in most circumstances can be safely secured with the harmonic scalpel using the variable setting. The adrenal vein may alternatively be controlled with titanium clips. If clips are used, the adrenal vein is cut such that two clips remain on the caval side. Alternatively, if the supra-adrenal area just medial to the inferior vena cava has been cleanly dissected, and the lateral border of the supra-adrenal IVC has been clearly identified, then an Endo-GIA vascular load can be used to secure all of the tissue medial to the adrenal and lateral to the IVC. This maneuver will result in the "taking" of the adrenal vein in the 3 cm line of vascular staples.

If preoperative staging suggests the tumor does not involve the adrenal gland, this structure may be spared. The upper medial border of the kidney is identified by incision of Gerota's fascia in this area. Once the renal parenchyma of the medial and anterior part of the upper pole is seen, an Endo-GIA stapler can be used to further define the margin of dissection from medial (i.e., IVC side) to lateral below the adrenal gland, thereby preserving the adrenal gland and adrenal vein.

Step 4: The Renal Hilum

Attention is then turned to the dissection of the right renal vein from the surrounding tissue. Lateral retraction with the PEER retractor held in position by the Endoholder can greatly facilitate hilar dissection by "opening" the operative field. If the IVC has been cleanly dissected, the take off of the renal vein is usually quite evident. Attention is usually turned to circumferential dissection of the renal vein. During laparoscopic nephroureterectomy, the CAT scan can be invaluable in helping determine the location of the renal artery. The artery is located posterior to the vein, but may be cephalad, caudad or directly posterior to this structure. Alternatively, with hand-assisted nephroureterectomy, the artery is localized by digital palpation. Mobilization of the renal artery must be adequate for comfortable placement of five 11-mm vascular clips. The artery is then divided between the second and third clips to leave three clips proximally. Alternatively, the artery can be controlled with a stapler (vascular load). The renal vein is then secured with an vascular stapler (3-cm load).

Occasionally, an adequate length of the renal artery cannot be exposed in the presence of the overlying renal vein. In this situation one or two clips can be applied across the artery to occlude the artery without transection. With the main renal artery occluded, the renal vein is divided with the Endo-GIA stapler. The artery is then further dissected and divided after five clips are applied as previously described. When using the stapler, it is imperative that the device not be deployed over titanium or plastic clips. Deploying the device on clips will cause it to "jam" such that it cannot be opened *(22)*.

If the Endo-GIA stapler should "jam" in this manner, the surgeon must fight the urge to pull the stapler as this will avulse the vessel within the jaws. The stapler can only be released by proximal dissection and application of another stapler. Alternatively, if proximal dissection in not possible, the patient should be converted to open surgery. Once the hilar vasculature has been controlled, the PEER retractor can be readjusted to further pull the specimen laterally, and the dissection should proceed medially to the specimen to identify the psoas muscle and the back wall of the abdomen. This maneuver facilitates clear separation and distinction between the specimen and the remaining stumps of the artery and vein, and prevents subsequent dissection from inadvertently involving these structures. If a laparoscopic ultrasound device is available, the use of the doppler setting can be used to confirm that renal arterial control is complete prior to transecting the renal vein.

Step 5: Distal Ureteral Dissection

The specimen, within Gerota'a fascia, is then freed from the retroperitoneum using the harmonic scalpel and blunt dissection. At this time, the lateral attachments of the kidney to the abdominal sidewall, which were kept intact at the beginning of the procedure, are incised freeing the renal specimen. The patient can be placed in the Trendelenberg position allowing gravity to facilitate the deep pelvic dissection. The ureter is grasped and gentle cephalad traction placed while the harmonic scalpel is used to dissect this structure from surrounding tissues. With hand-assisted technique this portion of the procedure is expedited by blunt finger dissection. The dissection proceeds caudally over the iliac vessels, toward the superior vesical vessels which should be identified to avert injury. Currently, at Columbia University, the distal ureteral dissection relies on good retraction with the PEER that had been inserted earlier at the time of the kidney dissection. In contrast to the standard laparoscopic nephrectomy, where the PEER is placed laterally in the mid-axillary line, between the two working trocars, the PEER is placed inferiorly, in line with the lower working trocar. The PEER's inferior position enables the surgeon to use it later in the case as a working site for dissection of the distal ureter. The PEER is best used for retracting bowel structures inferior and medially. An additional 5-mm trocar can be used by the assistant to grasp and place cephalad traction on the ureter, so the surgeon can dissect this distal components of this structure. Placing the table in a steep Trendelenberg position also may help maintain the bowel from obscuring the distal ureteral dissection.

Step 6: Excision of Distal Ureter and Bladder Cuff

There are several techniques for distal ureteral management which are reviewed in subsequent sections. The ureter is dissected free from its attachments into the pelvis toward the bladder. Once the superior vesical artery is identified it is ligated either with clips or with an energy device at the same level it crosses the dissected ureter. The ureter is dissected caudally until the detrusor muscle fibers at the ureterovesical junction are identified. Grasping forceps are passed through the lower anterior axillary-line port, and the ureter is retracted superiorly and laterally, tenting up the wall of the bladder at the ureterovesical junction. A 12-mm laparoscopic tissue stapler (Endo-GIA; Auto-Suture, Norwalk, CT or Endocutter, Ethicon Endosurgery, Cincinnati, OH) is used to simultaneously divide the distal ureteral stump, excise the bladder cuff and close the cystostomy *(23)*. Indigo carmine is administered intravenously to assure that the contralateral ureteral orifice has not been divided. The bladder is then filled with saline via a Foley catheter to rule out any extravasation. If there is a hole along the staple line, it is sutured closed, either manually or with a Lapra-Ty stitch (Ethicon Inc., Piscataway, NJ).

Alternatively, for patients with a long torso or who are very obese in which pelvic reconstruction in the flank position is very challenging, the Washington University technique for distal ureteral management may be applied *(24)*. The Washington University technique includes fine dissection of the distal ureter which will frequently allow some of the intramural ureter to be mobilized. A laparoscopic stapler (tissue load) is then applied to the distal ureter/bladder cuff to free the specimen. This technique can be facilitated by application of a stapler with a reticulating head. The reticulating stapler may improve staple deployment and simplify subsequent ureteral unroofing.

Step 7: Specimen Entrapment and Intact Extraction

The specimen is most easily controlled by grasping the ureter with the subcostal 12-mm trocar site. The patient is maintained in the Trendelenberg position and the kidney placed over the edge of the liver. The inferior trocar is then removed, and a 15-mm Endocatch II or a LapSac is introduced and opened just beneath the liver; the self-opening design of this entrapment sack facilitates the entrapment process. The Endocatch II entrapment sack deployment mechanism has a 15 mm diameter and cannot be passed through a 12-mm trocar. As such, the trocar is removed and the barrel of the 15-mm entrapment sack deployment mechanism is gently passed through the trocar incision site under direct endoscopic vision. We have found that deployment of the Endocatch through the trocar site is facilitated by slightly deploying the bag which gives the instrument a slightly less blunt tip.

For intact specimen removal during pure laparoscopy, the surgeon should fight the urge to "connect the dots" by extending or connecting existing trocar incisions. It is recommended to make a lower midline abdominal, Gibson, or a Pfannenstiel incision. Specimen extraction can also be preformed by extending the inferior working trocar site. Along with the Gibson and Pfannenstiel, another method for the hand-assisted technique is extending the hand port incision. In a study by Tisdale and colleagues, that compared extending the hand port incision with a Pfannenstiel incision for tumor extraction, they found a significant decrease in the post-operative analgesia requirement with the Pfannenstiel incision compared to an extended hand port incision. There was, however, no difference in operative time, hospital stay, and time to oral intake *(25)*.

Irrespective of the method, the specimen is then extracted intact within an entrapment sack. Although all attempts are made to minimize the extraction incision, only gentle traction should be placed on the specimen to avoid rupturing the entrapment sack. Once the specimen is extracted, the entire operative field is inspected for hemostasis. As the pneumoperitoneum is an effective form of venous tamponade, the insufflation pressure is reduced to 5 mmHg and the entire operative field inspected once again prior to closure of the abdominal incisions. If dilating trocars are used fascial closure of these sites is not required. With the hand-assisted technique, the incision is closed in a traditional fashion as per surgeon preference. All skin incisions are closed with subcuticular sutures.

STEP 8: IF THE DISTAL URETER HAS BEEN MANAGED WITH THE WASHINGTON UNIVERSITY TECHNIQUE, CYSTOSCOPIC MANAGEMENT OF THE DISTAL URETER/BLADDER CUFF IS PERFORMED

After wound closure, the patient is re-positioned into the cystolithotomy position and rigid cystoscopy is performed. If staples are visualized in the bladder, the area around the ipsilateral ureteral orifice is fulgurated and the procedure can be terminated. More commonly, the ureteral orifice is visualized and a ureteral catheter is gently placed into the remaining short intramural ureteral segment (Fig. 12a and b). An Orandi knife or alternatively a 1,000 μ holmium laser fiber is then used to "unroof" the intramural ureter over the ureteral catheter (Fig. 13a and b). Unroofing proceeds until the staples are identified. After staple identification, a resectoscope with a roller-ball electrode is introduced and the ureteral tunnel and surrounding urothelium are fulgurated for a radius of 1 cm around the site of unroofing (Fig. 14a and b). A Foley catheter is left to drain the bladder for 48 h.

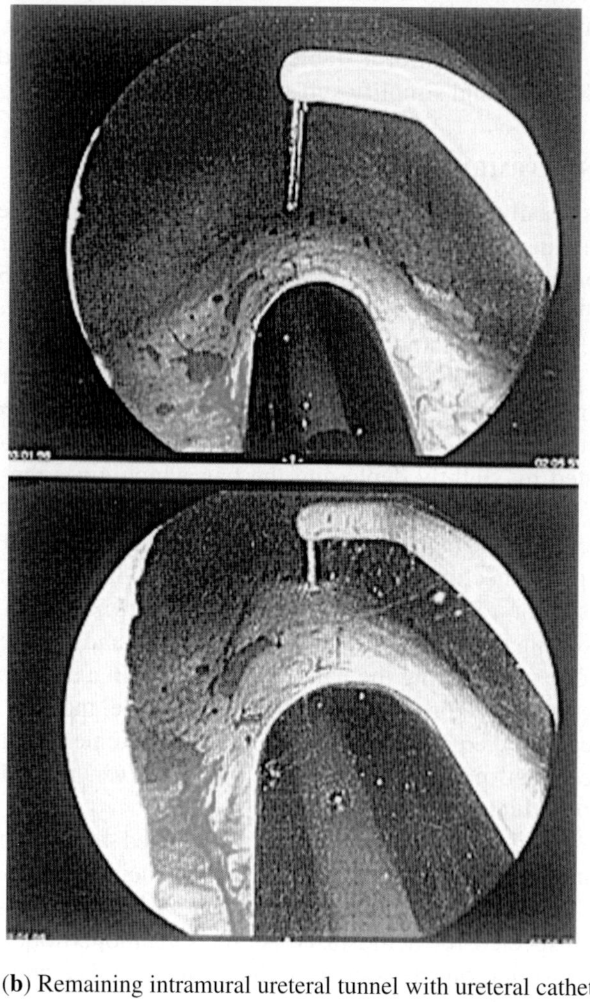

Fig. 12. (**a**) and (**b**) Remaining intramural ureteral tunnel with ureteral catheter in positon.

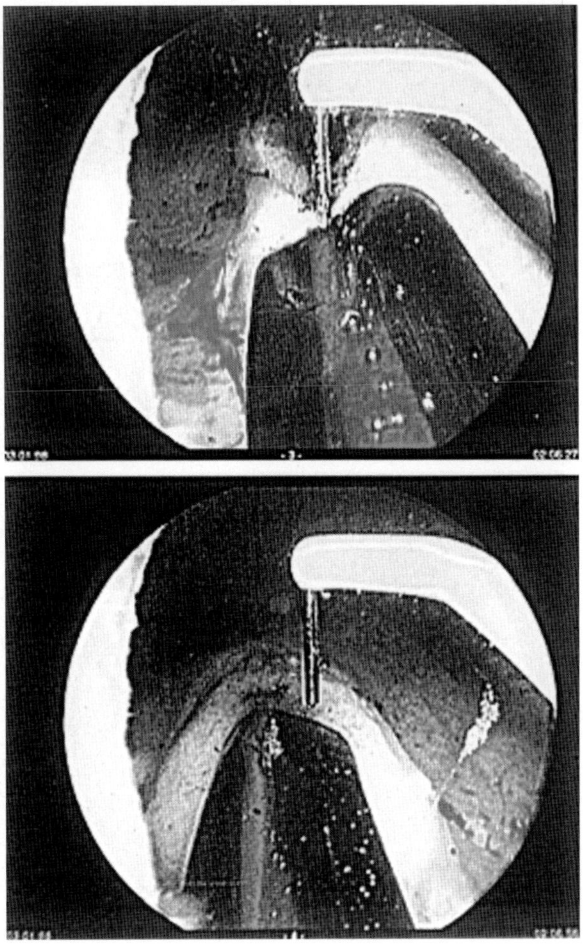

Fig. 13. (**a**) and (**b**) The Orandi knife is used to "unroof" the ureteral tunnel until staples from the Endo-GIA stapler used to transect the distal ureter are identified.

Left Side

After laparoscopic abdominal inspection, the outline of the left kidney within Gerota's fascia can commonly be identified beneath the descending colon.

STEP 1: PERITONEAL INCISIONS AND PARARENAL DISSECTION

The template for anatomic dissection of the left kidney assumes the configuration of an inverted cone (Fig. 15). The lateral side of the cone is formed by the line of Toldt that is incised from the pelvic brim, cephalad to the level of the diaphragm. On the left side, the colon should be mobilized from the iliac vessels to the diaphragm as previously described. However, even in the virgin abdomen, there are usually adhesions from the splenic flexure of the descending colon to the anterior abdominal wall; these attachments need to be released with the harmonic scalpel in order to carry the incision in the line of Toldt cephalad alongside the spleen and up to the diaphragm. This cephalad incision serves to release any splenophrenic attachments thereby mobilizing the spleen from the abdominal sidewall. The spleen should be mobilized such that it rotates medially by gravity away from the operative field. Adequate splenic mobilization early in the procedure opens the area of the renal hilum facilitating this dissection, and helps prevent inadvertent splenic injury. During this portion of the dissection excellent

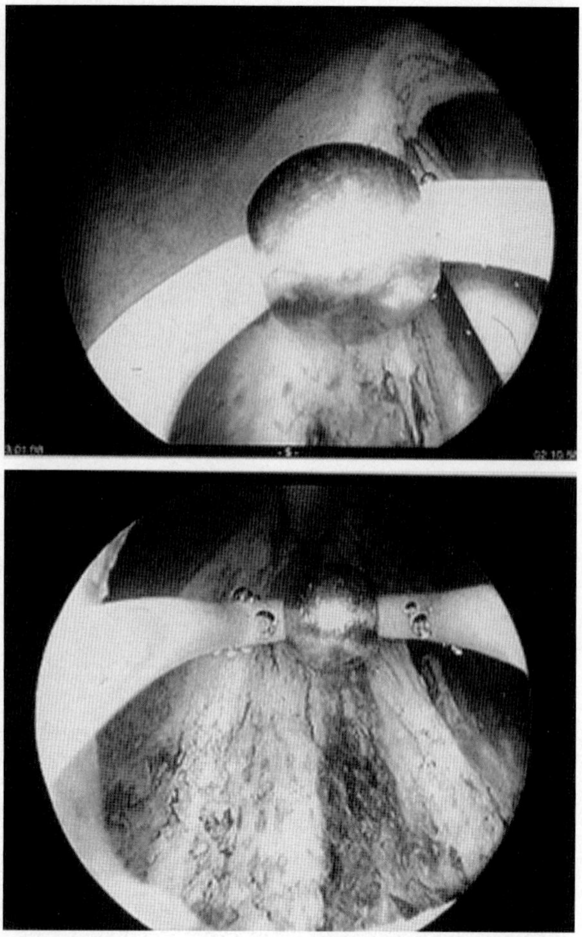

Fig. 14. (**a**) and (**b**) After staples have been identified, a roller-ball electrode is used to fulgurate the area around the ureteral orifice.

exposure can be gained by medial and inferior traction on the specimen with the PEER retractor. If the hand-assisted technique is employed, the surgeon's hand can gently retract the spleen superiorly and medially to further delineate the proper plane of dissection.

The medial aspect of the cone is then formed by retracting the peritoneal reflection of the descending colon medially and developing the plane between Gerota's fascia and the colonic mesentery. As with the right-sided dissection, this natural plane between the mesentery of the descending colon and Gerota's fascia is most easily identified and entered along the lower pole of the kidney or just inferior to the kidney.

The anterior upper curve of the cone is formed by the spleno-colic ligament, which is incised in order to fully mobilize the descending colon medially. The posterior upper curve of the cone is formed by the spleno-renal ligament that is incised to further release the spleen and thus precludes any inadvertent tearing of the splenic capsule. Incision of the splenorenal ligament may be difficult at this early stage of the procedure and, if need be, can be performed later in the procedure after the renal vessels have been secured. The dissection then follows the plane between the spleen and the superior portion of Gerota's fascia. At this point, the en bloc area of dissection has been defined and incorporates all of Gerota's fascia, the pararenal and perirenal fat, and the adrenal gland.

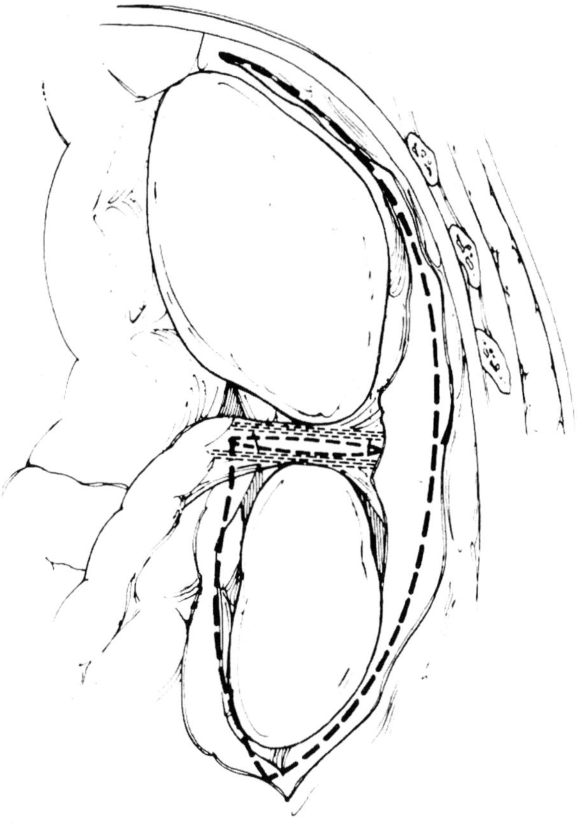

Fig. 15. Diagram demonstrating the inverted cone template for en bloc dissection during left laparoscopic nephroureterectomy. Unlike on the right side, the reflection of the colon comes to the lateral sidewall and thus an incision in the line of Toldt parallel to the kidney needs to be made; this incision is not carried deeply in an effort to hold the kidney lateral which helps somewhat with the hilar dissection.

Step 2. The Gonadal Vein

Identification and isolation of the left gonadal vein is useful as it reliably leads the surgeon to the renal vein. The gonadal vein can be most easily exposed inferiorly; it is then traced up to its entry into the renal vein. Anteriorly along the gonadal vein, there are no tributaries thereby providing the surgeon with a safe plane of dissection all the way up to the insertion of the gonadal vein into the main renal vein.

Step 3. Identifying the Proximal Ureter

The left ureter usually lies just posterior and lateral to the gonadal vein. It is carefully dissected from the retroperitoneal tissues and treated in the same manner as the right ureter was for a right nephroureterectomy. Again, lower pole mobilization helps to optimize access to the renal hilum by granting the surgeon access to both the inferior and lateral aspects of the renal artery and vein.

Step 4. Securing the Renal Hilum

After tracing the gonadal vein to its junction with the main renal vein, it is secured using the harmonic scalpel on the variable setting. Alternatively, if the vessel is robust (>4 mm), it can be secured with vascular clips and divided. Care should be taken to identify the posterior lumbar vein that may enter the renal vein posteriorly in the area of the gonadal vein or may even join the gonadal vein near its insertion into the renal vein. Thoughtful utilization of the 30° degree lens during renal vein dissection will allow the surgeon to visualize the area behind the renal vein. Thus, optical identification of lumber veins during the posterior dissection of the renal vein is possible. This maneuver helps avoid the unwelcome "surprise" of bleeding associated with blind dissection behind the renal vein. Lumbar veins can similarly be secured with the harmonic scalpel or with four clips and incised. The advantage of vascular control of small vessels with the harmonic scalpel is that there is no concern of clip entrapment with the laparoscopic stapler during hilar transection.

The superior border of the renal vein is then dissected from surrounding tissue. The adrenal vein is identified during this dissection, usually lying medial to the insertion of the gonadal vein on the renal vein. The adrenal vein is secured with the harmonic scalpel or with four vascular clips and divided. If clips are applied, the clips should be placed with consideration of subsequent safe placement of the laparoscopic vascular stapler across the renal vein.

Although the location of the renal artery usually becomes evident during the renal vein dissection, careful review of preoperative imaging (CAT scan or MRI) will suggest the location of the renal artery when it is not immediately evident (i.e., cephalad or caudad to the vein). With hand-assisted technique localization of the renal artery is simplified by digital palpation. The renal artery is dissected free, and five 11-mm titanium clips are applied. The artery is then transected between the second and third vascular clips leaving three clips proximally. Occasionally, the hilar dissection may seem simplified by the presence of a renal artery that is parallel or anterior to the renal vein. In this situation, extreme caution should be exercised as the superior mesenteric artery can easily be mistaken for the renal artery. If the "presumed" renal artery is not behind the renal vein, additional dissection of the vessel should be performed to clearly delineate the anatomy before vessel transection is performed.

Distal ureteral dissection, entrapment, specimen extraction, and cystoscopic management of the intramural ureteral tunnel are all identical to the description for the right side. The only exception is that the left kidney specimen is moved such that it rests on the anterior surface of the spleen just prior to entrapment.

Alternative Management Strategies for the Distal Ureter

There are several techniques for the laparoscopic handling of the distal ureter and only the methods most commonly performed will be discussed.

Methods for the Hand-Assisted Laparoscopic Technique

Open technique: This can be performed either by an extravesical or intravescial technique. Following nephrectomy, the ureter is mobilized just inferior to the pelvic brim. The hand port is extended. Extending a midline infraumbilical incision is muscle sparing and improves post-operative pain. Some authors modify the hand port position and use a Pfannenstiel incision, which too is muscle sparing. The specimen can then be removed en bloc through this incision after entrapment. The advantage of an extravesical approach is that it avoids opening the bladder and risking tumor seeding. When using an intravesical approach, it is crucial to make sure there are no lesions in the bladder by performing a cystoscopy and to clip the distal ureter before entering the bladder.

Flexible cystoscopy with electrode excision: Nadler and colleagues recently describe a technique using a flexible cystoscope *(26)*. Once the kidney and ureter have been freed to the level of the bladder wall, a flexible cystoscope is inserted through the urethra into the bladder. A 5F electrode (ACMI, Norwalk, CT) is used to incise a 2-cm circumferential cuff of bladder around the ureteral orifice. The surgeon's hand provides manipulation and traction of the ureter and periureteral tissues. The surgeon's finger also prevents extravasation of fluid from the bladder during cystoscopic ureteral dissection. A drain is left adjacent to the bladder to drain the pelvis and the bladder is not routinely close. A 20F urethral catheter is left for 7–10 days, and is removed following a negative cystogram. However, the authors prefer not to apply any technique that does not results in a formal closure of the bladder (suturing or stapling) due to concerns of tumor seeding.

Methods for the Pure Laparoscopic Technique

Pluck technique: Transurethral ureteral resection ("pluck" ureterectomy) is performed cystoscopically prior to the laparoscopic component of the procedure with the patient in a dorsal lithotomy position. The ureteral orifice, tunnel, and ureterovesical junction are transurethrally resected out to the perivesical fat. The ureter is thereby released from the bladder. Hemostasis is obtained and a urethral catheter is placed. Early in the laparoscopic portion of the procedure, the ureter is clipped to prevent further leakage of urine into the retroperitoneum. After laparoscopic dissection of the kidney, the surgeon can "pluck" the ureter cephalad, thereby precluding any pelvic dissection of the ureter. The major drawback of this approach is concern about leakage of malignant cell-laden urine into the retroperitoneum until the ureter is laparoscopically occluded. Indeed, instances of seeding after an open "pluck" procedure have now been reported by several urologists *(27–29)*.

Needlescopic (Cleveland Clinic) technique: Application of a needlescopic technique for management of the distal ureter was described by Gill and colleagues in 1999 *(30)*. The patient first undergoes cystoscopy to rule out a concomitant bladder tumor and to insure adequate bladder capacity. Diminished bladder capacity (less than 200 mL) increases the technical difficulty due to limited working space. Cystoscopy is performed with the patient in 30° Trendelenburg position. Two needlescopic trocars (2 mm) are inserted supra-pubically into the bladder under cystoscopic vision. A 2-mm Endoloop is inserted through the needlescopic trocar. A 6F ureteral catheter is passed through the loop and into the affected ureter with the assistance of a guidewire. A 24F continuous flow resectoscope is then passed into the bladder alongside the ureteral catheter. A Collins knife is used to electrosurgically score circumferentially the urothelium around the intramural ureter such that a 2–3-cm cuff is outlined.

Using a 2-mm grasper the ureteral orifice and hemitrigone are retracted anteriorly and a full-thickness incision is made with the Collins knife. In this manner, approximately 3–4 cm of ureter may be dissected free from surrounding tissues. The previously placed endoloop is then positioned over the ureter and closed tightly, occluding the lumen as the ureteral catheter is withdrawn. The tail of the Endoloop is then cut with 2-mm laparoscopic scissors. The bladder edges about the excised ureter are then coagulated. All instruments are removed from the bladder and a Foley catheter is left indwelling. The laparoscopic nephrectomy component of the procedure is then performed and the ureter is pulled up with the specimen via a 7–10 cm incision.

All patients, regardless of the technique should have at least a 7 mm Jackson–Pratt drain placed behind the bladder cuff. There is debate over the length of time necessary to keep the bladder catheterized. This decision can be made intra-operatively based on the surgeon's confidence in the integrity of the bladder closure. If there is truly a question concerning the adequacy of the bladder closure, it is reasonable to perform a cystogram before its removal.

Brown and colleagues reviewed 55 hand-assisted procedures using four different methods. This study included cystoscopic disarticulation with a Collins knife in 16 patients, stapled division in seven, open distal ureterectomy in three, and hand-assisted laparoscopic extravesical en bloc distal ureterectomy with bladder cuff in 29. The authors found that the cystoscopic TUR took the longest, secondary to patient repositioning and had the most complications, blood loss and open conversions *(31)*.

Post-operative Care

Patients receive 15 mg of ketorlac (Toradol) IV q6h as requested, for 36 h. Typically, patients will require supplemental analgesic control with an oral narcotic. Diet is resumed immediately with clear fluids and advanced as tolerated. Pneumatic compression boots remain on the patient and activated until the patient is ambulating well. Typically, the patient is ambulated on the first post-operative day. At Washington University, mean hospital stay for laparoscopic nephroureterectomy has been 3.3 and 4.5 days for laparoscopic and hand-assisted laparoscopic nephroureterectomy, respectively. The patient is discharged on oral narcotics as needed *(19)*. However, with extended experience, the authors have reduced the hospital stay to 2.2 days in their last 23 cases.

Complications

A review of the literature listed in Table 2, comparing open nephroureterectomy and laparoscopic nephroureterectomy, reveals a 10.4 and a 6.6% complication rate, respectively. The most common intra-operative complication was hemorrhage and the two most common post-operative complications were pneumonia, followed by ileus *(32)*. Other intra-operative complications include lacerations of the kidney, spleen, and bowel. These most often can be repaired laparoscopically, without necessitating conversion or significant post-operative sequelae. However, splenectomy, splenic injury requiring transfusions, and bowel laceration causing a prolonged ileus have also been reported *(33)*. Terranova and co-workers reported on wound complications of the hand port. Of 54 patients undergoing hand-assisted renal surgery, there was a 9.3% complication rate. Complications ranged from wound infections to one wound dehiscence *(34)*. Major long-term post-operative complications, include bowel obstructions secondary to adhesions, which required lysis and hernia from the hand port. As with open surgery and other laparoscopic procedures, systemic complications have occurred. These include cardiac, vascular, respiratory, sepsis, and even death.

TAKE HOME MESSAGES

1. Anatomic dissection following the described templates for the right and left nephrectomy component of the procedure will facilitate a safe dissection that is oncologically sound.
2. On the right side, the surgeon should actively "seek-out" the duodenum to identify and protect this structure during medial dissection of the renal specimen.
3. On the left side, identification of the gonadal vein helps expedite hilar dissection. The surgeon must remember the superior mesenteric artery if the "renal artery" is located anterior or parallel to the renal vein.
4. Preliminary data have demonstrated that the hand-assisted laparoscopic technique will expedite nephroureterectomy, and will likely have only a small impact on post-operative analgesic requirements and convalescence.

CONCLUSIONS

For localized TCC laparoscopic and hand-assisted laparoscopic nephroureterectomy have become accepted alternatives to open nephroureterectomy. Application of laparoscopic technique provides excellent oncologic control and minimizes the patient's post-operative discomfort and convalescence. Using the anatomic templates and techniques herein described and illustrated, the laparoscopic urologic surgeon can successfully extract the kidney and adrenal within Gerota's fascia as well as the ureter and a cuff of bladder.

REFERENCES

1. Clayman, R.V., Kavoussi, L.R., Figenshau, R.S., Chandhoke, P.S., and Albala, D.M.: Laparoscopic nephroureterectomy: Initial case report. J Laparoendosc Surg 1:343–349, 1991.
2. Shalhav, A.L., Dunn, M.D., Portis, A.J., Elbahnasy, A.M., McDougall, E.M., and Clayman, R.V.: Laparoscopic nephroureterectomy for upper tract transitional cell cancer: The Washington University experience. J Urol 163: 1100–1104, 2000.
3. Doehn, C., Fornara, P., Fricke, L., and Jocham, D.: Comparison of open and laparoscopic nephroureterectomy for benign disease. J Urol 159:732–734, 1998.
4. Keeley, F.X. and Tolley, D.A.: Laparoscopic nephroureterectomy: Making management of upper-tract transitional cell carcinoma entirely minimally invasive. J Endourol 12:139, 1998.
5. Gill, I.S., Sung, G.T., Hobart, M.G., Savage, S.J., Meraney, A.M., Schweizer, D.K., et al.: Laparoscopic radical nephroureterectomy for upper tract transitional cell carcinoma: The Cleveland Clinic experience. J Urol 164: 1513–1522, 2000.
6. Cummings, K.B.: Nephroureterecotmy: Rationale in the management of transitional cell carcinoma of the upper urinary tract. Urol Clin N Am 7:569–578, 1980.
7. Gittes, R.F.: Management of transitional cell carcinoma of the upper tract: Case for conservative local excision. Urol Clin N Am 7:559–568, 1980.
8. Nocks, B.N., Heney, N.M., Dally, J.J., Perrone, T.A., Griffin P.P., and Prout G.R. Jr.: Transitional cell carcinoma of renal pelvis. Urology 19:472–477, 1982.
9. Wagle, D.G., Moore, R.H., and Murphy, G.P.: Primary carcinoma of the renal pelvis. Cancer 33:1642–1648, 1974.
10. Wallace, D.M., Whitfield, H.N., Hendry W.F., and Wickham J.E.: The late results of conservative surgery for transitional cell carcinomaa. Br J Urol 53:537–541, 1981.
11. Lee, B.R., Jabbour, M.E., Marshall, F.F., Smith, A.D., and Jarrett T.W.: 13-year survival comparison of percutaneous and open nephroureterectomy approaches for management of transitional cell carcinoma of renal collecting system: Equivalent outcomes. J Endourol 13:289–294, 1999.
12. Stoller, M.L., Gentle, D.L., McDonald, M.W., Reese, J.H., Tacker, J.R., Carroll, P.R., et al.: Endoscopic management of upper tract urothelial tumors. Tech Urol 3:152–157, 1997.
13. Gerber, G.S. and Lyon, E.S.: Endourological management of upper tract urothelial tumors. J Urol 150:2–7, 1993.
14. Plancke, H.R.F., Strijbos, W.E.M., and Delaere, K.J.P.: Percutaneous endoscopic treatment of urothelial tumours of the renal pelvis. Br J Urol 75:736–739, 1995.
15. M.E. Jabbour, Desgrandchamps, F., Cazin, S., Teillac, P., Le Duc, A., and Smith, A.D.: Percutaneous management of grade II upper urinary tract transitional cell carcinoma: The long-term outcome. J Urol 163:1105, 2000.
16. M.C. Goel, Mahendra, V., and Roberts, J.G.: Percutaneous management of renal pelvic urothelial tumors: Long-term followup. J Urol 169:925–930, 2003.
17. Clayman, R.V., Kavoussi, L.R., Soper, N.J., Dierks, S.M., Meretyk, S., Darcy, M.D., et al.: Laparoscopic nephrectomy: Initial case report. J Urol 146:278, 1991.
18. Tan, B.J., Ost, M.C., and Lee, B.R.: Laparoscopic nephroureterectomy with bladder cuff resection: Techniques and outcomes. J Endourol 19:664–676, 2005.
19. Landman, J., Lev, R., Bhayani, S., Alberts G., Rehman J., Pattaras J.G., et al.: Comparison of hand-assisted and standard laparoscopic radical nephroureterectomy for management of localized transitional cell carcinoma. J Urol 167(6):2387–2391, 2002.
20. Rehman, J., Monga, M., Landman, J., Lee, D.I., Felfela, T., Conradaie, M.C., Srinivac, R., Sundaram, C.P., and Clayman, R.V.: Characterization of intrapelvic pressure during ureteropyeloscopy with the ureteral access sheath. Urology 61:713–718, 2003.
21. Landman, J., Kerbl, K., Rehman, J., Andreoni, C., Olweny, E., Collyer, W.C., et al.: Comparison of the LigaSure system, bipolar energy, ultrasound energy, and conventional vascular control techniques for laparoscopic vascular control in a porcine model. J Endourol 15(1):A1, 2001.
22. Chan, D., Bishoff, J.T., Ratner, L., Kavoussi, L.R., and Jarrett, T.W.: Endovascular gastrointestinal stapler device malfunction during laparoscopic nephrectomy: Early recognition and management. J Urol 164:319, 2000.
23. Jarrett, T.W., Chan, D.Y., Cadeddu, J.A., and Kavoussi, L.R.: Laparoscopic nephroureterectomy for the treatment of transitional cell carcinoma of the upper urinary tract. Urology 57(3):448–453, 2001.
24. McDougall, E.M., Clayman, R.V., and Elashry, O.: Laparoscopic nephroureterectomy for upper tract transitional cell cancer: The Washington University experience. J Urol Sep;154(3):975–979, 1995.
25. Tisdale, B.E., Kapoor, A. et al.: Intact specimen extraction in laparoscopic nephrectomy procedures: Pfannenstiel versus expanded port site incisions. Urology 69(2):241–244, 2007.
26. Vardi, I.Y., Stern, J.A., Gonzalez, C.M., Kimm, S.Y., Nadler, R.B.: Novel technique for management of distal ureter and en block resection of bladder cuff during hand-assisted laparoscopic nephroureterectomy, Urology Jan;67(1): 89–92, 2006.
27. Jones, D.R. and Moisey, C.U.: A cautionary tale of the modified "pluck" nephroureterectomy. Br J Urol 71:486–487, 1993.

28. Hetherington, J.W., Ewing, R., and Philip, N.H.: Modified nephroureterectomy: A risk of tumor implantation. Br J Urol 58:368–372, 1986.
29. Arango, O., Bielsa, O., Carles, J., and Galabert-Mas A.: Massive tumor implantation in the endoscopic resected area in modified nephroureterectomy. J Urol 157:1893–1896, 1997.
30. Gill, I.S., Soble, J.J., Miller, S.D., and Sung G.T.: A novel technique for management of the en bloc bladder cuff and distal ureter during laparoscopic nephroureterectomy. J Urol 161:430–434, 1999.
31. Brown, J.A., Strup, S.E., Chenven, E., Bagley, D., Gomella, L.G.: Hand-assisted laparoscopic nephroureterectomy: Analysis of distal ureterectomy technique, margin status, and surgical outcomes. Urology Dec;66(6):1192–1196, 2005.
32. Brown, J.A., Strup, S.E., Chenven, E., Bagley, D., and Gomella, L.G.: Hand-assisted laparoscopic nephroureterectomy: analysis of distal ureterectomy technique, margin status, and surgical outcomes. Urology 66: 1192–1196, 2005.
33. Wolf, J.S. Jr., Dash, A., Hollenbeck, B.K., Johnson, W.K. 3rd, Madii, R., Montgomery, J.S.: Intermediate followup of hand assisted laparoscopic nephroureterectomy for urothelial carcinoma: factors associated with outcomes. J Urol Apr: 173(4):1102–1107, 2005.
34. Terranova, S.A., Siddiqui, K.M., Preminger, G.M., Albala, D.M.: Hand-assisted laparoscopic renal surgery: Hand-port incision complications. J Endourol Oct;18(8):775–779, 2004.
35. Stifelman, M.D., Sosa, R.E., Andrade, A., Tarantino, A., and Shichman, S.: Hand-assisted laparoscopic nephroureterectomy for the treatment of transitional cell carcinoma of the upper urinary tract. Urology 56(5): 741, 2000.
36. Jarrett, T.W., Chan, D.Y., Cadeddu, J.A., and Kavoussi L.R.: Laparoscopic nephroureterectomy for the treatment of transitional cell carcinoma of the upper urinary tract. Urology 57(3):448–453, 2001.
37. Wolf, J.S. Jr., Dash, A., Hollenbeck, B.K., Johnston, W.K. 3rd, Madii, R., and Montgomery, J.S.: Intermediate followup of hand assisted laparoscopic nephroureterectomy for urothelial carcinoma: factors associated with outcomes, J Urol Apr;173(4):1102–1107, 2005.
38. Cannon, G.M. Jr., Averch, T., Colen, J., Morrisroe, S., Durrani, O., Hrebinko, R.L., Hand-assisted laparoscopic nephroureterectomy with open cystotomy for removal of the distal ureter and bladder cuff. J Endourol Oct;19(8): 973–975, 2005.
39. Kurzer, E., Leveillee, R.J., Bird, V.G.: Combining hand assisted laparoscopic nephroureterectomy with cystoscopic circumferential excision of the distal ureter without primary closure of the bladder cuff – is it safe? J Urol Jan;175(1):63–67, 2006.
40. Muntener, M., Nielsen, M.E., Romero, F.R., Schaeffer, E.M., Allaf, M.E., Brito, F.A., Pavlovich, C.P., Kavoussi, L.R., Jarrett, T.W.: Long-term oncologic outcome after laparoscopic radical nephroureterectomy for upper tract transitional cell carcinoma. Eur Urol Jun;51(6):1639–1644, 2007.
41. Shalhav, A.L., Dunn, M.D., Portis, A.J., Elbahnasy, A.M., McDougall, E.M., and Clayman, R.V.: Laparoscopic nephroureterectomy for upper tract transitional cell cancer: the Washington University experience. J Urol 163: 1100, 2000.
42. Seifman, B.D., Montie, J.E., and Wolf, J.S.: Prospective comparison between hand-assisted laparoscopic and open surgical nephrouretererctomy for urothelial cell carcinoma. Urology 57(1):133–137, 2001.
43. Keeley, F.X. and Tolley, D.A.: Laparoscopic nephroureterectomy: making management of upper-tract transitional cell carcinoma entirely minimally invasive. J Endourol 12: 139, 1998.
44. Hattori, R., Yoshino, Y., Gotoh, M., Katoh, M., Kamihira, O., Ono, Y.: Laparoscopic nephroureterectomy for transitional cell carcinoma of renal pelvis and ureter: Nagoya experience. Urology Apr;67(4):701–705, 2006.
45. Rassweiler, J.J., Schulze, M., Marrero, R., Frede, T., Palou Redorta, J., Bassi, P.: Laparoscopic nephroureterectomy for upper urinary tract transitional cell carcinoma: Is it better than open surgery?. Eur Urol Dec;46(6):690–697, 2004.
46. Roupret, M., Hupertan, V., Sanderson, K.M., Harmon, J.D., Cathelineau, X., Barret, E., Vallancien, G., and Rozet, F., Oncologic control after open or laparoscopic nephroureterectomy for upper urinary tract transitional cell carcinoma: A single center experience. Urology Apr;69(4):656–661, 2007.

Laparoscopic Live Donor Nephrectomy

David J. Hernandez, Adam W. Levinson, and Li-Ming Su

INTRODUCTION

Renal transplantation is acknowledged as the preferred method of renal replacement therapy, offering significant advantages for individuals with end-stage renal disease (ESRD) as compared to dialysis. In addition to improved overall survival and quality of life, renal transplantation remains the most cost-effective treatment; in fact, it remains one of the most cost-effective therapies in health care *(1)*. Due to the aging population, increasing frequency of predisposing conditions such as diabetes and hypertension as well as improved life-expectancy resulting from enhanced medical management of patients with ESRD, the incidence and prevalence of ESRD have increased dramatically. As a result, the growing number of patients with ESRD who would benefit from transplantation has overwhelmed the supply of cadaveric donor kidneys. The United Network for Organ Sharing (UNOS) and the Organ Procurement and Transplantation Network (OPTN) estimate that the number of patients awaiting transplantation in the United States will increase by approximately 3,000 per year *(2,3)*. Thus, the gap between supply and demand for renal allografts continues to grow such that 72,942 candidates are currently on the waiting list for a kidney and 48,176 (66%) have been on the list for over a year *(3)*. Though expanded criteria for cadaveric organs including using extremes of age and double kidney donation has increased supply, it still falls short of the continually increasing demand.

Living donor transplantation has been increasingly employed to enhance the supply of available allografts given that the supply of cadaveric kidneys remains inadequate. According to national statistics on kidney allografts in the United States maintained by UNOS and OPTN, the percentage of all renal allografts obtained from live donors steadily increased from 31.9% in 1988 to 52.9% in 2003 with an absolute increase from 1,817 to 6,473 in that time *(3)*. Though the number of donor allografts has remained stable thereafter, the percentage has declined to 47.3% in 2006 likely due to expanded criteria for cadaveric organ use *(3)*. The increase in living donor transplantation has been facilitated not only by the widespread use of minimally invasive donor nephrectomy but also by the increased use and success of living unrelated donors, paired living donors and other HLA-incompatible allografts *(2–12)*.

Over 50 years have passed since the first successful living donor renal transplantation *(13)*, and the method has shown significant superiority to that of cadaveric renal transplantation. In addition to superior graft function and survival, living donor renal transplantation is associated with shorter waiting times, reduced immunosuppression requirements and less recipient morbidity *(10,14,15)*. Even the ideal cadaveric allograft [in good condition with high human leukocyte antigen (HLA)-match] does not survive as long as the average living donor allografts, and neither do their recipients *(15)*.

From: *Current Clinical Urology: Essential Urologic Laparoscopy*
Edited by: S. Y. Nakada and S. P. Hedican, DOI 10.1007/978-1-60327-820-1_12

The advantages of living donor renal transplantation are believed to stem from shorter warm and cold ischemia times with a near absence of ischemic injury to the graft and a relative insensitivity to poor tissue matching. With improved immunosuppressive regimens, some groups are now reporting 5-year graft survival rates as high as 90% for living transplants being used for ABO incompatible recipients *(7)*. It stands to reason that living donor kidneys now comprise approximately 50% of all transplanted renal allografts *(2–6)*. The only disadvantage of live donor renal transplantation is the requirement of a healthy individual to accept the risks of major surgery and then live with a solitary kidney, with no direct medical benefit.

Until 1995, the standard approach for organ procurement was open donor nephrectomy through either a flank, subcostal or transabdominal incision. Due to the prolonged postoperative hospital stay and convalescence as well as the high levels of postoperative pain and poor cosmetic results generally associated with this invasive approach, there were considerable disincentives to potential organ donors. However, the paradigm of living renal transplantation was dramatically altered in 1995 when Ratner and Kavoussi performed the first laparoscopic live donor nephrectomy, an operation devised to reduce the disincentives to live kidney donation in hopes of increasing the pool of potential live kidney donors *(16)*. This approach, now standard at most institutions, has resulted in significantly less postoperative pain, shorter hospital stays, reduced postoperative convalescence, and improved cosmesis without jeopardizing either donor safety or the quality of allograft provided to the recipient *(10,16–32)*.

Since its inception, laparoscopic live donor nephrectomy has emerged as "the optimal form" of renal replacement therapy *(10)*. Notwithstanding the aforementioned advantages for the donor, recipient outcomes have been equivalent to those for conventional open donor nephrectomy *(10,16–32)*. With increased surgeon experience, recipient complications such as delayed graft function and ureteral stricture have declined *(25,28,29,33–36)*. Overall, the risks to the donor have decreased, with current morbidity and mortality rates similar to that of the open technique, approximately 8 and 0.03%, respectively *(10,25,28–33,37)*. In studies comparing living donors to their siblings, no increased risk of renal failure or hypertension has been found. Only 4% of living donors are dissatisfied in long-term surveys *(11,12,26,38,39)*. At our institution as at many others, laparoscopy is the preferred approach for the procurement of left and right kidneys with selection of the appropriate kidney for donation based on the criteria previously established for conventional open donor nephrectomy. If the kidneys appear to be equivalent in function and without anomaly, the left is excised preferentially over the right due to the longer left renal vein.

Herein we describe our current step-by-step technique for laparoscopic live donor nephrectomy, emphasizing a few key modifications in the modern era.

PREOPERATIVE ASSESSMENT

Patient Selection

All donor candidates require extensive medical and psychological evaluation in accordance with guidelines published by the American Society of Transplant Physicians *(40)* and by the International Forum on the Care of the Live Kidney Donor *(41)*. The transplantation team must carefully evaluate the donor's motivation, emotional stability, and general medical and mental health. In particular, the patient must not have morbid obesity, significant stone disease, active infection, uncontrolled diabetes or hypertension or a recent disqualifying malignancy *(41)*. All potential donors undergo screening chest X-ray and electrocardiogram. If over 40 years of age, a recent PAP smear and mammogram is recommended for female candidates as are a prostate-specific antigen and digital rectal examination for males. Additionally, donor candidates must undergo numerous laboratory studies (in addition to histocompatibility testing) to ensure that he/she will maintain adequate renal function following unilateral nephrectomy. Blood analyses include a complete blood count, serum chemistries, coagulation profile, ABO histocompatibility, HLA crossmatching, and serologies for hepatitis B and C, syphilis, human immunodeficiency virus (HIV), cytomegalovirus (CMV), Epstein-Barr virus (EBV), and varicella (VZV). Urine tests include urinalysis, urine culture and a 24-hour urine collection for creatinine clearance and protein.

Radiographic Evaluation

Laparoscopic donor nephrectomy requires accurate preoperative radiographic imaging, especially of the renal vasculature. Precise preoperative mapping of the renal vessels is paramount, as knowledge of their number and location (especially when aberrant vessels are present) is needed to plan the dissection and to minimize vascular complications. For this purpose, we use dual-phase spiral computed tomography (CT) with three-dimensional angiography in lieu of the previously accepted combination of standard angiography and intravenous pyelography with excretory urography. Three-dimensional CT angiography can accurately demonstrate subtleties in renal vascular anatomy and clearly characterizes the renal parenchyma, pelvis, and ureter. We find it valuable in planning both the donor and recipient operations, especially when multiple renal arteries or veins are identified (Fig. 1), and will display the films in the operating room at the time of surgery for reference. Specific attention should be paid to small accessory lower pole renal arteries, as these may be vital to ureteral blood supply.

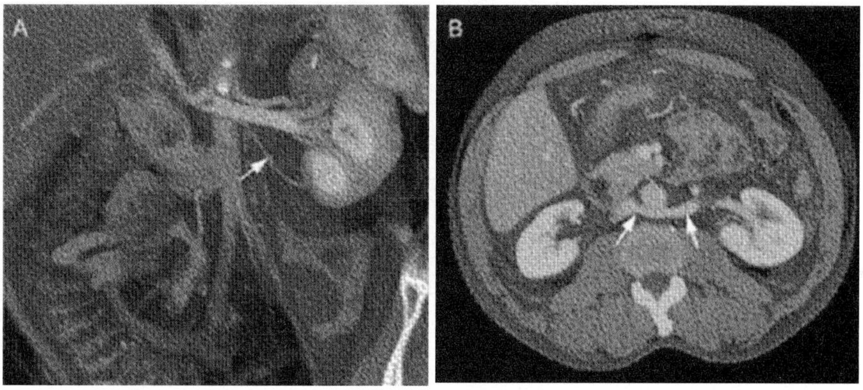

Fig. 1. Three-dimensional CT angiography demonstrates (**a**) an accessory left lower pole renal artery (*white arrow*) and (**b**) a retroaortic left renal vein (*white arrows*) in two separate donor patients.

Patient Preparation

Patients are advised to remain on a clear liquid diet the entire day prior to surgery. The patient is kept fasted after midnight the evening prior to surgery. No specific bowel preparation is required.

OPERATING ROOM SET-UP

Personnel and Equipment Configuration

In addition to the operating surgeon, laparoscopic live donor nephrectomy requires the following personnel: a surgical assistant, scrub technician, circulating nurse, and anesthesia team. Both the operating surgeon and assistant stand on the abdominal side of the patient, contralateral to the targeted kidney. The scrub nurse and equipment table are situated near the surgical team at the foot of the table. The operating table must be adjustable and allow for medial and lateral rotation. Two high-definition flat-panel color monitors are positioned at eye level on either side near the head of the table to allow the operating surgeon, assistant, and scrub technician to continuously monitor the surgical procedure. A light source and carbon dioxide (CO_2) insufflator are generally placed on the side opposite the operating surgeon. A high-definition digital video camera is attached to the laparoscope during the procedure and provides a sharp color image of the surgery, which is projected on both video monitors. A standard monopolar electrocautery unit is placed either in front or behind the operating surgeon. If the AESOP® (Intuitive Surgical, Inc., Sunnyvale, CA) robotic arm is employed to stabilize and control the laparoscope in lieu of the surgical assistant, it should be attached to the operating table on the surgeon's side and at the level of the patient's shoulders, taking great care to ensure that it does not come in contact with the patient's hands, arms or shoulder during maneuvering of the robotic arm. A typical operating room configuration for a left laparoscopic live donor nephrectomy is shown in Fig. 2.

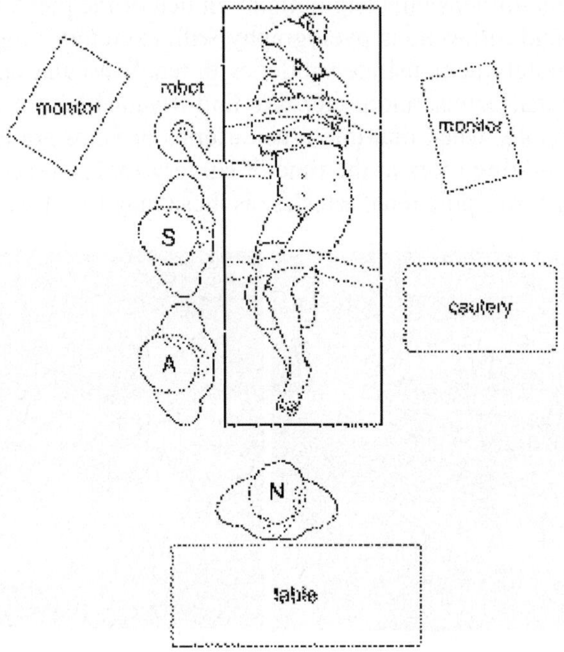

Fig. 2. Patient positioning and operating room configuration for left laparoscopic live donor nephrectomy: S = surgeon, A = assistant, N = scrub nurse/technician.

Patient Positioning

Prior to patient positioning, the entire operating table is padded to reduce the risk of neuromuscular injuries. After induction of general endotracheal anesthesia, the patient is given one dose of intravenous broad-spectrum antibiotics, and an orogastric tube and Foley catheter are placed to decompress the stomach and bladder, respectively. A marking pen is used to outline the location of the 5–6 mm Pfannenstiel incision for the eventual delivery site of the kidney (approximately 2–3 fingerbreadths above the pubic symphysis) prior to positioning the patient in the modified flank position in order to ensure symmetry when the incision is later created. Knee- or thigh-length compression stockings (TEDs) and sequential compression devices (SCDs) are placed on the lower extremities. The patient is then placed in a modified lateral decubitus position at a 45° angle with the operating table (with the flank ipsilateral to the donor kidney up). A cylindrical, gel-filled padding is placed posteriorly for support and the arms are kept outstretched on an arm board with sufficient padding placed under the arms. Alternatively, if the AESOP is to be used, the arms can be protected by crossing them over the chest and padding them with egg crate or pillows (Fig. 2). Neither an axillary roll nor flexion of the table is required. The hips are slightly rotated flat to allow exposure of the anterior lower abdomen and eventual delivery site of the renal allograft. The dependent leg is gently flexed at the knee and pillows are placed between the legs with strict attention to padding all pressure points. The patient is secured to the operating table with heavy cloth tape at the level of the shoulders and thighs. Additional egg crate sponge padding is placed over the shoulder and hips to prevent compression injuries as a result of the cloth tape. Prior to initiating the procedure, the operating room table is rotated to the extreme lateral limits to ensure that the patient is adequately secured to the table.

Trocar Configuration

Our technique of laparoscopic donor nephrectomy requires four trocars (5-, 12-, 12-, and 12-mm) as depicted in Fig. 3. We use an EndoTip™ (Karl Storz, Culver City, CA) 5-mm trocar at the subxiphoid position. A recent modification has been to place this trocar more laterally (i.e., toward the allograft) in order to maintain a more acute angle of dissection when freeing the upper pole of the kidney. With this modification, the 5-mm trocar is thus placed three fingerbreadths lateral to the abdominal midline, at a level halfway between the umbilicus and xiphoid process. A 12-mm trocar is placed at the level of the umbilicus just lateral to the rectus muscle to avoid injury to the epigastric vessels. These two trocars serve as the main working trocars. A 12-mm trocar placed at the umbilicus is utilized predominately for the laparoscope. A third 12-mm trocar is inserted in the middle of the planned Pfannenstiel incision and is used for retraction of the colon, mesentery, and small bowel. This trocar site is extended transversely on both sides to a total length of 5–6 mm to accommodate the renal allograft extraction at the end of the operation. In case of an obese patient, all trocars should be shifted laterally and towards the allograft in order to account for a large pannus and avoid problems with reach.

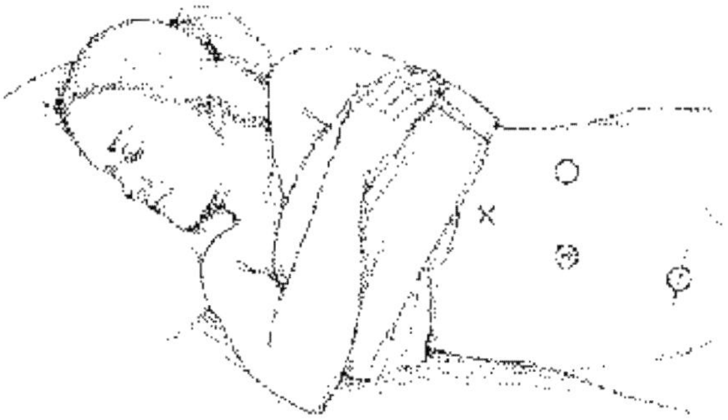

Fig. 3. Trocar configuration for left laparoscopic live donor nephrectomy: X = 5-mm trocar, O = 12-mm trocar. The kidney is delivered through a 5–6 mm Pfannenstiel incision (*dotted line*).

Instrumentation and Medications

In performing laparoscopic live donor nephrectomy, specific instrumentation is required. The following list outlines the necessary laparoscopic instruments and medications as well as optional equipment.

Instruments:

- Veress Needle
- Maryland dissector
- Suction–irrigation device and probe

- Monopolar electrocautery scissors
- Hand-held electrocautery device
- Visiport device (United States Surgical Corporation, Norwalk, CT)
- 5- and 10-mm vascular clip appliers
- 10-mm 0° and 30° laparoscopic lens
- Anti-fog lens solution and/or sterile hot water thermos
- 12-mm laparoscopic trocar *(3)*
- 5-mm EndoTip™ (Karl Storz, Culver City, CA) laparoscopic trocar *(1)*
- 15-mm Endocatch™ bag (United States Surgical Corporation, Norwalk, CT)
- 10-mm Endoscopic GIA stapling device™ (United States Surgical Corporation, Norwalk, CT)
- Endoscopic GIA vascular staple cartridges *(3–4)*
- Carter–Thomason® (Inlet Medical, Eden Prairie, MN) fascial closure device
- 2-0 polyglactin suture for trocar site fascial closure *(2)*
- 0-polyglactin suture to secure trocars to the skin *(4)*
- #1 polyglyconate suture for closure of the abdominal wall fascia at extraction site *(1–2)*
- No. 10 and 15 scalpel blades
- 16 French Foley catheter
- 16 French orogastric tube
- Sterile ice slush and container (to cool and transport renal allograft)
- One litre of ice-cold standard preservation solution (to perfuse harvested renal allograft prior to transplantation)
- Standard open nephrectomy tray and instrumentation with Bookwalter or Omni retractor (in case of open conversion)

Optional Equipment:

- AESOP® Robotic Arm (Intuitive Surgical, Inc., Sunnyvale, CA)
- Electrocautery hook
- Bipolar electrocautery forceps
- Ultrasonic shears or Harmonic scalpel (Ethicon Endo-Surgery, Cincinnati, OH)
- Ligasure™ vessel sealing system (Valleylab, Boulder, CO)
- 12-mm Endo Paddle retractor (United States Surgical Corporation, Norwalk, CT)
- Hem-o-lock clips (Weck, Research Triangle Park, NC)

Medications:

- Cephazolin (1 g i.v.)
- Protamine (30 mg i.v.)
- Furosemide (40 mg i.v.)
- Mannitol (12.5 g i.v. × two doses)
- Heparin (3,000 units i.v.)
- Papavarine (30 mg/ml solution, 10–20 ml total)

OPERATIVE TECHNIQUE

Laparoscopic procurement of the left kidney is preferred, primarily due to the longer renal vein obtained as compared to that of the right kidney, and therefore will be discussed first and in greater detail. The technique for right laparoscopic donor nephrectomy and methods to maximize renal vascular length will then be described. Finally, the technique of hand-assisted laparoscopic nephrectomy will be briefly described. Robot-assisted laparoscopic donor nephrectomy has also been reported *(42,43)* using the daVinci Surgical System (Intuitive Surgical Inc., Sunnyvale, CA). Some centers perform laparoscopic donor nephrectomy via a retroperitoneal approach, particularly for a right-sided technique *(44–52)*; however, as both the robot-assisted and retroperitoneal approach are less commonly performed and limited to a few institutions, neither will be presented herein.

Left Laparoscopic Live Donor Nephrectomy

Obtaining Access and Insufflating the Abdomen

In order to obtain access to the peritoneal cavity for insufflation of the abdomen, a Veress needle is inserted into the base of the umbilicus. For patients with prior abdominal surgery, other sites of access include the right or left upper quadrant, 2–3 fingerbreadths below the costal margin, or the right or left lower quadrant, lateral to the rectus muscles. Great care must be taken to lift up and stabilize the anterior abdominal wall during insertion of the Veress needle to prevent injury to intra- or retroperitoneal structures, including the bowel, liver, spleen, gallbladder, kidney, inferior vena cava, aorta, or iliac vessels, depending on the site of insertion. The Veress needle should be inserted directly perpendicular to the skin surface in a steady and deliberate manner. The insufflation tubing is connected to the end of the Veress needle and CO_2 gas is infused initially at a low flow rate. If the needle is in proper position, a reading of low intraperitoneal insufflation pressures (less than 10 mmHg) should be noted. If a high insufflation pressure is detected, the Veress needle should be immediately removed and the above steps repeated. Once proper positioning of the Veress needle is confirmed, the flow rate on the insufflator is increased to a high setting. If proper technique is used, a four-quadrant pneumoperitoneum is achieved. The peritoneal cavity is insufflated to a target pressure of 15 mmHg. When proper positioning is not achieved or in patients with extensive prior intra-abdominal surgery, a direct cut down (Hasson technique) should be utilized.

Trocar Placement

A No. 15 scalpel blade is used to create a 1-cm horizontal skin incision in the left lower quadrant, just lateral to the rectus muscle and at the level of the umbilicus. A 10-mm 0° laparoscopic lens is placed into the Visiport device with a preloaded 12 mm laparoscopic trocar. The Visiport is inserted into the incision staying perpendicular to the skin surface and access is gained into the peritoneal cavity under direct laparoscopic view by firing the trigger device, which deploys a small cutting knife at the tip of the Visiport. Steady forward pressure with rotational movement of the Visiport between each firing of the device can help define and incise separate layers of the abdominal wall as well as to help identify and avoid subcutaneous vessels. Once access is gained into the peritoneum, the insufflation tubing is connected to the 12-mm trocar. The abdomen and its contents are carefully inspected to identify any adhesions as well as to confirm atraumatic insertion of the Veress needle. The Veress needle is then removed.

The 0° lens is replaced with a 10-mm 30° lens, which is utilized during the remainder of the operation. Under direct laparoscopic vision, the second 12-mm trocar is inserted through the umbilicus, and the 5-mm trocar is inserted three fingerbreadths lateral to the midline half way between the umbilicus and xiphoid process. The final 12-mm trocar is inserted through the middle of the planned Pfannenstiel extraction site (see "Trocar Configuration"). Once in place, all trocars are secured to the skin with 0 polyglactin sutures on the side opposite the kidney to allow for optimum range of motion of the trocar without placing tension on the skin sutures.

Step 1: Reflecting the Colon

The operating table is maximally rotated towards the operating surgeon to allow the colon to fall medial and away from the kidney. With a Maryland dissector in the 5-mm trocar and laparoscopic monopolar electrocautery scissors placed in the left lower quadrant 12-mm trocar, the line of Toldt along the descending colon is sharply incised from the splenic flexure down to the pelvic inlet (Fig. 4).

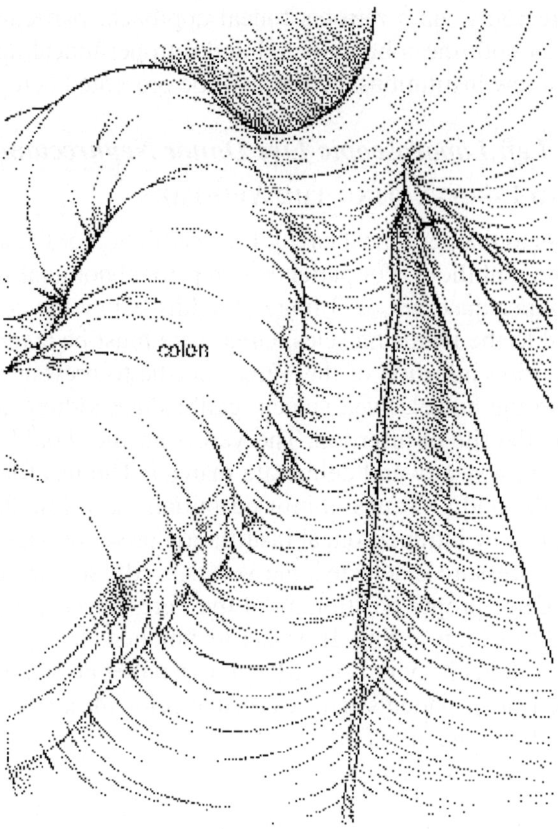

Fig. 4. Incising the line of Toldt along the descending colon.

Only the peritoneal attachments between the colon and lateral sidewall should be released at this time. Inadvertent release of the deeper lateral attachments of the kidney can cause the kidney to fall and rotate medially and obscure the renal hilum, making dissection of the renal vessels more difficult. Electrocautery should be minimized while reflecting the colon in order to avoid accidental thermal injury to the bowel. The colon is bluntly dissected with a suction–irrigation device in a medial direction, exposing Gerota's fascia overlying the kidney. Great care must be taken to develop the precise plane between Gerota's fascia and the mesentery of the colon. Dissecting too close to the colonic mesentery can result in inadvertent injury to the mesenteric vessels or creating a defect in the mesentery. Likewise, entering and dissecting within Gerota's fascia prematurely will result in excessive bleeding and may compromise exposure of the renal hilum. The mesenteric fat may oftentimes be difficult to distinguish from Gerota's fat, but is typically a brighter shade of yellow. If a defect within the mesentery is created, this should be closed laparoscopically with either 3-0 polyglactin sutures or clips to minimize the chance of an internal hernia.

A 15-mm Endocatch device may be placed at this time for retraction of the colon and small bowel (Fig. 5). To accomplish this, the 12-mm trocar located along the middle of the Pfannenstiel incision is removed and the tract bluntly dilated with the surgeon's index finger. This allows the 15-mm Endocatch device to fit snugly within the tract without continuous loss of pneumoperitoneum during the remaining steps of the operation. The purpose of the Endocatch device is two-fold. First, without deploying the bag (i.e., bag closed) this device is used during the initial steps of the operation as a blunt retractor to facilitate medial reflection of the colon and to provide optimum exposure of the renal hilum. Second,

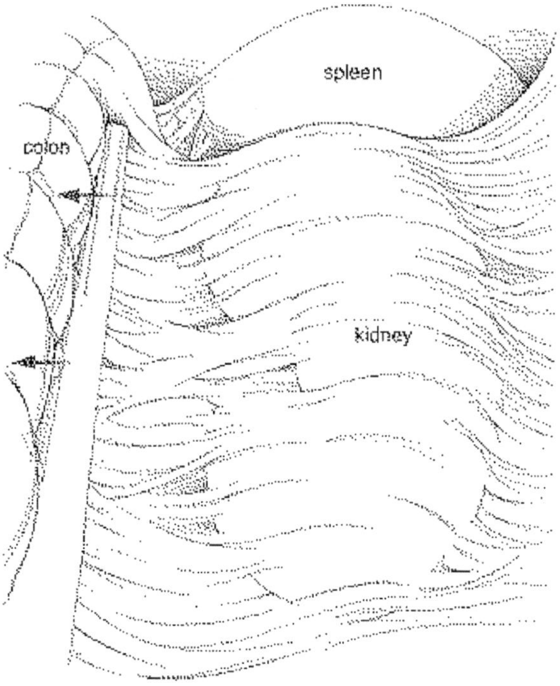

Fig. 5. Medial retraction of the colon and mesentery using a 15-mm Endocatch device (*bag closed*).

the Endocatch device can be left in place during the remaining steps of the operation until the end of the procedure at which time the bag is deployed, thus serving as the device for entrapment and delivery of the kidney. As an alternative to the Endocatch device, a 12-mm Endo Paddle retractor (United States Surgical Corporation, Norwalk, CT) may be placed through the 12-mm trocar and used to retract the bowels.

STEP 2: DISSECTING THE RENAL VEIN AND ARTERY

After medial reflection of the descending colon, the gonadal vein is identified running parallel and lateral to the aorta. The gonadal vein is traced cephalad to its insertion into the left renal vein and is therefore an important landmark for identification of the renal hilum and vessels. From the start of the operation, the patient should be aggressively hydrated to maintain a high intravascular volume status, optimize renal perfusion, and combat the effects of pneumoperitoneum on renal blood flow. Five to 6 l of crystalloid is routinely administered during the course of this operation. Mannitol (12.5 g) is administered intravenously prior to dissection of the renal pedicle to stimulate a brisk osmotic diuresis. As an indication of adequate hydration, the renal vein should appear plump and full prior to dissection of the renal vessels. At this stage, the lateral, posterior, and inferior (i.e., ureter) attachments to the kidney are still maintained creating a three-point fixation (Fig. 6). Leaving these attachments intact during the dissection of the renal hilum limits the mobility of the kidney and prevents the kidney from dropping medially and obscuring the renal vessels. This also prevents inadvertent kinking or torsion of the kidney about its vascular pedicle during the operation.

The renal pedicle is placed on gentle traction by elevating the ureteral packet and lower pole of the kidney, thus facilitating identification and dissection of the renal vein and artery (Fig. 7). The proper plane of dissection is along the relatively avascular plane directly on the advential wall of the renal artery and vein. Here, primarily blunt dissection should be used. Sharp dissection is used sparingly around the renal pedicle and is performed with great care in order to minimize the chance of iatrogenic

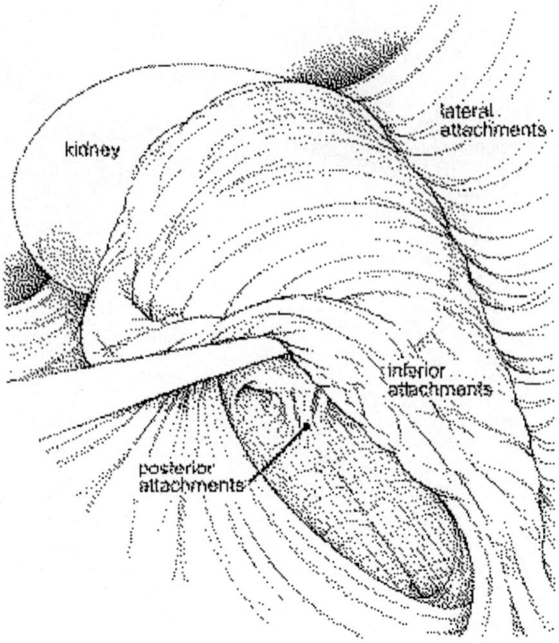

Fig. 6. The inferior, posterior, and lateral attachments of the kidney provide a three-point fixation of the kidney to the retroperitoneum.

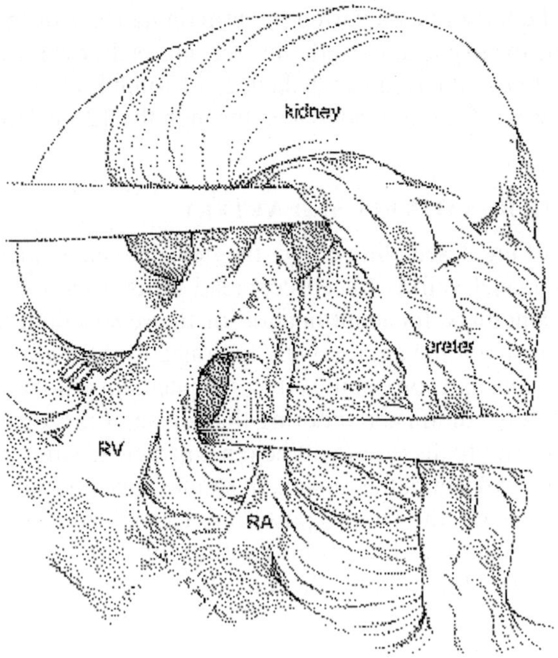

Fig. 7. Dissection of the renal vessels and perivascular connective tissue: RV = renal vein, RA = renal artery (left adrenal vein stump is seen clipped).

injury to the renal vessels and their branches. The renal vessels should be skeletonized of all of their surrounding perivascular connective tissue and lymphatics. The electrocautery hook, bipolar forceps, or ultrasonic scalpel may all be used to divide these perihilar connective tissues. Hemostatic clips are applied to the adrenal and any lumbar veins prior to transection. These clips should, however, be avoided specifically near the origin of the renal vessels as they may subsequently become entrapped within the endoscopic GIA stapler and cause misfiring of this device at the time of transection of the renal vessels. The renal artery is dissected completely to its origin with the aorta and the renal vein dissected as far medial beyond the adrenal vein as possible in order to achieve maximal renal vascular length. For optimal exposure of the renal vessels, the 15-mm Endocatch device or paddle retractor is utilized for medial retraction of the surrounding colon, mesentery, and small bowel. Topical papavarine (30 mg/mL) may be applied to the renal artery periodically using a laparoscopic needle-tipped applicator to minimize arterial vasospasm, which can be caused by excessive traction on the renal pedicle or aggressive dissection. At the end of the dissection of the renal vessels, furosemide (40 mg) and a second dose of mannitol (12.5 g) are administered intravenously.

If bleeding from the renal vessels or their branches occurs, direct pressure should be applied to the point of bleeding when possible using a laparoscopic instrument or 4 × 8-in. sterile gauze introduced through a 12-mm trocar. In addition, the insufflation pressure can be increased temporarily to help tamponade any ongoing bleeding. Small venous injuries will often subside with these two maneuvers; Surgicel or Gelfoam can then be placed and the operation continued. Larger venous or arterial injuries may require open conversion. Although certain vascular injuries may be managed laparoscopically, the author emphasizes the importance of having a low threshold for open conversion in efforts to both minimize donor morbidity and preserve renal allograft function. If open conversion is deemed necessary, pressure should be maintained at the point of bleeding with laparoscopic control until the necessary equipment is available and the proper incision is made exposing the renal hilum. Standard equipment and instrumentation used for an open donor nephrectomy procedure should always be kept available in the operating room. Either a standard flank or midline incision can be used for open conversion.

Step 3: Exposing the Upper Pole of the Kidney and Preservation of the Adrenal Gland

Gerota's fascia is incised sharply along the anteromedial aspect of the upper pole of the kidney and the renal capsule exposed. At this point, with a laparoscopic Maryland dissector in the left hand and a suction–irrigation device in the right hand, the upper pole is gradually freed from within Gerota's fascia using mainly blunt dissection. By dissecting along the medial border of the upper pole of the kidney, the adrenal gland is preserved and excluded from the field of dissection. Direct manipulation of the adrenal gland should be avoided as unnecessary bleeding can occur due to its vascular nature.

The dissection of the upper pole is facilitated by the aforementioned modification in the subxiphoid trocar placement (i.e., lateral shift of the 5-mm subxiphoid trocar). This modification allows the Maryland dissector to enter at a more acute angle of dissection to the upper pole. Without this modification, inadvertent entry into the upper pole renal parenchyma may occur due to the more shallow approach to the upper pole dissection using the Maryland dissector. While one instrument is used to elevate the upper pole, another is used to bluntly dissect the posterior upper pole attachments (Fig. 8). Great care must be taken to avoid injury to any upper pole renal vessels that may course in this location. As mentioned previously, preoperative three-dimensional CT angiography is helpful in identifying the presence of accessory renal arteries and veins. However, despite preoperative imaging, one must maintain vigilance during dissection to identify and spare any crossing vessels in this region. By the end of this step, the entire upper pole should be free of all perirenal attachments.

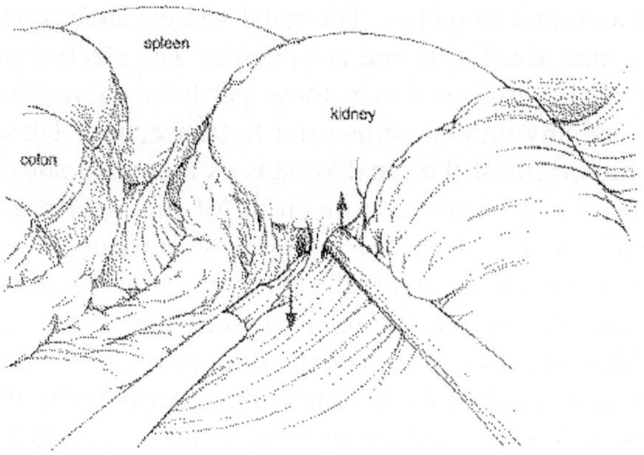

Fig. 8. Dissection of the upper pole of the kidney; as one instrument is used to elevate the upper pole, the second instrument is used to bluntly dissect the posterior attachments.

Step 4: Dissecting the Ureter

In efforts to avoid skeletonizing the ureter with resultant devascularization, a refinement in the technique of dissecting the ureter has been made. In this modified technique, a generous "V"-shaped packet of periureteral tissue (i.e., mesoureter) is maintained along with the ureter from the lower pole of the kidney down to the pelvic inlet (Fig. 9). Dissection is first carried out medial to the gonadal vein, bluntly sweeping this structure and the periureteral tissues in a lateral direction. Similar to the dissection of the upper pole of the kidney, one instrument is placed beneath the ureteral packet elevating it anteriorly while the other instrument bluntly dissects the posterior attachments. The fascia overlying the psoas muscle is an important landmark, which defines the posterior margin of the ureteral dissection. The plane between the ureteral packet and psoas fascia is often avascular. Great care must be taken to avoid dissecting beneath the psoas fascia, where bleeding from the psoas muscle is often encountered. Once the left abdominal sidewall is reached, this posterior dissection is continued superiorly towards the renal hilum and inferiorly to the iliac vessels. Hemostatic clips are applied to small perforating vessels and lymphatics. Electrocautery is used sparingly to prevent transmission of thermal injury to the ureter and its delicate blood supply. A conscious effort should be made to avoid

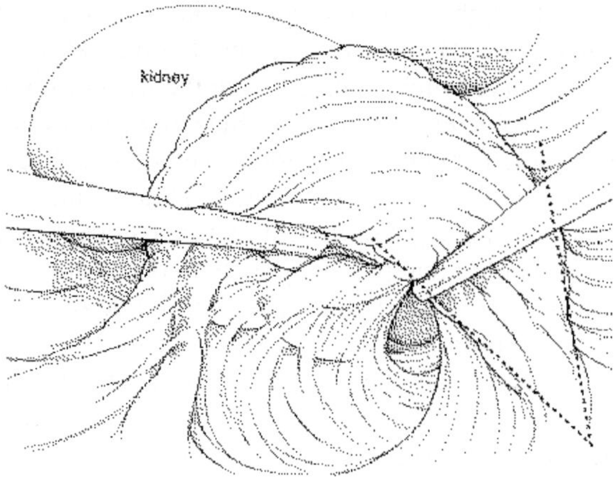

Fig. 9. Dissection of the ureter, maintaining a generous "V"-shaped packet of surrounding mesoureter (*dotted line*).

skeletonization or any direct manipulation of the ureter. Generally, the ureter should not be dissected or visualized until it crosses the iliac vessels. Staying medial to the gonadal vein ensures that the dissection is not too close to the ureter which could jeopardize its delicate blood supply. Because the only ureteral blood supply that remains intact in a transplanted kidney arises from the renal artery, dissection between the renal artery and proximal ureter should be avoided, and great diligence should be taken to prospectively identify and spare accessory lower pole arteries. At the end of this step the ureter is left intact and is not clipped or divided until the entire kidney and renal vessels are completely dissected. If divided early, continuous output of urine from the proximal end of the ureter will fill the abdominal cavity and operative field making dissection of the renal hilum more challenging.

Step 5: Releasing the Inferior, Lateral, and Posterior Renal Attachments

At this point the remaining inferior, lateral, and posterior attachments to the kidney can be safely released. A combination of sharp and blunt dissection is used to release Gerota's fascia from the lateral and posterior aspect of the kidney down to the renal capsule. The Ligasure™ device is a useful instrument for rapid release of these attachments. The Gerota's fat surrounding the lower pole and proximal ureter is left intact. It is important that the renal artery, vein, and ureter remain as the only attachments to the kidney at the end of this step (Fig. 10).

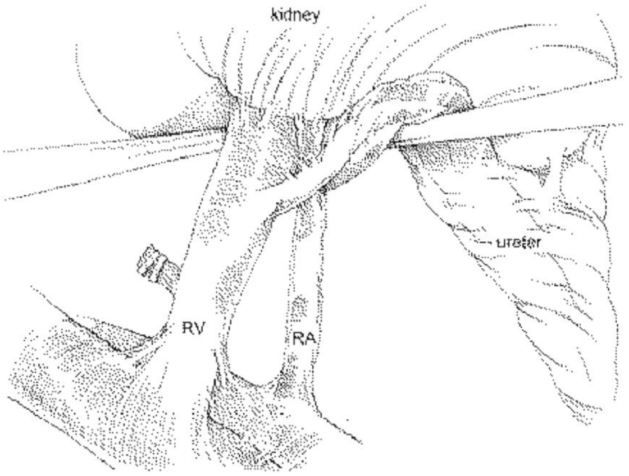

Fig. 10. Dissection of the kidney, ureter, renal vein (RV), and renal artery (RA).

Step 6: Preparing the Kidney Extraction Site

The extraction site of the kidney is prepared at this time by extending the previously marked Pfannenstiel incision transversely on either side of the Endocatch device to a total length of approximately 5–6 mm. A generous subcutaneous pocket is created cephalad and caudad just above the level of the anterior rectus fascia to provide sufficient room for extraction of the kidney. The rectus fascia and underlying peritoneum are left intact, thus preserving the pneumoperitoneum.

Step 7: Transecting the Gonadal Vessels and Ureter

After confirmation that the recipient transplantation team is prepared to receive the kidney, the gonadal vessels and ureter are transected distally at the level of the iliac vessels using either an endoscopic GIA stapler or hemostatic clips (Fig. 11). Preferably, the ureter is only clipped distally and is cut sharply without cautery. In a well-hydrated patient, urine is usually seen emanating from the proximal end of the ureter following transection.

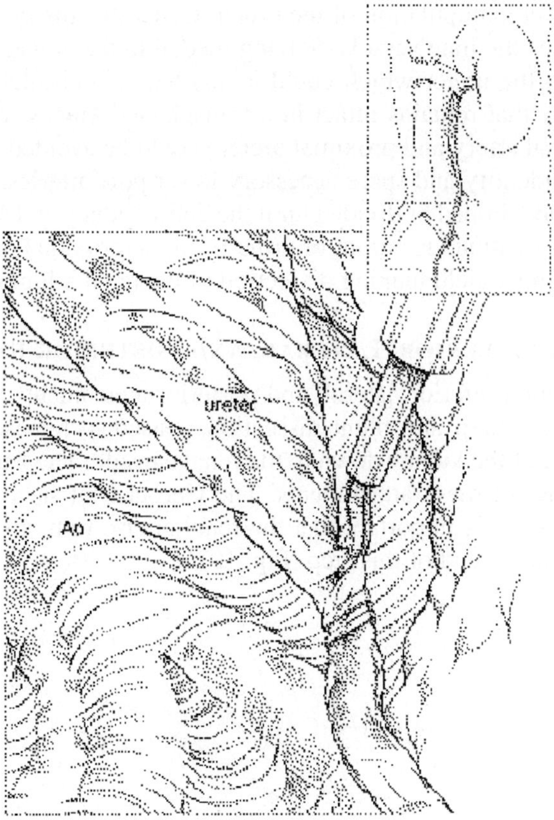

Fig. 11. Hemostatic clips are applied to the distal ureter at the level of the iliac vessels prior to transection; alternatively, an endoscopic GIA stapling device can be used. Ao = aorta.

Step 8: Transecting the Renal Vessels

Prior to transection of the renal artery and vein, the patient is given 3,000 units of intravenous heparin sulfate. The laparoscope is moved to the left lower quadrant trocar to allow the endoscopic GIA stapling device to be placed through the umbilical trocar. This provides the best angle of approach for transection of the renal vessels with the stapling device at a 90° angle, flush with the great vessels, thus maximizing allograft vessel length. With the renal vessels on gentle traction anterolaterally, the endoscopic GIA stapler is applied first to the renal artery (Fig. 12) followed immediately by the renal vein using a second vascular load in the stapling device. The renal artery is divided at its origin with the aorta and the renal vein is transected as far medial to the adrenal vein stump as possible to ensure maximum renal vascular length for transplantation. If multiple renal arteries are present, each should be transected prior to transection of the renal vein(s).

Others have reported alternative renal vessel ligation techniques, including the use of either an endovascular TA stapler, titanium clips, or a plastic, self-locking hemostatic clip [Hem-o-lok clips (Weck Closure Systems, Research Triangle Park, NC)] with or without additional metallic clips, followed by transection using laparoscopic scissors *(31,53,54)*. It must be noted, however, that Weck, the manufacturer of the Hem-o-lok clips, reported in 2006 that use of their product is contraindicated specifically during ligation of the renal artery during laparoscopic donor nephrectomy due to clip dislodgement and that more than one clip is recommended to ligate the renal artery in other procedures *(55,56)*. Though no current method of vascular control is perfect, stapler complications can typically be

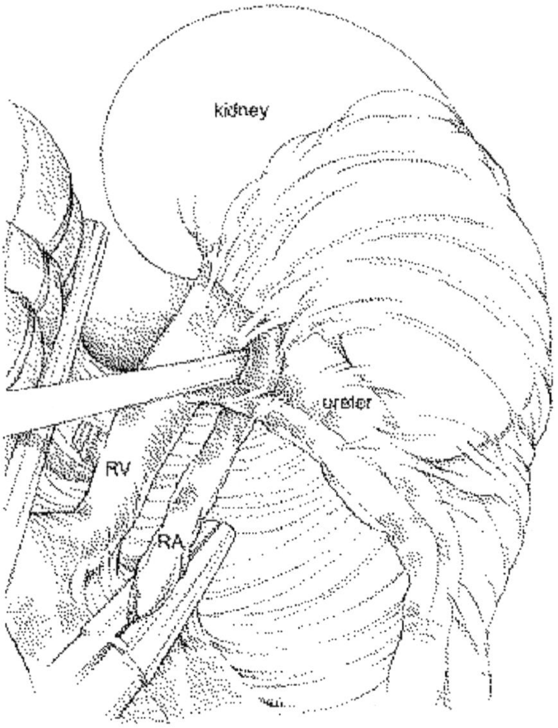

Fig. 12. Transection of the renal artery (RA) using an endoscopic GIA stapling device: RV = renal vein.

managed intraoperatively with laparoscopic techniques or rapid open conversion whereas Hem-o-lok failures often present in a delayed, potentially catastrophic fashion *(57)*. The endo-GIA also obviates the need to introduce scissors into the operative field during this critical part of the operation, when inadvertent vascular injury can occur due to the requirement for complex movements to be executed in rapid succession. Consequently, our preferred method of renal vascular ligation and transection is by endo-GIA stapler.

Step 9: Entrapment and Delivering of the Kidney

To facilitate entrapment, the kidney is placed above the spleen after transection of the renal vessels. The 15-mm Endocatch bag, which should already be placed within the delivery site (Pfannenstiel incision), is now deployed below the spleen and the kidney is gently placed within the bag (Fig. 13). After ensuring that the entire kidney and ureter are within the bag, the ring cord of the Endocatch device is pulled thus entrapping the kidney. A muscle-splitting longitudinal incision is made in the rectus fascia and underlying peritoneum along the linea alba using heavy scissors. The surgeon's hand is used to protect the intraperitoneal contents, taking great care not to injure either the bladder or bowel during this maneuver. The fascial incision should be made large enough to allow for atraumatic delivery of the kidney (Fig. 14). Once the kidney is delivered within the bag, it is passed off to the recipient transplantation team for immediate immersion in ice slush and perfusion with iced preservation solution.

Step 10: Inspecting the Renal Bed and Closing Abdominal Incisions

The patient is given 30 mg of intravenous protamine sulfate and the rectus fascia is closed with a running #1-polyglyconate suture. Pneumoperitoneum is reestablished and the renal bed and stumps of

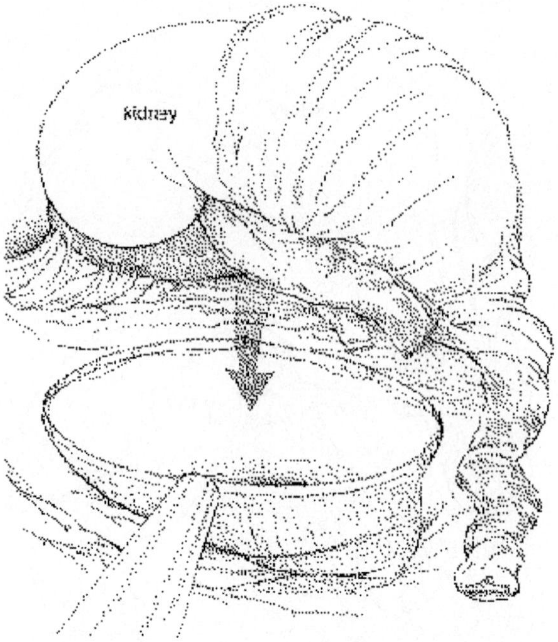

Fig. 13. Entrapment of the renal allograft using a 15-mm Endocatch bag; the kidney is placed above the spleen and lowered down into the bag to facilitate entrapment.

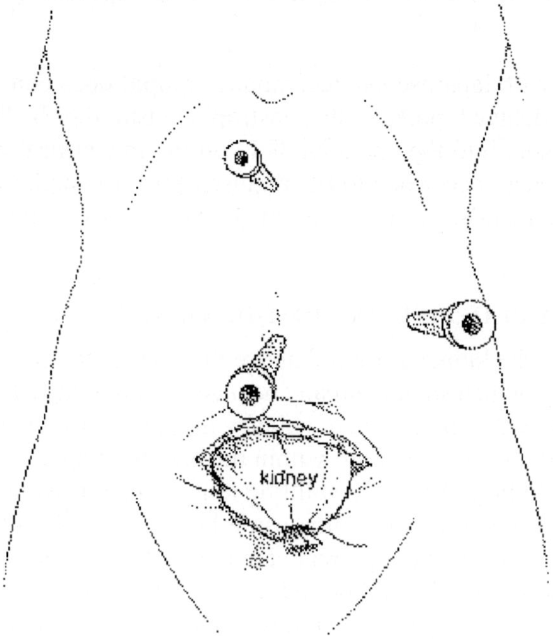

Fig. 14. Delivery of the renal allograft within the Endocatch bag through the Pfannenstiel incision; three trocars remain in place to allow for inspection of the renal bed after delivery of the kidney.

the renal vessels are inspected for bleeding under low insufflation pressure (e.g., 5–10 mmHg). The nephrectomy bed should be copiously irrigated using the suction–irrigation device with meticulous hemostasis achieved using either bipolar forceps or vascular clips. Identification of milky appearing lymphatic fluid within the operative field should prompt special attention to identifying leaky lymphatic channels that should be clipped in order to avoid a postoperative lymphocele or even chylous ascites. The colon and its associated mesentery, small bowel, spleen, and adrenal bed should be inspected closely for any bleeding or injuries. Once meticulous hemostasis is achieved, the 12-mm trocars are sequentially removed and the fascia closed with 2-0 polyglactin suture using the Carter–Thomason® fascial closure device (Inlet Medical, Eden Prairie, MN) under direct laparoscopic visualization. The 5-mm trocar site typically requires no fascial closure. The abdomen is desufflated of all CO_2 gas prior to removal of the last trocar.

Right Laparoscopic Live Donor Nephrectomy

Laparoscopic donor nephrectomy was initially reserved for the left side due to reduced renal venous length when procuring a right-sided kidney. Though we have become more comfortable with right laparoscopic live donor nephrectomy over time, we caution that it remains a technically challenging procedure best left to experienced laparoscopic surgeons. Common indications for right-sided donor nephrectomy include multiple left renal arteries or veins, smaller right kidney, right renal cysts, or ptosis of the right kidney. However, it should be noted that many recipient surgeons prefer two donor renal arteries with a long renal vein than a single artery and a shorter right renal vein *(58)*. Several high-volume transplant centers have published their right laparoscopic live donor nephrectomy experience with results equivalent to the left side *(58–62)*. In either case, the conventional rule holds true; the better functioning kidney should remain in the donor patient.

For a right-sided laparoscopic donor nephrectomy, trocar configuration is typically the mirror image of that used for a left-sided dissection. The steps used for dissecting the kidney are similar to that on the left, though Kocherization of the duodenum is also required. If additional liver retraction is needed, a blunt 5-mm laparoscopic grasper can be introduced through a trocar placed either below the xiphoid process or along anterior axillary line.

Herein we describe two possible modifications that should be considered in efforts to preserve maximum length of the anatomically shorter right renal vein. In the first modification, the placement of the endoscopic GIA stapling device is relocated so as to transect the right renal vein in a plane parallel to the inferior vena cava. In contrast to procurement of a left kidney, where the stapling device is placed in the umbilical trocar position, with procurement of a right kidney the stapling device is introduced into the right lower quadrant port located lateral to the rectus muscle. This angle of approach allows the stapling device to transect the right renal vein parallel to and flush with the inferior vena cava, thus preserving maximum length of the right renal vein. The kidney is subsequently delivered through a Pfannenstiel incision. This modification also permits use of a 10-mm fascial splitting EndoTip™ trocar in the umbilical laparoscope site, which does not need to be closed after removal. Note that when performing a left-sided technique, a 10-mm trocar may not be used at the umbilical site as the cannula is not large enough to permit passage of the endoscopic GIA stapler.

The second modification involves relocating the extraction site of the renal allograft in place of using an infra- or periumbilical incision. After completely dissecting the kidney, renal vessels, and ureter laparoscopically, a 5–6 mm transverse subcostal muscle-splitting incision is made directly overlying the renal hilum. This incision is used for open transection of the renal vessels and for delivery of the renal allograft as an alternative to a Pfannenstiel incision. To optimize the length of the right renal vein, a Satinsky clamp may be placed on the inferior vena cava, allowing the renal vein to be transected along with a cuff of vena cava. The vena cava is subsequently closed with a nonabsorbable, monofilament suture after delivery of the renal allograft.

Hand-Assisted Laparoscopic Live Donor Nephrectomy

Hand-assisted laparoscopy allows a right-handed operating surgeon to place the left hand in the abdomen through a 6–8-cm incision (depending on the size of the surgeon's hand), using a pneumatic sleeve device to preserve the pneumoperitoneum. The surgeon can thus use his left hand inside the abdomen in concert with his right, which controls conventional laparoscopic instrumentation outside of the abdomen. The intraperitoneal hand can be used to provide tactile sensation, expose, dissect, and retract tissues as well as secure hemostasis.

In performing hand-assisted laparoscopic donor nephrectomy, any of the commercially available hand-assistance port devices can be utilized. Selection of the proper incision site for placement of the hand-assist device is important. For a left-sided donor nephrectomy, either a periumbilical or infraumbilical midline incision can be used for the hand-assist device. A 30° laparoscopic lens is introduced through a 12-mm trocar placed along the anterior axillary line at the level of the umbilicus. The working trocar is placed lateral to the rectus muscle just below the level of the umbilicus. For a right-sided donor nephrectomy, the incision for the hand-assist device is made in the right lower quadrant along a muscle-splitting incision (i.e., Gibson incision) and the umbilicus serves as the working trocar. The laparoscope is placed in the abdominal midline, half way between the xiphoid process and umbilicus. For retraction of the liver, a blunt 5-mm laparoscopic instrument can be introduced through a trocar placed either below the xiphoid process or along anterior axillary line above the hand-assist device.

Dissection of the kidney and renal vessels is carried out in a similar fashion to conventional laparoscopic techniques. Instead of the Endocatch device, the left hand is used to reflect and retract the bowel contents. The intraperitoneal hand is useful in elevating the kidney during transection of the renal vessels, thus optimizing renal vascular length. After transection of the renal vessels, the kidney is delivered directly through the hand-assist port and does not require entrapment within a bag.

RESULTS

Laparoscopic live donor nephrectomy has had a substantial impact on the donor operation by providing a less invasive approach to kidney procurement as compared to open donor nephrectomy. This has resulted in less postoperative pain and shorter hospitalizations and postoperative convalescence for the donor patient while maintaining a high-quality allograft for the recipient *(10,16–32)*. A meta-analysis published in 2004 compared laparoscopic donor nephrectomy to conventional open donor nephrectomy and found that laparoscopic live donor nephrectomy was at least as safe and efficacious as the open technique in the short-term *(30)*. The open technique took significantly less time but donor pain, oral intake, hospital stay, and return to employment favored the laparoscopic approach. Delayed graft function, acute rejections, overall complication rates as well as patient and graft survival were similar in both groups, though the types of complications experienced differed between the two procedures. Open donors were more likely to experience pulmonary complications, deep venous thrombosis, fever, pain, and nausea, whereas the laparoscopic donors were more likely to experience mechanical (e.g., splenic or bowel injuries) and vascular complications *(30)*.

Overall risks to the donor have decreased to approximately 0.03% mortality and 8% morbidity *(10,25,28–33,37)*. In studies that have compared living donors to their siblings, there has been no increased risk of renal failure or hypertension. Donor complications have remained low (4–17%) and comparable to open donor nephrectomy series *(10,25,28–33,37,63,64)*. Ureteral complications have declined (0–7%) with modifications in surgical technique *(25,28,29,30,34–36,63,64)*. Immediate as well as long-term renal allograft function has paralleled that of kidneys procured by open surgical techniques *(10,18,20,28,30,32,58–71)*. One risk of note involves the method of ligation of the renal artery *(55)*. Three primary laparoscopic methods of arterial ligation have been described, namely, stapling devices, metallic clips, and self-locking plastic clips. Though many groups have reported success with all methods, it is important to recognize that all methods are liable to failure and may result in bleeding, morbidity, and death. Recently, use of Hem-o-lok clips has been reported as a contraindication during renal artery ligation specifically during laparoscopic donor nephrectomy *(56)*.

Hand-assisted laparoscopic live donor nephrectomy may reduce operative times and warm ischemia times as compared to pure laparoscopy *(30,72)*, though allograft function does not differ. A recent meta-analysis comparing laparoscopic versus hand-assisted live donor nephrectomy demonstrated shorter operative and warm ischemia times and decreased intraoperative bleeding; however, the donor and recipient complication rates and graft function was similar *(72)*. Most importantly, the hand-assisted technique serves as an intermediary between open and pure laparoscopic approaches and thereby may allow for more widespread implementation by surgeons with less laparoscopic proficiency and experience.

TAKE HOME MESSAGES

The technique of laparoscopic live donor nephrectomy requires substantial technical skill and knowledge of renal vascular anatomy in order to successfully procure a healthy, functioning renal allograft suitable for transplantation. Whether using conventional or hand-assisted laparoscopic techniques, adherence to the following four principles is important.

(1) **Maintaining the Renal Attachments During Dissection of the Renal Hilum:** In order to facilitate identification and dissection of the renal vessels, it is crucial that the lateral, posterior, and inferior renal attachments remain intact until the renal vein and artery are completely dissected. These three attachments fixate the kidney to the retroperitoneum, minimizing its mobility, and preventing the kidney from dropping medially and obscuring the renal hilum. These attachments also prevent kinking or torsion of the kidney about its renal pedicle.

(2) **Exposure of the Renal Hilum:** Just as in open surgery, proper exposure of the renal hilum for dissection of the renal vessels is crucial. Complete medial reflection of the ipsilateral colon is an important initial step in providing the necessary exposure of the renal hilum. Placement of the Endocatch device early on during the laparoscopic dissection of the kidney provides an excellent blunt retractor for medial retraction of the colon and further exposure of the renal hilum. However, the authors caution that the terminal end of the Endocatch device is not blunt and therefore should be used gently during retraction. In addition, great care must be taken to avoid contacting the Endocatch device when using cautery during the operation, as this device is not insulated and can therefore transmit electrical current to adjacent tissues. Alternatively, an insulated paddle retractor can be used for retraction of the bowels. With the exposure provided by either the Endocatch device or paddle retractor, the renal vessels are easily visualized and dissected back towards their origin with the great vessels. Inadvertent injury to these structures and their branches is thus minimized.

(3) **Dissection of the Renal Vessels:** Minimizing sharp dissection and electrocautery around the renal hilum is important in preventing inadvertent injury to the main renal vessels. Blunt dissection along the advential wall of the renal vessels is preferable. When dissecting the perivascular tissue, hemostatic clips should be used judiciously. Excessive use of clips especially around the origin of the renal vessels can pose significant problems when it comes time to transect the renal vessels. These clips can become lodged within the endoscopic GIA stapling device resulting in misfiring of the staple line and incomplete transection of the renal vessels. This can result in significant bleeding, often requiring emergent open conversion. As an alternative, the electrocautery hook, bipolar electrocautery, or ultrasonic shears can be used instead of clips to transect the often abundant perivascular lymphatic and connective tissues. The renal artery and vein should be skeletonized and dissected back to their origin with the aorta and vena cava, respectively, to optimize renal vascular length.

(4) **Dissection of the Ureter:** The blood supply to the transplant ureter is based solely upon branches of the renal artery. Therefore, maintaining abundant mesoureter and minimizing ureteral dissection espe-

cially between the renal artery and proximal ureter are important principles for optimizing the vascular integrity of the ureter and minimizing postoperative ureteral complications. Lower pole accessory renal arteries should be spared whenever possible. The use of electrocautery around the ureter, as well as, direct manipulation of the ureter itself should be avoided. Blunt dissection is predominately used starting medial to the gonadal vein, sweeping this structure along with the ureter and mesoureter in a lateral and anterior direction. Ultimately a "V"-shaped packet of tissue should be maintained surrounding the ureter from the lower pole to the iliac vessels. The ureter should not be directly manipulated or even visualized until it crosses the iliac vessels, where it can be safely clipped and then transected.

ACKNOWLEDGEMENTS

The authors would like to acknowledge Louis R. Kavoussi, M.D. and Lloyd E. Ratner, M.D. for their pioneering contributions in the development and dissemination of the laparoscopic live donor nephrectomy technique.

We also thank Felipe Pedrinho, M.D. and Jeffrey Piacitelli, P.A. for their assistance in the creation of the video.

REFERENCES

1. Karlberg I, Nyberg G: Cost-effectiveness studies of renal transplantation. Int J Technol Assess Health Care 1995;11: 611–622.
2. http://www.unos.org, accessed 8/30/07
3. http://www.optn.org/latestData/rptData.asp, accessed 8/30/07
4. 2006 Annual Report of the U.S. Scientific Registry of Transplant Recipients and the Organ Procurement and Transplantation Network: Transplant Data 1990–1999. Rockville, MD and Richmond, VA: HHS/HRSA/OSP/DOT and UNOS. Retrieved August 30, 2007 from http://www.optn.org/data/annualReport.asp
5. Danovitch GM, Cohen DJ, Weir MR, et al. Current status of kidney and pancreas transplantation in the United States, 1994–2003. Am J Transplant 2005;5:904–915.
6. Delmonico FL, Dew MA. Living donor kidney transplantation in a global environment. Kidney Int 2007;71:608–614.
7. Ishida H, Miyamoto N, Shirakawa H, et al. Evaluation of immunosuppressive regimens in ABO-incompatible living kidney transplantation-single center analysis. Am J Transplant 2007;7:825–831.
8. Gill JS, Gill J, Rose C, Zalunardo N, et al. The older living kidney donor: part of the solution to the organ shortage. Transplantation 2006;82:1662–1666.
9. Ugarte R, Kraus E, Montgomery RA, et al. Excellent outcomes after transplantation of deceased donor kidneys with high terminal creatinine and mild pathologic lesions. Transplantation 2005;80:794–800.
10. Rettkowski O, Hamza A, Markau S, et al. Ten years of laparoscopic living donor nephrectomy: retrospect and prospect from the nephrologist's point of view. Transplant Proc 2007;39:30–33.
11. Ball AJ, Colonna JO, Fabrizio MD, et al. Expanding the criteria for renal transplant donation. AUA Update Series 2005, Lesson 20;24:174–179.
12. AUA Specialty Course Board Preparation 2006; 2:17–34.
13. Merrill JP, Murray JE, Harrison JH, et al. Successful homotransplantations of the human kidney between identical twins. JAMA 1956;160:277–282.
14. Cecka JM. Living donor transplants. Clin Transpl 1995;363–377.
15. Cecka JM, Terasaki PI. Living donor kidney transplants: superior success rates despite histocompatibilities. Transplant Proc 1997;29:203.
16. Ratner LE, Ciseck LJ, Moore RG, et al. Laparoscopic live donor nephrectomy. Transplantation 1995;60:1047–1049.
17. Ratner LE, Kavoussi LR, Sroka M, et al. Laparoscopic assisted live donor nephrectomy – a comparison with the open approach. Transplantation 1997;63:229–233.
18. Lee BR, Chow GK, Ratner LE, et al. Laparoscopic live donor nephrectomy: outcomes equivalent to open surgery. J Endourol 2000;14:811–819.
19. Ratner LE, Montgomery RA, Kavoussi LR. Laparoscopic live donor nephrectomy: the four year Johns Hopkins University experience. Nephrol Dial Transplant 1999;14:2090–2093.
20. Ratner LE, Montgomery RA, Maley WR, et al. Laparoscopic live donor nephrectomy: the recipient. Transplantation 2000;69:2319–2323.
21. Sosa JA, Albini TA, Powe NR, et al. Laparoscopic vs. open live nephrectomy: a multivariate patient outcome analysis. Transplantation 1998;65:S85.

22. Flowers JL, Jacobs S, Cho E, et al. Comparison of open and laparoscopic live donor nephrectomy. Ann Surg 1997;226:483–489.
23. London E, Rudich S, McVicar J, et al. Equivalent renal allograft function with laparoscopic versus open live donor nephrectomies. Transplant Proc 1999;31:258–260.
24. Odland MD, Ney AL, Jacobs DM, et al. Initial experience with laparoscopic live donor nephrectomy. Surgery 1999;126:603–606.
25. Jacobs SC, Cho E, Foster C, et al. Laparoscopic donor nephrectomy: the University of Maryland 6-year experience. J Urol 2004; 171: 47–51.
26. Rodrigue JR, Cross NJ, Newman RC, et al. Patient-reported outcomes for open versus laparoscopic living donor nephrectomy. Prog Transplant 2006;16:162–169.
27. Engen DE. Transplantation update. AUA Update Series 1997;16(27):210–215.
28. Simforoosh N, Basiri A, Tabibi A, et al. Comparison of laparoscopic and open donor nephrectomy: a randomized controlled trial. BJU Int 2005;95:851–855.
29. Su LM, Ratner LE, Montgomery RA, et al. Laparoscopic live donor nephrectomy: trends in donor and recipient morbidity following 381 consecutive cases. Ann Surg 2004;240:358–363.
30. Tooher RL, Rao MM, Scott DF, et al. A systematic review of laparoscopic live-donor nephrectomy. Transplantation 2004;78:404–414.
31. Melcher ML, Carter JT, Posselt A, et al. More than 500 consecutive laparoscopic donor nephrectomies without conversion or repeated surgery. Arch Surg 2005;140:835–839.
32. Paul A, Treckmann J, Gallinat A, et al. Current concepts in transplant surgery: laparoscopic living donor of the kidney. Langenbecks Arch Surg 2007;392:501–509.
33. Breda A, Veale J, Liao J, et al. Complications of laparoscopic living donor nephrectomy and their management: the UCLA experience. Urology 2007;69:49–52.
34. Philosophe B, Kuo PC, Schweitzer EJ, et al. Laparoscopic versus open donor nephrectomy: comparing ureteral complications in the recipients and improving the laparoscopic technique. Transplantation 1999;68:497–502.
35. Dunkin BJ, Johnson LB, Kuo PC. A technical modification eliminates early ureteral complications after laparoscopic donor nephrectomy. J Am Coll Surg 2000;190:96–97.
36. Kuo PC, Cho ES, Flowers JL, et al. Laparoscopic living donor nephrectomy and multiple renal arteries. Am J Surg 1998;176:559–563.
37. Matas AJ, Bartlett ST, Leichtman AB, et al. Morbidity and mortality after living kidney donation, 1999–2001: survey of United States transplant centers. Am J Transplant 2003;3:830–834.
38. Dahm F, Weber M, Muller B, et al. Open and laparoscopic living donor nephrectomy in Switzerland: a retrospective assessment of clinical outcomes and the motivation to donate. Nephrol Dial Transplant 2006;21:2563–2568.
39. Giessing M, Reuter S, Deger S, et al. Laparoscopic versus open donor nephrectomy in Germany: impact on donor health-related quality of life and willingness to donate. Transplant Proc 2005;37:2011–2015.
40. Kasiske BL, Ravenscraft M, Ramos EL, et al. The evaluation of living renal transplant donors: clinical practice guidelines. Ad Hoc Clinical Practice Guidelines Subcommittee of the Patient Care and Education Committee of the American Society of Transplant Physicians. J Am Soc Nephrol 1996; 7:2288–2313.
41. Delmonico F; Council of the Transplantation Society. A report of the Amsterdam forum on the care of the live kidney donor: data and medical guidelines. Transplantation 2005;79:S53–66.
42. Renoult E, Hubert J, Ladriere M, et al. Robot-assisted laparoscopic and open live-donor nephrectomy: a comparison of donor morbidity and early renal allograft outcomes. Nephrol Dial Transplant 2006;21:472–477.
43. Horgan S, Galvani, Gorodner MV, et al. Effect of robotic assistance on the "learning curve" for laparoscopic hand-assisted donor nephrectomy. Surg Endosc 2007;21:1512–1517.
44. Yashi M, Yagisawa T, Ishikawa N, et al. Retroperitoneoscopic hand-assisted live-donor nephrectomy according to the basic principle of transplantation in donor kidney selection. J Endourol 2007;21:589–594.
45. Narita S, Inoue T, Matsuura S, et al. Outcome of right hand-assisted retroperitoneoscopic living donor nephrectomy. Urology 2006;67:496–500.
46. Ruszat R, Sulser T, Dickenmann M, et al. Retroperitoneoscopic donor nephrectomy: donor outcome and complication rate in comparison with three different techniques. World J Urol 2006;24:113–117.
47. Wadstrom J. Hand-assisted retroperitoneoscopic live donor nephrectomy: experience from the first 75 consecutive cases. Transplantation 2005;80:1060–1066.
48. Yoshimura K, Takahara S, Kyakuno M, et al. Retroperitoneoscopic living related-donor nephrectomy: clinical outcomes of 50 consecutive cases and comparison with open donor nephrectomy. J Endourol 2005;19: 808–812.
49. Tanabe K, Miyamoto N, Ishida H, et al. Retroperitoneoscopic live donor nephrectomy (RPLDN): establishment and initial experience of RPLDN at a single center. Am J Transplant 2005;5:739–745.
50. Tsuchiya N, Iinuma M, Habuchi T, et al. Hand-assisted retroperitoneoscopic nephrectomy for living kidney transplantation: initial 44 cases. Urology 2004;64:250–254.
51. Ng CS, Abreu SC, Abou El-Fettouh HI, et al. Right retroperitoneal versus left transperitoneal laparoscopic live donor nephrectomy. Urology 2004;63:857–861.

52. Hoznek A, Olsson LE, Salomon L, et al. Retroperitoneal laparoscopic living-donor nephrectomy. Preliminary results. Eur Urol 2001;40:614–618.
53. Meng MV, Freise CE, Kang SM, et al. Techniques to optimize vascular control during laparoscopic donor nephrectomy. Urology 2003;61:93–97.
54. Baumert H, Ballaro A, Arroyo C, et al. The use of polymer (Hem-o-lok) clips for management of the renal hilum during laparoscopic nephrectomy. Eur Urol 2006;49:816–819.
55. Meng MV. Reported failures of the polymer self-locking (Hem-o-lok) clip: review of data from the Food and Drug Administration. J Endourol 2006;20:1054–1057.
56. Weck Hem-o-lok Regulatory Affairs correspondence from D.D. Maurer, Vice President, Regulatory Affairs, Teleflex Medical. June 1, 2006.
57. Steinberg PL, Pobi K, Axelrod DA, et al. Re: Herve Baumert, Andrew Ballaro, Carlos Arroyo, Amir V. Kaisary, Peter F.A. Mulders and Ben C. Knipscheer. The use of polymer (Hem-o-lok) clips for management of the renal hilum during laparoscopic nephrectomy. Eur Urol 2007;51:572–573.
58. Mandal AK, Cohen C, Montgomery RA, et al. Should the indications for laparoscopic live donor nephrectomy of the right kidney be the same as for the open procedure? Anomalous left renal vasculature is not a contraindication to laparoscopic left donor nephrectomy. Transplantation 2001;71:660–664.
59. Diner EK, Radolinski B, Murdock JD, et al. Right laparoscopic donor nephrectomy: the Washington Hospital Center experience. Urology 2006;6:1175–1177.
60. Kay MD, Brook N, Kaushik M, et al. Comparison of right and left laparoscopic live donor nephrectomy. BJU Int 2006;4:843–844.
61. Liu KL, Chiang YJ, Wu CT, et al. Why we consistently use the left donor kidney in living related transplantation: initial experience of right laparoscopic donor nephrectomy and comparison with left nephrectomy. Transplant Proc 2006;38:1977–1979.
62. Husted TL, Hanaway MJ, Thomas MJ, et al. Laparoscopic right living donor nephrectomy. Transplant Proc 2005;37:631–632.
63. Montgomery RA, Kavoussi LR, Su LM, et al. Improved recipient results after 5 years of performing laparoscopic donor nephrectomy. Transplant Proc 2001;33:1108–1110.
64. Novotny MJ. Laparoscopic live donor nephrectomy. Urol Clin North Am 2001;28:127–135.
65. Ratner LE, Fabrizio M, Chavin K, et al. Technical considerations in the delivery of the kidney during laparoscopic live-donor nephrectomy. J Am Coll Surg 1999;189:427–430.
66. Fabrizio MD, Ratner LE, Montgomery RA, et al. Laparoscopic live donor nephrectomy. Urol Clin North Am 1999;26:247–256.
67. D'Alessandro AM, Sollinger HW, Knechtle SJ, et al. Living related and unrelated donors for kidney transplantation: a 28-year experience. Ann Surg 1995;222:353–362.
68. Johnson EM, Remucal MJ, Gilligham KJ, et al. Complications and risks of living donor nephrectomy. Transplantation 1997;64:1124–1128.
69. Streem SB, Novick AC, Steinmuller DR, et al. Flank donor nephrectomy: efficacy in the donor and recipient. J Urol 1989;141:1099–1101.
70. Waples MJ, Belzer FO, Uehling DT: Living donor nephrectomy: a 20-year experience. Urology 1995;45:207–210.
71. Dunn JF, Nylander WA Jr, Richie RE, et al. Living related kidney donors. A 14-year experience. Ann Surg 1986;203:637–643.
72. Kokkinos C, Nanidis T, Antcliffe D, et al. Comparison of laparoscopic versus hand-assisted live donor nephrectomy. Transplantation 2007;83:41–47.

Laparoscopic and Robotic Pyeloplasty

Sean P. Hedican and Murali K. Ankem

INTRODUCTION

Laparoscopic pyeloplasty as a treatment option for the obstructed ureteropelvic junction (UPJ) combines the advantage of an open reconstruction under direct magnified vision with the low morbidity of an endoscopic approach. First described as a minimally invasive treatment option by Schuessler and colleagues in 1993 *(1)*, there are several large published series with extended follow-up confirming long-term patency rates of 96–100% *(2)*. These results parallel the outcomes of the prior gold standard approach (i.e., open pyeloplasty) and exceed what is observed with endoscopic incisional operations. As demonstrated with other minimally invasive operations, patients undergoing laparoscopic pyeloplasty have reduced analgesic requirements, hospital stays, and time until return of full activities compared to their open surgery counter-parts *(3)*. The recovery as compared to endopyelotomy is less clear. Though technically challenging, thc low incidence of failure combined with reduced postoperative morbidity has made this an increasingly popular treatment option at institutions offering this approach.

The introduction of robotic surgical platforms has greatly enhanced the performance of complex extirpative and reconstructive urologic procedures. The da Vinci Surgical System (Intuitive Surgical Inc., Sunnyvale, CA) was developed and popularized to minimize the difficulties with conventional laparoscopy. The da Vinci system offers a three-dimensional view, instruments with an articulated wrist and seven degrees of freedom, tremor filtering, and motion scaling all of which significantly improve intra-corporeal suturing for the less experienced laparoscopist. Therefore, the da Vinci system has proven to be a useful adjunct in performing laparoscopic pyeloplasty.

PATIENT SELECTION

As with most laparoscopic procedures, there are few contraindications to laparoscopic pyeloplasty. It has been utilized in the treatment of secondary, as well as, primary UPJ obstructions. Prior failed treatment approaches in patients with secondary UPJ obstructions undergoing successful laparoscopic pyeloplasty have included incisional and open operations. This technique is particularly advantageous in the reconstruction of the obstructed UPJ due to anterior crossing vessels because the low angle, 10- to 15-fold magnification aids in the delicate dissection around these structures. This procedure has also been successfully performed in patients with additional associated anomalies such as a horseshoe kidney, duplication, or nephroptosis.

The strongest relative contraindications to this approach are patients with a very small intra-renal pelvis. This later condition limits mobility of the pelvis and requires intra-hilar dissection making

From: *Current Clinical Urology: Essential Urologic Laparoscopy*
Edited by: S. Y. Nakada and S. P. Hedican, DOI 10.1007/978-1-60327-820-1_13

laparoscopic, as well as open, reconstruction difficult. In such patients, an incisional procedure may be the preferred initial treatment option. Preoperative recognition of this condition is best made by careful inspection of the intravenous pyelogram, CT urogram or ultrasound. A retrograde pyelogram is often less helpful in judging the amount of extra-renal pelvis, since it does not outline the location of the parenchyma relative to the collecting system. Patients who have failed a prior open or laparoscopic pyeloplasty are often best approached with an incisional procedure if the resultant area of stenosis is limited *(4)*. Other conditions which are somewhat more controversial include pre-pubertal children, due to the delicate dimensions of the UPJ and the low morbidity of a posterior lumbotomy approach although use of the robot or standard laparoscopic approaches have been advocated with excellent success rates by several groups *(5)*.

OPERATING ROOM SET-UP

The side on which the patient's UPJ obstruction exists determines the variables in the operating room set-up. The patient is placed in a semi-flank position as described below with the affected side up. The operating surgeon and first assistant stand on the contralateral side of the pathology facing the patient's abdomen while the second assistant and scrub nurse (or technician) stand on the opposite side of the table facing the primary surgeon (Fig. 1). This positioning facilitates direct passage of equipment by the scrub personnel across the table to the operating surgeon so he or she does not have to reach behind, or to their side, to receive instruments. It is valuable to have a second assistant for the later portion of the procedure, especially in larger patients, because the spread of the trocars can lead to shoulder fatigue in the first assistant trying to maintain the camera while operating instruments from the lateral port site. Tower or boom-arm monitors should be positioned at approximately the location of the patient's shoulders and angled slightly toward the feet with screens at a comfortable eye level to the surgeons. The exact angulation and position is ultimately adjusted to the visual preference of the operating surgeon. The tower containing the insufflator, light source, and camera plug-in should be across from the primary surgeon to facilitate visual monitoring of the pressure recordings. The irrigation fluids are hung on one of the anesthetic poles at the head of the operative table. The harmonic and electrocautery generator units are located near the patient's feet on the same side of the table as the operating surgeon. The nurse places his or her working table directly over the patient's lower legs. The back equipment tables are positioned in an L-configuration just foot-ward of the working table extending toward the scrub nurse to allow easy access to the equipment.

RoboticModifications: The da Vinci robot is brought into position posterior to the patient's flank with the camera arm centered at the umbilical port and the fourth arm retracted and inactivated. We prefer to use the robot for preparing and performing the anastomosis only whereas other authors have advocated its use for the entire procedure *(6)*. Therefore, the robot is brought into position and docked following incision of the UPJ (Section "Incision of the Ureteropelvic Junction"). To make room for the robot the nurse or scrub technician stands on the same side as the operating surgeon and positions his or her back equipment tables in an L-configuration extending toward the same side. The da Vinci console can be placed behind the robot or toward the foot of the patient depending upon the size and shape of the operating room.

PATIENT PREPARATION AND POSITIONING

It is of great advantage to prepare the patient for this procedure by stenting their obstructed ureter at least 1 week prior to laparoscopic pyeloplasty. This allows for passive dilation of the UPJ and ureter, which will aid in performing the reconstruction. A stent that is at least one size (2 cm) longer than would normally be inserted based upon the patient's height is selected. This additional length reduces

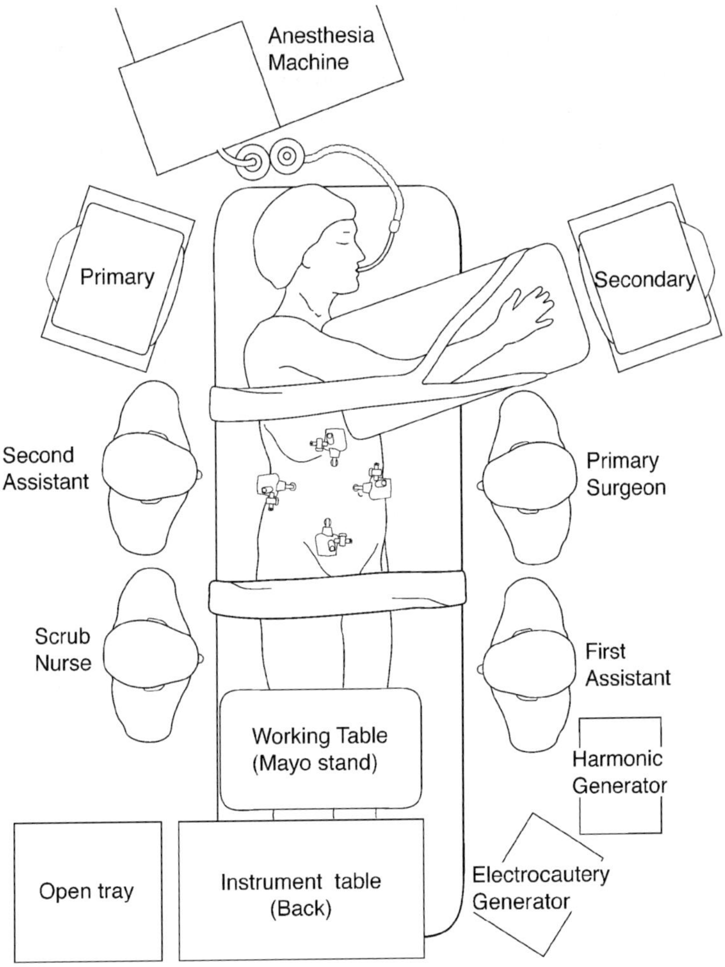

Fig. 1. Schematic representation of the operating room set-up and personnel arrangement for a right laparoscopic pyeloplasty. A mirror image arrangement is utilized for a left-sided procedure. The first assistant operates the camera while the second assistant manipulates instruments from the lateral-most trocar. Alternatively, an adjustable instrument holder arm can be secured to the table at the position of the first assistant and utilized to hold the laparoscopic camera. The first assistant then takes the position shown for the second assistant who is no longer required for the procedure.

the risk of pulling the stent into the distal ureter during its laparoscopic manipulation. A smaller stent caliber (i.e., 6 Fr) is also utilized since it provides a greater amount of space between the stent and the urothelium of the ureteral wall. This facilitates needle placement during suturing and improves urine flow around the stent following completion of the anastomosis.

There are several additional imaging studies that may be of value in the preoperative assessment of a particular patient. Attempts to radiographically demonstrate the presence of crossing lower pole vessels via computed tomography or magnetic resonance imaging with vascular reconstructions are not critical if the laparoscopic approach is pre-ordained. If there is any question regarding the degree of recoverable function within the obstructed renal unit or the degree of obstruction from an asymptomatic narrowing, it is valuable to obtain a nuclear renal scan with diuretic washout. This study helps to identify patients who may be more appropriately treated with a nephrectomy for a poorly functioning kidney, or patients without significant obstruction who may be observed. It also establishes baseline functional and drainage values for the patient against which postoperative studies can be compared. A retrograde pyelogram can be performed at the time of stent placement if a prior contrast study has not adequately defined the anatomy of the UPJ and distal ureter. This information is particularly important in defining the length of the scarred segment following previous failed procedures.

The patient is prepared for transperitoneal laparoscopy utilizing a standard bowel cleansing of magnesium citrate and a clear liquid diet the day prior to their operation. Preparation of the bowels is important because it facilitates visualization by decompressing the colon, reduces the risk of fecal soiling thus enabling a laparoscopic repair should an intraoperative bowel injury occur, and reduces the severity of postoperative ileus following the operation. At the beginning of the procedure, an oro- or nasogastric tube is placed to decompress the stomach and a Foley catheter is inserted to drain the bladder. Sequential compression devices are applied to the lower extremities to decrease lower extremity venous pooling noted during prolonged laparoscopy and the risk of resultant deep venous thrombosis. A 3-in. foam pad is placed on the operative table beneath the patient to assist in securing their surgical positioning with a minimum of pressure points.

Once the anesthetic has been induced, the patient is placed in a semi-flank position (angled back approximately 15° from vertical) with their kidney over the break in the table. The table is flexed slightly to increase the space between the rib cage and the iliac crest. Significant elevation of the kidney rest is discouraged as it can lead to myonecrosis or sensory nerve injury due to the duration of the operation. The down leg is flexed with foam padding placed beneath the knee, ankle, and foot. The upper leg is kept straight and three or more pillows are positioned between the legs at right-angles to the upper leg. Right-angle positioning of the pillows between the legs reduces the chance that the upper leg will roll off the pillows and bring the knees into prolonged contact. A quantity of pillows sufficient to keep all portions of the lower extremities from touching without significant abduction is recommended (Fig. 2).

Two arm boards are positioned side-by-side with slight cephalad elevation at the level of the patient's shoulder on the side they are facing. A soft foam or gel pad axillary roll is positioned perpendicular to the patient two finger-breadths below the axilla contacting the table. One pillow is placed beneath the down arm and three or more pillows are placed between the arms to support the upper extremity. The pillows should be inserted parallel to the arms and the proximal end placed deep into the upper axilla. A sufficient number of pillows should be used to prevent the shoulder from sagging while avoiding elevation of the upper arm above the shoulder. In-line placement of the pillows between the arms is important since perpendicular placement will limit the movements of laparoscopic instruments, especially as the surgeon's hands or robotic arms are brought toward the patient's head (Fig. 2).

The safety strap is moved to the lower portion of the operating table and is brought across the patient's lower legs in the mid-region. A cautery pad is adhesed just above the TED hose of the patient's upper leg. A towel is placed at the hip just cephalad to the cautery pad and 3-in. cloth tape is brought from table edge to table edge over the towel to secure the patient to the table. A second towel is folded in half, lengthwise, to cover from the patient's elbow to across the shoulder. Two to three strips of 3-in. cloth tapes are passed across this towel securing the patient's torso and upper extremities to the table. The tape is split once it is brought past the elbow and is placed on either side of the arm board. A gel pad roll is covered by a towel, placed behind the patient's lumbar spine and secured using a jointed support arm secured to the operative table. The operating surgeon must be confident that the patient is adequately secured to allow airplaning of the table without shifting of position or padding. A foam ring or gel pad may be required to support the patient's head in a neutral orientation following final positioning.

The anesthesiologist should be encouraged to replace fluid deficits and adequately hydrate the patient prior to creation of the pneumoperitoneum to limit the hemodynamic effects that are enhanced by volume depletion. Nitrous oxide inhalational agents should be avoided to reduce bowel distention. As with many laparoscopic operations, oliguria is common and vigorous fluid bolusing regardless of

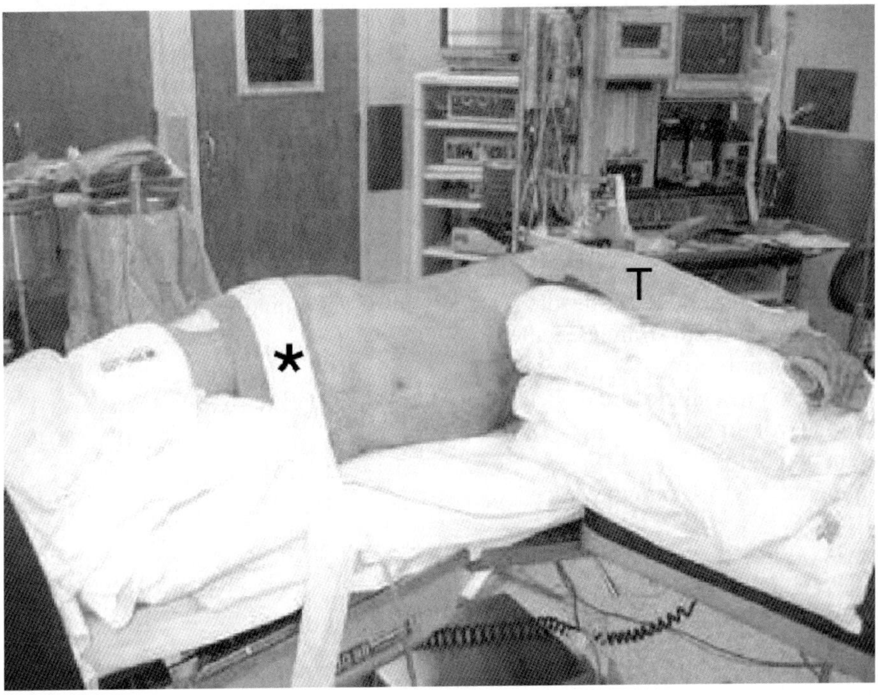

Fig. 2. Semi-flank positioning and padding of a patient undergoing a right laparoscopic pyeloplasty. Note the minimal amount of flexion applied to the operating room table at the level of the kidneys. Pillows are placed perpendicular to the legs to prevent them from rolling off the table, but are aligned parallel to the arms to maximize the amount of room for cephalad movement of the instruments. A quantity of pillows sufficient to prevent shoulder sagging without abduction above the joint is utilized. A folded towel (T) is placed across the shoulder to beyond the elbow and at the hip to protect the skin from the 3-in. wide cloth tape (∗) used to secure the patient to the operative table.

pressure or heart rate changes is to be avoided. Intravenous lines or monitoring devices (e.g., blood pressure cuff) that the anesthesiologist wishes to have quick access to should be placed on the upper arm. A pneumatic warming device may be adhered to the upper chest down to the level of the xiphoid process. The entire abdomen and back is shaved if necessary from the midline to the posterior axillary line and from xiphoid to pubis. Providone-iodine (Betadine) or a similar preparation solution is painted onto the abdomen with special care to make certain the umbilicus is adequately prepped.

RoboticModifications: Identical to above description.

NECESSARY EQUIPMENT

1. 10-mm laparoscope (0 and 30°)
2. Laparoscopic needle drivers
3. Maryland dissector *(2)*
4. Laparoscopic right-angle dissector
5. Right-angle electrocautery hook and generator cord
6. Diamond Flex Triangle retractor (Genzyme Surgical Products, Tucker, GA)
7. Martin arm or similar instrument holding device (Right-sided procedures)
8. Laparoscopic injecting needle
9. Veress needle
10. 10-mm non-bladed trocars (Maximum quantity 3)

11. 5-mm non-bladed trocars (Maximum quantity 2)
12. 10-mm Optiview introducing cannula (Ethicon Endo-Surgery, Inc., Cincinnati, OH)
13. Endoshears
14. 5-mm Harmonic Shears (Ethicon Endo-Surgery, Inc., Cincinnati, OH)
15. Endostitch Autosuturing Device (Covidien, Norwalk, CT) (Fig. 3)
16. Polysorb 4-0 autosuture (Covidien, Norwalk, CT). Quantity #15
17. Irrigator–aspirator with 5 mm wand
18. Umbilical tape
19. 2-0 Vicryl suture (Quantity 4)
20. 4-0 Vicryl or Monocryl on RB-1 needle (Quantity to be determined)
21. 3-0 Nylon suture on Keith straight needle
22. 0 Vicryl ties (Quantity 3)
23. Carter–Thomason fascial closure device (Inlet Medical, Eden Prairie, MN)
24. 15 Fr round Davol drain
25. Grenade suction bulb
26. Skin stapling device to secure the drapes
27. Benzoin
28. Steri-strips (1/4 in.)
29. Band-Aids (Quantity 3)
30. Standard open tray for flank surgery including preferred retractor

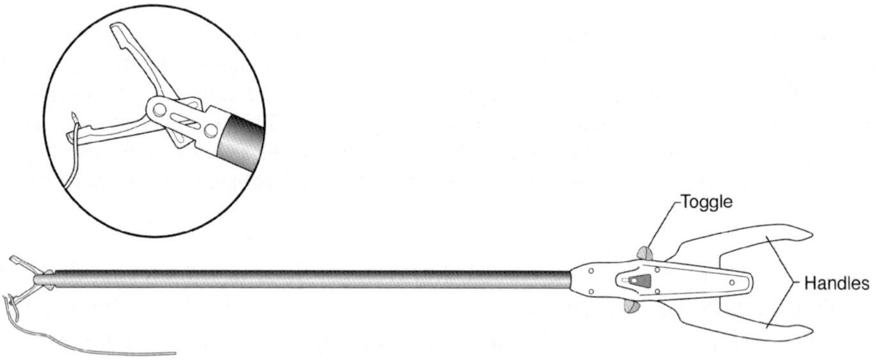

Fig. 3. The Endostitch Autosuturing Device (Covidien, Norwalk, CT) and a close-up of the jaws with mounted needle (*inset*). The suture attaches to the mid-portion of the short straight needle which passes from jaw-to-jaw as the handles of the device are squeezed and the toggle is flipped up or down out of neutral position.

The Endostitch Autosuturing Device (Covidien, Norwalk, CT) is an automated instrument which passes a suture attached to a small straight needle from jaw-to-jaw through the tissues (Fig. 3). This was designed to assist with rapid intra-corporeal suturing (Fig. 4) and knot-tying *(7)* (Fig. 5). The most delicate suture available for this instrument is the 4-0 Polysorb (Covidien, Norwalk, CT) which should be utilized when performing pyeloplasties in adult patients. As with all laparoscopic equipment, it is imperative that the operating surgeon understands the technique of loading and unloading the suturing device. Briefly, the suture is placed flat on the table in its plastic loading scaffolding and the jaws of the Autosuturing Device are closed over each end of the suture-loaded needle. The handles are squeezed and both arms of the needle toggle are drawn simultaneously toward the handle. The jaws are kept closed on the needle and the suture material is drawn out and cut to the desired length. The ideal suture length is 12 cm, which enables placement and efficient tying of two intra-corporeal sutures. Longer lengths allow for placement of more sutures, however, the additional length is cumbersome and results in inefficient knot-tying and prolonged operative times.

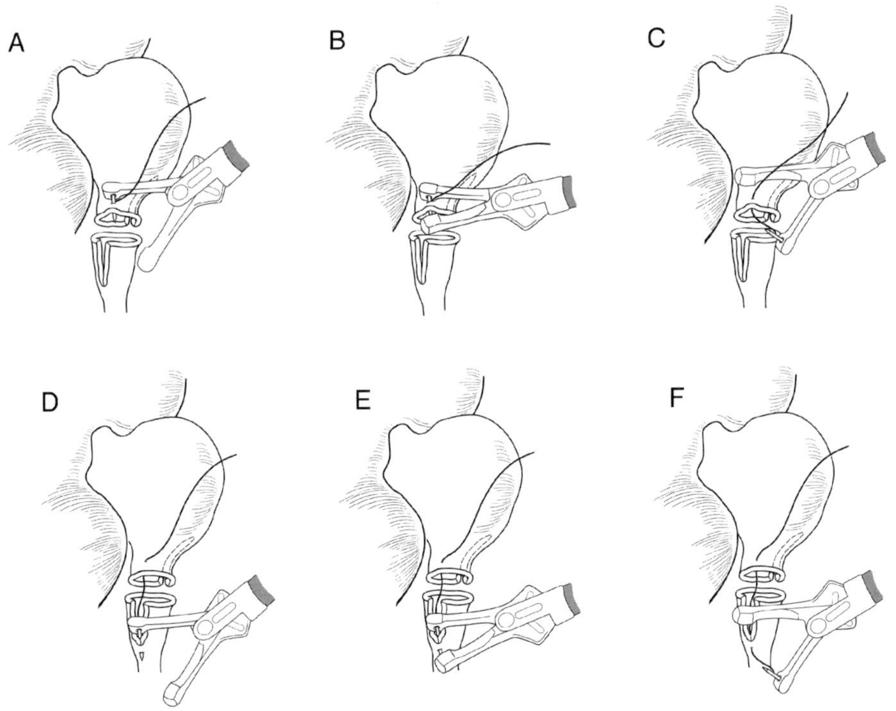

Fig. 4. Intra-corporeal placement of the lateral corner stitch during right laparoscopic pyeloplasty utilizing the Endostitch Device. The ureter has been spatulated laterally and the pelvis medially. (**A**) The suture-mounted needle is passed from outside-to-inside on the lateral flap of the pelvis. (**B**) The jaws of the device are closed by squeezing the handle. (**C**) The toggle of the Endostitch is then flipped and the handle is released transferring the needle to the opposite jaw, which is pulled through the tissue of the pelvis along with the suture. (**D**) The needle is then passed from inside-to-outside in the deepest point of the ureteral spatulation taking care to include mucosa. (**E**) The jaws of the Endostitch Device are closed by squeezing the handle. (**F**) The toggle is then flipped and the handle is released transferring the needle to the opposite jaw, which is pulled through the tissue of the ureter. The corner stitch is now ready to be tied.

RoboticModifications: Additional Equipment

1. 12-mm da Vinci laparoscope (0 and 30° lens)
2. 10–12-mm non-bladed trocar (2)
3. 8-mm robotic ports (2)
4. Scissors curved monopolar [Intuitive Ref#400179] (Quantity 1)
5. Scissors Potts endo [Intuitive Ref#400001] (Quantity 1)
6. Forceps Maryland bipolar [Intuitive Ref#400172] (Quantity 1)
7. Needle driver large [Intuitive Ref#400006] (Quantity1)
8. Suture cut needle driver [Intuitive Ref#400209] (Quantity 1) (Fig. 6)

The suture cut needle driver has a cutting element located proximal to the flat jaws of the driver adjacent to the hinge allowing the operating surgeon to cut their own suture (Fig. 6), thus eliminating the need for numerous instrument exchanges by the assistant surgeon. This is particularly helpful when interrupted suturing is performed due to the need for frequent cutting of suture. Care must be utilized when using this device to perform a running suture, since grasping of the suture deep in the jaw of the driver will result in inadvertent transection.

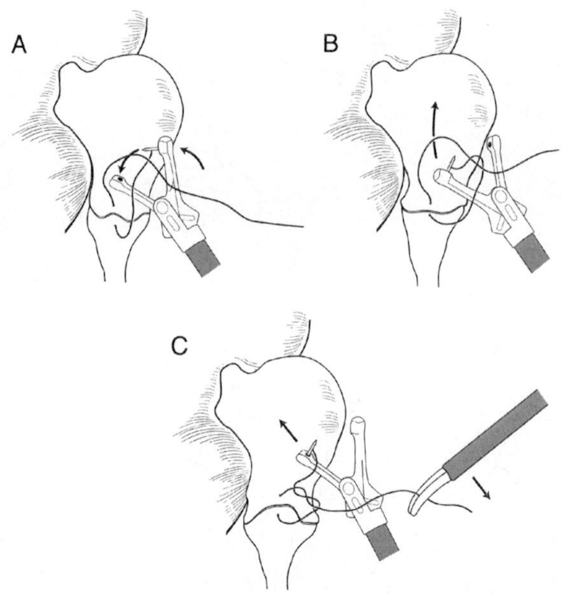

Fig. 5. Rapid intra-corporeal knot-tying using the Endostitch Device. (**A**) A square-knot is formed by passing the suture-mounted needle through the internal loop formed by crossing the free end of the suture over the more proximal end that is draped over the lower jaw of the Endostitch. The jaws of the device are then closed and the needle transferred through the loop to the jaw located on the opposite side. (**B**) Once transferred, the needle and attached suture are pulled further through the loop. The first knot of each suture placed during a laparoscopic pyeloplasty should be a surgeon's knot to prevent loosening and separation of the tissues. Passing the needle back through the same loop a second time prior to tightening forms this knot. (**C**) The throw is completed by pulling the two ends in opposite directions while making certain the knot lies down square.

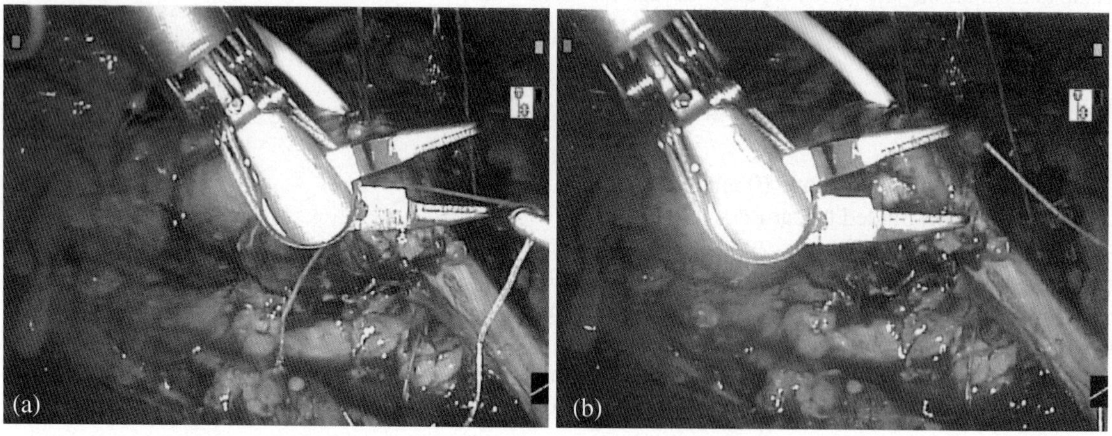

Fig. 6. Suture cut needle driver utilized during a robotic pyeloplasty. (**A**) The suture is introduced deep into the hinge of the jaws of the needle driver. (**B**) Closure of the jaws performs an efficient cut of the suture and the needle can then be used again or removed from the peritoneum.

OPERATIVE PROCEDURE – STANDARD LAPAROSCOPIC PYELOPLASTY

Port Placement

An initial 1 cm incision for introduction of the Veress needle and 10 mm camera port is placed midway between the umbilicus and the superior iliac crest just lateral to the rectus muscle. A small curved clamp is used to spread the subcutaneous tissues down to the level of the fascia and the Veress needle is introduced. Typically, the first popping sensation indicates puncturing of the fascia and the second denotes entry into the peritoneal cavity. Saline injected into the hub of the Veress needle should flow easily into the peritoneal cavity and aspiration should not yield any gas, blood, or bowel contents. The abdomen is insufflated to 15 mmHg pressure and initial pressure readings should be below 10 mmHg pressure to indicate presence within the peritoneal cavity.

All 10 mm ports are introduced using the OptiView non-bladed introducer and the tip should be directed slightly toward the kidney. The non-bladed trocar splits the fascia along the course of the fibers thereby reducing the risk of postoperative hernia formation. A second 10 mm port is placed at the superior lateral margin of the umbilicus and the third port is placed just lateral of the midline halfway between the xiphoid process and the umbilicus. This third trocar can be either a 5 mm (left pyeloplasty: right-handed surgeon/right pyeloplasty: left-handed surgeon) or a 10 mm port (left pyeloplasty: left-handed surgeon/right pyeloplasty: right-handed surgeon) depending on the side and the dominant hand of the operating surgeon (Fig. 7). Care must be taken to angle this port so it enters lateral to the Falciform Ligament to prevent entrapment of the instruments by this structure as they are introduced through the trocar. Internally, the ports are pulled back until they are just far enough in to fully expose the insufflation hole. They are rotated until the stop-cock is furthest away from the kidney. All three trocars can be secured to the abdomen using 2-0 Vicryl suture tied at the skin and around the stop-cock due to the frequent introduction and withdrawal of instruments which can result in port dislodgment. Contemporary laparoscopic port designs include outer fascial stabilization ridges which often obviate the need for securing sutures.

Exposure of the Retroperitoneum

The camera is inserted via the lower quadrant port and held by the assistant surgeon while the operating surgeon manipulates instruments inserted via the epigastric and umbilical trocars. The harmonic shears are utilized to rapidly incise the line of Toldt and peri-colonic attachments. The extent of the dissection and medial colonic mobilization can be tailored somewhat depending upon the position and ease of exposure of the UPJ. It is advantageous to have complete exposure of the pelvis and upper ureter to minimize the interference of bowel and adjacent structures during the suturing process. Unlike the laparoscopic nephrectomy, however, extensive dissection and exposure of the hilar vessels, or cephalad portions of the kidney, are unnecessary. On the left side, it may be adequate to simply release the Line of Toldt and carry the dissection around the splenic flexure between the colon and spleen if the colon is mobile and the UPJ lies in a more lateral position. In other cases where the UPJ is located more medially, it may be necessary to completely release the spleen together with the bowel and roll the spleen, bowel, and tail of the pancreas medially to expose the retroperitoneum. On the right, the peritoneal incision is carried around the hepatic flexure and the underlying duodenum can be left in situ in many cases as it is often displaced medially by the dilated pelvis.

Once the colon is reflected medially, a fourth and final trocar (5 mm) is introduced midway between the tip of the 12th rib and the superior iliac crest. It is usually unnecessary to maintain constant elevation of the liver when performing a right-sided pyeloplasty since the UPJ tends to lie well below the liver edge. If liver elevation is required the irrigator–aspirator can be inserted via the lateral-most trocar or the Diamond Flex Triangle retractor (Genzyme Surgical Products, Tucker, GA) can be utilized.

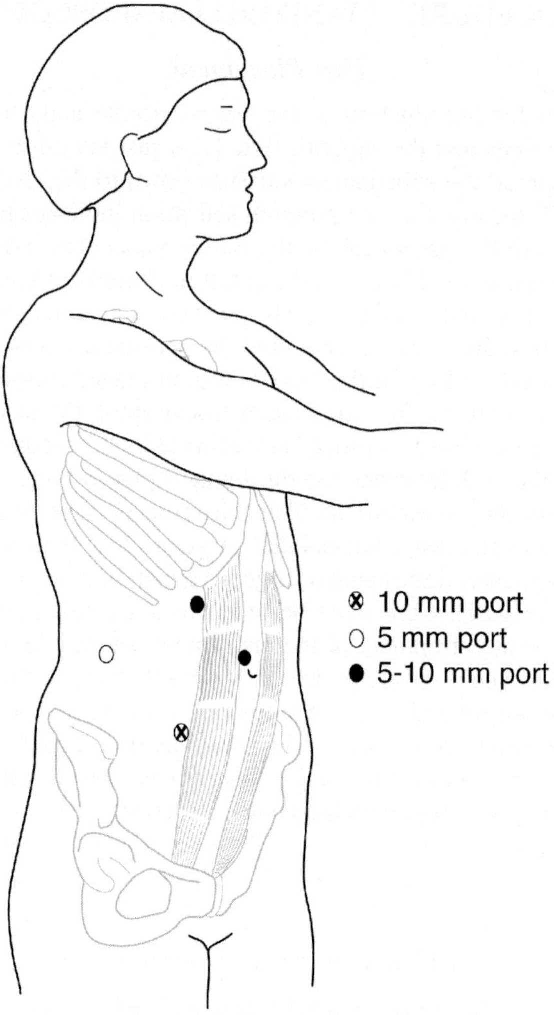

Fig. 7. Standard port arrangement for a right laparoscopic pyeloplasty. A mirror image distribution is used for a left laparoscopic pyeloplasty. The trocar placed in the epigastrium, midway between the umbilicus and xiphoid, can be either a 5 or a 10 mm port depending upon the side of the obstruction and the dominant hand of the operating surgeon. In general, the Endostitch Device is held in the surgeon's dominant hand and must be inserted via a 10 mm port. This gives the left-handed surgeon performing a right pyeloplasty, and the right-handed surgeon performing a left-pyeloplasty, the option of using a 5 mm port at this upper location.

Dissection of the Retroperitoneum

After mobilization of the colon, the next step is to identify the upper extent of the ureter. Opening Gerota's fascia over the lower pole of the kidney and incising the fascia medially facilitates this maneuver. Once this area is fully exposed, a laparoscopic instrument is gently drawn from lateral to medial across the presumed location of the ureter. Due to the presence of the stent, there is usually enough tactile feedback via the instrument to indicate the presence of a firm band-like structure running in a cranial–caudal direction in the retroperitoneum. The gonadal vein can provide another aid to identification of the ureter, since the ureter usually lies lateral and slightly deep to the gonadal vein when the patient is in a semi-flank position. When a tubular structure is identified and there is a question of whether or not it represents ureter, gentle contact with an instrument will usually produce a peristaltic reaction. Once identified, the ureter is then elevated and traced to the area of the UPJ. Full circumferential dissection is limited to the first 3–4 cm of upper ureter in an effort to preserve as much ureteric vasculature as possible. This maneuver is facilitated by placing the curve of the Maryland Dissector (non-dominant hand) just below the surface of the ureter, elevating it, and bluntly teasing away the underlying fat using the harmonic shears to coagulate all small feeding vessels (dominant hand). A 4-in. cut segment of umbilical tape is then passed around the ureter and its ends grasped to facilitate elevation and retraction of the upper ureter.

As the dissection is carried cephalad toward the renal pelvis, it is important to be cautious in examining the area for the presence of anterior crossing vessels which can be present in 57–76% of cases of adult UPJ obstruction *(2)*. If identified, these vessels must be meticulously isolated from the renal pelvis above, UPJ beneath, and upper ureter below. Usually a paired artery and vein are identified in this location but any combination of vessels can be seen. The right-angle cautery hook is an ideal instrument for gently elevating and separating the tissues between the UPJ and the vessels. The back of the instrument can be used to peel apart the tissues and the tip to create planes between the two structures. Obviously, care must be taken to use the lowest effective setting on the cautery and to avoid puncturing the vessels, ureter, or pelvis, with the tip of the instrument. The assistant elevates the upper ureter utilizing the umbilical tape and the dissection is initially completed posterior staying on the ureter, then UPJ, and finally pelvic surface. This helps define the anatomy and location of the pelvis. Once identified the fat is teased and separated from the surface of the pelvis until the glistening surface is exposed above the vessels.

Unlike the ureter, the pelvis can be gently grasped during the dissection as long as care is taken to avoid grasping near the region of the planned reconstruction. If a pelvic reduction is planned, the region to be excised is the best area to grasp. Another alternative to assist in elevating and freeing up the pelvis is to pass a 3-0 Nylon mounted on a Keith straight needle through the abdominal wall directly over the region of the hilum, through the renal pelvis, and back out the abdominal wall. The suture ends are then secured with a straight clamp as they exit the abdominal wall and the suture can be raised and lowered as desired. The dissection must be carried out until a right-angle clamp can be passed freely behind the vessels and traction on the pelvis draws the area of the UPJ above the level of the vessels.

In cases of secondary UPJ obstruction, or significant prior inflammatory episodes, there may be a thick fibrous rind surrounding the UPJ and pelvis. The pelvis, UPJ, and upper ureter need to be freed from the confines of this tissue as much as possible prior to transecting the UPJ, because the dissection planes often become less distinct once the pelvis is fully decompressed and urine is constantly draining into the operative field.

Incision of the Ureteropelvic Junction

Circumferential incision of the UPJ should be made directly at the juncture of the ureter with the pelvis even in cases, where an anterior crossing vessel appears to be the source of the pathology. In the presence of a crossing vessel, this maneuver can be facilitated by gentle downward traction through the underlying window in the periureteric soft tissue using the non-dominant hand (Fig. 8) or by grasping and retracting the umbilical tape segment. The curved Endoshears are the ideal instrument for making this initial incision and great care should be exercised not to cut the indwelling ureteral stent. Prior to making the incision, it is important to note a surface landmark on the ureter such as a vessel, or attachment of soft tissue, which will help the operating surgeon quickly identify the anterior wall of the ureter after it is transected. It is crucial to maintain correct orientation once it becomes time to spatulate the ureter. The assistant surgeon should utilize the irrigator–aspirator to slowly drip saline on the ureter as it is transected and to aspirate urine and blood from the lumen of the ureter which obscure visualization of the stent. Once the ureter is opened adequately to expose the underlying stent,

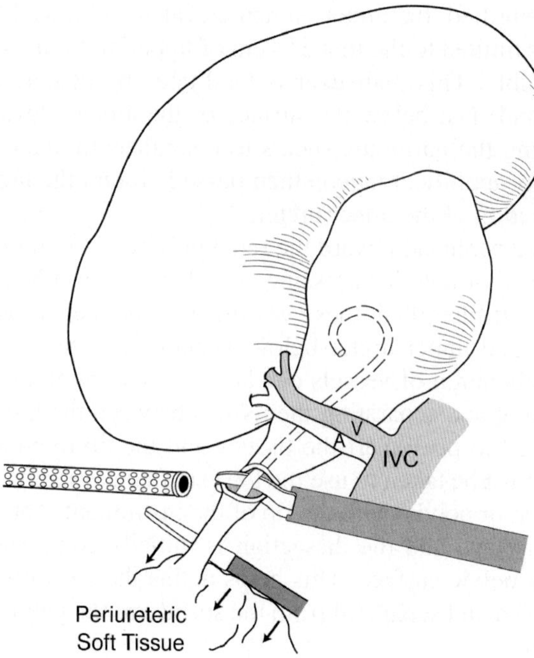

Fig. 8. Transection of the posterior wall of an obstructed UPJ due to lower pole crossing vessels. A Maryland dissector, held in the non-dominant hand of the operating surgeon, is placed in the periureteric soft tissue window created by circumferential dissection of the upper portion of the ureter. Downward retraction with the Maryland draws the UPJ below the vessels to allow unimpeded transection. Once the anterior wall is cut, exposing the indwelling stent, the upper jaw is passed beneath the stent to transect the posterior wall. The assistant utilizes the irrigator-aspirator device to help maintain exposure of the stent.

the lower jaw of the shears can be inserted into the lumen so the anterior wall lies between the jaws of the shears while the stent is protected beneath the back of the lower jaw. After completing this anterior incision, the upper jaw is passed between the stent and the posterior wall to complete transection of the posterior ureteric wall (Fig. 8). The stent is then grasped just above its exit point from the ureter as the upper portion is drawn out of the renal pelvis. It is important to avoid pulling out the portion of the stent contained within the ureter during manipulations as this can result in the distal pigtail being withdrawn through the ureteral orifice into the intravesical tunnel.

Preparation of the Anastomosis

If lower pole crossing vessels are present, the pelvis is elevated cephalad by gently grasping the upper portion of the pelvis and lifting until it relocates anterior to the vessels. Often additional fibrous attachments to the pelvis remain which inhibit its tension-free anterior positioning. These must be transected using the harmonic shears or electrocautery hook. Once tension-free anterior positioning is established, the Endoshears are used to spatulate the ureter laterally. Caution should be exercised to avoid spiraling the incision. The gentle curve of the Endoshears facilitates this lateral based cut by using only the tips of the shears to cut with the concavity of the shear facing anteriorly. The previously established landmark on the anterior surface of the ureter also assists in maintaining orientation during this maneuver. The assistant utilizes the irrigator–aspirator to continuously drip saline on the tissues when bleeding obscures visualization. The length of the spatulation can vary depending on the size of the patient's ureter and whether or not the edges of the spatulated ureter need to be excised. Usually, the spatulation is approximately the length of the metallic jaws on the Endoshears (approximately a 12 mm cut). We try to minimize the amount of tissue removed by performing the spatulation first prior to excision. This enables a closer inspection of the health of the mucosa and muscular layer of the ureter. Most often there is sufficient tactile feedback when incising the ureter to gauge the length of the fibrotic ring, if present, that needs to be trimmed off of the ureteral and pelvic side of the anastomosis. The pelvis is spatulated medially and, if it is sufficiently redundant, tissue can be excised regardless of the length of the ureteral spatulation since the pelvis can be closed to itself to insure a dependent cone-shaped reconstruction. All excised tissue should be sent for pathologic inspection to rule out the possibility of an unsuspected malignancy as the cause of obstruction. Once the spatulations are completed the segment of umbilical tape is removed from the peritoneal cavity.

Performing the Anastomosis

The Endostitch device is used to place a corner stitch at each of the spatulations with care taken to include adequate amounts of muscular wall as well as full thickness mucosa. The knots should be placed on the outside of the anastomosis. It is advisable to pass the lateral corner stitch from outside-to-inside on the renal pelvis side and from inside-to-outside on the ureter side as this insures that an adequate bite of ureter with underlying mucosa is included in the depth of the ureteral spatulation (Fig. 4). The medial corner stitch is performed in a mirror image fashion passing from outside-in on the ureter side and from inside-out in the depth of the renal pelvis spatulation. A total of four knots should be placed in each stitch with the first being a surgeon's knot; care is taken to make certain each knot lays down square as it is tied (Fig. 5). The ureteral stent should be kept anterior to the pelvis and between, but not entrapped within the corner stitches. The ends of the corner sutures are both left long by throwing only one stitch from the entire 12-cm length of suture. This allows the ends to be grasped and passed behind the ureter to expose the posterior edges of the anastomosis. Alternatively, laparoscopic needle drivers can be utilized and a 4-0 Vicryl cut to 6 in. in length and mounted on an RB-1 needle. We prefer standard laparoscopic intra-corporeal suturing when the tissues appear delicate or the straight needle of the Endostitch device does not allow proper suture placement.

After completion of the corner stitches, a right-angle grasper is passed lateral-to-medial behind the ureter and is used to grasp the medial corner stitch. This stitch is then pulled lateral (behind the ureter) as the lateral corner stitch is retracted medially (in front of the ureter) to expose the posterior edges of the anastomosis (Fig. 9). On occasion, the anatomy of the reconstruction is such that less tension is placed on the anastomosis, and better exposure of the posterior edges is obtained, by pulling the lateral corner stitch behind the ureter medially. This determination can only be made intraoperatively. Regardless of which corner stitch is passed behind the ureter, the first assistant is asked to grasp the lateral-most corner stitch to allow placement of the posterior row of sutures.

We prefer using interrupted sutures with each consecutive suture placed to divide the unsutured regions that remain rather than immediately adjacent to one another. Each undivided segment is then further divided working lateral-to-medial. As each suture is placed, the assistant holds the tag of the lateral suture and the operating surgeon holds the medial suture, of the segment being divided, in their non-dominant hand as the suture is placed using the dominant hand. A total of two sutures can be obtained from each 12-cm length of Polysorb stitch. Therefore, the first posterior row suture is placed midway between the corner sutures dividing it into two equally long unsutured segments. The next suture divides the more lateral half into two segments (quarters), and the next divides the more lateral quarter into eighths, and so on (Fig. 10). This approach is advantageous because it prevents bunching of the anastomosis with associated narrowing that can occur with a running stitch. It also (1) facilitates visualization of both ureteral and pelvic mucosa during suture placement, (2) prevents undue continued tension on any one section of the anastomosis, and (3) rapidly reapproximates the pelvis and ureter using the minimum number of sutures to achieve a water tight seal. As the operating surgeon completes the final knot of each stitch, the assistant surgeon exchanges their graspers for the

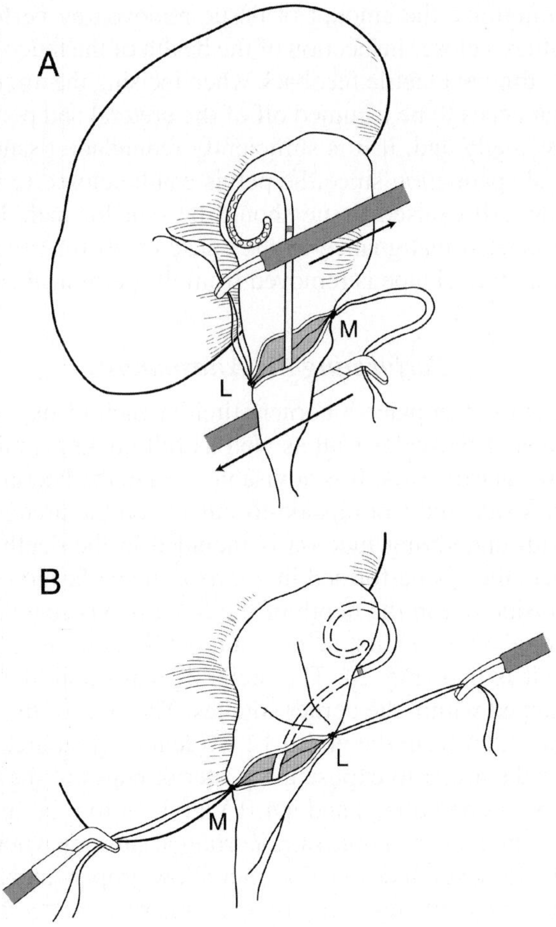

Fig. 9. Exposure of the posterior edges of the anastomosis. (**A**) The right-angle dissector is passed behind the ureter from lateral-to-medial and the medial corner stitch (M) is grasped and pulled behind the ureter laterally. At the same time, the lateral corner stitch (L) is retracted medially over the anterior surface of the UPJ using the Maryland dissector. (**B**) The posterior edges of the anastomosis are exposed anteriorly for suturing and the stent is displaced on the anterior surface of the pelvis, which now faces posteriorly.

Endoshears and cuts the end of the suture attached to the Endostitch device leaving the other free end long. This suture end is then grasped to assist in placement of the next stitch. Similar to the corner stitches, standard laparoscopic needle drivers and 4-0 Vicryl suture mounted on an RB-1 needle, but cut to 5 in. in length can be utilized whenever the Endostitch device does not allow easy and acceptable needle placement. This slightly smaller length is optimum for placement of 2 stitches using the same suture. We do not place a specific number of sutures, but tailor the anastomosis based on the length of the spatulations.

After completion of the posterior row, all remaining extra lengths of suture are trimmed to appropriate size and the right-angle clamp is passed behind the ureter, directly opposite the way it was passed initially, to replace the corner stitch in its normal position. At this point, the upper pigtail of the stent should be reinserted into the pelvis. This can be a difficult maneuver laparoscopically due to the memory of the pigtail and concerns about pulling the stent from the ureter or placing tension on the newly completed posterior anastomosis. The most effective way of performing this step is to have the assistant grasp the stent just as it emerges from the ureter. The operating surgeon uses a Maryland

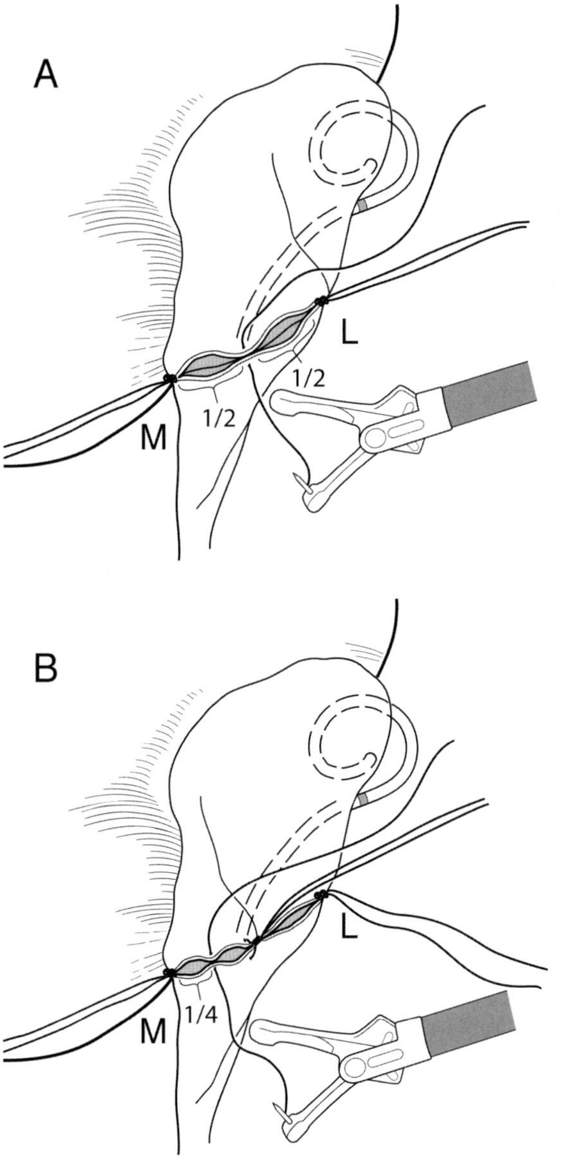

Fig. 10. Closing the posterior row of the anastomosis with each interrupted suture dividing the unsutured segments from lateral-to-medial. The posterior edges of the anastomosis have been exposed by retracting the medial corner stitch (M) behind the ureter laterally, and the lateral corner stitch (L) medially. (**A**) The first stitch is placed midway between the two corner stitches (held on tension) to divide the posterior row into two equal-sized, unsutured half segments. (**B**) The laterally located medial corner stitch (M) and midway stitch are then held on tension and the next suture divides the unsutured lateral half into quarters.

dissector in their non-dominant hand to grasp midway up the exposed straight length of the stent while a right-angle clamp is used in the dominant hand to grab the stent approximately 0.5 cm back from its tip. The right-angle clamp is then rotated in a counter-clockwise direction on the left, or clockwise direction on the right, to uncoil the pigtail and the end is then inserted as far as the cut edge of the pelvis will allow. The straight portion of the stent is grasped with the Maryland dissector just above the assistant's grasper and the assistant gently releases their grip on the stent as it is elevated into the pelvis with the Maryland dissector. The assistant then re-grips the stent tightly as the primary surgeon then releases their grip on the stent first with the right-angle followed by the Maryland dissector (Fig. 11). It is important to make certain the stent has passed into the pelvis and not through the posterior suture line prior to placing the anterior sutures. The anterior row of interrupted sutures is then placed using the Endostitch device or laparoscopic needle drivers in similar fashion to what was performed on the posterior row with each consecutive suture dividing unsutured segments from lateral-to-medial.

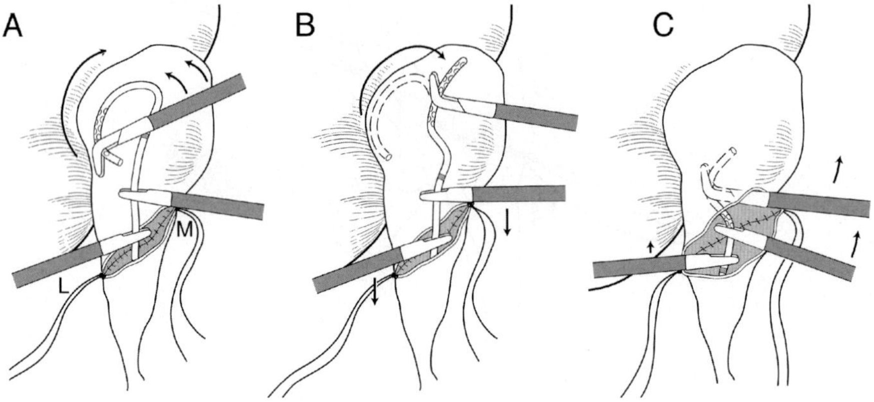

Fig. 11. Reinsertion of the upper pigtail of the stent into the renal pelvis prior to placement of the anterior row of sutures. (**A**) The assistant grasps the stent as it emerges from the ureter to prevent its upward movement. The operating surgeon uses a right-angle dissector to uncoil the pigtail in a clockwise direction while grasping midway up the exposed straight length of the stent. (**B**) After the pigtail is straightened, the stent is advanced down into the ureter to minimize the exposed length. (**C**) The right-angle dissector is utilized to insert the tip of the stent into the renal pelvis as far as the lower edge will allow. The assistant relaxes their grip on the stent while the primary surgeon elevates the stent into the pelvis as the jaws of the right-angle dissector are slowly opened to allow re-formation of the pigtail within the pelvis.

Final inspection should reveal a dependent anastomosis with no lines of tension observed on the anastomosed pelvis (Fig. 12). No areas of significant urine leakage should be observed. All suture ends are trimmed including the two corner stitches. It is unusual to have significant disparity between the ureteral and pelvic spatulations requiring separate closure of the pelvis unless excess pelvis was initially excised. Any residual pyelotomy can be closed using a running 4-0 Polysorb after completion of the anastomosis. If anterior crossing vessels have been transposed posteriorly, they should not be under tension and the lower pole should appear well-perfused. If duskiness is noted and there is no apparent tension on the transposed vessels, the artery may be in spasm. This can be relieved with the topical application of vasodilators such as papaverine or lidocaine via a laparoscopic injecting needle.

Exiting the Abdomen

The area of dissection is inspected under reduced insufflation pressures of 8 mmHg and all areas of bleeding are controlled using the harmonic shears or electrocautery. Once adequate hemostasis has been achieved, the pressure is increased and figure-of-eight fascial closure sutures of 0-Vicryl are placed at each of the 10 mm port sites using a grasping needle device such as the Carter–Thomason. The ports are left in place temporarily to assist in positioning a 15 Fr round Davol drain in the retroperitoneum. The spike is cut from the drain and a clamp is placed across the end to prevent escape of the pneumoperitoneum. The perforated end is then fed into the abdomen via the lateral 5 mm port and positioned in the retroperitoneum so it does not directly contact the anastomosis. The port is pulled off of the drain tubing after momentarily releasing the clamp and the drain is secured to the flank using a 2-0 Nylon suture. It is important to position the drain in the retroperitoneum away from the anastomosis so it does not apply suction directly to the suture line. Each port is removed under vision

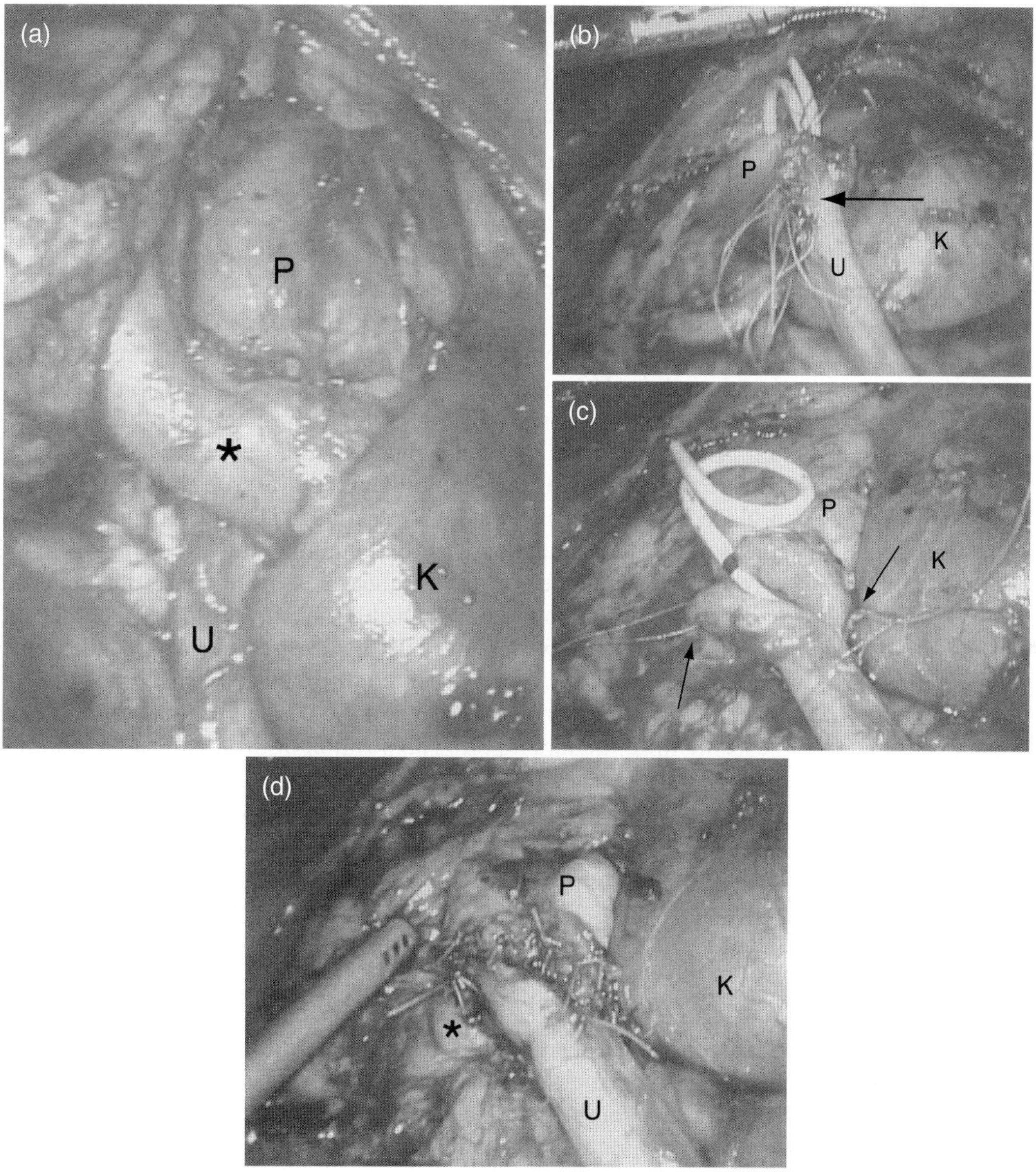

Fig. 12. Left laparoscopic pyeloplasty to reconstruct a UPJ obstructed by lower pole crossing vessels. (**A**) Anterior vessels (∗) crossing the area of the UPJ to supply the lower pole of the left kidney (K) with the renal pelvis (P) visible above the vessels and the ureter (U) below. (**B**) After transection, spatulation, and transposition of the UPJ anterior to the vessels, the completed posterior row (*arrow*) can be easily seen as the medial corner stitch is rolled laterally in the jaws of the Maryland dissector. (**C**) The stent is now ready to be re-inserted into the pelvis following completion of the posterior row of sutures and relocation of the corner stitches (*arrows*) into their normal location. (**D**) The completed cone-shaped, dependent anastomosis with the lower pole crossing vessels (∗) now residing posteriorly.

and the closure suture tied leaving the lower quadrant port until the end. The pneumoperitoneum is released and the fascial suture is elevated while withdrawing the final port from the abdomen leaving the laparoscope in the peritoneal cavity. The laparoscope is removed slowly while making sure the peritoneal contents fall away from the fascia as it exits.

After tying down the final fascial suture, the drain is cut to an appropriate length and placed to bulb suction. The port sites are irrigated with antibiotic solution and closed using a running 4-0 Monocryl suture. Benzoin, steri-strips, and a standard band-aid are applied to each of the port-sites. A dry, sterile gauze dressing is placed at the drain site completing the operation.

OPERATIVE PROCEDURE – ROBOTIC LAPAROSCOPIC PYELOPLASTY

Port Placement

An identical ipsilateral lower quadrant incision as that described for a standard laparoscopic pyeloplasty is made midway between the umbilicus and the superior iliac crest at least 8 cm away from the umbilicus. The incision is made large enough to allow insertion of an 8 mm robotic port, the subcutaneous tissues are spread, and the Veress needle is inserted. Needle position is tested and the pneumoperitoneum is created as described above. Since the robotic ports do not allow direct visualization of the tissue layers on insertion and cannot be attached to the insufflator, we leave the Veress needle in position and make a 12 mm insertion at the umbilicus then insert a 10–12 mm port at this site using the OptiView non-bladed introducer as previously described. The area of entry of the Veress needle is inspected, the needle is then removed and the insufflation tubing transferred to the 10–12 mm port. An 8 mm robotic port is then inserted at the prior site of the Veress needle insertion using a back-and-forth twisting motion under direct vision until the port sheath is advanced several centimeters into the peritoneal cavity and the obturator is removed. Care must be taken to enter perpendicular to the abdominal surface without angulation to allow a proper fulcrum to be established once the robot is docked to the ports. A second 8 mm robotic port is inserted at least 8 cm above the periumbilical port in the same approximate line as the lower quadrant port. The position of this port can be modified and placed slightly more medial when performing a right-sided pyeloplasty in an effort to avoid proximity to the liver margin. A 10–12 mm assistant port is introduced in the midline between the periumbilical and either the upper or lower robotic port. The upper location tends to afford wider spacing of the ports and less concern regarding interaction of introduced instruments and the bowel (Fig. 13). An additional 5 mm port can be inserted between the 12th rib and iliac crest to allow retraction of the liver margin when required.

Exposure of the Retroperitoneum

We prefer to expose and dissect the retroperitoneum using standard laparoscopic instruments in a fashion identical to what has already been described above. Our rational for not using the robot to perform these steps of the dissection is that it is somewhat more cumbersome for executing the relatively broad cranio-caudad movements required. When operating through ports inserted for a robotic procedure, the insufflation tubing is attached to the assistant port, a 10 mm 0° laparoscopic lens is inserted via the umbilical port and instruments are inserted through the robotic ports. Each robotic port has an attached seal reducer plug allowing introduction of 5 mm instruments without loss of the pneumoperitoneum.

When the liver obscures the right kidney and UPJ, a lateral 5 mm port and Diamond Flex Triangle retractor can be inserted for sustained retraction of the liver margin to facilitate exposure. This can be secured utilizing a multi-jointed instrument holder (i.e., Martin arm) which bolts to the operating table. The robotic arms will pass over this device once they are docked to the ports, thus minimizing the chance of collisions.

Dissection of the Retroperitoneum

This step is performed identical to what was described for standard laparoscopic pyeloplasty (Section "Dissection of the Retroperitoneum").

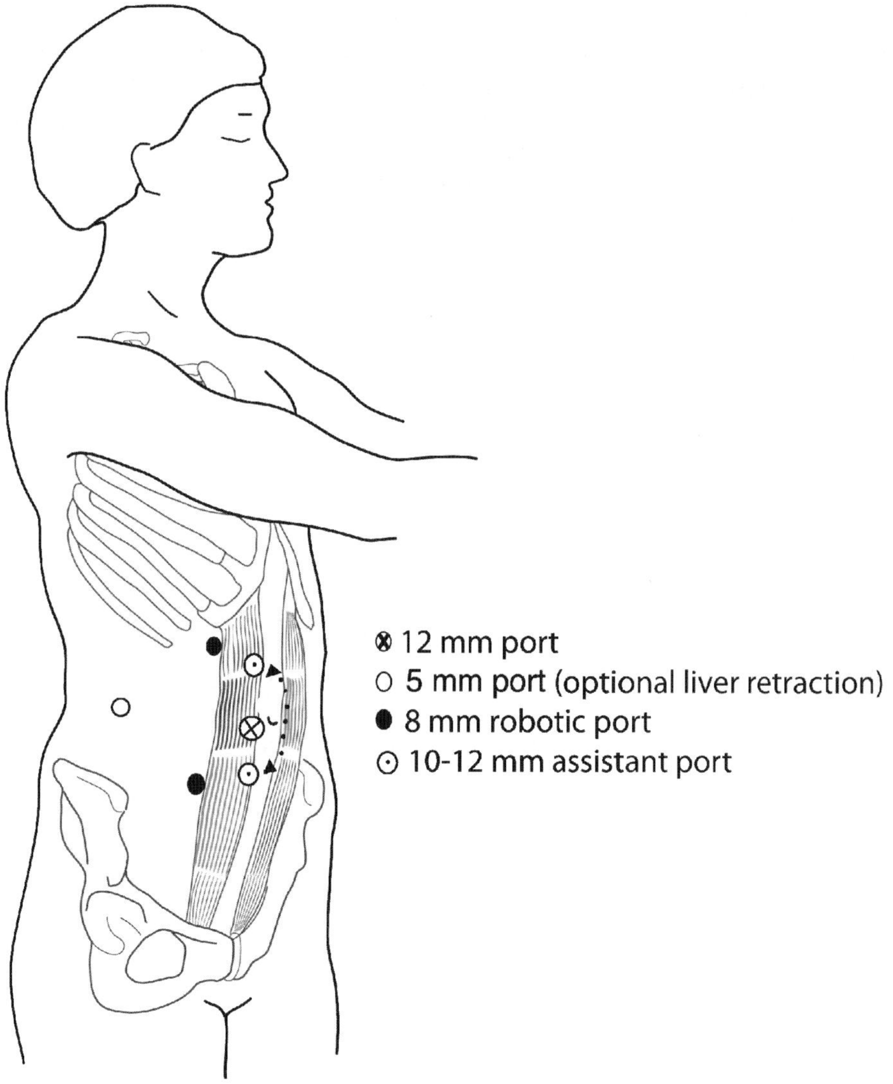

Fig. 13. Standard port arrangement for a robotic laparoscopic pyeloplasty. A mirror image distribution is utilized for a left robotic pyeloplasty. The 10–12 mm assistant port can be inserted between the periumbilical and epigastric or the right lower quadrant robotic port as illustrated by the *dotted arrows*.

Incision of the Ureteropelvic Junction

This step is also performed identical to what was described for standard laparoscopic pyeloplasty (Section "Incision of the Ureteropelvic Junction").

Preparation of the Anastomosis

After incising the UPJ and transposing the renal pelvis anterior to the lower pole crossing vessels when present, the da Vinci robot is brought into position for docking. Prior to removal of the laparoscope, the robotic ports are inspected to make sure they are advanced into the peritoneal cavity until the second marked line is visualized. The seal reducers are uncapped and the laparoscope is removed. The main support post of the robot is centered at the umbilical port and advanced into position perpendicular to the patient by the circulating personnel. The robotic arms are docked into position and secured to their corresponding ports. The 0° da Vinci laparoscope is introduced and the Maryland bipolar forceps are inserted via the upper port and the curved shears via the lower port for the pelvic spatulation and pyelotomy. These instruments are then switched when performing the ureteral spatulation to facilitate extending the incision caudad.

As described for the standard laparoscopic pyeloplasty, care must be exercised not to spiral the ureteral incision. The ureter is spatulated laterally prior to excision of any tissue from the region of the UPJ and the operating surgeon must rely on visual inspection of the mucosa and cut edge of the ureter to decide whether the tissue is fibrotic and needs to be excised. The medial pelvic spatulation with or without pelvic reducing excision is performed identical to what was described above (Section "Preparation of the Anastomosis"). The Potts endo scissors provide a much more delicate tip for performing spatulations in tightly fibrotic or pediatric ureters.

Performing the Anastomosis

The suture cut needle driver is attached and inserted via the robotic port corresponding to the surgeon's non-dominant hand and the standard large needle driver via the robotic port controlled by the dominant hand. The assistant surgeon introduces a 4-0 Vicryl suture cut to 6 in. in length and mounted on an RB-1 needle. Once the suture is grasped, the assistant utilizes the irrigator–aspirator to irrigate the tissues when necessary to expose the edges of the spatulation for proper needle placement. Corner stitches are placed identical to what was described for a standard laparoscopic approach. As the first corner stitch is tied down carefully the assistant applies downward traction on the kidney using the irrigation wand to keep tension from the anastomosis until the second stitch is placed.

The posterior row of the anastomosis is closed using a maneuver identical to what was used during standard laparoscopic pyeloplasty. This is facilitated by the articulations of the endo-wrist to pass the lateral corner stitch behind the ureter while the medial corner stitch is retracted laterally. To maintain stable position of the anastomosis as the sutures are placed, the assistant grasps and retracts the lateral-most stitch. We prefer to place interrupted sutures as described for standard laparoscopic pyeloplasty with each subsequent stitch dividing the lateral-most segment until a watertight closer is appreciated. This can usually be accomplished with the assistant having to re-grasp a new suture end only twice, switching first to the middle dividing stitch once the lateral half of the anastomosis is completed, and then switching to the quarter-mark suture after completion of the lateral three quarters of the posterior row. Both of the suture tags should be left long to allow the assistant to grasp the end and position the suture so it does not interfere with the robotic ports. All other suture tags are cut short to prevent their interference and incorporation into subsequent knots as they are being tied down.

If bleeding and fluid at the edge of the anastomosis obscures visualization during needle placement, the operating surgeon can hold one of the lateral tag sutures while the assistant irrigates the area of the anastomosis. Alternatively, the backside of the curved portion of the needle can be used to wipe blood and fluid away from the tissues to expose the edges of the reconstruction. This latter approach does not require the assistant to release their grip on the anastomotic suture. On occasion one of the edges of the anastomosis will tuck down beneath the other. This can be appropriately everted for suturing by inserting the open jaw of the driver into the gap and drawing it out slowly.

Once the posterior row of the anastomosis is completed in a water-tight dependent fashion, the corner stitches are re-located to their normal anatomic position. The ureteral stent is then re-inserted into the abdomen which is a maneuver greatly facilitated by the increased degrees of freedom provided by the robot's endo-wrists relative to standard laparoscopy. The Suture-Cut needle driver is utilized to grasp the stent as it emerges from the lumen of the ureter, while the standard needle driver is used to grab and unwind the exposed pigtail. Once it is unwound the tip is inserted beneath the edge of the pelvis side of the anastomosis and advanced into the renal pelvis as much as its cut edge will allow.

The stent is slowly released and the robotic needle driver is withdrawn. We then insert the irrigator aspirator device into the renal pelvis via the unclosed anterior row of the anastomosis to irrigate it free of blood clots and to check the integrity of the posterior closer.

The same interrupted suturing technique is then utilized to close the anterior portion of the anastomosis with interrupted sutures. Often this requires minimal to no retraction by the assistant of the suture tags. After completion of the anastomosis, all of the suture tags including those of the corner stitches are cut and removed by the assistant.

Exiting the Abdomen

At this point we undock the da Vinci robot and back the system away from the operative table. A 5-mm standard laparoscope is introduced via the periumbilical port and the areas of the dissection are inspected under standard and low insufflation pressures. All bleeding points are controlled using the electrocautery and harmonic shears when indicated. The camera is then transferred to the lower quadrant robotic port if the assistant's port was inserted near the epigastrium or via the epigastric robotic port if a low midline location was utilized. The Carter–Thomason needle closure device is utilized to place a 0-Vicryl simple full thickness stitch incorporating the fascia, muscle, and peritoneum to prevent hernia formation at each of the 10–12 mm port sites.

A 15-French round Davol drain with the spike removed is inserted via the lower quadrant robotic port or the lateral port on the right side if a liver retractor was utilized. The port through which the drain is inserted is removed over the drain which is secured to the skin using a 2-0 nylon suture. The remaining ports are removed under direct inspection and the corresponding fascial closure sutures are tied down. The wounds are irrigated with antibiotic solution, injected with 0.25% Marcaine, and subcuticular skin closures are performed using 4-0 Monocryl suture. Benzoin and steri-strips are then applied followed by Band-Aids.

FOLLOW-UP

The patient is placed on a clear liquid diet which is advanced as tolerated. The Foley catheter is left in place for 24 h and then removed unless drain outputs remain greater than 50 cc per 8 h shift with a fluid creatinine value greater than the serum level. Once the Foley is removed the patient is encouraged to void every 2 h to prevent reflux up the stent. The drain output is monitored for another 4–6 h and if the outputs do not increase the drain is removed and the patient is discharged home.

The patient is sent out on low-dose antibiotic prophylaxis until the stent is removed in the office 6 weeks following their operation. We do not perform imaging studies before or at the time of stent removal, since the early appearance of the anastomosis is often difficult to interpret. An intravenous pyelogram is performed 6 weeks after stent removal and a diuretic renal scan at 3, 12, and 18 months after the operation. Patients are discharged from follow-up clinic visits if they remain asymptomatic and without signs of radiographic obstruction or declining renal function at their 18 month appointment.

RESULTS

To date, this author (S.P.H.) has performed laparoscopic pyeloplasty in 107 renal units of 104 patients. Twelve were performed for secondary UPJ obstructions having failed a prior endoscopic approach. Dismembered reconstructions were performed in 103 renal units and Heineke-Mikulicz with suture tacking of crossing vessels in four. Anterior lower pole crossing vessels were identified in 68% of the renal units. Clinical freedom from associated episodes of pain and radiographic patency rates have been confirmed in 96% of patients who are at least 3 months from surgery at the time this manuscript was prepared including the three patients who underwent reconstruction of both renal units. Four patients demonstrated recurrent radiographic obstruction with or without associated clinical symptoms requiring a secondary procedure at a mean of 8 months (range 5–10) after their pyeloplasty. Minor peri-operative complications occurred in seven patients with two suffering a prolonged post-operative ileus, two urinary tract infections, one chronic obstructive pulmonary disease exacerbation, one encrusted ureteral stent, and one with a transient elevation of their creatinine.

The Johns Hopkins Hospital published its large single institution series of 100 laparoscopic pyeloplasties performed by their group of surgeons in 99 patients between August 1993 and January 1999 *(2)*. A total of 17 patients had secondary UPJ obstructions and 57 patients were found to have crossing lower pole vessels. Dismembered reconstructions were performed in 71 cases, Y-V plasty in 20, Heineke-Mikulicz in eight, and a Davis intubated ureterotomy in one case. Mean clinical and radiographic follow-up was 2.7 and 2.2 years, respectively, with radiographic patency confirmed in 96% of patients. All reported failures occurred within the first year of the patients operation and the overall complication rate was 13%.

Dr. Patel published his single institution series of 50 robotic laparoscopic pyeloplasties performed in 50 patients between 2002 and 2004 *(6)*. A total of five patients had secondary UPJ obstructions and 45 patients were found to have crossing lower pole vessels. The mean operative time was 122 min. Dismembered reconstructions were performed in all cases. Mean clinical and radiographic follow-up was 11.7 months with no patient demonstrating clinical or radiographic evidence of obstruction.

TAKE HOME MESSAGES

(1) Laparoscopic pyeloplasty with or without da Vinci robot assistance is an excellent minimally invasive treatment option for the obstructed UPJ with patency rates equivalent to the open approach.
(2) All forms of primary and secondary UPJ obstruction can be treated using this technique including anterior crossing lower pole vessels.
(3) The only significant relative contraindication to laparoscopic pyeloplasty is a small, intra-renal pelvis.
(4) The procedure is technically demanding, but the Endostitch device and da Vinci robot facilitate the intra-corporeal suturing and knot-tying required during this operation.

REFERENCES

1. Schuessler WW, Grune MT, Tecuanhuey LV, et al.: Laparoscopic dismembered pyeloplasty. *J Urol* 150: 1795, 1993.
2. Jarrett TW, Chan DY, Charambura TC, et al.: Laparoscopic pyeloplasty: the first 100 cases. *J Urol* 176: 1253, 2001.
3. Chen RN, Moore RG, Kavoussi LR: Laparoscopic pyeloplasty. Indications, technique, and long-term outcome. *Urol Clin N Amer* 25: 323, 1998.
4. Varkarakis IM, Bhayani SB, Allaf ME, et al.: Management of secondary ureteropelvic junction obstruction after failed primary laparoscopic pyeloplasty. *J Urol* 172: 180, 2004.
5. Lee RS, Retik AB, Borer JG, Peters CA: Pediatric robot assisted laparoscopic dismembered pyeloplasty: comparison with a cohort of open surgery. *J Urol* 175: 683, 2006.
6. Patel V: Robotic-assisted laparoscopic dismembered pyeloplasty. *Urology* 66: 45, 2005.
7. Cadeddu JA, Kavoussi LR: Laparoscopic pyeloplasty using an automated suturing device. In: Olsson CA (ed.). *Current Surgical Techniques in Urology*. Wilmington: Medical Publications, Inc; 1997; Vol. 10 (Issue 3).

Laparoscopic Adrenalectomy

Stuart S. Kesler, Grant I.S. Disick, and Ravi Munver

INTRODUCTION

The surgical approach to the adrenal gland was historically described via an open technique. Recently, the laparoscopic approach has become the preferred method for removal of the adrenal gland when affected by a variety of pathologic disorders. Since laparoscopic adrenalectomy was described by Gagner et al. *(1)*, numerous reports and comparative studies have demonstrated laparoscopic adrenalectomy to be superior to open adrenalectomy with regards to blood loss, cosmesis, analgesic requirements, hospital stay, and recovery time *(1–4)*. Laparoscopic adrenalectomy is efficacious and safe and has become the standard for the majority of surgical adrenal disorders.

INDICATIONS AND CONTRAINDICATIONS

The indications for laparoscopic adrenalectomy may be classified into several categories (Table 1). These include functional tumors, non-functional symptomatic tumors, indeterminate cysts, solitary metastatic lesions, malignant lesions, and incidental adrenal lesions with features such as large size, rapid growth rate, and indeterminant radiographic characteristics.

Functional adrenal adenomas that secrete hormones such as aldosterone and cortisol are among the most common indications for surgical excision of the adrenal gland. These benign lesions are optimal for laparoscopic excision due to their location and small size. While the exact size of an adrenal lesion prompting surgical exploration is controversial, most authorities agree that lesions greater than 4–5 mm should be removed because of the higher likelihood of malignancy. Smaller lesions are commonly benign and thus are frequently followed radiographically.

Laparoscopic excision of adrenal lesions larger than 10 mm or of adrenal carcinomas is controversial. While some experienced surgeons have approached these lesions laparoscopically, many authorities consider these to be contraindications to laparoscopic adrenalectomy *(5–9)*. These cases can be exceedingly complex, with high complication rates and more frequent conversions to an open procedure. Large lesions or those with potential for local invasion are recommended to be managed using an open approach.

Relative contraindications to laparoscopic adrenalectomy include significant adhesions from prior surgery, morbid obesity, uncorrected coagulopathy, and cardiopulmonary disease that precludes hypercapnea that is associated with pneumoperitoneum. These cases must be evaluated on an individual basis, and the surgeon's experience and comfort level must be taken into consideration.

From: *Current Clinical Urology: Essential Urologic Laparoscopy*
Edited by: S. Y. Nakada and S. P. Hedican, DOI 10.1007/978-1-60327-820-1_14

Table 1
Indications/contraindications for laparoscopic adrenalectomy

Indications
Aldosterone producing adenoma
Cortisol producing adenoma
Bilateral adrenal hyperplasia
Pheochromocytoma
Non-functioning adenoma > 4–5 mm
Symptomatic cyst
Symptomatic myelolipoma
Solitary adrenal metastasis
Contraindications
Large tumor > 10 mm (relative)
Morbid obesity (relative)
Uncorrected coagulopathy (relative)
Pyelonephritis (relative)
Adrenocortical carcinoma (relative)
Malignant pheochromocytoma (relative)
Significant abdominal adhesions (relative)
Severe cardiopulmonary disease (relative)
Local invasion (absolute)
Venous involvement (absolute)
Pregnancy (absolute)

PREOPERATIVE EVALUATION

A complete history and physical examination is mandatory in the evaluation of a patient with an adrenal mass. While a complete discussion of the metabolic evaluation of adrenal lesions is beyond the scope of this chapter, a distinct effort to rule out the diagnosis a pheochromocytoma is crucial, as dire consequences may result from a misdiagnosis. This can be accomplished by evaluating the patient's plasma free metanephrines, along with confirmatory urinary catecholamine and metanephrine levels if necessary. A complete endocrinologic evaluation should also include measurement of serum electrolytes, serum hormone levels, and urine levels of steroid hormones and their metabolites. The exact tests ordered will depend on the observed clinical signs and symptoms as well as the patient's history and physical exam. In addition, stimulation studies such as the low- and high-dose dexamethasone suppression tests and measurement of plasma renin and aldosterone levels can be obtained if clinically warranted. A review of the recommended work-up for the incidental adrenal lesion may be found in the NIH Consensus and State-of-the-Science Statement "Management of the Clinically Inapparent Adrenal Mass" *(10,11)*.

Radiographic imaging is essential in the evaluation of an adrenal mass. While a pathologic evaluation can yield a definitive diagnosis, invaluable information can be obtained from a properly performed radiographic study. Computed tomography (CT) scans with and without intravenous contrast, with thin 2–5 mm cuts, are vital in assessing adrenal lesions. Lipid-rich adenomas are commonly homogeneous lesions that measure less than 10 Hounsfield units on non-contrast CT, while lipid-poor adenomas may be differentiated by measuring levels of enhancement or percent contrast washout. Lymphadenopathy and local invasion are features that are more consistent with a malignant lesion.

Magnetic resonance imaging (MRI) scans are also commonly obtained in the evaluation of adrenal masses. This study can provide additional information such as identifying adipose tissue within lesions and can improve the identification of invasion into surrounding structures. Metaiodobenzylguanidine (MIBG) scans have poor spatial resolution and play a limited role in the evaluation of adrenal lesions. However, this study can be helpful in localizing small pheochromocytomas. This is especially true for those patients with multiple endocrine neosplasia (MEN) syndromes, who are high risk for extra-adrenal pheochromocytomas. Additionally, MIBG scans are useful in suspected cases of malignant or bilateral pheochromocytomas *(12)*.

Once an adrenal lesion is determined to require removal, standard preoperative evaluation and preparation are required. Patients diagnosed with a pheochromocytoma require a more thorough preoperative assessment. This includes alpha blockade for 2 weeks prior to surgery, along with the addition of beta blockers to treat tachycardia or arrhythmias if present. Beta blockers should only be given once complete alpha blockade is achieved. Furthermore, these patients also require cardiac consultation for the evaluation of occult cardiomyopathy.

RELEVANT ANATOMY

Adrenal arterial supply is highly variable. The adrenal glands typically draw their blood supply from arterial cascades arising from the inferior phrenic artery, aorta, and renal artery. Adrenal venous drainage also displays great variability. On the right side, a short adrenal vein typically provides drainage into the posterolateral aspect of the vena cava. On the left side, the adrenal vein usually drains into the left renal vein. Not uncommonly, accessory adrenal veins are present near the superior and medial diaphragmatic attachments and provide additional drainage into the inferior phrenic vein. Meticulous dissection and appreciation of retroperitoneal anatomy is required in order to avoid inadvertent vascular injury.

PATIENT PREPARATION, OPERATING ROOM SET-UP, AND PATIENT POSITIONING

Informed consent with explanation of pertinent risks is obtained prior to the procedure. Patients are instructed to maintain a clear liquid diet for 12–24 h prior to surgery and administer a bowel preparation consisting of 300 ml of magnesium citrate on the prior day. Sequential compression devices are placed on the lower extremities and a single dose of intravenous antibiotics is given 60 min prior to surgical incision. After induction of general anesthesia, an orogastric tube and Foley catheter are placed to decompress the stomach and bladder, respectively. Bilateral intravenous access may be beneficial as upper extremity exposure is limited once positioning is completed. Administration of nitrous oxide can lead to bowel distention and should be avoided.

For cases of pheochromocytomas, invasive arterial monitoring, large bore intravenous access or central line placement is recommended. These patients must be aggressively hydrated prior to surgery, as hypotension is frequently encountered after the induction of anesthesia. Anesthetic agents such as propofol, ketamine, and halothane should be strictly avoided *(13)*.

The patient is placed in a modified lateral decubitus position (45–60°) with the flank situated over the kidney rest. The table may be flexed to increase the area between the iliac crest and costal margin. A bean bag or large gel rolls are used to support the patient in this position. Pillows are placed between the legs and the dependent leg is flexed at the knee while the opposite leg is placed straight. The arms are placed parallel onto well padded arm boards. The ankles, knees, dependent hip, shoulders, and brachial plexus are adequately padded. After verifying that all areas prone to pressure injury are well padded, the patient is secured to the operating table using 3" cloth tape across the shoulder and arm as well as across the hip. Figure 1 demonstrates proper patient positioning for left laparoscopic

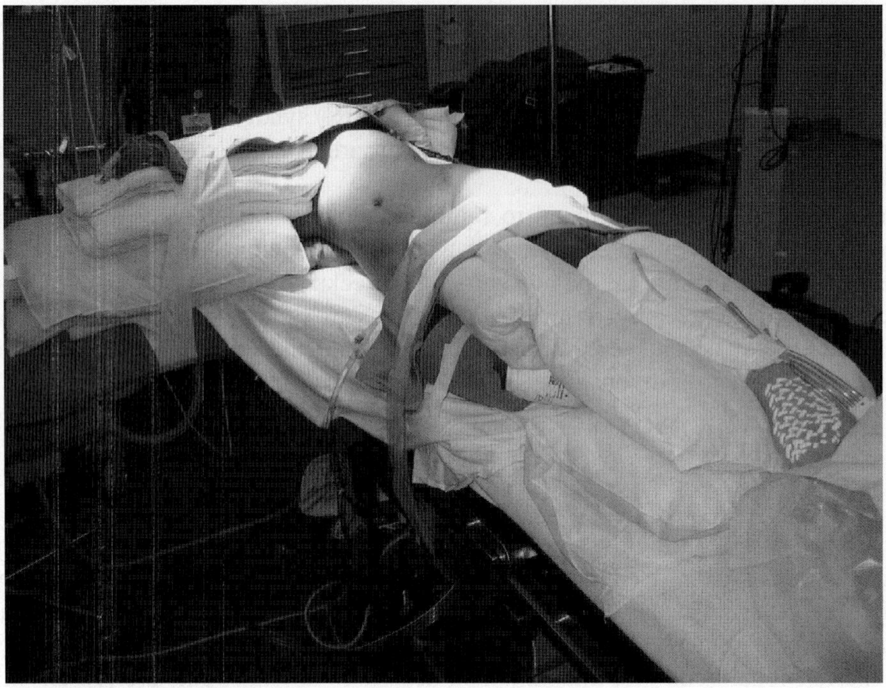

Fig. 1. Patient positioning for left-sided laparoscopic adrenalectomy.

adrenalectomy. Positioning for right laparoscopic adrenalectomy is the mirror image of that for the left side. Furthermore, some surgeons have reported using a needlescopic technique which employs 2–3-mm trocars.

INSTRUMENTATION

The instrumentation and setup for laparoscopic adrenalectomy is similar to that for laparoscopic renal surgery, and consists of a video tower with a color monitor, video system, and CO_2 insufflator. Both 0 and 30° lenses are commonly used. A liver retractor is useful for right sided procedures, and several types of retractors are commercially available. The liver retractor is held in place by an assistant or a self retaining device that is attached to the operating table. The surgeon utilizes an atraumatic grasper, laparoscopic Kittner, or suction-irrigator in the non-dominant hand and a dissecting instrument in the surgeon's dominant hand. A variety of laparoscopic thermal energy devices are available. Ultrasonic shears are useful for colon mobilization and adrenal vein dissection. A bipolar device has excellent hemostatic properties and is our preferred instrument for performing the adrenal dissection. This device has been shown to significantly decrease blood loss and operative time during adrenal dissection compared to other devices *(14)*. Furthermore, we routinely use this device to ligate and divide the adrenal vein, which obviates the need for hemostatic clips. Intraoperative ultrasound has also shown to be helpful in localizing small adrenal lesions, especially in obese individuals with extensive amounts of retroperitoneal adipose tissue. A laparoscopic specimen retrieval bag is required. A list of commonly used instruments is shown in Table 2.

Table 2
Instrumentation for laparoscopic adrenalectomy

- Veress needle
- 5 or 10 mm, 0 and 30° laparoscopic lens
- Laparoscopic liver retractor
- Ultrasonic shears
- Bipolar device
- Curved dissecting scissors
- Laparoscopic atraumatic forceps
- Laparoscopic right angle
- Laparoscopic Kittner
- Maryland dissector
- Laparoscopic ultrasound probe
- Laparoscopic stapling device
- Polymer or titanium hemostatic clips (5 or 10 mm)
- Suction/irrigator device
- Laparoscopic retrieval bag

SURGICAL TECHNIQUE

The adrenal gland can be removed laparoscopically by a variety of approaches. These include the lateral transperitoneal, anterior transperitoneal, lateral retroperitoneal, posterior retroperitoneal, and transthoracic approach. The majority of laparoscopic adrenalectomies are performed using the lateral transperitoneal technique *(15)*.

Right Transperitoneal Laparoscopic Adrenalectomy

A skin incision is made 2 mm superior to and 2 mm lateral to the umbilicus, just to the right of the midline. A Veress needle is introduced into the abdominal cavity through this incision and the peritoneal cavity is insufflated to 15 mmHg. A 12-mm trocar is placed at this site and a 5 mm laparoscope with a 30° lens is used to inspect the abdominal contents. A 5-mm trocar is placed in the midline, 2 mm below the xiphoid process. A 12-mm trocar is placed at the mid-clavicular line (MCL), 2 mm above the level of the umbilicus. An accessory 5-mm trocar is placed at the anterior axillary line (AAL), below the costal margin. The laparoscope is then placed through the sub-xiphoid 5-mm trocar, ultrasonic shears are introduced through the periumbilical 12-mm trocar, atraumatic forceps are introduced through the MCL 12-mm trocar, and a liver retractor is placed through AAL 5-mm trocar. This trocar configuration is illustrated in Fig. 2a. Another commonly used trocar configuration for right transperitoneal laparoscopic adrenalectomy is illustrated in Fig. 2b.

The right triangular ligament is divided using ultrasonic in order to mobilize the liver adequately for exposure of the adrenal gland. The posterior peritoneum is divided close to the liver edge and this incision is carried from the inferior vena cava (IVC) to the abdominal side wall. Extensive liver mobilization is required such that the superior aspect of the adrenal gland is visible, as seen in Fig. 3. Mobilization of the colon is rarely needed. A Kocher maneuver is performed to mobilize the duodenum medially to expose the IVC. Exposure of the IVC is essential, as its medial border can be traced cephalad to identify the adrenal vein.

The superior border of the kidney is identified and Gerota's fascia is entered using ultrasonic shears. The adrenal gland is localized along the supero-medial aspect of the kidney. Dissection begins along the supero-medial aspect of the adrenal gland, just lateral to the IVC. If inferior phrenic arterial branches are encountered, they are clipped and divided. Lateral traction of the adrenal gland is

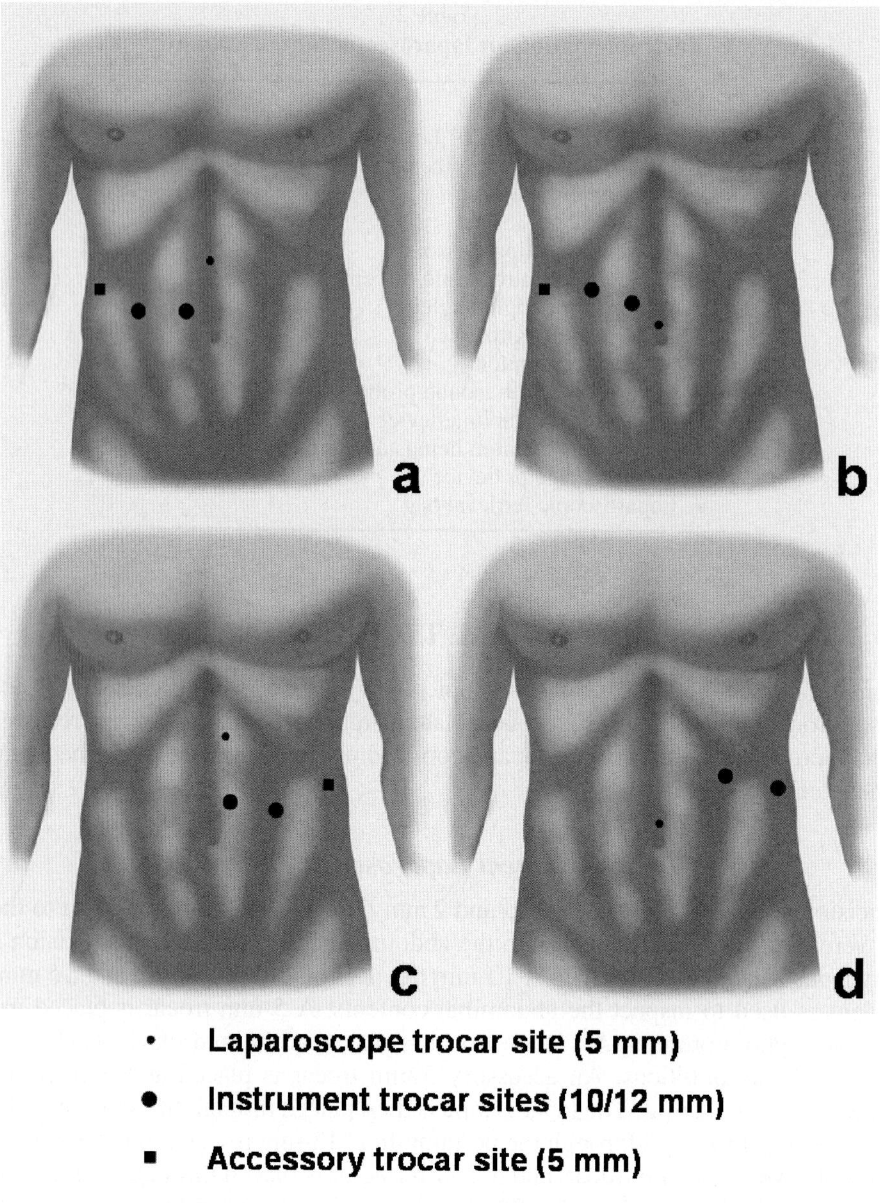

Fig. 2. (**a**) Trocar configuration for right transperitoneal laparoscopic adrenalectomy. (**b**) Alternate trocar configuration for right transperitoneal laparoscopic adrenalectomy. (**c**) Trocar configuration for left transperitoneal laparoscopic adrenalectomy. (**d**) Alternate trocar configuration for left transperitoneal laparoscopic adrenalectomy.

accomplished using a laparoscopic Kittner or a suction–irrigator device. An atraumatic grasper should not be used to retract the adrenal as it can fracture the adrenal parenchyma or cause bleeding in the surrounding adipose tissue. The right adrenal vein is identified and dissected from surrounding tissues as seen in Fig. 4. The vein is doubly ligated with hemostatic polymer clips and divided using laparoscopic scissors. Alternatively, the adrenal vein can be ligated and divided with a bipolar vessel sealing device. Care must be taken when manipulating the right adrenal vein due to its short length and insertion into the IVC.

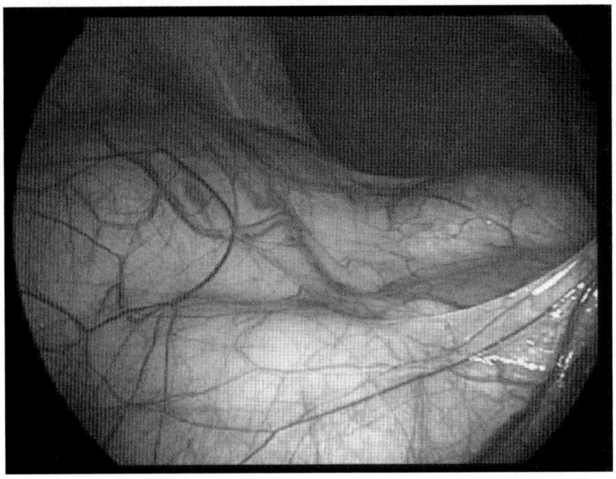

Fig. 3. Mobilization of the liver allows visualization of the right adrenal gland, kidney, and IVC.

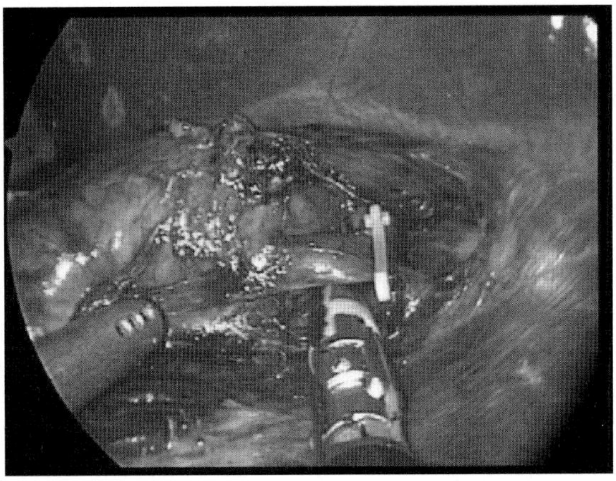

Fig. 4. The right adrenal vein is dissected from surrounding tissues and ligated with hemostatic polymer clips.

Dissection continues circumferentially around the adrenal gland in a clockwise fashion. As bleeding is easily encountered, this dissection is best accomplished using a bipolar device. The lateral attachments of the adrenal gland should be divided last, as they prevent the gland from medial mobilization, thus obscuring the dissection. Once the gland is completely dissected from surrounding structures, it is placed into the laparoscopic retrieval bag. The pneumoperitoneum pressure is lowered to 5 mmHg and the area is inspected for bleeding. The specimen is removed by enlarging a 10-mm trocar site as necessary. Trocar sites 10 mm or larger are closed with a fascial closure device and skin incisions are closed with subcuticular sutures or skin staples.

Left Transperitoneal Laparoscopic Adrenalectomy

A skin incision is made 2 mm superior to the umbilicus and to the left of the midline. A Veress needle is introduced into the abdominal cavity through this incision and the peritoneal cavity is insufflated to 15 mmHg. A 12-mm trocar is placed at this site and a 5-mm laparoscope with a 30° lens is used to inspect the abdominal contents. A 5-mm trocar is placed to the left of the midline, 2 mm below the xiphoid process. A 12-mm trocar is placed at the MCL, 2 mm above the level of the umbilicus. An accessory 5-mm trocar is placed at the AAL, below the costal margin. The laparoscope is introduced through the sub-xiphoid 5-mm trocar, atraumatic forceps are introduced through the periumbilical 12-mm trocar, and ultrasonic shears are introduced through the MCL 12-mm trocar. The AAL 5-mm trocar is used to assist with retraction of the kidney and as an additional site for the laparoscope during certain maneuvers. This trocar configuration is illustrated in Fig. 2c. Another commonly used trocar configuration for left transperitoneal laparoscopic adrenalectomy is illustrated in Fig. 2d.

The descending colon is mobilized along the white line of Toldt using ultrasonic shears or an alternate thermal energy device. The superficial peritoneal attachments between the colon and lateral sidewall should be released initially. Lateral renal attachments to the sidewall should not be released as this will result in medial mobilization of the kidney. This maneuver will obscure the renal hilum and interfere with further dissection. The colon is further dissected medially using the suction-irrigator device, exposing the plane between the colonic mesentery and Gerota's fascia. Recognition of this plane is important, as inadvertent entry into the mesentery can lead to bleeding as well as mesenteric defects with potential for internal herniation. Premature entry into Gerota's fascia can create bleeding and limit visualization of the renal hilum. The dissection is carried cephalad towards the upper pole of the kidney. Extensive splenic mobilization is required to provide adequate exposure of the upper pole of the kidney and adrenal gland, as seen in Fig. 5. This is one of the most critical parts of the operation, and with adequate mobilization, the spleen should fall medially without requiring active retraction.

Following splenic mobilization, some surgeons elect to approach the adrenal gland at its supero-medial aspect and then proceed inferiorly along its lateral border. Our preference is to begin dissection at the infero-medial aspect. The renal hilum is first identified, along with the insertion of the left adrenal vein into the renal vein, as seen in Fig. 6a. The left adrenal vein is dissected free from surrounding structures and is doubly ligated with hemostatic clips and divided with laparoscopic scissors. Alternatively, the adrenal vein can be ligated and divided with a bipolar device, obviating the need for clip application, as seen in Fig. 6b.

Once the adrenal vein is divided, the adrenal gland is gently retracted medially and meticulous dissection between the adrenal gland and the upper pole of the kidney is carried out, as seen in Fig. 7. The use of clips, ultrasonic shears, or a bipolar device is beneficial in this area due to the highly vascular nature of the adrenal gland. If bleeding is encountered in this area, the application of gentle pressure is usually effective in obtaining hemostasis. If inferior phrenic arterial branches are encountered, they

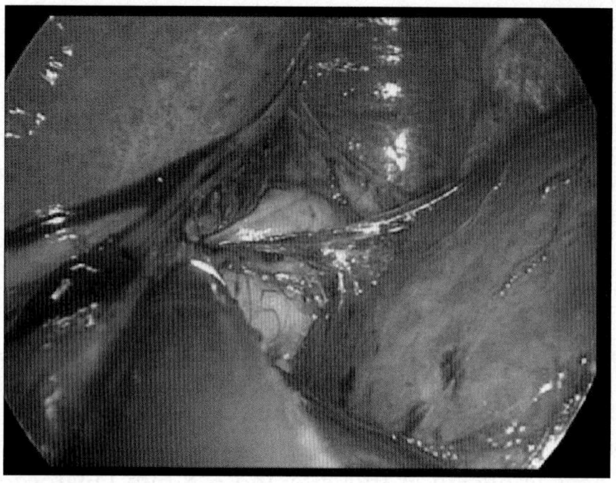

Fig. 5. Extensive splenic mobilization is required to provide adequate exposure of the upper pole of the kidney and left adrenal gland.

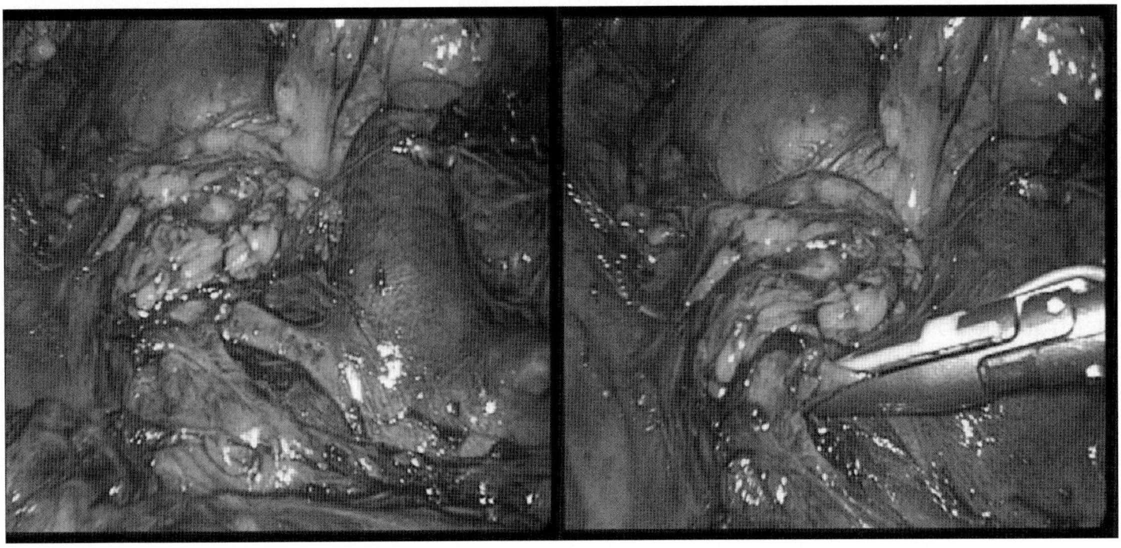

Fig. 6. (**a**) After medial mobilization of the colon, the renal hilum is exposed and the insertion of the left adrenal vein into the renal vein is identified. (**b**) The left adrenal vein is ligated and divided with a bipolar device.

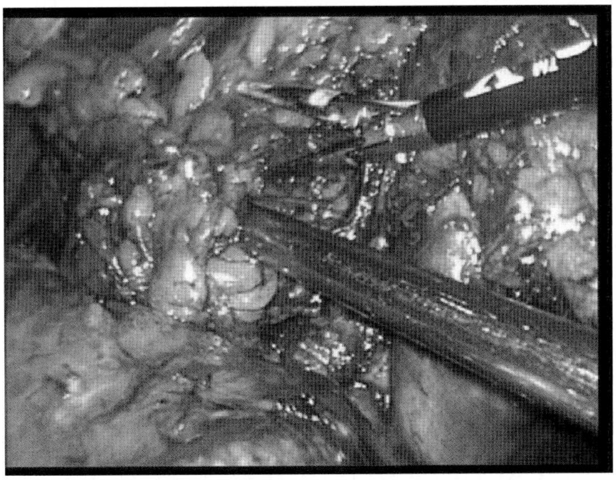

Fig. 7. The left adrenal gland is gently retracted medially and meticulous dissection between the adrenal gland and the upper pole of the kidney is carried out. The use of clips, ultrasonic shears, or a bipolar vessel sealing device is beneficial in this area due to the highly vascular nature of the adrenal gland.

are clipped and divided. In addition, renal arterial branches between the upper pole of the kidney and adrenal gland are not uncommonly encountered during this portion of the dissection, and one should be careful about inadvertent vascular injury. The remaining attachments are divided superiorly and the specimen is placed into a laparoscopic retrieval bag. The pneumoperitoneum pressure is lowered to 5 mmHg and the area is inspected for bleeding. The specimen is removed by enlarging a 10-mm trocar site as necessary. Trocar sites 10 mm or larger are closed with a fascial closure device and skin incisions are closed with subcuticular sutures or skin staples.

Retroperitoneal Approach

A 1.5-cm skin incision is made in the mid-axillary line 2 mm below the costal margin. The underlying muscles are split bluntly to access the retroperitoneum. Digital dissection is used to create a small space by retracting the peritoneum medially. The retroperitoneal space is developed in a nontraumatic fashion by employing a commercially available dissecting balloon. The balloon is inserted and directed laterally and posterior to Gerota's fascia. A laparoscope can be placed through the dissecting balloon and allows direct visualization as the retroperitoneal working space is developed. The balloon is inflated and maintained for several minutes to establish hemostasis. Alternatively, the working space may be developed with finger dissection alone. On occasion, small perforating vessels that enter from the posterior wall may be disrupted during this dissection. These vessels can easily be controlled with electrocautery or ultrasonic shears. After the retroperitoneal working space is developed, the balloon is deflated and replaced with a 10-mm Hassan trocar. The retroperitoneal space is insufflated to 15 mmHg. A 30-degree laparoscope is placed through the initial trocar. Additional trocars are placed under direct vision or with digital guidance. A variety of trocar configurations may be used. Our preference is to place two additional trocars (5 and 12 mm) approximately 3–4 mm cephalad to the initial trocar in the posterior and AALs. An additional 5-mm trocar may be placed for additional retraction or for suction and irrigation purposes. In order to confirm appropriate dissection, the psoas muscle should be identified posteriorly and the kidney should be displaced anteriorly and medially. Proper trocar placement for right retroperitoneal laparoscopic adrenalectomy is seen in Fig. 8. The configuration for left retroperitoneal laparoscopic adrenalectomy is the mirror image of that used for the right side.

The retroperitoneal approach is more difficult than its transperitoneal counterpart due to the paucity of anatomic landmarks and abundance of retroperitoneal adipose tissue. Reflecting the peritoneum medially is a critical maneuver that allows medial reflection of the liver and ascending colon during right adrenalectomy, and of the spleen and descending colon during left adrenalectomy. Moreover, this maneuver exposes the psoas muscle and develops the working space. The renal hilum, located medial to the psoas muscle, is often identified by the pulsation of the renal artery. Surgical dissection is performed with minimal manipulation of the adrenal gland. Identification and control of the adrenal vein prior to mobilization of the adrenal gland is of critical importance. This is especially crucial for pheochromocytoma, although Bonjer et al. reported performing retroperitoneal laparoscopic adrenalectomy in 19 patients with pheochromocytoma in whom the vein was controlled at the end of the dissection without adverse sequela *(16)*.

RIGHT RETROPERITONEAL LAPAROSCOPIC ADRENALECTOMY

Removal of the right adrenal gland begins with identification of the psoas muscle and IVC, located medial to the psoas muscle. Blunt dissection of the posterolateral aspect of the vena cava leads to identification of the main adrenal vein which is meticulously isolated, ligated, and divided. Anomalous vessels that are encountered must be controlled, clipped, and divided. The medial and inferior surfaces of the adrenal gland are dissected off the renal vein and the vena cava with the ultrasonic shears or dissecting forceps. Small arteries can be controlled using ultrasonic shears, hemostatic clips, or bipolar device. If inferior phrenic vessels are encountered, they are clipped and divided. The inferior surface of the adrenal gland is dissected off of the upper pole of the kidney. The lateral surface is the final portion that is dissected. Once the specimen is completely free from its surrounding tissues, it is placed into a laparoscopic retrieval bag. The pneumoperitoneum pressure is lowered to 5 mmHg and the area is inspected for bleeding. The specimen is removed by enlarging the 12-mm trocar site as necessary. Trocar sites 10 mm or larger are closed with a fascial closure device and skin incisions are closed with subcuticular sutures or skin staples.

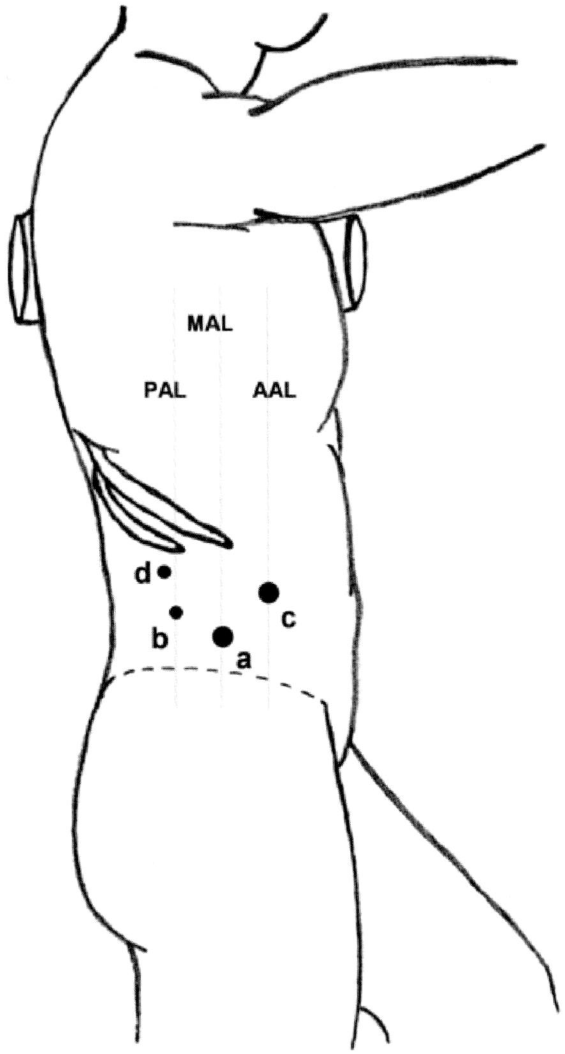

Fig. 8. Trocar placement for right retroperitoneal laparoscopic adrenalectomy. (**a**) 10-mm trocar; (**b**) 5-mm trocar; (**c**) 12-mm trocar; (**d**) 5-mm accessory trocar. MAL = mid axillary line; AAL = anterior axillary line; PAL = posterior axillary line.

Left Retroperitoneal Laparoscopic Adrenalectomy

Removal of the left adrenal gland begins with the identification of the renal hilum. Blunt dissection and caudal retraction of the left renal artery leads to identification of the left adrenal vein, which is meticulously isolated, ligated, and divided. The superior aspect of the adrenal gland is dissected from the diaphragm using ultrasonic shears or an alternate thermal energy device. Inferior phrenic vessels, if encountered, require vascular control as well. The lateral surface of the adrenal gland is then dissected off of the kidney. Cephalad retraction allows dissection of the inferior surface of the gland using ultrasonic shears. The medial surface of the adrenal gland is the final portion that is dissected. Once the specimen is completely free from its surrounding tissues, it is placed into a laparoscopic retrieval bag. The pneumoperitoneum pressure is lowered to 5 mmHg and the area is inspected for bleeding.

Table 3
Large contemporary series of laparoscopic adrenalectomy

Series	*Year*	*Number of cases*	*Approach*	*Operative time (min)*	*Blood loss (ml)*	*Length of stay (days)*	*Conversion rate (%)*	*Complication rate (%)*	*Mortality rate (%)*
Miccoli et al. *(17)*	2002	137	N/A	111	N/A	3.8	4.3	3.9	0
Porpiglia et al. *(18)*	2002	125	N/A	139	100	4	3.2	11.2	0.8
Del Pizzo et al. *(19)*	2002	100	LTA	164	178	3.1	2	6	0
Chiu et al. *(20)*	2003	120	Ret.	100–210	20–100	2	5	N/A	0
O'Boyle et al. *(21)*	2003	172	TA	65	80	3	7	5	0
Zeh et al. *(22)*	2003	100	TA	N/A	N/A	1	13	6	0
Prager et al. *(23)*	2004	102	TA	N/A	N/A	N/A	5	9	0
Poulouse et al. *(24)*	2005	100	TA	150	NR	2.6	1	14	1
Naya et al. *(25)*	2005	127	TA	179	53	N/A	0	N/A	0
Ramacciato et al. *(26)*	2005	104	TA/Ret.	108	106	N/A	5	5	0
Lifante et al. *(27)*	2005	179	–	N/A	N/A	7.6	11	8	2
Castillo et al. *(28)*	2006	164	N/A	83	N/A	2.5		6	
Walz et al. *(29)*	2006	560	Posterior	55	10	N/A	2	7	0
Nocca et al. *(30)*	2007	131	LTA	N/A	N/A	2.5	2	5	0

The specimen is removed by enlarging the 12-mm trocar site as necessary. Trocar sites 10 mm or larger are closed with a fascial closure device and skin incisions are closed with subcuticular sutures or skin staples.

POSTOPERATIVE MANAGEMENT

The orogastric tube is removed at the completion of the procedure. A chemistry panel and complete blood count are obtained in the recovery room and on the first postoperative day. The Foley catheter is removed on the first postoperative day. A clear liquid diet is started on the first postoperative day and the diet is advanced as tolerated. Serum cortisol levels are evaluated to assure that no element of adrenal insufficiency requires supplementation. Most patients may be discharged on the first postoperative day.

PUBLISHED RESULTS

While there have been no prospective randomized studies comparing open versus laparoscopic adrenalectomy, numerous reports and case-controlled studies have validated the benefits of the laparoscopic approach. The majority of surgeons utilize the lateral transperitoneal technique; however, many approaches have been reported in the literature, showing no distinct advantage of any specific technique.

Laparoscopic adrenalectomy has been consistently shown to have improved cosmesis, reduced hospital length of stay, decreased analgesic requirements, and a shorter convalescent period. A summary of large contemporary series of laparoscopic adrenalectomy is shown in Table 3 *(17–30)*.

Bleeding is the most common complication during and after laparoscopic adrenalectomy, accounting for 40% of complications *(31)*. The next most common complication is injury to surrounding organs such as the liver, spleen, colon, pancreas, and diaphragm, accounting for less than 5% of all complications. Approximate rates for overall complications, conversion to open, and mortality are 2.6–16%, 0.8–7%, and 0.0–1.3%, respectively. Laparoscopic adrenalectomy has evolved since it was initially described. Refinement in technique and increased experience have resulted in decreased operative times, post operative pain, blood loss, and shortened convalescence. As such, laparoscopic adrenalectomy is recognized as the current standard for surgical removal of the adrenal gland.

TAKE HOME MESSAGES

1. Laparoscopic adrenalectomy is considered the standard of care for excision of small adrenal masses. Controversy still exists regarding the optimal management of malignant lesions or large adrenal masses.
2. Transperitoneal and retroperitoneal laparoscopic approaches are safe and efficacious, but neither has been proven superior. Surgeon preference and experience are most important when selecting the surgical approach.
3. Complete mobilization of the spleen or right hepatic lobe is essential in order to achieve adequate exposure of the adrenal gland.
4. Adrenal gland localization and identification of suprarenal anatomy may be facilitated by use of laparoscopic ultrasonography.

REFERENCES

1. Gagner M, Lacroix A, Bolte E. Laparoscopic adrenalectomy in Cushing's syndrome and pheochromocytoma. *N Engl J Med* 1992; 327: 1033.
2. Prinze R. A comparison of laparoscopic and open adrenalectomies. *Arch Surg* 1995; 130: 489–492.
3. Smith C, Weber C, Amerson J. Laparoscopic adrenalectomy: a new gold standard. *World J Surg* 1999; 23: 389–396.

4. Gill I. The case for laparoscopic adrenalectomy. *J Urol* 2001; 166: 429–436.
5. Henry J, Sebag F, Iacobone M, et al. Results of laparoscopic adrenalectomy for large and potentially malignant tumors. *World J Surg* 2002; 26: 1043–1047.
6. Moinzadeh A, Gill IS. Laparoscopic radical adrenalectomy for malignancy in 31 patients. *J Urol* 2005; 173: 519–525.
7. MacGillivray D, Whalen G, Malchoff C, et al. Laparoscopic resection of large adrenal tumors. *Ann Surg Oncol* 2002; 9: 480–485.
8. Kebebew E, Siperstein A, Clark O, et al. Results of laparoscopic adrenalectomy for suspected and unsuspected adrenal neoplasms. *Arch Surg* 2002; 137: 948–953.
9. Gonzalez R, Shapiro S, Sarlis N, et al. Laparoscopic resection of adrenal cortical carcinoma: a cautionary note. *Surgery* 2005; 138: 1078–1085.
10. NIH state-of-the-science statement on management of clinically inapparent adrenal mass ("incidentaloma"). *NIH Consen State Sci Statements* 2002; 19: 1–23.
11. Munver R, Fromer D, Watson R, Sawczuk I. Evaluation of the incidentally discovered adrenal mass. *Curr Urol Rep* 2004, 5(1):73–77.
12. Miskulin J, Shulkin B, Doherty G, et al. Is preoperative iodine 123 MIBG scintigraphy routinely necessary before initial adrenalectomy for pheochromocytoma? Surgery 2003; 134: 918–922.
13. Zacharias M, Haese A, Jurczok A, et al. Transperitoneal laparoscopic adrenalectomy: outline of the preoperative management, surgical approach, and outcome. *Eur Urol* 2006; 49: 448–459.
14. Munver R, Lombardo S, Ilbeigi P. et al. Advances in the minimally invasive treatment of benign and malignant adrenal lesions: laparoscopic adrenalectomy using a novel vessel-sealing system – a combined experience (Abstract). *J Urol* 2006, 175(4); 347.
15. Assalia A, Gagner M. Laparoscopic adrenalectomy. *Br J Surg* 2004; 91: 1259–1274.
16. Bonjer H, Sorm V, Berends F, et al. Endoscopic retroperitoneal adrenalectomy: lessons learned from 111 consecutive cases. *Ann Surg* 2000, 232 (6): 796–803.
17. Miccoli P, Raffaelli M, Berti P, et al. Adrenal surgery before and after the introduction of laparoscopic adrenalectomy. *Br J Surg* 2002; 89; 779–782.
18. Porpiglia F, Destefanis P, Fiori C, et al. Does adrenal mass size really affect safety and effectiveness of laparoscopic adrenalectomy? *Urology* 2002; 60: 801–805.
19. Del Pizzo J, Shichman S, Sosa E. Laparoscopic adrenalectomy: the New York-Presbyterian Hospital experience. *J Endourol* 2002; 16, 591–597.
20. Chiu A. Laparoscopic retroperitoneal adrenalectomy: clinical experience with 120 consecutive cases. *Asian Journal of Surgery* 2003; 26: 139–144.
21. O'Boyle C, Kapadia C, Sedman P, et al. Laparoscopic transperitoneal adrenalectomy. *Surg Endosc* 2003; 17: 1905–1909.
22. Zeh H, Udelsman R. One hundred laparoscopic adrenalectomies: a single surgeon's experience. *Ann Surg Oncol* 2003; 10(9); 1012–1017.
23. Prager G, Heinz-Peer G, Passler C, et al. Applicability of laparoscopic adrenalectomy in a prospective study in 150 consecutive patients. *Arch Surg* 2004; 139: 46–49.
24. Poulose B, Holzman M, Lao O, et al. Laparoscopic adrenalectomy: 100 resections with clinical long term follow-up. *Surg Endosc* 2005; 19: 379–385.
25. Naya Y, Suzuki H, Komiya A, et al. Laparoscopic adrenalectomy in patients with large adrenal tumors. *Int J Urol* 2005; 12: 134–139.
26. Ramacciato G, Paolo M, Pietromaria A, et al. Ten years of laparoscopic adrenalectomy: lesson learned from 104 procedures. *Am Surg* 2005: 71: 321–325.
27. Lifante J, Cenedese A, Fernandez Vila J, et al. Impact of laparoscopy on the management of adrenal diseases: a retrospective study of 220 patients. *Ann Chirug* 2005; 130: 547–552.
28. Castillo O, Cortes O, Kerkebe M, et al. Laparoscopic surgery in the treatment of adrenal pathology: experience with 200 cases. *Actas Urol Esp* 2006; 30(9): 926–932.
29. Walz M, Alesina P, Wenger F, et al. Posterior retroperitoneoscopic adrenalectomy – results of 560 procedures in 520 patients. *Surgery* 2006; 140: 943–950.
30. Nocca D, Aggarwal R, Mathieu A, et al. Laparoscopic surgery and corticoadenomas. *Surg Endosc* 2007; 21: 1373–1376.
31. Gumbs A, Gagner M. Laparoscopic adrenalectomy. *Best Practice Res Clin Endocrinol Metab* 2006; 20(3); 483–499.

Laparoscopic Retroperitoneal Lymph Node Dissection for Nonseminomatous Germ Cell Tumors

Ernesto Reggio, Kevin Smith, and Louis Kavoussi

INTRODUCTION

Testicular cancer is one of the most curable solid cancers. The dramatic improvement in survival is a result of the efficient staging techniques and multimodal treatment. Even some patients with metastatic retroperitoneal disease can be cured by surgical excision.

Treatment of stage I nonseminomatous germ cell tumors (NSGCT) remains controversial. Proponents of surveillance argue that 70–75% of such patients are already cured. The overall survival rate in studies of men with stage I NSGCT is 98% *(1)*. Nevertheless, surveillance is not advised in the presence of unfavorable testis histology. Three cycles of chemotherapy are necessary, but 7–10% of patients who develop recurrence may not be salvaged with chemotherapy *(2)*. Cisplatin-based chemotherapeutic regimens achieve high-cure rates, however, are ineffective against teratoma, decrease fertility, and the long-term consequences of chemotherapy are unknown *(3)*.

Retroperitoneal lymph node dissection (RPLND) was first described by Donohue in 1977 *(4)*. Since then several modifications have been made to the original technique in an effort to reduce morbidity. RPLND provides accurate staging, cures small volume cancer and, with the mapping studies and development of modified retroperitoneal lymphadenectomy, preserves antegrade ejaculation in up to 98% of patients *(5)*.

Laparoscopic retroperitoneal lymph node dissection (LRPLND) was first performed in 1992 *(6)*. Initially it was performed only for staging purposes, with no dissection of nodes posterior to the lumbar vessels. Currently, LRPLND is performed as an exact replication of the open RPLND at select centers. Technological advances in hemostasis, suturing, and instrumentation allow a full duplication of the open technique, even with retrocaval and retroaortic dissection, which leads to decreased morbidity and enhanced oncological efficacy. LRPLND demands considerable experience in laparoscopic surgeries and dissection of the great vessels.

PREOPERATIVE ASSESSMENT AND PATIENT PREPARATION

LRPLND has been used for diagnosis and treatment of clinical stage I of NSGCT. The ideal patient would be slender, has not had multiple abdominal surgeries, has no history of peritonitis, does not show evidence of metastatic disease, and fulfills biochemical and radiological criteria to be classified

From: *Current Clinical Urology: Essential Urologic Laparoscopy*
Edited by: S. Y. Nakada and S. P. Hedican, DOI 10.1007/978-1-60327-820-1_15

as stage I of NSGCT. More recently, clinical stage II and persistent retroperitoneal disease following chemotherapy for stages IIB and IIC have been also treated by LRPLND *(7)*

Patients must be fully informed and counseled about other treatment options and potential complications, such as bleeding, injury to intra-abdominal structures, conversion to open procedure, lymphatic leak, and retrograde ejaculation. Preoperative sperm banking and autologous blood donation are recommended.

The day before the operation the patient is placed on a clear liquid diet and undergoes a mechanical bowel preparation. Prophylactic broad-spectrum intravenous antibiotics are administered. Sequential pneumatic compression devices are used throughout the procedure.

SURGICAL TECHNIQUE

General anesthesia is established while the patient is in the supine position. Nasogastric tube and Foley catheter are inserted and secured. The patient is placed in a supine position with both arms tucked. The patient is carefully taped to the operation table across the chest, hips, and legs, allowing the surgeon to rotate the patient into a lateral position if necessary. The patient's abdomen is prepped and draped in a sterile fashion from the nipples to mid thigh.

Standard laparoscopic instruments are used throughout the procedure, such as 10-mm 30° laparoscope, Veress needle, atraumatic grasping, scissors, clip appliers, and irrigation/suction device. Specific equipment is as follows:

- laparoscopic paddle retractor
- radiolucent polypropylene clips (Hem-o-Lock, Weck Closure Systems, Triangle Park, NC)
- Needle driver loaded with 4-0 Prolene suture
- Oxidized cellulose (Surgicel, Ethicon, Piscataway, NJ)
- Bipolar coagulation

The operating room set-up for a left LRPLND is shown in Fig. 1.

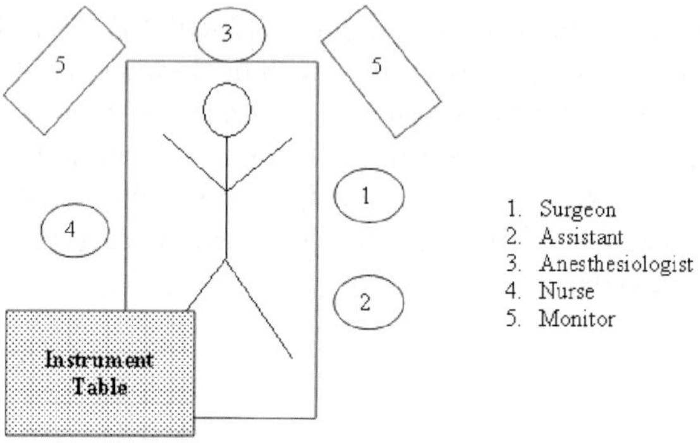

Fig. 1. Operation theater set-up.

Access and Trocar Placement

Pneumoperitoneum is established using a 14-gauge Veress needle, placed in the inferior umbilical crease, up to 20 mmHg pressure. Each potential port side is injected with 0.25% bupivacaine prior to any incision. A variety of port placements will allow successful LRPLND. Our transperitoneal approach involves placement of four equidistant 10/12 trocars in the midline beginning 2–4 mm

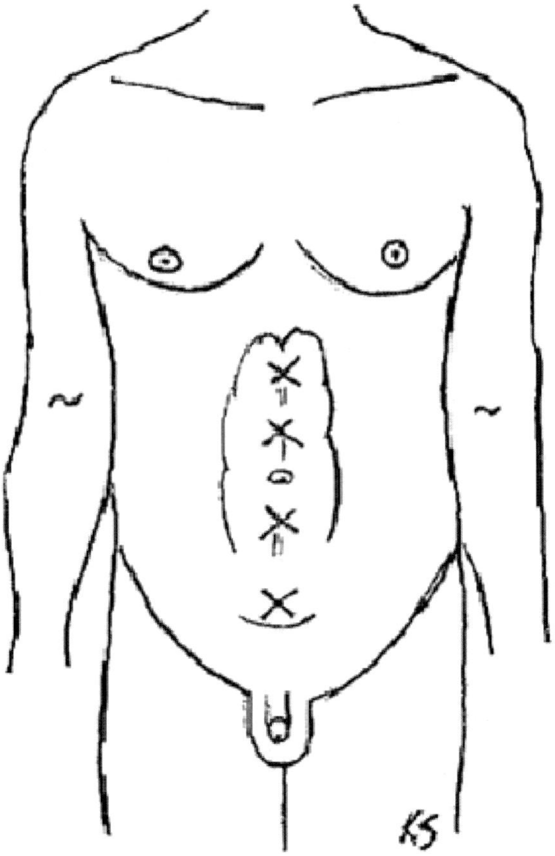

Fig. 2. Diagram demonstrating port sites for LRPLND.

below the xiphoid process (Fig. 2). All secondary trocars are placed under endoscopic control and anchored with 2-0 silk sutures to prevent inadvertent dislodgment during the procedure. If needed a 5-mm port may be placed in the mid-axillary line, halfway between the iliac crest and ribs for additional retraction.

A 10-mm 30° laparoscope is inserted through the umbilical port. The lower port is used to retract the bowel medially in order to expose the great vessels. This maneuver is usually done by the assistant, using the laparoscopic paddle retractor. The surgeon uses the ports above the umbilicus.

Retroperitoneal Dissection

We use the limits of the dissection of LRPLND as proposed by Donohue et al. *(5)* for the open RPLND: on the right the limits are the ureter, the renal vessels, the aorta, and the common iliac artery; on the left the limits are the ureter, the vena cava, the common iliac artery, and the renal vessels (Fig. 3). In both templates the inferior mesenteric artery is spared. The removal of tissue behind the aorta and vena cava is controversial since some authors state there is no evidence that this tissue is landing site for metastatic disease *(8)*. We believe, however, the removal of this tissue is an exact replication of the open RPLND and potentially provides a better outcome for these patients.

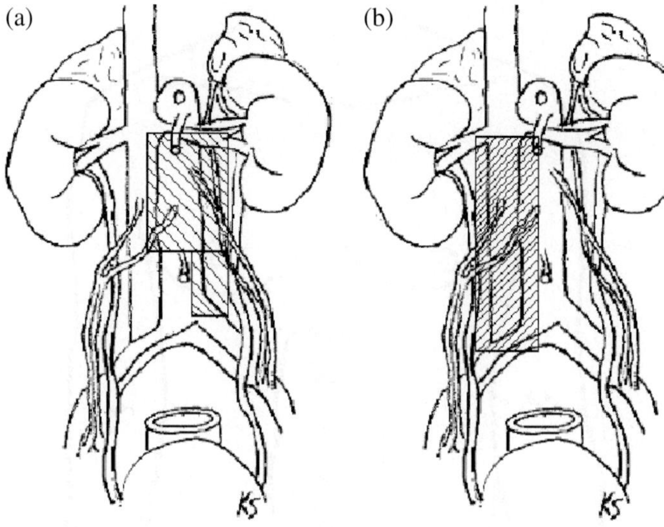

Fig. 3. (**a**) and (**b**) templates for right- and left-sided LRPLND.

Right-Side Procedure

Wide access to the retroperitoneum is necessary for LRPLND. Dissection starts by incising the line of Told from the iliac vessels to the hepatic flexure and the colon is mobilized away from the abdominal wall. Care must be taken to avoid injury of the mesenteric vessels. On the right side, the surgeon defines the duodenum and Kocher's maneuver is carried out. This reflects the head of pancreas medially and allows adequate exposure of the anterior surfaces of the inferior vena cava and both renal veins.

After the colon mobilization, the internal ring is identified; the spermatic cord remnant from the previous radical inguinal orchiectomy is dissected and completely excised. Then, the gonadal vein is dissected from the internal ring to the inferior vena cava and then excised. Special care must be taken on the right side when the gonadal vein opens into the inferior vena cava due to the risk of avulsion. The spermatic artery is clipped and transected at its crossing over the vena cava. The ureter is found as it crosses the iliac vessels.

All the lymphatic tissue between the ureter and the great vessels is excised, using the "split/roll" technique. The tissues overlying precaval/preaortic are split laterally from cranial to caudal, superiorly to the renal vein and inferiorly to the common iliac vessels. The lateral nodal tissue is lifted and blunt dissection is carried down to the lumbar vessels, which are clipped and transected. The underlying psoas fascia is separated. At this point, the lower pole renal arteries may be encountered and should not be confounded with lumbar vessels.

Cephaled to the inferior mesenteric artery, the dissection is continued along the left margin to the aorta. The interaortocaval tissue is cautiously dissected, taking care of all vascular branches off the great vessels. The right renal artery and left renal vein must always be identified. Small blood and lymphatic vessels are clipped. The entire package is gently dissected off the surface of the great vessels using the irrigation/suction device. Special care must be taken when dissecting posteriorly to the inferior vena cava since the efferent sympathetic nerves fibers may be injured.

We perform the retrocaval dissection as an exact replication of open RPLND. The inferior vena cava is lifted with atraumatic instruments and all lymphatic tissue is teased off the retrocaval space. Posterior lumbar vessels are clipped and transected (Fig. 4).

The caudal point of dissection is the point where the ureter crosses the iliac vessels. At this point the entire nodal package is clipped distally and can be removed.

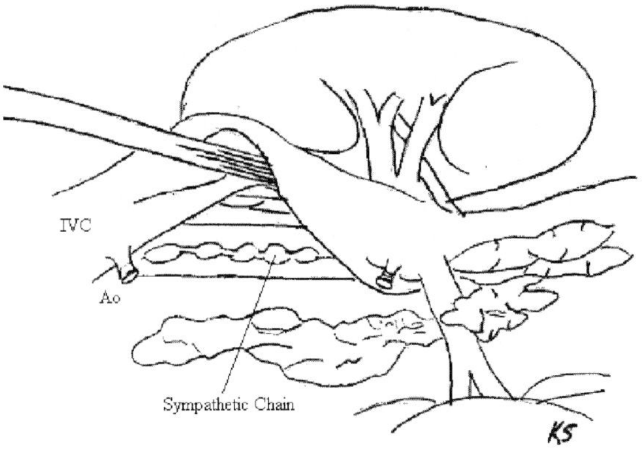

Fig. 4. Retrocaval dissection: lumbar vessels were clipped and sympathetic chain was spared.

Left-Side Procedure

On the left side the peritoneum is incised along the line of Told from the iliac vessels to the splenic flexure. The splenocolic and phrenicocolic ligaments are divided. Then, the colon is mobilized medially until the anterior surface of the aorta and vena cava are exposed.

The spermatic vein is identified and proximally dissected toward to the left renal vein, where it is clipped. The left renal artery is then identified, paying close attention to the lumbar vein draining into the left renal vein, which can be injured. The spermatic artery is clipped at its origin from the aorta and transected. The ureter is identified and separated. The nodal package is dissected free in a similar way as to the right side, according to the template limits. Retroaortic dissection is performed as in the open RPLND. Care must be taken with the lumbar arteries during this step. The sympathetic chain must be identified and spared.

The specimen is entrapped and removed using an Endocatch device (US Surgical, Norwalk, CT). Intra-abdominal pressure is lowered to 5 mmHg in order to evaluate possible bleeding. A drain is not routinely placed. Port sides are endoscopically closed under direct vision.

COMPLICATIONS AND PREVENTION

The major complication during LRPLND is hemorrhage. Careful dissection of the great vessels and their branches, along with the advent of new equipments allow the prevention of bleedings. Furthermore, the magnification provided by the laparoscope facilitates the tissue dissection, preventing injuries. Anatomical landmarks, potential risks of injury and the maneuvers to prevent and treat some complications are described as follows:

- Lumbar vessels can be injured mainly during retrocaval and retroaortic dissection. The vessels encountered must be carefully ligated and divided. An important point is to leave a long vessel stump, in case a clip dislodges, making bleeding control easier. Hemorrhage from retroperitoneal muscles can be managed with a figure-of-eight stitch placed deep into the muscle.
- Accessory lower pole renal arteries may be found and should not be confounded with lumbar vessels. The right renal artery and left renal vein should also not be confused with lumbar vessels at the interaortocaval dissection.
- Lacerations of the inferior vena cava and aorta do not demand open conversion. As in open surgery, acute bleeding, mainly from venous bleeding, can be stopped by direct pressure applied with a surgical

sponge. Most venous bleeding can be stopped with the help of fibrin glue. Clips, bipolar cautery, or intracorporeal suturing, using 3-0 monofilament nonabsorbable sutures, may be used to control arterial bleeding.

- On the right side, dissection of the duodenum and the head of the pancreas must be gentle, using sharp movements and avoiding thermal energy.
- Meticulous ligation of lymphatic channels throughout the procedure can minimize the risk of postoperative lymphocele formation. Use of ultrasound shears is not recommended since the sealing of large lymphatic channels is improbable.
- Retrograde ejaculation has been reported at a rate similar to that seen with open RPLND, using the template introduced by Donohue and colleagues. Efferent sympathetic nerve fibers, passing posteriorly to the inferior vena cava, should be identified and carefully dissected. On the left side the dissection is limited to a level 5 mm inferior to the renal vessels to spare the lumbar splanchnic nerves.

POSTOPERATIVE CARE

The nasogastric tube is removed in the operation room and the urethral catheter is removed as soon as the patient is alert and oriented. Postoperative pain can be managed with oral analgesics. Diet is restarted immediately with clear fluids and advanced as tolerated. Most patients are ready to discharge on postoperative day 2 and can resume normal activity between 10 and 20 days.

RESULTS

LRPLND was first used as a staging procedure. Some centers of excellence still perform it for this purpose with high rate of success *(9)*. Retrocaval and retroaortic dissection have allowed the true duplication of open RPLND. Consequently, LRPLND can be considered in this way as a therapeutic procedure, limiting relapses outside the template, analogous to the open counterpart.

Nevertheless, despite the wide excision of lymphatic tissue, some medical oncology departments routinely give two cycles of chemotherapy for all patients with positive nodes. This practice makes the oncological comparison between open and laparoscopic RPLND complex. However, if the LRPLND did not remove as much tissue from the retroperitoneum as the open procedure, some nodes could be missed and retroperitoneal recurrence would be expected for stage I patients. Our experience and the recent results from University of Washington *(10)*, however, have shown no recurrence. Therefore, we believe that LRPLND can replicate the advantages of open RPLND, with potential reduction in morbidity, shorter length of stay and recovery time, and avoidance of a large incision.

A review of the recent literature, despite the different surgical purposes, demonstrates high success rates. A summary of the results is presented in Table 1. Recurrences have been described outside the template. Among the patients with clinical stage I NSGCT, laparoscopic RPLND has been performed safely without open conversion in 88–100% of patients. Antegrade ejaculation has been maintained in 97–100% of patients.

LRPLND AFTER CHEMOTHERAPY

RPLND after chemotherapy has been complementary in the overall prospect of curing high-volume stage II and stage III testicular cancer. Cisplatin-based therapy provides a 60–80% complete response in patients with advanced germ cell tumor *(11)*. However, one-third of the patients will require RPLND for any residual mass. Pathologic analysis of resected specimen shows 40% of patients will have necrosis, 40% teratoma, and 20% a viable tumor. In addition, there is a risk of malignant transformation of a mature teratoma to adenocarcinoma or sarcoma.

Table 1
A review of the recent results from literature

					Recurrence (%)		*Complication rate (%)*	
Author	*No. of patients*	*Success rate (%)*	*Mean blood loss (ml) range*	*Mean hospital stay (days) range*	*Local*	*Distant*	*Minor*	*Major*
Gerber et al. *(17)*	20	90	250	3	0	10	20	0
Nelson et al. *(18)*	29	93	389	2.6	0	6.9	6.9	0
Rassweiler et al. *(19)*	34	88	–	–	0	5.9	8.8	5.9
Janetschek et al. *(1)*	125 (stage I, 76; stage II, 49)	98	–	3.3; 3.5	1.3; 0	0, 0	10	0
Permpongksol et al. *(7)*	16 (stage II, 13; stage III, 3)	87.5	903	2 (median)	0	1	25	3

Surgical excision of retroperitoneal nodes allows an accurate detection of residual tumor with complete removal of all lymphatic tissue. Nevertheless, RPLND can add considerable morbidity to those patients who already received chemotherapy. In this scenario, LRPLND is an attractive alternative to reduce morbidity associated with the procedure. However, in comparison to stage I RPLND, the postchemotherapy procedure has shown a much higher morbidity and mortality, even for open RPLND *(12)*. Fibrosis often obliterates the natural tissue planes and desmoplastic reaction can be encountered around large vessels, making the dissection difficult. The Indiana experience reported an overall complication rate of 20.7% and a mortality rate of up to 0.8% after open RPLND *(12)*.

We perform LRPLND for stage II tumors using the same technique described above for clinical stage I of NSGCT, according to the templates defined by Donahue *(5)*. Retrocaval and retroaortic tissue was not removed in our early series *(13)*. However, with the experience acquired from our previous results, these tissues were also included in the dissection in our later series *(7)*. Major complications can occur, usually involving vascular injuries. Adequate hemostasis is of crucial importance to provide a bloodless surgical field. Chylous ascites has been associated with LRPLND, possibly since the oral intake occurs much earlier, increasing the production and flow of lymph *(14)*.

Our initial experience with LRPLND in a small series of patients *(7)* has described the most common complication as vascular injury. Rassweiler et al. *(15)* have shown that LRPLND is feasible for stage I tumors, albeit they did not recommend this technique for stage IIB and IIC tumors due to their personal experience and high rate of open conversion. Janetschek et al. *(16)* performed LRPLND on 35 patients following initial chemotherapy for stage IIB (unilateral metastasis no larger than 5 mm before chemotherapy) and 14 patients with stage IIC tumors. In these cases there was not a single conversion to open surgery. Intraoperative hemorrhage occurred in nine patients but was managed lasparoscopically in all cases. Thus far, 47 patients have been followed for at least 6 months (mean follow-up 35 months) and not a single relapse has been observed. However, as laparoscopy permits only unilateral dissection, the authors have restricted the procedure for stage IIB tumors.

On the basis of our experience, we believe that LRPLND is a technically feasible procedure in the postchemotherapy setting that should be only be attempted at institutions with considerable laparoscopic expertise and that open conversion should be considered when fibrosis is encountered.

CONCLUSION

Laparoscopic RPLND currently duplicates the open technique for stage I NSGCT, with excellent results. It requires technical expertise in laparoscopic surgery. Preliminary results are very promising. Prospective randomized studies would be the ideal method to convince all of the advantages.

TAKE HOME MESSAGES

- LRPLND is a technically advanced procedure usually carried out in young men in the most productive years of their lives.
- The procedure demands considerable experience in laparoscopic dissection of the great vessels.
- Some centers of excellence perform the surgery as staging procedure.
- Technological advances in hemostasis, suturing, and instrumentation allow a full duplication of the open technique.
- LRPLND is a technically feasible procedure in the postchemotherapy setting that as with open surgery has a higher complication rate.

REFERENCES

1. Sogani, P.C., Fair, W.R.: Surveillance alone in the treatment of clinical stage I nonseminomatous germ cell tumor of the testis (NSGCT). hSemin Urol. 1988 Feb;6(1):53–56.
2. Thompson, P.I., Nixon, J., Harvey V.J.: Disease relapse in patients with stage I nonseminomatous germ cell tumor of the testis on active surveillance. J Clin Oncol;6(10):1597–1603.
3. Grossfeld, G.D., Small, E.J.: Long-term side effects of treatment for testis cancer. Urol Clin North Am. 1998 Aug; 25(3):503–515.
4. Donohue, J.P.: Retroperitoneal lymphadenectomy: the anterior approach including bilateral suprarenal-hilar dissection. Urol Clin North Am. 1977 Oct;4(3):509–521.
5. Donohue, J.P., Thornhill, J.A., Foster, R.S., Rowland, R.G., Birhle, R.: Retroperitoneal lymphadenectomy for clinical stage A testis cancer (1965 to 1989): modifications of technique and impact on ejaculation. J Urol. 1993 Feb;149(2): 237–243.
6. Rukstalis, D.B., Chodak, G.W.: Laparoscopic retroperitoneal lymph node dissection in a patient with stage 1 testicular carcinoma. J Urol. 1992 Dec;148(6):1907–1909; discussion 1909–1910.
7. Permpongkosol, S., Lima, G.C., Warlick, C.A., Allaf, M.E., Varkarakis, I.M., Bagga, H.S., et al.: Postchemotherapy laparoscopic retroperitoneal lymph node dissection: evaluation of complications. Urology. 2007 Feb;69(2):361–365.
8. Holtl, L., Peschel, R., Knapp, R., Janetaschek, G., Steiner, H., Rogatsch, H., Hittmair, A., et al.: Primary lymphatic metastatic spread in testicular cancer occurs ventral to the lumbar vessels. Urology. 2002 Jan;59(1):114–118.
9. Albgami, N., Janetschek, G.: Laparoscopic retroperitoneal lymph-node dissection in the management of clinical stage I and II testicular cancer. J Endourol. 2005 Jul-Aug;19(6):683–692; discussion 692.
10. Fong, B., Chan, D., Porter, J.: Laparoscopic retroperitoneal lymph node dissection. In: Smith's Textbook of Endourology, 2nd edition, B.C. Decker, Hamilton, ON, ANO:589–594.
11. Williams, S.D., Birch, R., Einhorn, L.H., Irwin, L., Greco, F.A., Loehrer, P.J.: Treatment of disseminated germ-cell tumors with cisplatin, bleomycin, and either vinblastine or etoposide. N Engl J Med. 1987 Jun 4;316(23):1435–1440.
12. Baniel, J., Foster, R.S., Rowland, R.G., Birhle, R., Donohue, J.P.: Complications of post-chemotherapy retroperitoneal lymph node dissection. J Urol. 1995 Mar;153(3 Pt 2):976–980.
13. Palese, M.A., Su, L.M., Kavoussi, L.R.: Laparoscopic retroperitoneal lymph node dissection after chemotherapy. Urology. 2002 Jul;60(1):130–134.
14. Janetschek, G., Hobisch, A., Hittmair, A., Holtl, L., Peschel, R., Bartsch, G.: Laparoscopic retroperitoneal lymphadenectomy after chemotherapy for stage IIB nonseminomatous testicular carcinoma. J Urol. 1999 Feb;161(2):477–481.
15. Rassweiler, J.J., Seeman, O., Henkel, T.O., Stock, C., Frede, T., Alken, P.: Laparoscopic retroperitoneal lymph node dissection for nonseminomatous germ cell tumors: indications and limitations. J Urol 1996 Sep;156(3):1108–1113.
16. Janetschek, G., Peschel, R., Hobisch, A., Bartch, G.: Laparoscopic retroperitoneal lymph node dissection. J Endourol. 2001 May;15(4):449–453; discussion 453–455.
17. Gerber, G.S., Bissada, N.K., Hulbert, J.C., Kavoussi, L.R., Moore, R.G., Kantoff, P.W., Rukstalis, D.B.: Laparoscopic retroperitoneal lymphadenectomy: multi-institutional analysis. J Urol. 1994 Oct;152(4):1188–1191; discussion 1191–1192.
18. Nelson, J.B., Chen, R.N., Bishoff, J.T., Oh, W.K., Kantoff, P.W., Donehower, R.C., Kavoussi, L.R.: Laparoscopic retroperitoneal lymph node dissection for clinical stage I nonseminomatous germ cell testicular tumors. Urol. 1999 Dec;54(6):1064–1067.
19. Rassweiler, J.J., Frede, T., Lenz, E., Seemann, O., Alken, P.: Long-term experience with laparoscopic retroperitoneal lymph node dissection in the management of low-stage testis cancer. Eur Urol. 2000 Mar;37(3):251–260.

Laparoscopic Cystectomy and Urinary Diversion

David Canes and Ingolf A. Tuerk

INTRODUCTION

Over the past 15 years, initial skepticism for laparoscopic radical cystectomy (LRC) has given way to enthusiasm. At specialized centers LRC is already offered as a feasible alternative *(1)* to open cystectomy, the reference standard *(2)*. Progress in the field of LRC has been measured, slowly and deliberately. Among genitourinary cancers, transitional cell carcinoma is unforgiving of surgical missteps. Positive margins and urine spillage for organ-confined disease are unacceptable – negatively impacting disease-specific survival *(3)*. Slow progress is therefore appropriate, indicating that irrational exuberance for technological advances have been tempered by dedicated pioneers who are intent on duplicating open oncological principles in this arena.

The goals of this chapter are threefold: (1) to place the surgical technique within its historical context; (2) to provide practical technical descriptions of LRC and urinary diversion; and (3) to stress oncological principles over global technique. We emphasize throughout the text that patients should receive the most appropriate procedure for their pathology, whether open, laparoscopic, or robotic. A particular surgeon's familiarity with a given technique must not influence surgical decision making. LRC with urinary diversion is technically challenging, requires advanced laparoscopic training, and should only be undertaken by those with appropriate experience. While urinary diversion for benign disease will be mentioned, the focus of this chapter is LRC and urinary diversion for cancer.

HISTORICAL BACKGROUND: CYSTECTOMY AND URINARY DIVERSION

We have witnessed profound strides in laparoscopic reconstructive urology since 1992 when Parra et al. performed the first laparoscopic cystectomy for recurrent pyocystis in a 27-year-old paraplegic woman who already had an ileocolonic reservoir with a continent stoma created 5 months earlier *(4)*. That same year the first laparoscopic ileal conduit was reported by Kozminski and Partamian, where a cystectomy was not performed *(5)*. Sanchez de Badajoz et al. reported the first laparoscopic radical cystectomy (LRC) for bladder carcinoma in a 64-year-old woman in 1995 *(6)*. Since then, substantial evolution of both extirpative and reconstructive laparoscopy has occurred. Increasing familiarity with laparoscopic radical prostatectomy, combined with the incorporation of laparoscopic staplers for vascular pedicle control, brought cystectomy within reach.

The period between 2000 and 2004 was marked by pioneering efforts to perform completely intracorporeal extirpative cystectomy including reconstructive urinary diversion *(7–10)*. Enthusiasm has waned for complete intracorporeal techniques, owing to complications related to laparoscopic bowel

From: *Current Clinical Urology: Essential Urologic Laparoscopy*
Edited by: S. Y. Nakada and S. P. Hedican, DOI 10.1007/978-1-60327-820-1_16

work *(11)*, as well as prolonged operative times. Most contemporary surgeons perform LRC intracorporeally, with urinary diversion through a mini-laparotomy incision *(12)*.

Virtually all forms of urinary diversion have now been completed laparoscopically, including ileal conduit *(5,8,10,13)*, rectosigmoid pouch *(7)*, orthotopic neobladder *(9,14–16)*, ileovesicostomy *(17,18)*, appendicovesicostomy *(19,20)*, Miami pouch *(21)*, and cutaneous ureterostomy *(22,23)*.

INDICATIONS: RADICAL CYSTECTOMY

The indications for laparoscopic cystectomy are the same as open cystectomy, including tumors with invasion of the muscularis propria, carcinoma in situ refractory to intravesical therapy, and recurrent, multifocal, or high grade superficial disease refractory to intravesical therapy. Contraindications are more relevant for the laparoscopic approach. Multiple prior abdominal surgeries portend extensive adhesions and may complicate laparoscopic access. On an individual basis, however, prior surgery is only a relative contraindication. One is often surprised by lack of correlation between the degree of intraperitoneal adhesions and the extent of prior abdominal surgery. Obesity must also be evaluated in each individual case. For instance, the exact distribution of subcutaneous abdominal fat differs amongst individuals. In cases where the fat is heavily distributed in the lower abdominal and suprapubic regions, excessive traction on trocars to obtain optimal instrument angles may be a limiting factor.

INDICATIONS: URINARY DIVERSION

Following radical cystectomy, and in certain cases for benign conditions, the flow of urine is directed either through a conduit, the so-called noncontinent diversion, or a continent reservoir. The latter includes continent reservoirs with catheterizable stomas in which a low-pressure reservoir is fashioned from a detubularized bowel segment. When the urethra is not involved with cancer, appropriate patients may have an orthotopic neobladder, where a reservoir is attached to the native urethra. The latter is the gold standard urinary diversion for patients undergoing radical cystectomy for muscle invasive bladder cancer.

General guidelines for choosing the type of laparoscopic urinary diversion, best suited to each patient, do not differ from their open surgical indications. There are technical advantages specific to certain laparoscopic procedures, however, particularly in regards to bowel fixation and ease of suturing. The choice of bowel segment is made with careful consideration of expected metabolic disturbances as they interact with existing medical conditions, as with open surgery. In all cases, a particular surgeon's comfort level with the laparoscopic versus open approach to a given urinary diversion should not guide the decision process. Sound oncologic principles and the creation of an appropriate urinary diversion suited to the individual patient take precedence.

The most common indication for any form of urinary diversion is following radical cystectomy for bladder cancer. In cases of locally advanced pelvic malignancy, urinary diversion may be indicated without cystectomy. The remainder of patients includes those with neurogenic bladder with chronic catheterization, refractory hemorrhagic cystitis, or other conditions in which the bladder may be left in situ while urinary flow is diverted.

Complex reconstructive laparoscopic surgery begins with careful patient selection. In cases where urinary diversion is required following radical cystectomy, exclusion criteria for the cystectomy portion of the procedure will generally dominate the decision process. However, common exclusion criteria for laparoscopic surgery in general will apply. As in open surgery, significant obesity may prevent adequate creation of an everted stoma without excessive mesenteric tension. Prior abdominal or pelvic radiation therapy is also a relative contraindication to laparoscopic urinary diversion, but may influence the choice of bowel segment.

TECHNIQUE: LAPAROSCOPIC RADICAL CYSTECTOMY

Table 1 lists relevant instrumentation and equipment.

Table 1
Equipment for laparoscopic radical cystectomy and urinary diversion

Instruments
Veress needle
Trocars, 5 and 12 mm
Laparoscopic 10 mm lenses, 0 and 30°
Tissue graspers
Scissors, with monopolar electrocautery attachment
Bipolar forceps
Harmonic scalpel
Needle holders
Fan retractor
Vascular Endo-GIA stapler with reloads
Clip appliers
Impermeable specimen retrieval bags (15 and 10 mm)
Carter–Thomason needle
Open surgical tray on standby
Hardware
High-flow carbon dioxide insufflator
Bipolar and monopolar electrocautery unit
Camera
Light source
Video recorder
Suction/irrigator device
Harmonic scalpel generator

Access, Port Placement

With the patient in the supine Trendelenberg position, pneumoperitoneum is obtained through as standard Veress needle technique. A five-port fan-shaped transperitoneal approach is employed (Fig. 1). A central 12 mm trocar accommodates a zero degree 10 mm optical lens. On the left (primary surgeon side), a medial 12 mm for most right-handed applications, and lateral 5 mm are placed. On the right (assistant side), two 5 mm trocars suffice. A previously marked stoma site away from the desired trocar sites should not compromise optimal port placement. If a stoma site coincides with a useful trocar location, it should of course be used.

Posterior Dissection

We prefer to leave the bladder in its native position as long as possible. The peritoneum is incised at the rectovesical cul-de-sac. Vasa and seminal vesicles are left en bloc with the specimen, but their limited dissection aids in isolating the pedicles. Denonvillier's fascia is incised and the rectum is mobilized to the apex of prostate.

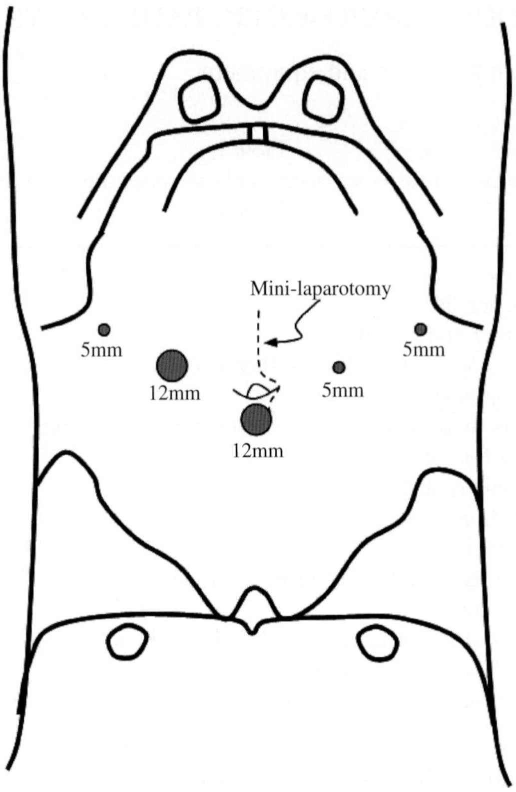

Fig. 1. Port placement, and location of mini-laparotomy incision.

Ureteral Dissection

Ureters are identified as they cross-over the iliac bifurcation. They are dissected with care to preserve periureteral soft tissue. Ureters are clipped at the detrusor hiatus, transected, and marked with colored 4-0 vicryl holding sutures for easy identification and manipulation during diversion. A distal ureteral frozen section is sent at the surgeon's discretion. Some advise clipping the proximal cut end of ureter to allow for hydrodistension prior to urinary diversion. We have not found this to be necessary.

Vascular Pedicles, Anterior Dissection

The vascular pedicles to the prostate and bladder are taken with successive firings of an Endo-GIA laparoscopic vascular stapler (usually five or six) (Fig. 2). The bladder is then dissected free from the anterior abdominal wall, endopelvic fascia is incised, and the dorsal vein complex is suture ligated. The apical dissection proceeds much like laparoscopic prostatectomy. The urethra is transected and the apex of the prostate is closed with a figure-of-eight suture to avoid urine spillage. The specimen is immediately placed in an endocatch bag to avoid spillage, and put aside for later retrieval through an abdominal incision through which the urinary diversion is created.

Female Cystectomy

The patient is positioned in lithotomy. Preoperatively, the vagina is tightly packed with betadine-soaked sponges for two reasons: (1) aids in identification of landmarks intraoperatively and

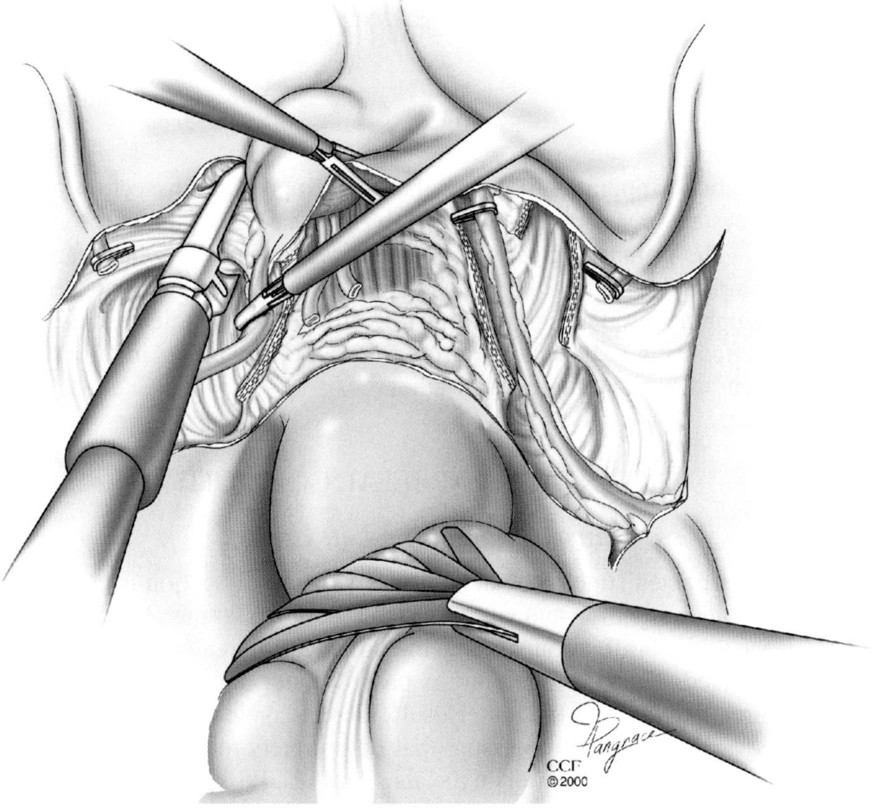

Fig. 2. Endovascular GIA stapler securing the left vascular pedicle.

(2) pneumoperitoneum is not lost following incision of the vaginal wall. Having a colleague dissecting the urethra circumferentially from a simultaneous vaginal approach is helpful.

The uterus is retracted anteriorly, and the sigmoid retracted out of the pelvis to expose the retrovesical cul-de-sac. The gonadal vessels are transected with vascular staplers. If the vagina is to be spared, a retrovesical peritoneotomy is made and the anterior vaginal wall released from the bladder. For standard anterior exenteration, the anterior vaginal wall is taken with the specimen. The vesical pedicles are taken with vascular staples, as in the male. The remainder of the procedure proceeds as described above, with appropriate minor modifications. Technical details of uterus, fallopian tube, and ovary-sparing cystectomy have also been described in the literature *(24)*.

TECHNIQUE: LAP EXTENDED LYMPH NODE DISSECTION

Increasing evidence exists for the diagnostic and therapeutic benefits of extended lymphadenectomy *(25–27)*. Extended lymphadenectomy is performed after the cystectomy because of improved working space and ureteral mobilization, which facilitates expeditious dissection along the common iliac arteries. Dissection includes bilateral external iliac, hypogastric, and obturator lymph nodes, as well as pre-sacral and common iliac nodes. Proximally the dissection extends onto the aortic bifurcation, and can feasibly reach the inferior mesenteric artery, just as in open surgery. Small lymphatics are sealed with bipolar electrocautery, and larger channels with Hem-o-Lock clips. The boundaries are as follows:

- Lateral: genitofemoral nerve
- Medial: bladder itself (i.e., includes perivesical nodes)
- Posterior: obturator nerve
- Distal: Cloquet's node
- Proximal: aortic bifurcation

Reasonable expectations for operative time are that the lymph node dissection often takes just as long as the extirpative cystectomy itself (approximately 1.5 h). We recommend sending each packet to pathology separately. The primary surgeon may find dissection easier when standing on the contralateral side of the lymph node dissection, which means switching to the opposite side of the table to remove left-sided lymph nodes. The surgeon must be prepared to handle vascular bleeding. While bipolar electrocautery effectively seals small arteriotomies and venotomies in the great vessels, a 3-0 vicryl stitch should be cut to size and ready at all times.

TECHNIQUE: LAP ILEAL CONDUIT

Transposition of the Left Ureter

The sigmoid colon is retracted superiorly and anteriorly. Blunt dissection is used to develop a tunnel posterior to the sigmoid mesocolon and anterior to the sacrum. Having already performed a lymph node dissection over the aortic bifurcation, and having already placed a holding suture, ureteral transposition is greatly facilitated. The holding suture is passed under the sigmoid mesocolon anterior to the sacrum, limiting direct handling of the ureter itself, thereby avoiding unnecessary vascular injury. Ureteral length is once again confirmed to assure that both ureters reach the proximal portion of the ileal segment in order to avoid undue tension on the anastomoses. Proximal dissection of the left ureter will provide the further length needed to reach the urinary diversion.

Harvesting Small Bowel

When a right-sided trocar site coincides with the desired stoma site, the trocar site is extended to 4.5 cm. When the stoma site is separate from all trocars, a 4.5 cm infraumbilical incision is made. The specimen is retrieved. The color-coded ureteral holding sutures are exteriorized. A 15 cm segment of ileum is selected with care to spare 15–20 cm proximal to the ileocecal junction. The efferent limb should reach the previously marked stoma site without undue tension or mesenteric kinking. The segment of bowel is delivered through the incision and isolated with a GIA stapler by transecting proximally and distally. The mesentery is divided below with care to preserve the major mesenteric vasculature. The isolated segment is dropped posteriorly.

Restoring Bowel Continuity

The stapled edges of the distal and proximal ileum are removed sharply. Applications of a GIA 55-mm stapler are used to create a side-to-side, functional end-to-end anastomosis along the antimesenteric border of the small bowel. The open end of the anastomosis is then closed using a TA 55-mm stapler. The end staple line is imbricated with interrupted, absorbable suture. The window through the mesentery is then closed with interrupted absorbable suture to prevent internal herniation.

Ureteroileal Anastomoses

Gentle traction on the ureteral holding sutures pulls the distal ureters into the operative field. The ureters are gently spatulated for approximately 1 cm. Bilateral ureteral 6 Fr. single "J" stents are passed into the renal pelvis. The ureters are sequentially implanted into the proximal end of the ileal segment in a standard Bricker fashion. The apices are fixed to the bowel using three interrupted 4-0 poliglecaprone sutures. The remainder of the ureteral implantation is performed using a running 4-0 poliglecaprone suture. The proximal end of the ileal conduit is replaced into the abdominal cavity. The ureteral stents are exteriorized through the ileal segment.

Creation of Ileal Stoma

The rectus fascia is partially closed, leaving space through which the conduit passes. The ileal segment is secured to the fascia using interrupted 2-0 polyglactin sutures. The stoma is matured in the standard open fashion. In the obese patient, ureteroileal anastomoses performed through an incision may require excessive proximal ureteral mobilization. In these cases, the stoma is matured first, and the ureteroileal anastomoses are performed completely intracorporeally.

Closure and Drains

The ureters and ileal diversion are inspected for any undue tension. Once meticulous hemostasis is assured, a flat Jackson–Pratt drain is placed through a lateral 5-mm trocar site into the small pelvis. The port sites are closed in the usual fashion with fascial closure for all sites 10 mm and greater under direct vision with 0-polyglactin.

Post-operative Period

Postoperatively, patients receive mechanical and chemo-prophylaxis for deep venous thrombosis, and they ambulate on the first postoperative day. The nasogastric tube is removed upon awakening from anesthesia, and the diet advanced on the first or second postoperative day accordingly. The drain is removed with diminished output (usually day 3 or 4). The patient is discharged between day 5 and 7. Stents are removed on day 10–12, with the urethral foley catheter removed the following day.

TECHNIQUE: LAP ORTHOTOPIC NEOBLADDER

We prefer the Studer ileal neobladder. Intuitively, the particular choice of neobladder assumes less importance for an open-assistance technique that relies less on intracorporeal suturing. A 65 cm segment of ileum is chosen and marked intracorporeally, sparing the terminal ileum, being sure to verify that the midportion easily reaches the urethral stump. This is delivered through a 5–7 cm lower midline incision and isolated with a GIA stapler. Bowel continuity is restored with a stapled side-to-side anastomosis. The proximal 10 cm are preserved as a Studer limb, and the remainder is incised along its anti-mesenteric border. The posterior plate is fashioned with running absorbable suture, followed by the anterior plate. The anterior enterotomy is left open for 3 cm at its inferior portion for the urethral anastomosis. The neobladder is reintroduced into the abdominal cavity and anterior rectus fascia at the midline incision is closed to reestablish pneumoperitoneum. The urethral anastomosis is performed intracorporeally in a running fashion (Fig. 3).

For the ureteroneovesical anastomosis, the following two options are available: (1) reopen the infraumbilical incision, deliver the Studer limb extracorporeally, and perform the anastomosis in an open fashion or (2) particularly in obese patients, bilateral anastomoses are performed completely intracorporeally. Bilateral 6F single "J" stents are passed into the renal pelvis and exteriorized through the neobladder and out on of the lateral 5-mm port sites. A flat Jackson–Pratt drain is placed through the contralateral 5-mm port.

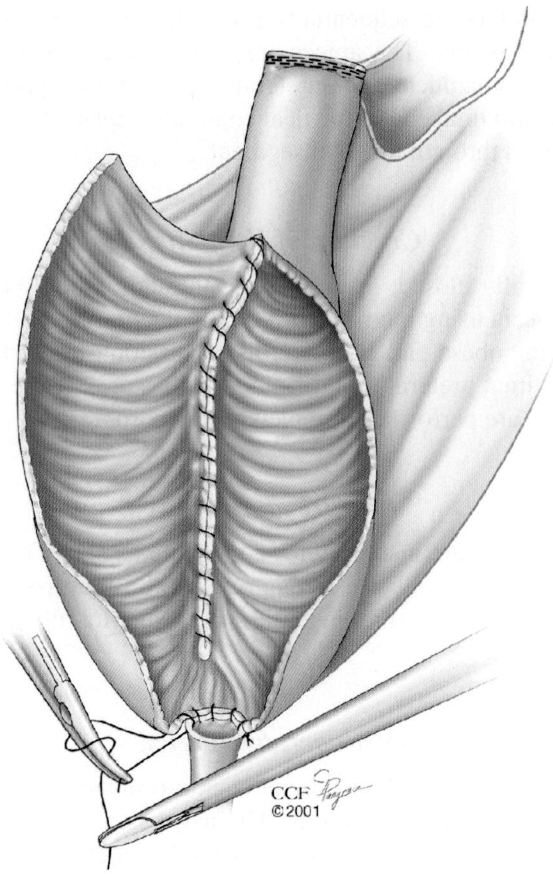

Fig. 3. The urethero-ileal anastomosis is being completed with a running suture.

OUTCOMES

The potential to decrease perioperative morbidity is the impetus for pursuing a minimally invasive approach. Such an approach may be offered if the following is true: (1) the procedure is technically feasible; (2) morbidity is comparable or improved compared to the open approach; (3) oncologic principles are respected; and (4) the procedure is not cost prohibitive. To date, over 800 LRC have been performed worldwide (Haber and Gill, personal communication). Early experience suggests that LRC satisfies these criteria.

MORBIDITY: PERIOPERATIVE OUTCOMES

Aggregate mean EBL from available minimally invasive cystectomy series is 350 mL (range <150–1,000) *(28)*. Experienced laparoscopic surgeons corroborate their impression that pneumoperitoneum results in decreased blood loss. When subject to rigorous prospective analysis in one study, perhaps plagued by small sample sizes that included the learning curve, these differences failed to reach significance. Basilotte compared 13 laparoscopic-assisted cystectomies with 11 open cases and blood loss was not statistically different *(29)*. Of note, mean blood loss in the laparoscopic group was 1,000 mL, the highest of published series. In this same comparison, the laparoscopic-assisted group had significantly lower postoperative analgesic requirements, faster resumption of oral intake

(2.8 versus 5 days), shorter hospital stay (5.1 days), and no difference in complication rates. Another recent prospective nonrandomized study *(30)* similarly found that the laparoscopic group had reduced analgesic consumption and earlier return of bowel function. Castillo and colleagues reported a multi-institutional retrospective study of 59 patients undergoing LRC, in which mean EBL was 488 mL, operative time was 337 min *(31)*. Postoperative major and minor complications occurred in 30% of patients, with 3.3% mortality. Worldwide data are summarized in Table 2.

ONCOLOGICAL OUTCOMES

Oncologic follow-up data for LRC are immature. Early results suggest that it provides comparable oncologic control. Haber et al. reported actuarial 5-year cancer-specific survival rate of 92% in a series of 37 patients with mean follow-up of 31 months *(11,32)*. If patients lost to follow-up were assumed to have passed from metastatic disease, re-calculated 5-year cancer-specific survival was 68%, which still compares favorably with open historical controls *(2)*.

In the author's review of worldwide cystectomy series through 2005, only one positive margin was reported out of 105 pooled patients *(33)*. Since that time, minimally invasive techniques have been applied to all patients previously considered candidates only for open cystectomy, and positive margin rates are comparable. A recent report by Wang et al. included a prospective comparison of robotic to open cystectomy *(34)*. Positive margins in each group occurred at statistically equivalent frequency ($p = 0.2$), and in patients with locally advanced, lymph node positive disease. Three patients undergoing open cystectomy (pT2N2), and two in the robotic group (pT3N1) had positive margins.

A unique theoretical risk of LRC is port site metastasis. Only one case report exists of port site seeding after RARC in a patient with high-grade disease *(35)*. Certain technical maneuvers are essential in this regard: (1) sutured closure of the urethra on the specimen immediately following transection and (2) immediate specimen entrapment in an impermeable bag for extraction. Local recurrence has been reported in one study following LRC, in which two pelvic recurrences were reported *(1)*.

Lymph node yields commensurate with open surgery can be achieved with a laparoscopic approach. The Bladder Cancer Collaborative Group has suggested that a minimum of 10–14 lymph nodes should be examined following radical cystectomy by any approach *(36)*. Finelli et al. demonstrated that this was indeed possible laparoscopically, reporting a median of 21 lymph nodes sampled during laparoscopic-extended lymphadenectomy *(37)*. No such data are yet available for the robotic approach.

It is clear that follow-up longer than 5 years is necessary to finally determine if oncological outcomes are equivalent between LRC and ORC. Instead, surrogate and intermediate endpoints (margin status, local recurrence, lymph node clearance), must be used instead. Large series with longer follow-up are required to confirm equivalence with open surgery, but these early surrogate measures are reassuring.

COST

No direct cost comparison has been made between open, laparoscopic, and robotic cystectomy. One would reasonably expect cost comparisons for prostatectomy to provide insight into cost differences that are likely to apply for cystectomy. In a 2004 analysis, open prostatectomy was the most cost effective, followed closely by laparoscopic (additional $487), taking into account length of stay. The robotic approach was the least cost effective, by margins of $1,155 and $1,726 over the laparoscopic and open approaches, respectively *(38)*. Maintenance fees and equipment costs account for some of this differential, and apply similarly in the case of robotic cystectomy.

Table 2
Selected series of minimally invasive radical cystectomy

Lead author	*Year*	*N*	*Male/female*	*Extracorporeal Assistance*	*OR time (h)*	*No. of ports*	*EBL*	*Pos margins*	*Urinary diversion*	*Firsts*
Kozminski *(5)*	1992	1	–	No	6.3	5	–	N/A	Ileal conduit	First lap ileal conduit
Puppo *(39)*	1995	5	F	Yes	6–9	5	–	NR	Cutaneous ureterostomy (1) ileal conduit (4)	
Bajadoz *(6)*	1995	1	F	Yes	8	5	–	NR	Ileal conduit	First LRC and diversion
Denewer *(40)*	1999	10	M (9)/F (1)	Yes	3.6	4	NR	NR	Sigmoid Pouch	
Gill *(8)*	2000	2	M	No	10–11.5	6	1–1.2L	None	Ileal Conduit	First LRC, ileal conduit, complete intracorporeal
Tuerk *(7)*	2001	5	M (3)/F (2)	No	7.4	6	245	None	Mainz II	First LRC, intracorporeal continent urinary diversion
Peterson *(41)*	2002	1	M	Yes	7.0	5	750	None	Ileal conduit	Only report of hand-assisted LRC

Gill *(9)*	2002	3	M (2)/F(1)	No	7–10.5	6–7	200–400	None	Studer orthotopic neobladder	First LRC, neobladder, complete intracorporeal
Abdel-Hakim *(14)*	2002	9	M (8)/F(1)	Yes	8.3	5–6	150–500	None	Ileal orthotopic neobladder (modified Camey II)	
Hemal *(42)*	2003	10	M (9)/F (1)	Yes	6.5	5–6	300–900	1	Ileal conduit	
Menon *(28)*	2003	17	M (14)/F (3)	Yes	4.3–5.1	6	<150	None	Ileal conduit (3), W pouch (10), Double chimney (2), T pouch (2)	
Deger *(43)*	2004	20	M (14)/F (6)	No	8.1	5–6	200	None	Rectosigmoid pouch (12), Neobladder (5), Ileal conduit (3)	
Cathelineau *(1)*	2005	84	M (71)/F (13)	Yes	4.3	6	550	NR	Neobladder (51), Ileal conduit (33)	
Castillo *(31)*	2006	59	M (46)/F (13)	No	5.6	5	488	NR	Neobladder (25), Indiana Pouch (4)	

While primary considerations should and will continue to be based on oncological efficacy, safety, and quality, the fact remains that in 2007, the robotic approach is accompanied by the largest short-term economic burden. This issue remains unresolved.

SUMMARY, FUTURE DIRECTIONS

LRC, with its robotic counterpart, is being performed at specialized centers around the world. Technical feasibility is well established, and perioperative variables of morbidity appear favorable. Five-year oncologic data support the conclusion that oncologic outcomes at this benchmark are similar to historical open controls. As a community, we still require well designed prospective trials are needed in this arena to rigorously define the role of LRC going forward. If we define clear standards up front, rather than being seduced by new technology, our patients will benefit.

REFERENCES

1. Cathelineau X, Arroyo C, Rozet F, Barret E, Vallancien G. Laparoscopic assisted radical cystectomy: the Montsouris experience after 84 cases. Eur Urol 47:780–784, 2005.
2. Stein JP, Lieskovsky G, Cote R, et al. Radical cystectomy in the treatment of invasive bladder cancer: long-term results in 1,054 patients. J Clin Oncol 2001, 19:666–675.
3. Dotan Z, Kavanagh K, Yossepowitch O, et al. Positive surgical margins in soft tissue following radical cystectomy for bladder cancer and cancer specific survival. J Urol. 2007 Dec;178(6):2308–2313.
4. Parra RO, Andrus CH, Jones JP, Boullier JA. Laparoscopic cystectomy: initial report on a new treatment for the retained bladder. J Urol. 1992 Oct;148(4):1140–1144.
5. Kozminski M, Partamian KO. Case report of laparoscopic ileal loop conduit. J Endourol 1992; 6: 147–150.
6. Sanchez de Badajoz E, Gallego Perales JL, Reche Rosado A, Gutierrez de la Cruz JM, Jimenez Garrido A. Laparoscopic cystectomy and ileal conduit: case report. J Endourol. 1995 Feb;9(1):59–62.
7. Tuerk I, Deger S, Winkelmann B, et al. Laparoscopic radical cystectomy with continent urinary diversion (rectal sigmoid pouch) performed completely intracorporeally: the initial 5 cases. J Urol. 2001; 165: 1863–1866.
8. Gill IS, Fergany A, Klein EA, et al. Laparoscopic radical cystoprostatectomy with ileal conduit performed completely intracorporeally: the initial 2 cases. Urology 2000; 56: 26–29.
9. Gill IS, Kaouk JH, Meraney AM, et al. Laparoscopic radical cystectomy and continent orthotopic ileal neobladder performed completely intracorporeally: the initial experience. J Urol. 2002; 168: 13–18.
10. Balaji KC, Yohannes P, McBride CL, Oleynikov D, Hemstreet GP 3rd. Feasibility of robot-assisted totally intracorporeal laparoscopic ileal conduit urinary diversion: initial results of a single institutional pilot study. Urology. 2004 Jan;63(1):51–55.
11. Haber GP, Gill IS. Laparoscopic radical cystectomy for cancer: oncological outcomes at up to 5 years. BJU Int. 2007 Jul;100(1):137–142.
12. Cathelineau X, Jaffe J. Laparoscopic radical cystectomy with urinary diversion: what is the optimal technique? Curr Opin Urol. 2007 Mar;17(2):93–97.
13. Potter SR, Charambura TC, Adams JB 2nd, Kavoussi LR. Laparoscopic ileal conduit: five-year follow-up. Urology. 2000 Jul;56(1):22–25.
14. Abdel-Hakim AM, Bassiouny F, Abdel Azim MS, Rady I, Mohey T, Habib I, Fathi H. Laparoscopic radical cystectomy with orthotopic neobladder. J Endourol. 2002 Aug;16(6):377–381.
15. Beecken WD, Wolfram M, Engl T, Bentas W, Probst M, Blaheta R, Oertl A, Jonas D, Binder J. Robotic-assisted laparoscopic radical cystectomy and intra-abdominal formation of an orthotopic ileal neobladder. Eur Urol. 2003; 44:337–339.
16. Gaboardi F, Simonato A, Galli S, Lissiani A, Gregori A, Bozzola A. Minimally invasive laparoscopic neobladder. J Urol. 2002 Sep;168(3):1080–1083.
17. Hsu TH, Rackley RR, Abdelmalak JB, Tchetgen MB, Madjar S, Vasavada SP. Laparoscopic ileovesicostomy. J Urol. 2002 Jul;168(1):180–181.
18. Abrahams HM, Rahman NU, Meng MV, Stoller ML. Pure laparoscopic ileovesicostomy. J Urol. 2003 Aug;170 (2 Pt 1):517–518.
19. Casale P, Feng WC, Grady RW, Joyner BD, Lee RS, Mitchell ME. Intracorporeal laparoscopic appendicovesicostomy: a case report of a novel approach. J Urol. 2004 May;171(5):1899.
20. Jordan GH, Winslow BH. Laparoscopically assisted continent catheterizable cutaneous appendicovesicostomy. J Endourol. 1993 Dec;7(6):517–520.

21. Pomel C, Castaigne D. Laparoscopic hand-assisted Miami Pouch following laparoscopic anterior pelvic exenteration. Gynecol Oncol. 2004 May;93(2):543–545.
22. Loisides P, Grasso M, Lui P. Laparoscopic cutaneous ureterostomy: technique for palliative upper urinary tract drainage. J Endourol. 1995 Aug;9(4):315–317.
23. Puppo P, Ricciotti G, Bozzo W, Pezzica C, Geddo D, Perachino M. Videoendoscopic cutaneous ureterostomy for palliative urinary diversion in advanced pelvic cancer. Eur Urol. 1995;28(4):328–333.
24. Moinzadeh A, Gill IS, Desai M, et al; Laparoscopic radical cystectomy in the female. J Urol. 2005. 173:1912–1917.
25. Herr HW, Bochner BH, Dalbagni G, et al; Impact of the number of lymph nodes retrieved on outcome in patients with muscle invasive bladder cancer. J Urol. 2002 Mar;167(3):1295–1298.
26. Konety BR, Joslyn SA, O′Donnell MA. Extent of pelvic lymphadenectomy and its impact on outcome in patients diagnosed with bladder cancer: analysis of data from the Surveillance, Epidemiology and End Results Program data base. J Urol. 2003 Mar;169(3):946–950.
27. Stein JP, Cai J, Groshen S, Skinner DG. Risk factors for patients with pelvic lymph node metastases following radical cystectomy with en bloc pelvic lymphadenectomy: concept of lymph node density. J Urol. 2003 Jul;170(1):35–41.
28. Menon M, Hemal AK, Tewari A, Shrivastava A, Shoma AM, El-Tabey NA, Shaaban A, Abol-Enein H, Ghoneim MA. Nerve-sparing robot-assisted radical cystoprostatectomy and urinary diversion. BJU Int. 2003 Aug;92(3):232–236.
29. Basillote JB, Abdelshehid C, Ahlering TE, Shanberg AM. Laparoscopic assisted radical cystectomy with ileal neobladder: a comparison with the open approach. J Urol. 2004 Aug;172(2):489–493.
30. Porpiglia F, Renard J, Billia M, Scoffone C, Cracco C, Terrone C, Scarpa RM. Open versus Laparoscopy-Assisted Radical Cystectomy: Results of a Prospective Study. J Endourol. 2007 Mar;21(3):325–329.
31. Castillo OA, Abreu SC, Mariano MB, et al. Complications in laparoscopic radical cystectomy. The South American experience with 59 cases. Int Braz J Urol. 2006 May-Jun;32(3):300–305.
32. Haber GP, Colombo JR, Aron M, Ukimura O, Gill IS. Laparoscopic radical cystectomy and urinary diversion: status in 2006. Eur Urol. 2006 Jul; S5: 950–955.
33. Canes D, Triaca V, Tuerk I. Laparoscopic radical cystectomy with continent urinary diversion. Curr Urol Rep. 2005 Mar;6(2):109–117.
34. Wang GJ, Barocas DA, Raman, JD, Scherr, DS. Robotic vs. open radical cystectomy: prospective comparison of perioperative outcomes and pathological measures of early oncological efficacy. BJU Int. 2007 Sep 20 [Epub ahead of print].
35. El-Tabey NA, Shoma AM. Port site metastases after robot-assisted laparoscopic radical cystectomy. Urology. 2005 Nov;66(5):1110.
36. Herr H, Lee C, Chang S, Lerner S; Bladder Cancer Collaborative Group. Standardization of radical cystectomy and pelvic lymph node dissection for bladder cancer: a collaborative group report. J Urol. 2004 May;171(5):1823–1828.
37. Finelli A, Gill IS, Desai MM, Moinzadeh A, Magi-Galluzzi C, Kaouk JH. Laparoscopic extended pelvic lymphadenectomy for bladder cancer: technique and initial outcomes. J Urol. 2004 Nov;172(5 Pt 1):1809–1812.
38. Lotan Y, Cadeddu JA, Gettman MT. The new economics of radical prostatectomy: cost comparison of open, laparoscopic and robot assisted techniques. J Urol. 2004 Oct;172(4 Pt 1):1431–1435.
39. Puppo P, Perachino M, Ricciotti G, Bozzo W, Gallucci M, Carmignani G. Laparoscopically assisted transvaginal radical cystectomy. Eur Urol. 1995;27(1):80–84.
40. Denewer A, Kotb S, Hussein O, El-Maadawy M. Laparoscopic assisted cystectomy and lymphadenectomy for bladder cancer: initial experience. World J Surg. 1999 Jun;23(6):608–611.
41. Peterson AC, Lance RS, Ahuja S. Laparoscopic hand assisted radical cystectomy with ileal conduit urinary diversion. J Urol. 2002 Nov;168(5):2103–2105.
42. Hemal AK, Singh I, Kumar R. Laparoscopic radical cystectomy and ileal conduit reconstruction: preliminary experience. J Endourol. 2003 Dec;17(10):911–916.
43. Deger S, Peters R, Roigas J, et al; Laparoscopic radical cystectomy with continent urinary diversion (rectosigmoid pouch) performed completely intracorporeally: an intermediate functional and oncologic analysis. Urology. 2004 Nov;64(5):935–939.

Laparoscopic Radical Cystectomy and Urinary Diversion with Handport Assistance

Marklyn J. Jones, J. Kyle Anderson, and Kenneth S. Koeneman

INTRODUCTION

Radical cystectomy is the standard of care for muscle invasive bladder cancer in the United States. Since the first reported simple laparoscopic cystectomy in 1992, multiple authors have reported on the use of laparoscopy for radical cystectomy *(1)*. Gill et al. reported the first two cases of laparoscopic radical cystoprostatectomy with ileal conduit done completely intracorporeally in 2000 *(2)*. A case report documented the use of the hand-assisted laparoscopic (HAL) technique for radical cystectomy with ileal conduit construction extracorpeally through the hand port for the first time *(3)*. Since the first reported HAL cystectomy, two series reports for HAL cystectomy included seven and eight patients *(4,5)*. Taylor et al. demonstrated in a prospective, non-randomized comparison that HAL cystectomy resulted in less blood loss (637 vs. 957 cc, $p=0.23$), decreased postoperative pain (31 vs. 149 mg morphine, $p=0.01$), shorter hospital stays (6.4 vs. 9.8 days, $p=0.06$) and decreased time to resumption of a regular diet (4.5 vs. 7.9 days, $p=0.05$) compared to open cystectomy. The immediate oncologic outcomes appear comparable in most laparoscopic cystectomy series, but long-term results are not available.

HAL cystectomy may have distinct advantages over standard laparoscopic cystectomy. Because of the need for intact specimen removal with urothelial cancer of the bladder, the hand port provides an ideal location for specimen removal, and may aid in less tumor spillage. In addition, the hand port allows tactile feedback during resection, fast and reliable retraction, an ideal instrument for blunt dissection, as well as an incision for creation of an ileal conduit urinary diversion. HAL cystectomy compared to laparoscopic cystectomy may also provide an easier transition for surgeons early in their laparoscopic experience. Current case reports and series are small, and larger prospective surgical series will be needed to confirm the oncologic effectiveness of HAL cystectomy, this relatively new surgical technique is a viable alternative for patients with invasive bladder cancer.

PATIENT SELECTION

The indications for radical cystectomy are well known and will therefore not be reviewed in this chapter. In general, patients who are considered medically fit for open radical cystectomy, can also be considered candidates for HAL cystectomy. Absolute contraindications for laparoscopic surgery include uncorrectable coagulopathy, intestinal obstruction, abdominal wall infection, hemoperitoneum, and peritonitis *(6)*. Relative contraindications include extensive prior abdominal or

From: *Current Clinical Urology: Essential Urologic Laparoscopy*
Edited by: S. Y. Nakada and S. P. Hedican, DOI 10.1007/978-1-60327-820-1_17

pelvic surgery, pelvic fibrosis, organomegaly, ascites, and larger aortic or iliac aneurysms *(6)*. Obesity is a relative contraindication to HAL cystectomy as difficulty can be encountered with the hand port, laparoscopic ports, and instrument angles due to the large abdominal pannus. Additionally, oxygenation may be more difficult when the patient is placed in the Trendelenburg position required for HAL cystectomy *(7)*. Patients with severe chronic obstructive pulmonary disease (COPD) may need additional preoperative work-up if laparoscopic surgery is to be considered. Large and locally advanced bladder tumors (stage $\geq$ T3b) are more difficult with the laparoscopic or HAL approach, especially managing the bladder pedicles, and a conventional open procedure may provide the most judicious course for surgical treatment.

PREOPERATIVE ASSESSMENT

The preoperative assessment for patients undergoing laparoscopic or hand-assisted cystectomy is similar to that done for open cystectomy. This usually includes a meticulous history and physical, laboratory assessment (basic metabolic panel, complete blood count, liver and function studies, coagulation studies), and imaging studies (chest CT scan or X-ray, computerized tomography scan of the abdomen and pelvis, and rarely bone scan). A bimanual examination under anesthesia should be routinely performed on patients prior to the initial transurethral resection of a bladder tumor to determine the need for neoadjuvant chemotherapy in muscle invasive bladder cancers. Patients with transurethral resection and imaging stage $\leq$T3a are likely the best candidates for HAL cystectomy approach, but higher stage tumors can be approached using this technique. In patients with a history of gastrointestinal (GI) disease, a thorough evaluation by a gastroenterologist is recommended prior to surgery. Patients with COPD may benefit from preoperative pulmonary function testing and arterial blood gas determination in order to evaluate the pulmonary fitness of the patient.

PREOPERATIVE PREPARATION

Patients perform a bowel preparation on the day prior to surgery. A mechanical preparation can be undertaken with oral polyethylene glycol or oral sodium phosphate, with care taken to follow the labeling instructions and contraindications. Antibiotic bowel preparation with neomycin and erythromycin base, or metronidazole is advocated by some. The patient should have a blood type and screen at a minimum, but generally two units of cross-matched packed red blood cells should be available if blood transfusion becomes necessary intraoperatively. The patient should have bilateral sequential compression devices on and functioning prior to anesthesia induction to reduce the risk of deep venous thrombosis. Some prefer to use subcutaneous heparin or low-molecular weight heparin which is given 2 h preoperatively.

LAPAROSCOPIC SPECIFIC INSTRUMENTATION

Surgical instrumentation is primarily based on surgeon preference and familiarity. Below is listed basic outline:

- 10 mm 0 and 30° lens/laparoscope
- Three to five 12 mm laparoscopic ports, usually blunt type
- At least one 5 mm laparoscopic port
- One laparoscopic hand-assisted device (GelPort – Applied Medical, Rancho Santa Margarita, CA or LAP DISC – Ethicon Endo-Surgery, Cornelia, Georgia)
- One 5 mm electrosurgical monopolar scissors

- One 5 mm electrosurgical hook
- Two 5 mm atraumatic forceps (bowel clamps)
- One 5 mm right-angle dissector
- One 10 mm right-angle dissector
- One 5 or 10 mm laparoscopic retractor
- Two large clip applicators with clips (either standard metal type, or Weck – Teleflex Medical, Research Triangle Park, NC or similar)
- Two needle drivers
- One 12 mm articulating Endo-GIA vascular stapler with multiple reloads (Autosuture – US Surgical, Norwalk, Connecticut or Ethicon Endo-Surgery, Cornelia, GA)
- One 10 mm bipolar cutting forceps (Gyrus ACMI, Maple Grove, Minnesota or Ligasure – Valleylab, Boulder, Colorado)
- One 5 mm irrigator/suction device
- One 15 mm laparoscopic specimen bag

PATIENT POSITION

The patient position is supine on a standard operating room table with legs abducted. Additional padding should be placed beneath the heels, legs, hips, and scapula. The patient should be properly secured to the table for the anticipated Trendelenberg position. After HAL and standard laparoscopic ports are placed, the patient is placed into a 20–30° Trendelenberg position.

OPERATING ROOM SET-UP

A right-hand dominant surgeon, could be positioned on the patient's right side. The non-dominant hand is traditionally placed into the HAL port, which leaves the dominant hand free to manipulate laparoscopic instruments. The assistant/camera operator should be positioned on the patient's left side. Monitors should be placed on both sides of the patient at level of the pelvis to allow the surgical team to view the procedure. For surgeons more comfortable with non-dominant hand laparoscopic instrument use, the positioning can be reversed.

PORT PLACEMENT

Prior to insufflation and port placement, a catheter should be inserted into the bladder and naso-gastric tube into the stomach. The hand-assisted port should be placed in midline with its inferior extent just below the umbilicus and extending superiorly in length as specified by manufacturer and surgeon's hand size. The laparoscopic port configuration includes a 12-mm port at approximately the level of the umbilicus in the midclavicular line (Fig. 1). Typically the right side 12-mm port site can be placed in the preoperatively marked stoma site (Fig. 2). Additional operating/assisting ports are placed 2 mm medial and superior to the anterior superior iliac spine bilaterally (12 mm on both sides, or for right-side 12 mm, and 5 mm on left-side).

HAND-ASSISTED LAPAROSCOPIC RADICAL CYSTECTOMY TECHNIQUE

With surgeon's hand for exposure and counter traction, the lateral white line of Toldt is incised bilaterally, reflecting the colon medially in order to expose the retroperitoneum. A wide incision is made in the peritoneum at the level of the rectovesical pouch. The vasa deferentia are identified, dissected,

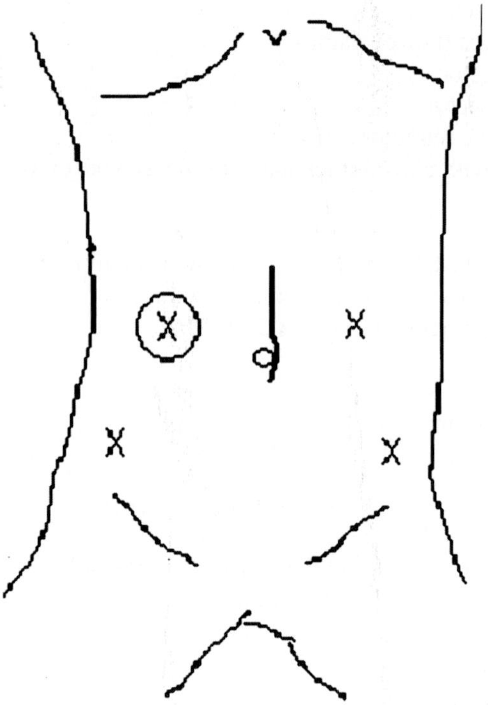

Fig. 1. Possible schema of laparoscopic port configuration.

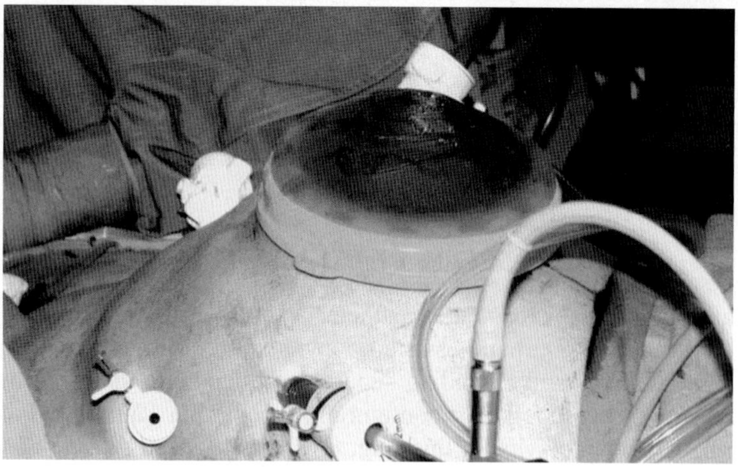

Fig. 2. Laparoscopic and hand device port placement.

and divided. The plane between the bladder/seminal vesicles/ampulla of vas deferens/prostate and the rectum is developed with the aide of blunt dissection using the hand. Denonvillier's fascia must be incised in order to allow dissection caudally to the prostate apex. The ureters are identified crossing the external iliac vessels. The ureters should be mobilized from the level of the sacral promontory distally to bladder (Fig. 3). The ureters are then clipped proximal and distal, divided, and tagged with long sutures or endoscopic loops for ease of identification (Fig. 4). The left ureter is delivered under

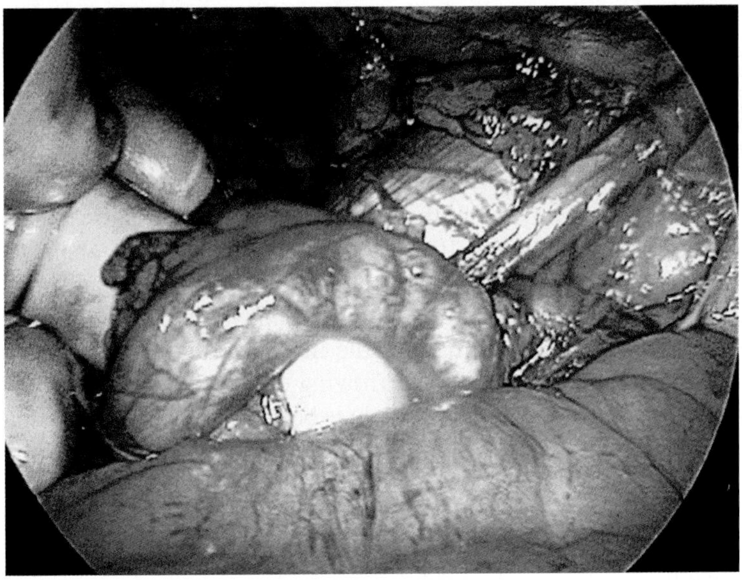

Fig. 3. Ureteral dissection.

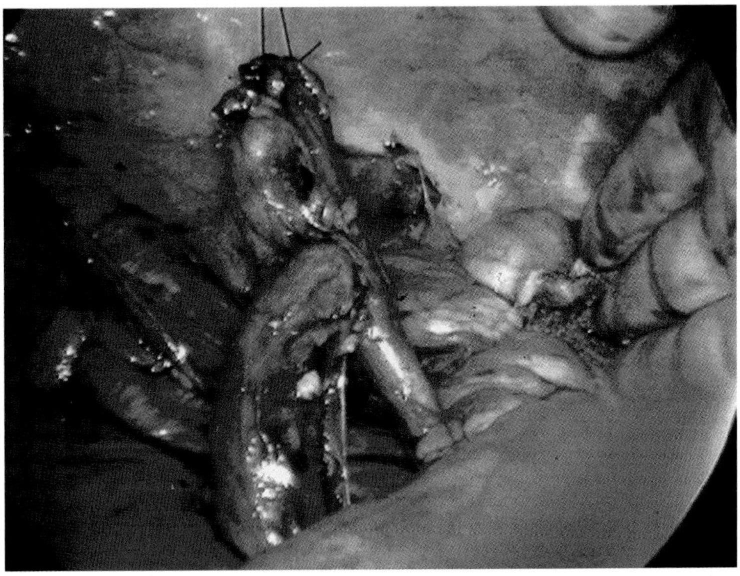

Fig. 4. Ureteral dissection and mobilization.

the sigmoid with a two-finger breadth hiatus at the sacral promontory. The two tagged ureters are secured to the abdominal wall when bringing the sutures through a small 1 mm incision in the right lower quadrant using a Carter–Thomlinson device, and prolene suture, or "endo-loop" device.

The prevesicle space of Retzius is now entered by extending the peritoneal incisions lateral to medial umbilical ligaments cephalad to the umbilicus. Bipolar cautery is employed when dividing the medial umbilical ligaments and urachus. The prevesical space should be developed until the pubic rami are exposed in the pelvis. The anterior prostatic fat is dissected away exposing the endopelvic fascia bilaterally. The endopelvic fascia is then incised, developing the plane between the prostate and levator muscle fibers. This plane should be dissected from the base to the apex of the prostate so that the deep dorsal venous complex (DVC) and the neurovascular bundles are exposed. The DVC is controlled with a 12 mm Endo-GIA vascular stapler, or a 2-0 Vicryl suture with a CT-1 or SH needle.

With the aide of the previous dissection, the lateral vesicle pedicles are isolated with the hand and divided with endovascular stapler reloads. If a nerve-sparing procedure is planned, care must be taken to stay medial to the neurovascular pedicles. The pedicles supplying the bladder and prostate are taken while progressing towards the prostate apex. With the endovascular stapling device, these pedicles can usually be secured from the bladder base to the mid prostate, or even to the prostatic apex. At times the apical prostatic pedicles (because of narrowing of working space) need to have clips placed. During nerve sparing surgeries, the prostatic pedicle is best taken with laparoscopic clips and then use sharp cautery-free dissection while incising the lateral prostatic fascia and reflecting the neurovascular pedicle laterally.

The cystoprostatectomy specimen should now be completely freed except for the urethra at the prostatic apex. With the foley catheter still in place, dissect the urethra with precision while avoiding the neurovascular bundles. A laparoscopic clip is applied to the prostatic urethral stump to prevent tumor spillage. The hand can assist specimen removal by compressing the urethra, hopefully facilitating absence of tumor spillage. For specimen retrieval, remove the right peri-umbilical 12-mm port and insert the 15-mm endocatch bag through this fascial defect. The specimen is secured inside the endocatch bag with the aide of the hand. Once bagged, the specimen can now be removed through the hand port.

Laparoscopic pelvic lymph node dissection is now performed. A full bilateral dissection should include the obturator fossa, the internal/external/common iliacs up to 2 mm below the aortic bifurcation. Alternatively, pelvic lymph node dissection may be completed prior to performing the cystectomy – this has the advantage of "skeletonizing" the vessels, in case quick vascular control is needed during cystectomy (transient internal iliac clamping can facilitate a less bloody field). Additionally, pre-cystectomy lymph node dissection can even allow for ease in visualizing the vesical branches of the internal iliac, making more precise hemostasis with metal clips. Hemostasis is confirmed prior to completion of the laparoscopic portion of the procedure. Lowering the intra-abdominal pressure to 0–5 mmHg for a few minutes, aids in the identification of bleeding which may be obscured by the normal working pneumoperitoneum pressure of 15 mmHg.

URINARY DIVERSION WITH HAND PORT

The hand-assist device port is removed and a Balfour retractor or similar retractor is placed within the midline incision (Fig. 5). The distal ileum is delivered through this incision and 20 mm segment is harvested approximately 15 mm proximal to ileocecal valve (to spare the ileocecal arterial blood supply). Standard open conduit construction is utilized with GIA staplers. The ureters can now be grasped from the securing suture placed during the laparoscopic portion of the procedure. A Bricker-type or similar spatulated end to side ureteral anastomosis is performed with placement of ureteral stents. Once completed, the ileal conduit is delivered out of the preoperatively selected stoma site (Fig. 6).

A Jackson–Pratt drain or Blake type drain is placed into the pelvis through the left lower quadrant 5-mm port. The midline fascial incision is closed, followed by the skin. Additional port sites are closed as needed and skin incisions are closed with absorbable suture (Fig. 7).

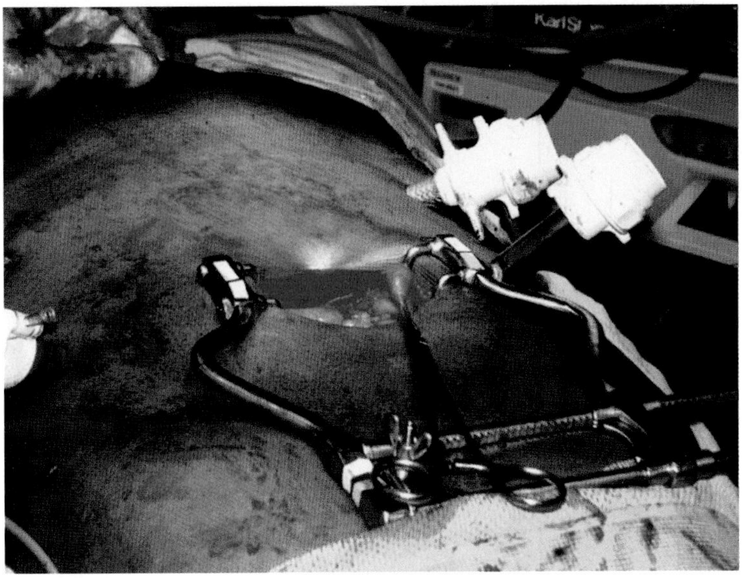

Fig. 5. Midline port site as access for ileal conduit creation.

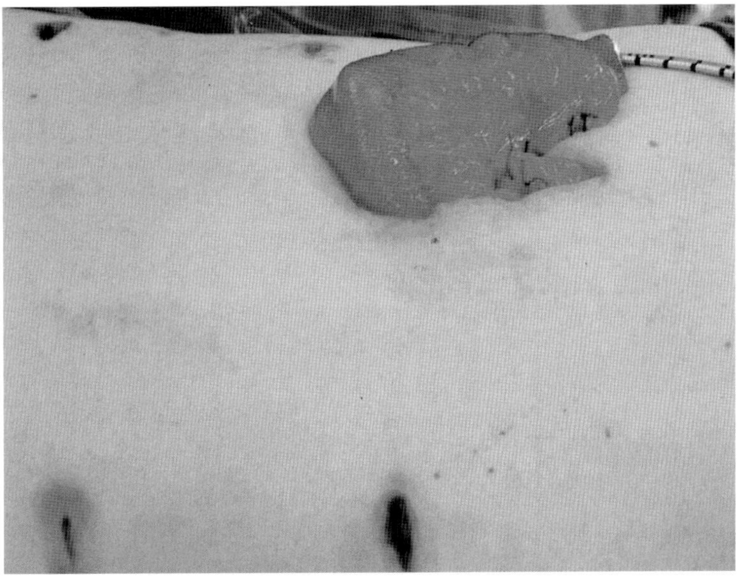

Fig. 6. Ileal conduit construction.

RESULTS

With only 17 cases of HAL cystectomy reported to date, the utility and benefit of this procedure relative to open cystectomy is not well established (Table 1), however, initial results or the technique are encouraging. As previously noted, oncologic efficacy needs further trials and longer follow-up. Taylor et al. presented the only prospective, non-randomized series comparing HAL cystectomy to open with eight patients in each group *(5)*. This study demonstrated a statistically significant benefit of the HAL

Table 1
HAL cystectomy literature review

	Case number	Path stage	Margins	EBL (ml)	Mean OR time (h)	Mean LOS (days)	Mean morphine requirement (mg)	Local recurrences	Complications	Conversion to open
Peterson et al. *(3)*	1	Not reported	Negative	750	7	7	Not reported	None	None	None
McGinnis et al. *(4)*	7	2 – TaN0M0 and CIS; 2 – T2aN0M0; 2 – T3aN1M0; 1- T3bN0M0 and CIS	Positive one (CIS at one ureteral margin)	420	7.6	4.6	28.8	2 (T3b with pelvic recurrence 9 months, T2a with rectal recurrence 18 months)	None	One
Hemal et al. *(8)*	1	T3b, N2, M0	Positive (left perivesical margin)	500	4.3	7	35	None (25 months)	None	None
Taylor et al. *(5)*	8	3 – T0; 1 – T2aN0M0; 1 – T3aN0M0; 1 – T3bN2M0; 2 – T4aN0M0	Positive in one (T4a patient)	637.5	6.7	6.4	30.9	None	Upper GI bleed; rectal injury and ileus	None

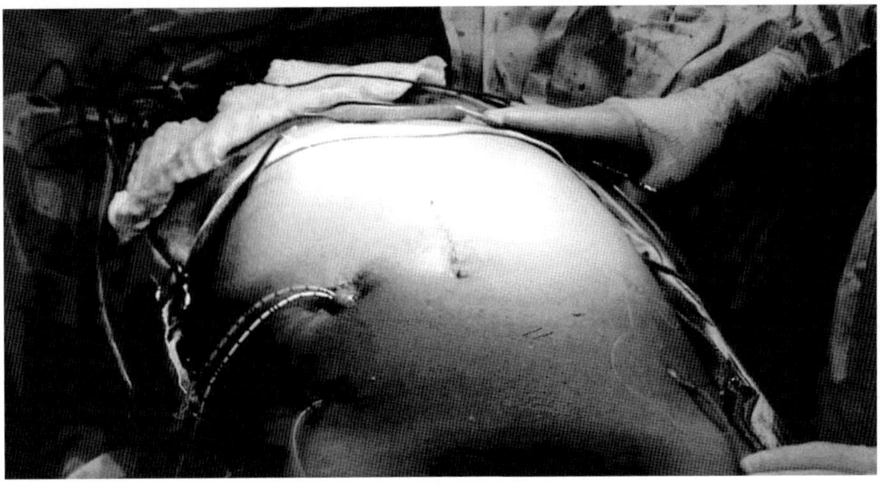

Fig. 7. Intraoperative stent and drain placement.

cystectomy over open cystectomy when comparing postoperative narcotic use (31 vs. 149 mg morphine, $p=0.01$) and postoperative resumption of regular diet (4.5 vs. 7.9 days, $p=0.05$), although this study has many limitations. A direct comparison with a prospective, randomized trial comparing open, vs. some form of laparoscopic technique comparison (pure laparoscopic, HAL, and/or robotic-assisted laparoscopic cystectomy) would be the optimal venue to make meaningful evidence-based conclusions. Perhaps the most pertinent question regarding the optimal technique for radical cystectomy is: which technique affords optimal construction of an orthotopic neobladder, continent catherizable pouch, or ileal conduit diversion?, yet still maintains oncologic efficacy. The hand-assisted approach offers the possibility of retraction, palpation, speed, and relatively minimal or equivalent morbidity, but surgical approach should depend on surgeon expertise, experience, and comfort *(4,9)*.

REFERENCES

1. Parra RO, Andrus CH, Jones JP, Boullier JA (1992) Laparoscopic cystectomy: initial report on a new treatment for the retained bladder. J Urol 148: 1140–1144.
2. Gill IS, Fergany A, Klein EA, Kaouk JH, Sung GT, et al. (2000) Laparoscopic radical cystoprostatectomy with ileal conduit performed completely intracorporeally: the initial 2 cases. Urology 56: 26–29; discussion 29–30.
3. Peterson AC, Lance RS, Ahuja S (2002) Laparoscopic hand assisted radical cystectomy with ileal conduit urinary diversion. J Urol 168: 2103–2105; discussion 2105.
4. McGinnis DE, Hubosky SG, Bergmann LS (2004) Hand-assisted laparoscopic cystoprostatectomy and urinary diversion. J Endourol 18: 383–386.
5. Taylor GD, Duchene DA, Koeneman KS (2004) Hand assisted laparoscopic cystectomy with minilaparotomy ileal conduit: series report and comparison with open cystectomy. J Urol 172: 1291–1296.
6. McDougal EM, Finley D, Clayman RV, Winfield HN, Gill IS, Nakada SY, Shalhav AL, Babayan RK, Sosa RE (2005) Basic Urologic Laparoscopy. Linthicum, MD: American Urologic Association. 85p.
7. Meininger D, Byhahn C, Mierdl S, Lehnert M, Heller K, et al. (2005) Hemodynamic and respiratory effects of robot-assisted laparoscopic fundoplication in children. World J Surg 29: 615–619; discussion 620.
8. Hemal AK, Singh I (2004) Hand assisted laparoscopic radical cystectomy for cancer bladder. Int Urol Nephrol 36: 191–195.
9. Cathelineau J (2007) Laparoscopic radical cystectomy and urinary diversion: what is the optimal technique? Curr Opin Urol 17(2): 93–97.

Laparoscopic and Robotic-Assisted Laparoscopic Radical Prostatectomy

Chandru P. Sundaram, Carl K. Gjertson, and Michael O. Koch

INTRODUCTION

There have been significant advances in laparoscopic skills and instrumentation since Schuessler and colleagues performed the first laparoscopic radical prostatectomy (LRP) in 1991 *(1)*. Only nine LRPs were performed between 1991 and 1995. However, the surgery was difficult, with long operating times, and the laparoscopic approach for the treatment of prostate cancer was believed to offer no advantage over open surgery. In 1998, Guillonneau and colleagues reported their initial experience with the surgery with early results of the transperitoneal approach comparable to contemporary series of open radical prostatectomy *(2)*. Since then, a number of centers have performed the LRP in increasing numbers with early results comparable to open surgery. However, LRP has not gained widespread popularity among urologists, owing to its technical demands, long operating times, and long learning curves.

The da Vinci Surgical System (Intuitive Surgical) is a master/slave device, where specially designed "wristed" laparoscopic instruments are manipulated by a surgical platform (the "robot") controlled by a surgeon at a remote console. The robotic-assisted laparoscopic radical prostatectomy (RALP) has rapidly become more popular than the laparoscopic radical prostatectomy. The RALP has similar benefits to the patient as LRP, but is considered easier to use and may allow an experienced open surgeon without extensive laparoscopic experience an easier transition to minimally invasive prostate surgery. It is estimated that 35–50% of radical prostatectomies performed in the United States are now performed robotically *(3,4)*. Although, the vast majority of centers in the United States have adopted robotic assistance, LRP without robotic assistance is still relevant when the da Vinci System is unavailable or during the unlikely event of robotic malfunction. Most surgical steps described in the section on robot-assisted radical prostatectomy may also be used for surgery without robotic assistance.

Preoperative Assessment

Indications for a RALP are identical to those for an open radical retropubic prostatectomy (RRP). Nerve sparing is generally recommended if the patient is potent and the surgeon determines that the patient is at relatively low risk for extracapsular extension based upon tumor volume, Gleason score, and clinical stage. Nerve sacrifice is generally recommended for patients with a predominance of Gleason pattern 4 or greater in their biopsy specimen, particularly if high volume. A pelvic lymph node dissection (PLND) can be safely performed in all patients, though we often omit node dissection for patients with Gleason ≤ 6 and cT1C disease.

From: *Current Clinical Urology: Essential Urologic Laparoscopy*
Edited by: S. Y. Nakada and S. P. Hedican, DOI 10.1007/978-1-60327-820-1_18

During a surgeon's initial experience with the LRP, patients may be selected with low-grade, low-stage cancers that do not require laparoscopic pelvic lymph node dissection. This helps limit the operating time, which is likely to be prolonged during a surgeon's early experience. The first 25 patients we selected had prostate-specific antigen (PSA) levels less than 10 and a Gleason score of 6 or below.

Factors that can adversely affect the prostatic dissection include obesity: a large (>80 g) or small (<20 g) prostate; a history of radiotherapy to the prostate; transurethral resection of the prostate; pelvic surgery; laparoscopic inguinal herniorrhaphy; and neoadjuvant hormonal therapy. The nerve-sparing technique is difficult during a surgeon's early experience, and can further add to the operating time. A large median lobe can make bladder neck preservation difficult and would necessitate bladder neck reconstruction. Virtually all patients who are candidates for open surgery can be approached laparoscopically after the surgeon has gained adequate experience.

Preoperative Preparation

Our standard preoperative tests include complete blood count, serum electrolytes, BUN and creatinine, electrocardiogram, chest X-ray, and urine culture. Patients discontinue aspirin or other antiplatelet medications 10–14 days prior to surgery. A "mini-" bowel preparation is performed: a clear liquid diet the day before; and an oral cathartic.

All patients receive prophylactic antibiotics intravenously, usually a first generation cephalosporin such as Cefazolin, as a single dose immediately after the induction of anesthesia. Sequential compression stockings are used for DVT prophylaxis. We do not routinely use subcutaneous heparin unless patients have a previous history of thrombosis. Surgery is performed under general anesthesia with endotracheal intubation and muscle relaxation. Intravenous fluids are limited to2 l for the duration of the case.

LAPAROSCOPIC RADICAL PROSTATECTOMY

Transperitoneal Approach

OPERATIVE TECHNIQUE

The Montsouris team in Paris reported the operating technique described in this chapter. Details of the technique have been modified, based on our experience. This approach differs from the principles of the open approach in that the dissection of the bladder neck and prostatic pedicles is performed before transection of the dorsal venous complex (DVC) and division of the urethra. Difficulties faced during our early experience will be mentioned. Bipolar coagulation and the laparoscopic scissors or the Harmonic Scalpel may be used throughout the operation depending on the surgeon's preference. We have used the Harmonic Scalpel during most of the prostatic dissection because there is less spread of heat and possibly less damage to the neurovascular bundles (NVBs). However, during dissection of or near the NVBs the scissors is used without any thermal energy, despite some bleeding.

INSTRUMENTATION

- Electrocautery unit set on auto-cut with a 40 W, max., 50 W for auto-coagulation and 40 W for bipolar coagulation.
- Five trocars: Two (or three) 12-mm trocars and three (or two) 5-mm trocars.
- A 0° 10 mm laparoscope, 30° 10 mm laparoscope, and a 30° 5 mm laparoscope should also be available.
- Harmonic Scalpel and generator (LCS; laparoscopic coagulating shears, Ethicon Endosurgery).
- Two 5 mm bipolar electrosurgical forceps: broad-tipped and fine-tipped
- 5 mm locking grasping forceps, Microfrance (Xomed) or Jarit.
- Two 5 mm needle holders (Ethicon Endosurgery). Self-righting needle holders should not be used.
- 5 mm curved electrosurgical scissors.

- Laparoscopic entrapment sack, 10 mm (Endo catch gold, Autosuture)
- 5 mm suction/irrigation unit with a long suction tip(Karl Storz or Stryker).
- Laparoscopic Kittner (Ethicon).
- Sutures (Ethicon):
  - #0 dyed polyglactin 910 suture on a 36 mm CT-1 needle.
  - 2-0 dyed polyglactin 910 suture on a #26, SH, or RB-1 needle.
- Carter–Thomason suture passer and Pilot 10–12 mm suturing guide (Inlet Medical).
- 24 Fr curved metal urethral sound.
- 1 in. cervical dilator. May be used as a rectal bougie during early experience.
- 20 Fr Foley catheter with a 30 cc balloon
- 18 Fr Foley catheter with a 5 cc balloon
- 10 mm Blake drain

Patient Positioning

Pneumatic compression boots are used as prophylaxis against deep vein thrombosis. The patient is positioned supine with his legs on spreader bars or in a low lithotomy position with Allen stirrups (Allen Medical Systems, Acton, MA). The abdomen is prepped from the xiphisternum to the perineum, including the genitalia. Adhesive tape is used to secure the patient to the table with both arms tucked at his side. Adhesive tape over foam strips strap the chest to the table, or padded shoulder supports can be used. Care should be taken not to impede breathing with the chest straps, or to cause pressure injury with the shoulder supports, though it must also be secure enough to prevent patient movement with the 30–40° Trendelenburg position during surgery. The thighs and lower extremities are also secured. All bony prominences are padded with foam or gel pads to minimize pressure injury. A 20 Fr Foley catheter is inserted per urethra and an orogastric tube placed. The anus is exposed during patient draping for insertion of a rectal bougie. During the early experience, the rectal bougie assists in identification of Denonvillier's fascia during posterior prostatic dissection.

Operating Room Set-Up

The surgeon stands on an elevated platform adjacent to the left shoulder of the patient, facing the pelvis. A second assistant stands on the patient's right, to the left of the first assistant, to hold the laparoscope. The scrub nurse is positioned beside the patient's left lower extremity. The video monitor is placed between the patient's feet, at the surgeon's eye level. Two ceiling-mounted video monitors placed just above each lower extremity may be used. A single monitor between the legs is also acceptable.

Trocar Configuration

Five laparoscopic ports are used: two (or three) 10–12 mm ports and three (or two) 5 mm ports. A Veress needle is used to establish pneumoperitoneum at the umbilicus. A 10–12 mm port is then inserted at that site using a visual obdurator and a 0° 10 mm laparoscope. After examining the abdominal contents for injury, the second 10–12 mm port is inserted between the umbilicus and the left anterior superior iliac spine. The third 10–12 mm port is inserted at the lateral border of the right rectus abdominis muscle, two fingerbreadths below the umbilicus. The third trocar can be 5 mm, but then cannot be used to introduce the needle during anastomosis. The entrapment sack also requires a 10–12 mm port. The fourth 5 mm port is inserted between the third port and right anterior superior iliac spine. The fifth 5 mm port is inserted between the umbilicus and pubic symphysis in the midline (Fig. 1, left). Urachal tissue may need to be held up to the abdominal wall with a grasper during introduction of the fifth trocar. The surgeon operates through the two ports on either side of the umbilicus.

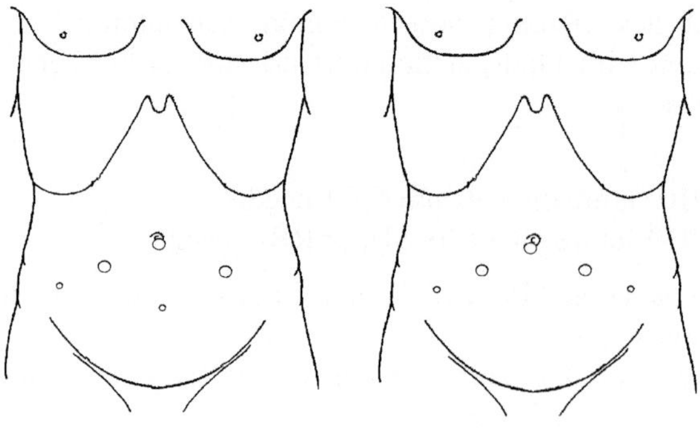

Fig. 1. (*left* and *right*) Diagrams depicting two variations in port placement for LRP.

In tall patients, the lateral 10–12 mm port positions are moved about 3 cm caudally to allow the instruments to reach the prostatic apex and urethra.

The fan configuration is the other alternative for trocar position, where two ports are placed on each side between the umbilical port and the anterior superior iliac spine (Fig. 1, *right*). With port placement in the fan configuration, the surgeon operates through the two left-sided ports and the assistant uses the two on the right.

Seminal Vesicle Dissection

The patient is placed in a 30–40° Trendelenburg position. The assistant via the right lateral port retracts the sigmoid colon superiorly using the suction irrigator or a fan retractor. To facilitate retraction of the sigmoid, a stay suture can be placed through the appendix epiploicae of the colon and brought out of the abdominal wall using the Carter–Thomason device. During the subsequent dissection, the assistant uses the suction irrigator through the lower midline port. There are two peritoneal arches anteriorly in the recto-vesical pouch. The vasa deferentia and seminal vesicles (SVs) are located deep to the lower peritoneal arch (Fig. 2). The peritoneum overlying the posterior bladder is held anteriorly by the assistant using a locking grasper to better expose the cul-de-sac. A transverse incision is made

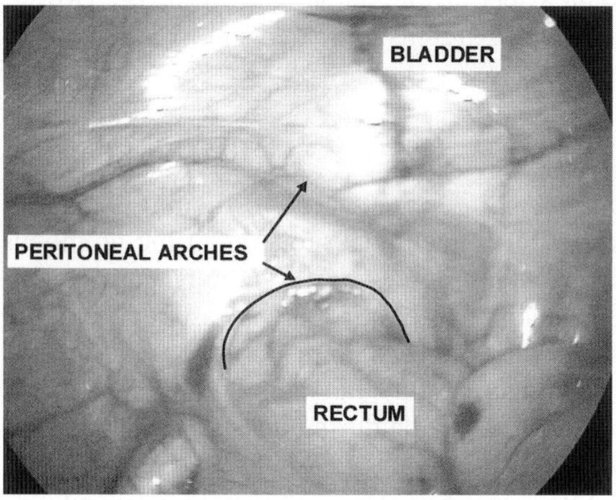

Fig. 2. The peritoneal arches in the retrovesical region are identified after cephalad retraction of the rectosigmoid colon.

at the lower arch to identify and dissect the vas deferens. The vas is coagulated with bipolar cautery or clipped and divided. The assistant then holds the vasa anteriorly, exposing the SVs on either side. Each SV is dissected circumferentially from the base to the apex, taking care to control the vessels to the SV.

If the vasa or SVs are not readily apparent after incision of the peritoneum in the pouch of Douglas, the vas deferens is identified more laterally along the lateral pelvic wall and followed posteriorly towards the prostate. During the dissection of the SVs, it is essential to remain close to the SV to prevent damage to the NVBs. In some instances, if the seminal vesicle dissection is particularly difficult or time consuming, one may choose to complete the SV dissection later via an anterior approach, after the bladder neck dissection is complete.

Incision of Denonvillier's Fascia

The fibers of Denonvillier's fascia are stretched and identified when the assistant holds the completely dissected SVs anteriorly. Denonvillier's fascia is transversely incised in the midline about 3 mm posterior to the base of the SVs. The perirectal fat is now visualized (Fig. 3). The complete dissection of the vasa and SVs is important to enable correct identification of Denonvillier's fascia. Dissection can now be carried out in the perirectal plane towards the prostatic apex. If the proper plane is not apparent during the incision of Denonvillier's fascia, an assistant's finger in the rectum or a rectal bougie can help to identify the rectal wall and avoid injury. Should injury to the rectal wall become apparent, it can be primarily closed in two layers after thorough irrigation of the pelvis, provided there is no gross fecal contamination.

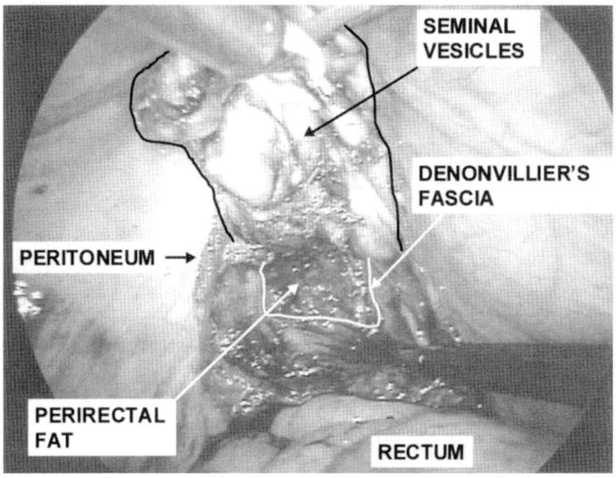

Fig. 3. Dissection of seminal vesicles: the vasa deferentia and seminal vesicles are dissected and held anteriorly. The Denonvillier's fascia is incised to expose the perirectal fat.

Retropubic Dissection

The bladder is distended with 150 cc of sterile saline or air via the Foley catheter to help visualize the bladder margins. With extensive surgical experience, distension of the bladder can be omitted. An inverted U-shaped peritoneal incision is made from one medial umbilical ligament to the other (Fig. 4). The peritoneal incision should be as high as possible on the anterior abdominal wall as it approaches the midline in order to prevent inadvertent injury to the dome of the bladder. Dissection begins just lateral to each medial umbilical ligament until the loose retropubic areolar tissue is identified and the pubic bone is felt. This plane is relatively avascular and copious bleeding could suggest dissection into the bladder wall. This dissection continues medially to the urachus. Both medial umbilical ligaments

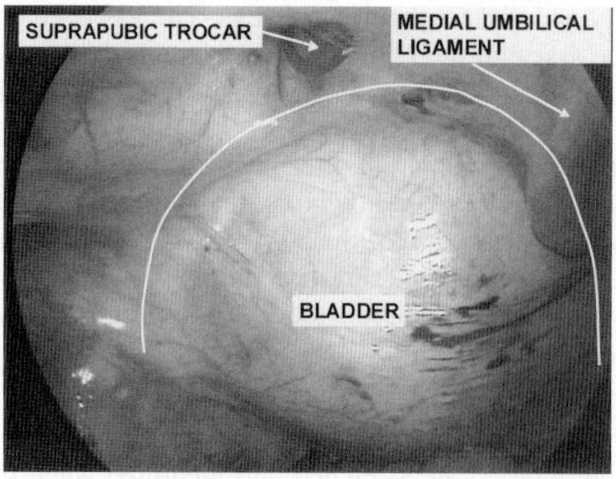

Fig. 4. The contour of the bladder is visible through the overlying peritoneum. The line of the planned incision in the peritoneum is outlined.

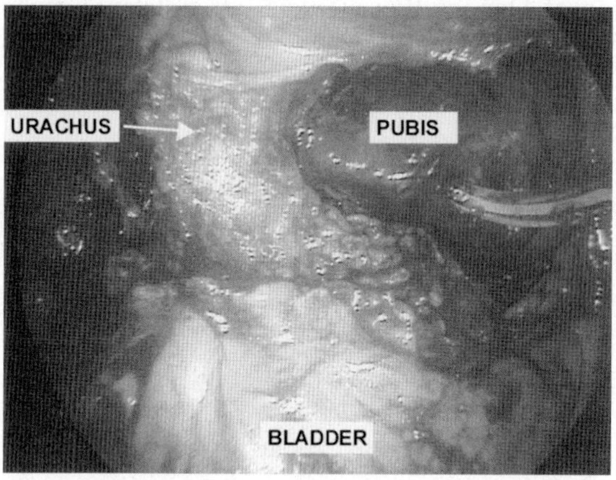

Fig. 5. Retropubic dissection is performed between the right medial umbilical ligament and the urachus. Entry into this avascular plane exposes the pubic bone.

and the urachus are individually divided after bipolar coagulation (Fig. 5). Bladder injury occurred in one patient in our experience, and was primarily closed without conversion to an open approach.

Dissection of the Endopelvic Fascia

The bladder is emptied by using the suction irrigator to evacuate urine from the Foley catheter. Gravity drainage is not adequate to empty the bladder in a steep Trendelenburg position. Blunt dissection with a laparoscopic Kittner eliminates overlying fat and exposes the endopelvic fascia. The superficial dorsal vein is coagulated and divided before the puboprostatic ligaments are exposed (Fig. 6). The endopelvic fascia is incised with endoshears just lateral to the prostatic surface along the lateral pelvic wall (Fig. 7). Precise bipolar electrocoagulation assures hemostasis. The lateral surface of the prostate is separated from the levator muscle with a laparoscopic Kittner dissector. The puboprostatic ligaments are divided close to their attachment to the pubic bone. The apex of the prostate is visualized before the DVC is ligated.

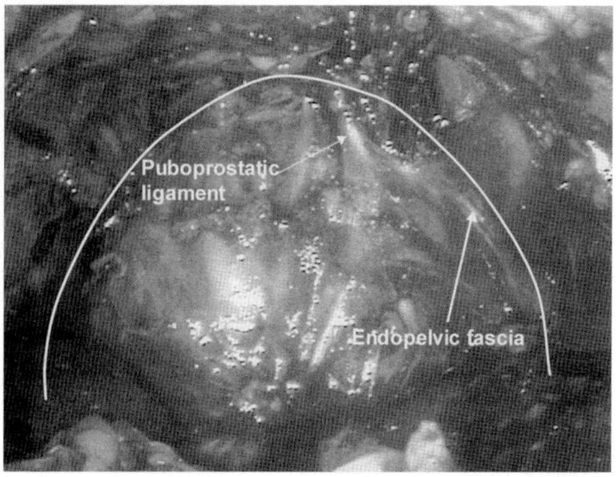

Fig. 6. Blunt dissection exposes the endopelvic fascia and the puboprostatic ligament.

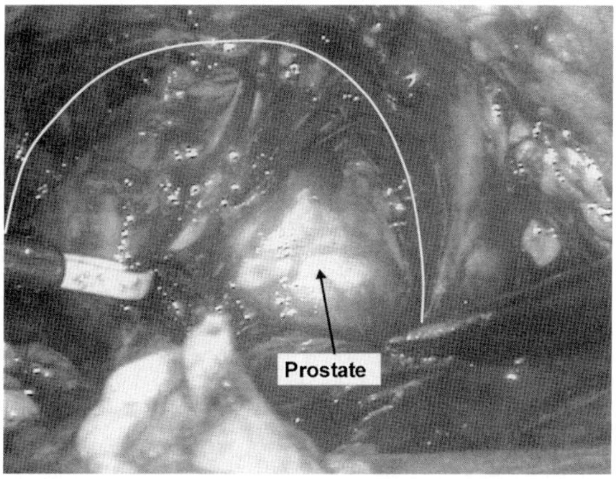

Fig. 7. The endopelvic fascia is incised on the right and the lateral aspect of the prostate exposed.

Ligation of the Dorsal Venous Complex

The DVC is ligated (Fig. 8) with a figure of eight stitch of 0- or 2-0 polyglactin 910 on a 36 mm CT-1 needle (Ethicon). Preliminary dissection near the apex of the prostate to sweep away the muscle fibers of the sphincteric complex will help identify the location for insertion of the needle posterior to the DVC but anterior to the urethra. The curve of the needle is made parallel to the curve of the pubic arch and the needle is passed posterior to the DVC with the right-handed needle holder. A second back-bleeding stitch can be applied on the anterior surface of the prostate to identify the base of the prostate to help with bladder neck dissection. This second stitch is not essential, as the vessels can be controlled during bladder neck dissection. The DVC is not divided until later in the operation.

Bladder Neck Dissection

The demarcation between the base of the prostate and the bladder neck is more accurately determined with increasing experience. The margin of the perivesical fatty tissue helps identify the plane of dissection (Fig. 9). The difference between the floppy bladder wall and the solid prostatic surface can be visualized. Movement of the urethral bougie or a Foley catheter within the bladder can also help. The prostatic base is separated from the bladder neck with blunt and sharp dissection. The Harmonic

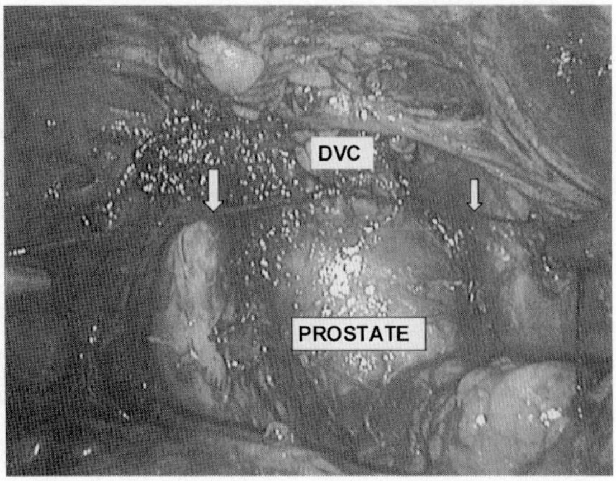

Fig. 8. The deep dorsal venous complex is ligated with 0 Polyglactin (*arrows*).

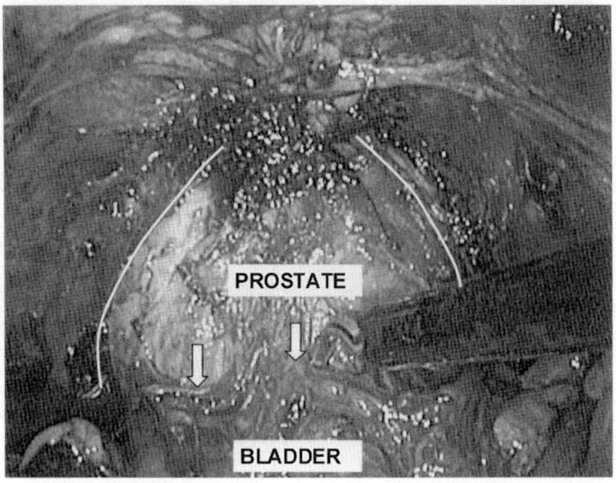

Fig. 9. The demarcation between the prostatic base and the bladder neck is visualized (*arrows*), before bladder neck dissection is begun.

Scalpel or scissors with the bipolar forceps can be used. The dissection is continued posteriorly on either side of the prostatic urethra (Fig. 10). The anterior bladder neck is incised in the midline with endoshears, exposing the metal bougie. Coagulation is not used during this maneuver because of the potential damage to the bladder mucosa in the presence of a metal bougie. After the anterior bladder neck is divided, the metal bougie is brought out through this opening and the base of the prostate retracted anteriorly. Alternatively, a urethral catheter can be inserted and its tip retracted anteriorly by the assistant with a grasping forceps. The posterior bladder neck is divided and retracted cranially with a laparoscopic grasper. Vertically directed dissection is performed in the plane between the posterior bladder neck and the base of the prostate. Dissection can inadvertently be intracapsular if the correct plane is missed. If bladder neck preservation is possible, the ureteral orifices are normally at a safe distance from the bladder neck. If not, intravenous indigo carmine can assist in identification of the ureteral orifices. For a large median lobe, the median lobe is retracted anteriorly prior to transection of the posterior bladder neck. Bladder neck preservation may not be possible in this case.

Completion of the posterior bladder neck dissection exposes the previously dissected vasa and SVs (Fig. 11), because Denonvillier's fascia was opened during the retrovesical dissection. After the metal

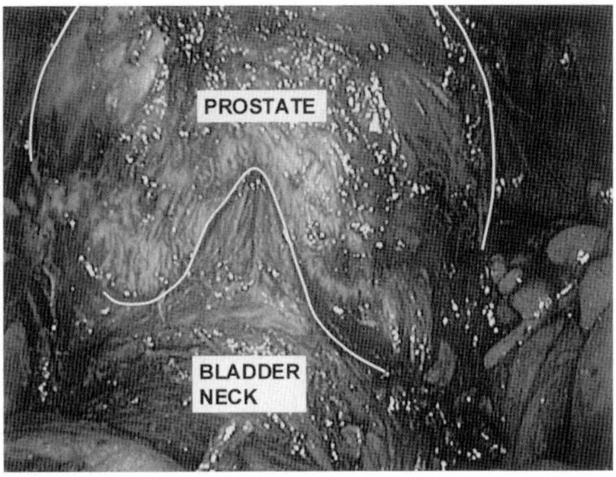

Fig. 10. The anterior bladder neck dissection is completed, exposing the vertical fibers of the bladder neck.

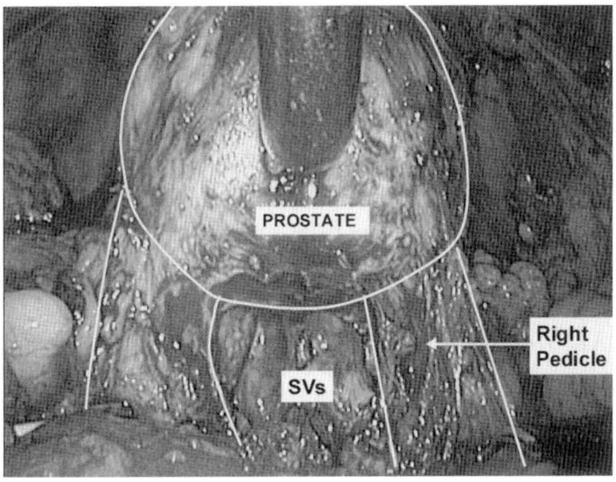

Fig. 11. The posterior bladder neck dissection is completed. The seminal vesicles are visualized through the opening that was previously made in the Denonvillier's fascia.

bougie or catheter is removed, the assistant holds the vasa and SVs with a locking atraumatic grasper and provides anterior retraction.

Control of the Prostatic Pedicles

As the assistant holds up the vasa and SVs, the prostatic pedicles are exposed (Fig. 12). The Harmonic Scalpel can be used for division of the pedicles, because it causes less lateral thermal damage and may be less likely to injure the NVBs. The periprostatic fascia on the lateral aspect of the prostate is carefully incised and the NVBs dissected off of the prostatic capsule. Maintaining dissection close to the prostate will allow for division of the prostatic pedicles and minimize damage to the NVB. After nerve-sparing transection of the prostatic pedicle is completed bilaterally, the base of the prostate should be free. Remnants of Denonvillier's fascia are divided to free the posterior aspect of the prostate.

Venous bleeding that occurs during the nerve-sparing portion of the procedure usually stops spontaneously during the remaining prostatic dissection. The intraperitoneal pressure may be increased to 20 mmHg for a few minutes to assist with hemostasis. Active bleeding can be controlled with

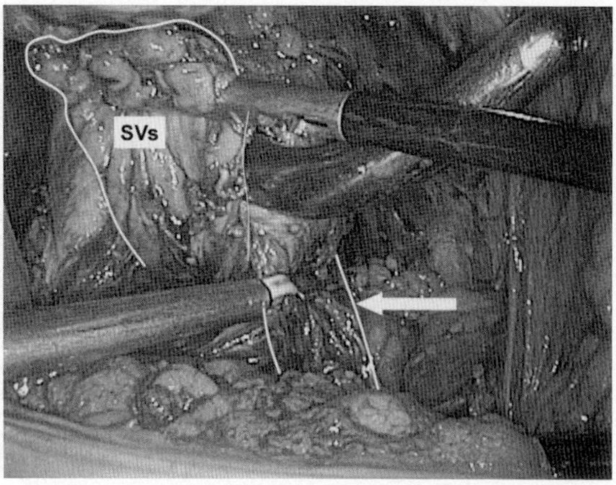

Fig. 12. The seminal vesicles are held up to place the prostatic pedicles (*arrow*) on stretch. The pedicles are controlled close to the prostate with bipolar coagulation or Harmonic scalpel without damage to the neurovascular bundles.

accurate bipolar coagulation using fine-tipped forceps. The nerve-sparing technique is especially difficult during the surgeon's early experience, and can add up to an hour of additional operating time. The narrow-tipped bipolar forceps can be used successfully for nerve sparing. For an athermal nerve-sparing technique, the 10 mm Hem-o-Lok polymer locking clip can be used for the prostatic pedicle. The dissection of the NVB can be performed sharply with the scissors, with the acceptance of some bleeding. The articulating vascular white Endo-GIA stapler (US Surgical) can be used for the pedicles during the non-nerve-sparing technique.

Division of the Dorsal Venous Complex

The deep DVC that was previously ligated is now divided using endoshears or the Harmonic Scalpel. Manipulation of the urethral bougie displaces the prostate posteriorly and stretches the DVC. The previously placed stitch may become dislodged during DVC division. Bleeding from the complex is controlled with a combination of increasing the intra-abdominal pressure and precise bipolar coagulation of the bleeding vessels. Occasionally, a figure-of-eight hemostatic stitch of 2-0 polyglactin 910 on a 36 mm CT-1 needle or 26 mm SH needle is applied.

Division of the Urethra

The prostatic apical dissection is completed to maximize the length of the urethral stump, without violation of the apical tissue. The anterior wall of the urethra is divided with endoshears or a laparoscopic knife, and the metal bougie within the urethra exposed. The bougie is then delivered through this opening, and the posterior urethral wall divided. The rectourethralis muscle is divided, without damage to the NVBs. The prostate along with the SVs is now entirely free if the previous posterior dissection was complete. Occasionally, remnants of Denonvillier's fascia will need to be divided. Care should be taken during these steps to avoid rectal injury. The prostate is placed in a 10 mm entrapment sack (Endo catch gold, Autosuture), which is closed and left in the abdomen for retrieval at the end of surgery (Fig. 13). The preserved NVBs can be visualized in the prostatic bed (Fig. 14).

Bladder Neck Reconstruction

The size of the bladder neck lumen and urethral stump lumen are usually similar if bladder neck preservation was successful; bladder neck reconstruction is therefore not required. If bladder neck preservation was not possible or not performed because of surgeon preference, the bladder neck may be

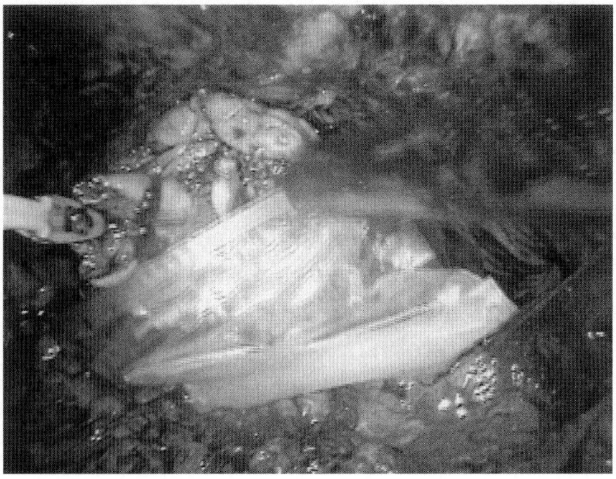

Fig. 13. The prostate is placed in the 10-mm Endocatch bag.

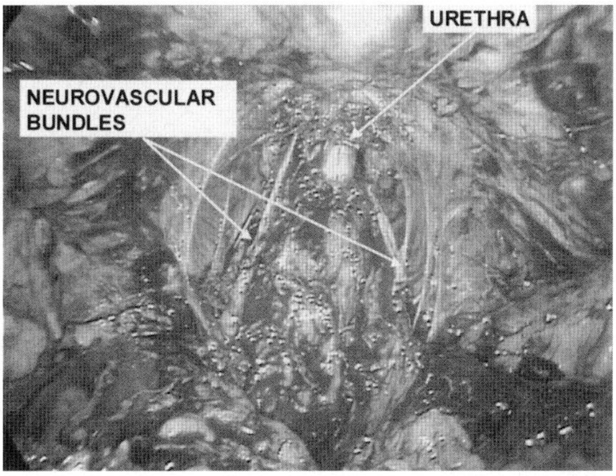

Fig. 14. The neurovascular bundles are visualized on both sides in the prostatic bed.

reconstructed with a racquet-handle technique. Posterior reconstruction may be required if the ureteral orifices are very close to the bladder neck margin. Alternatively, the parachute technique may be employed where sutures are more closely placed on the urethra compared to the bladder neck. We do not evert the bladder neck mucosa and rely on mucosal apposition during a watertight vesicourethral anastomosis. Before the anastomosis begins, the intra-abdominal pressure is decreased to 5 mmHg to confirm that there is no significant bleeding. Bleeding from the prostatic bed after the anastomosis is complete will be difficult to accurately control.

Vesicourethral Anastomosis

Good-quality needle holders are essential during this procedure. Ethicon needle holders inserted through two ports on either side of the umbilicus are used. Self-righting needle holders should not be used because the needle should be held at different angles, depending on the particular anastomotic suture. Interrupted 2-0 dyed polyglactin 910 sutures on a 26 mm SH needle with intracorporeal knot tying has been described. The 17.45 mm RB1 needle can also be used (Ethicon). All knots are tied with the intracorporeal technique; the first knot is a surgeon's knot. A total of three knots are tied for each stitch. The suture is 6 in. long for each interrupted stitch. However, as experience is gained, a

9 in. suture can be used for two or three interrupted stitches. Six to 12 interrupted sutures are placed, depending on the size of the bladder neck and the urethra. The assistant handles the metal bougie within the urethra, which helps guide the needle through the full thickness of urethra. A sponge stick is occasionally used to exert pressure on the perineum to help visualize the urethral stump clearly.

The first suture, at the 5 o'clock position, is placed inside-out on the urethra and outside-in on the bladder with a right-hand forehand approach. The second stitch at the 6 o'clock position is placed right-hand forehand inside-out on the urethra and left-hand forehand outside-in on the bladder ad tied within the lumen. The third stitch is at 7 o'clock: right-hand forehand inside-out on the urethra and left-hand forehand outside-in on the bladder (Fig. 15). These sutures are tied within the lumen of the anastomosis. There have not been problems with calcifications owing to the intraluminal knots. All other sutures are placed with extraluminal knot tying. The lateral sutures on the right side are placed right-hand forehand outside-in on the bladder and right-hand backhand inside-out on the urethra. On the left side, the sutures are placed left-hand forehand outside-in on the bladder and right-hand backhand inside-out on the urethra (Fig. 16). The anterior stitches are placed at the 1 o'clock and 11 o'clock positions using similar technique: right-hand forehand outside-in on the urethra and right-hand

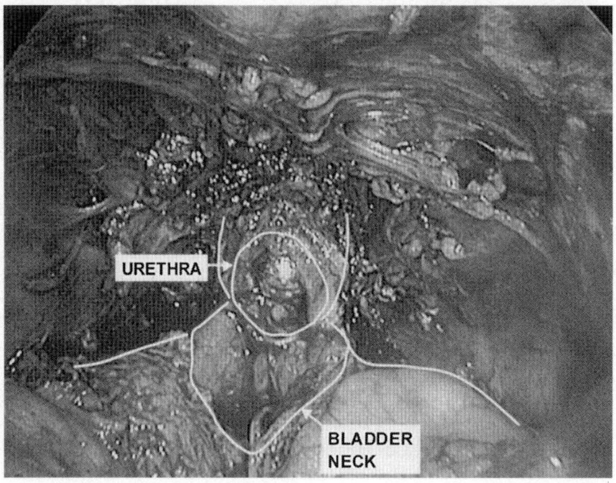

Fig. 15. The posterior layer of the urethrovesical anastomosis is complete. Bladder neck reconstruction is not required since bladder neck preservation was successful.

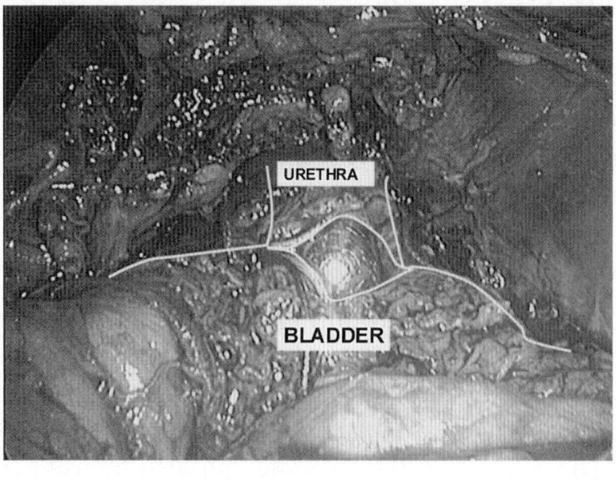

Fig. 16. The urethra-vesical anastomosis is almost complete. The metal bougie is then removed and the anastomosis completed over a catheter.

forehand inside-out on the bladder. The last two stitches are not tied until the 18 Fr Foley catheter is passed into the bladder across the anastomosis. The catheter balloon is inflated with 10 cc of water and the last two stitches are tied. After the anastomosis is complete, the catheter is irrigated to ensure that the anastomosis is watertight.

During the initial experience, the vesicourethral anastomosis is the most time-consuming and challenging part of the operation. However, with experience, suturing is predictable and precise. In our experience, there were four anastomotic leaks in our first eight patients, and all were treated conservatively with continued Foley catheter drainage. None of our subsequent patients have had an anastomotic leak. A continuous suture has also been described for vesicourethral anastomosis, one for the posterior suture line and another continuous suture for the anterior suture line *(5)*. The technique described in the section on robot-assisted radical prostatectomy may also be used and could be faster.

DRAIN INSERTION, PORT SITE CLOSURE, AND SPECIMEN EXTRACTION

A 10 Fr Blake drain is inserted through the right lateral 5 mm port site and placed in the region of the anastomosis. A #0 dyed polyglactin 910 suture is inserted across each 10–12 mm port site for closure using a Carter–Thomason suture passer and Pilot 10-12 mm suturing guide (Inlet Medical). If non-bladed dilating trocars are used, closure of the fascia is not required after removal of the trocars. After removal of the trocars under vision, the umbilical incision is extended and the prostate within the specimen bag is extracted. Care is taken not to exert too much traction on the specimen bag which could cause it to rupture.

POST-OPERATIVE RECOVERY

Patients are typically discharged home on the first post-operative day. The patient is on a clear liquid diet on the day of surgery and advanced to a regular diet the next morning. Compression stockings are used for the duration of hospitalization. The Foley catheter is typically removed on the sixth or seventh post-operative day. With increasing experience, the integrity of the anastomosis is secure and the duration of catheterization decreases considerably *(5)*.

Extraperitoneal Approach

Preservation of the peritoneal integrity and the elimination of the potential for intraperitoneal injury are obvious benefits of the extraperitoneal approach. There is, however, less operating space than the transperitoneal approach and the bladder may be less mobile at the time of vesicourethral anastomosis. Results suggest that this approach may be comparable to the transperitoneal approach with similar complication rates, duration of catheterization, positive margin rates, and continence *(6,7)*.

RESULTS

Laparoscopic radical prostatectomy is presently being performed by selected surgical teams with advanced laparoscopic skills (see Table 1). The learning curve is long and steep. Since the surgical technique has now been established, the learning curve should become shorter. Furthermore, as urologists at several centers become proficient at the surgery, colleagues and residents will be trained in the procedure. This can be achieved by an experienced surgeon assisting a novice surgeon. Operating time can be shortened by practicing suturing on a pelvic trainer. In several centers, teams previously performing the LRP have switched to performing the surgery with robotic assistance because of several advantages that are described in the chapter on robot-assisted LRP. Robot assistance will become even more widespread in future with greater advances in instrumentation and decrease in manufacturing expenses and costs.

The average time in the first 50 patients in multiple series was between 4.2 and 5.5 h *(7,10,11)*. With even more experience the mean time drops to approximately 3 h for the transperitoneal approach *(12)*.

Table 1
Short-term biochemical progression-free survival data for LRP

			Positive margins (%)				*Three-year biochemical progression free survival (%)*			
Authors	*N*	*Median f/u*	*pT2a*	*pT2b*	*pT3a*	*pT3b*	*pT2a*	*pT2b*	*pT3a*	*pT3b*
Guillonneau *(8)*	1,000	12 mo	6.9	18	30	32	91.8	88	77	44
Rassweiler *(9)*	500	40 mo	2.1	9.9	25.2	42	95.2 (all pT2)		74.1	69.0 (and T4)[a]

[a]Received immediate adjuvant androgen deprivation therapy mo, months.

Multiple non-randomized comparisons of LRP to open radical prostatectomy have shown less blood loss and less analgesia requirement with laparoscopy, though longer operating times. Complication rates, margin positivity, and continence have been similar *(13–15)*.

Short-term biochemical progression-free survival data are now available for LRP (Table 1) and are comparable to what has been reported for open radical prostatectomy. Complications for 1,228 LRPs performed by 13 surgeons at six European centers included: conversion to open surgery in 26 (2%), rectal or bowel perforation in 15 (1.2%), ureteral injuries in 12 (1%), anastomotic leak in 69 (5.6%), and thromboembolic complications in two patients. Major bleeding from the epigastric artery occurred in three patients. Twenty-three patients (1.9%) had additional surgery; for port-site hernias in ten, ureteral injuries in five, bleeding in five, and anastomotic leak in three *(16)*.

Advantages of the Laparoscopic Approach

Blood loss and transfusion rates are significantly less with the laparoscopic approach. The tamponade effect of the pneumoperitoneum is one factor that results in decreased bleeding. The antegrade approach to the prostatectomy where the pedicles are controlled early may also be a contributing factor. In most laparoscopic series the estimated blood loss was less than 500 cc compared to about 1,000 cc in many open series *(17)*. Urinary continence following surgery appears satisfactory *(18)*. Erectile function may not completely recover for 1–2 years after surgery. Magnification and the better visualization provided during laparoscopy may result in more accurate dissection during preservation of the NVBs.

ROBOTIC-ASSISTED LAPAROSCOPIC RADICAL PROSTATECTOMY

Transperitoneal Approach

Instrumentation

- da Vinci surgical system (Intuitive Surgical Inc.) with four arms
- Robotic instruments:
  - 0 and 30° binocular telescope
  - EndoWrist PK dissecting forceps or Maryland bipolar graspers
  - EndoWrist Prograsp forceps
  - EndoWrist monopolar scissors
  - Two EndoWrist needle drivers
- Three 8 mm robotic trocars
- Two 12 mm laparoscopic trocars
- PK generator with footswitch (Gyrus-ACMI)
- Standard electrocautery generator

- Veress needle
- 5 mm Suction irrigator with long cannula
- Laparoscopic grasping forceps
- Laparoscopic scissors
- Laparoscopic needle driver
- Laparoscopic entrapment sack, 10 mm (Endo catch gold, Autosuture)
- 18 Fr Foley catheter with 30 cc balloon and 18 Fr Foley catheter with 5 cc balloon
- Sutures:
  - #1 polyglactin 910 suture on a CT needle
  - Two 3-0 poliglecaprone 25 sutures on RB-1 or SH needles, one undyed and one dyed
  - 0-polydioxanone suture on a CT-2 needle
  - 4-0 poliglecaprone 25 suture on a PS-2 needle

Operating Room Set-up

The room must be large enough to accommodate the robot and its sterile draping and still have access to the patient during induction. The technique described here uses a "four-arm" da Vinci system: one arm controlling the telescope, and three surgical arms, one on the right and two on the left. The assistant surgeon stands at the patient's right side. The scrub nurse stands at the patient's left and the instrument table is at the patient's left foot. Two monitors are positioned at the foot, one on each side for the assistant and scrub nurse. If a three-arm system is used, an additional assistant will be required to stand on the left.

Patient Positioning

The patient is in modified low dorsal lithotomy position to accommodate the robot which is placed between the legs. Both arms are copiously padded and tucked at the patient's side. Most of the case will require 30–40° of Trendelenberg; and appropriately secured to prevent slippage. The abdomen is prepped from the xiphisternum to the perineum, including the genitalia. After sterile draping is complete, an 18 Fr Foley catheter with a 30 cc balloon is placed. Meanwhile, the anesthesiologist places an orogastric tube and connects to low wall suction.

Trocar Configuration

Five or six ports are used (Fig. 17): two 12 mm laparoscopic ports, three 8 mm robotic ports, and an optional 5 mm laparoscopic port. Pneumoperitoneum at 15 mmHg is established with a Veress needle through a horizontal incision just superior to or through the umbilicus, and a 12 mm trocar inserted at this site. The visual obturator cannot be used with the da Vinci laparoscope. The first trocar is therefore inserted blindly. The fascia at the site of the primary trocar insertion can be scored with diathermy to enable trocar entry without considerable force and indentation of the abdominal wall. The 30° telescope is inserted and the abdominal contents inspected for injury. The additional trocars are then placed under laparoscopic guidance. The second and third ports, both 8 mm robotic trocars, are placed at a point 8 cm lateral to the midline on each side and 14 cm from the pubic symphysis. A fourth 12 mm laparoscopic trocar is placed on the right side, 8 cm lateral to and in the same line as the second port. A fifth 8 mm robotic trocar is placed on the left side, 8 cm lateral to and in the same line as the third port. Care should be taken that neither of the lateral ports are lateral to nor too close to the anterior superior iliac spine. An optional sixth 5 mm laparoscopic port can be placed on the right side, between ports 1 and 2 and slightly superior to the umbilicus, which will be an additional port for the assistant surgeon.

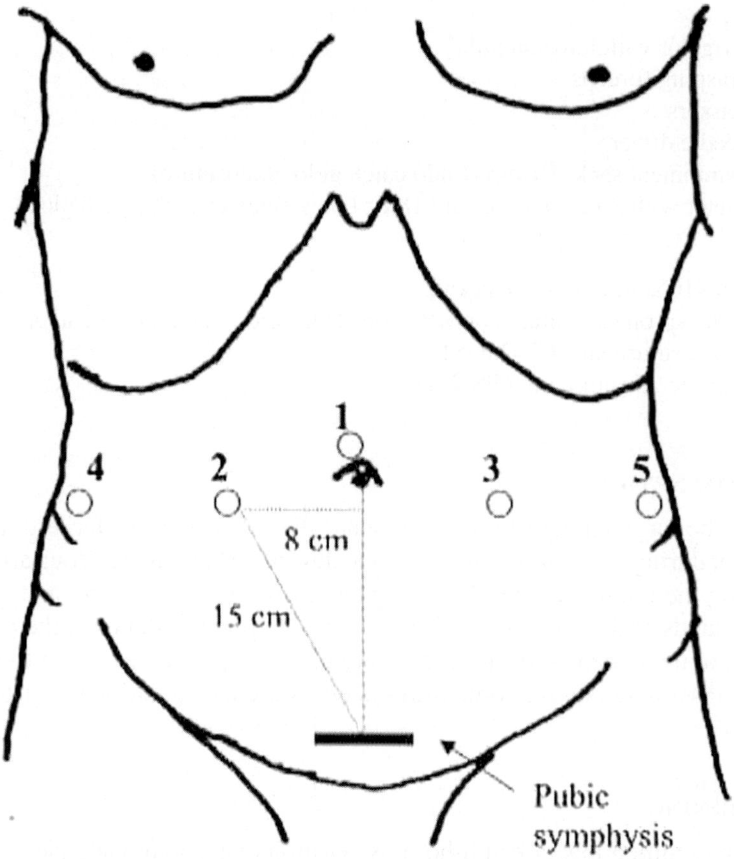

Fig. 17. Diagram depicting port placement for RALP. *Dashed lines* indicate measurements after the abdomen is insufflated. (1) 12 mm laparoscopic port, for telescope; (2) 8 mm robotic port, for instrument; (3) 8 mm robotic port, for instrument; (4) 12 mm laparoscopic port, for assistant's instruments; (5) 8 mm robotic port, for Prograsp.

Entry into the Extraperitoneal Space

After port placement is completed, the table is placed in maximum Trendelenberg, approximately 30–40°. The robot is docked and a 30° upward telescope positioned in the center port. The robotic fourth arm is attached to the most lateral trocar on the left and a Prograsp forceps inserted. In the robotic right arm is a monopolar scissors, and in the robotic left arm the PK dissector or a bipolar Maryland grasper. The assistant surgeon manipulates the suction irrigator placed through the most lateral right trocar. The insufflation tubing is connected to the most lateral left trocar rather than the camera port to reduce fogging of the lens. Pneumoperitoneum is maintained at 15 mmHg. Any adhesions of the sigmoid colon to the left abdominal wall and posterior bladder are taken down to adequately expose the left inguinal ring and the vas deferens as it crosses the iliac vessels. An inverted U-shaped incision into the peritoneum is started just lateral to the medial umbilical ligaments but medial to the inguinal rings and proceeds superiorly, anterior to the bladder. Injecting air into the Foley catheter can help to visualize the bladder. Identification of the vas deferens medial to its entry into the internal inguinal ring provides the most posterior extent of the peritoneal incision. At this point the vas can be coagulated with bipolar cautery and divided. The pubic bone is identified as the posterior aspect of the incision is deepened with blunt dissection, and care must be taken not to inadvertently damage the iliac vessels, which lie just slightly lateral. The plane between the bladder and the pubic bone and anterior abdominal wall should be avascular. Dissecting in a plane close to the anterior abdominal wall will prevent bladder injury. The medial umbilical ligaments and urachus are treated with bipolar cautery and then divided close to the anterior abdominal wall, and the space of Retzius is entered as the bladder is dissected posteriorly off the anterior abdominal wall.

Incision of the Endopelvic Fascia

The Prograsp in the robotic fourth arm is now activated to grasp the urachus and/or the perivesical tissue and pull cephalad to provide some traction on the bladder and improve exposure. The superficial dorsal vein is easily visualized between the two puboprostatic ligaments and it is cauterized and divided. This allows the fat to be removed from the anterior surface of the prostate using bipolar cautery and suction. The endopelvic fascia is then incised lateral to the prostate and the muscle fibers (levator ani) of the pelvic floor swept laterally (Figs. 18 and 19) until the dorsal vein complex and external rhabdosphincter are exposed. The puboprostatic ligaments are preserved and the deep dorsal venous complex is divided later during the apical dissection. We do not ligate or divide the dorsal vein at this time.

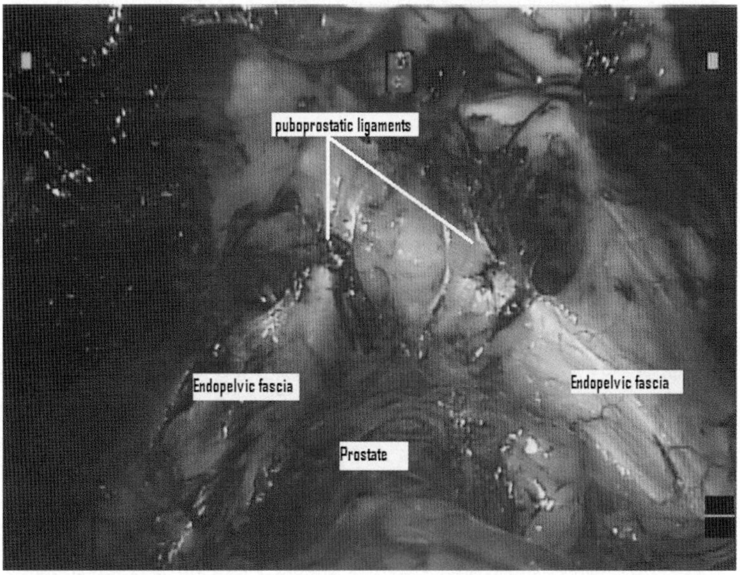

Fig. 18. The prostate is defatted and the endopelvic fascia exposed.

Bladder Neck Dissection

The telescope is changed to a 30° downward lens. The Prograsp in the fourth arm continues to provide traction on the bladder. The bipolar forceps and monopolar scissors are replaced in the left and right robotic arms, respectively. The assistant moves the Foley catheter in and out of the urethra. The movement of the balloon facilitates identification of the bladder neck. The plane between the anterior bladder neck and the prostatic base is developed. This plane should be relatively avascular, but bipolar coagulation is often required. Bladder neck fibers running vertically in the midline to the prostatic urethra can be identified when the dissection is complete. The anterior wall of the bladder neck is divided about 1 mm from the base of the prostate, exposing the Foley catheter (Fig. 20). When the anterior bladder neck incision is complete, the Foley balloon is deflated and the tip of the catheter withdrawn into the prostatic urethra. Dissection of the bladder neck on either side of the midline assists with precise posterior bladder neck dissection. The posterior bladder neck is incised in the midline with

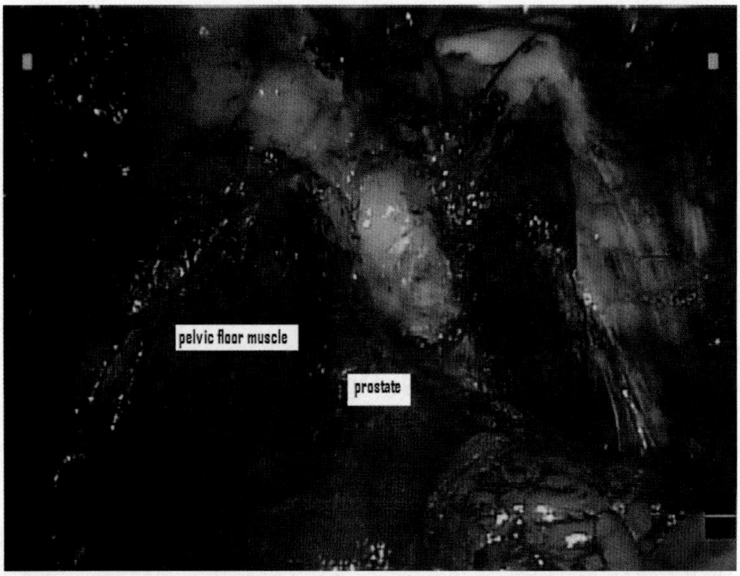

Fig. 19. The endopelvic fascia is opened and the muscle fibers of the pelvic floor swept laterally.

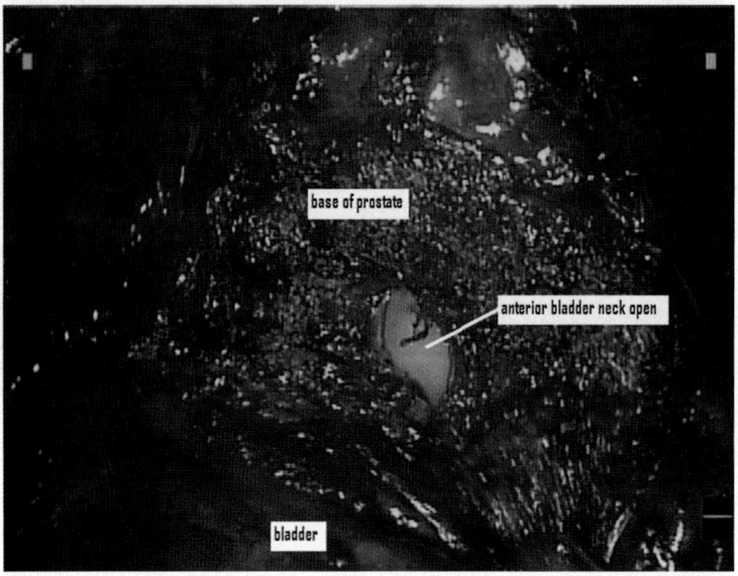

Fig. 20. The anterior bladder neck is opened to expose the Foley catheter.

cold scissors or monopolar cautery. To aid in the dissection, the tip of the Foley catheter is pushed out of the prostatic urethra and grasped with the fourth arm. Anterior traction with the fourth arm and clamping the external part of the catheter to the drape improves exposure of the posterior bladder neck (Fig. 21). The surgeon should inspect the posterior bladder neck to determine the angle relative to the base of the prostate and to determine if there is a median lobe. If there is a median lobe, the proper incision is under the median lobe and then anterior traction of the lobe. The lip of the posterior bladder neck can then be held in the midline to assist with dissection between the posterior bladder

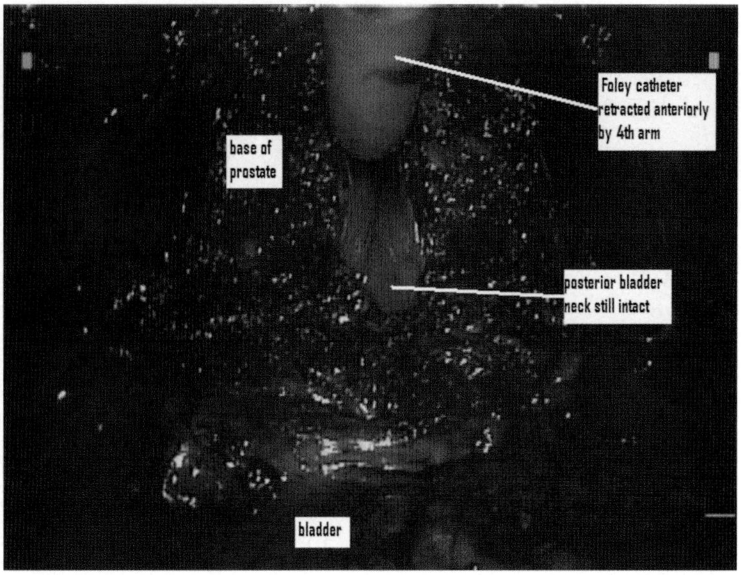

Fig. 21. Anterior retraction of the catheter aids in exposure of the posterior bladder neck.

neck and the posterior base of prostate. Care is taken not to cut into the prostate or to undermine the posterior bladder neck. This can be accomplished by dissecting at right angles to the base of prostate, posteriorly. There are other tips to help stay in the correct plane. The assistant's suction can retract the bladder neck in a cephalad direction as the plane is developed. The relative mobility of the posterior bladder neck and the immobility of the prostate are also helpful. Finally, bladder neck muscle fibers can be visualized before they are divided at the base of the prostate. The bladder mucosa is inspected to see if the ureteral orifices are nearby. When the bladder neck incision is complete, the anterior layer of Denonvillier's fascia should be exposed with the vasa deferentia and seminal vesicles immediately behind (Fig. 22).

Vas Deferens and Seminal Vesicle Dissection

The Prograsp in the fourth arm continues to hold the tip of the catheter and provide anterior traction on the prostate. The anterior layer of Denonvillier's fascia is incised transversely and each vas exposed. Further dissection of the vas is accomplished by incising the tissue parallel and just off its wall. After an adequate length has been dissected posteriorly, each vas is coagulated with bipolar cautery and divided about 5 cm from the base of the prostate. Adequate dissection of the vas helps with later dissection of the seminal vesicles. The fourth arm can then release the catheter tip and grasp both vasa to provide anterior traction (Fig. 23). The vessels supplying the seminal vesicle lie between the vas and the seminal vesicles and need to be divided to expose the clean plane overlying the seminal vesicles. Both seminal vesicles are similarly exposed and their blood supply controlled with bipolar cautery (Fig. 24). It is important to stay on the wall of the seminal vesicle and dissect from the medial to lateral surface. Cautery should be avoided at the tip and especially lateral to the seminal vesicle to prevent injury to the proximal neurovascular plate.

Posterior Dissection

The telescope is switched to a 0° lens. Both vasa and both seminal vesicles are grasped with the fourth arm and retracted anteriorly. If the seminal vesicles are too large for all four structures to be grasped simultaneously, one can alternate grasping the seminal vesicle and vas of each side as the

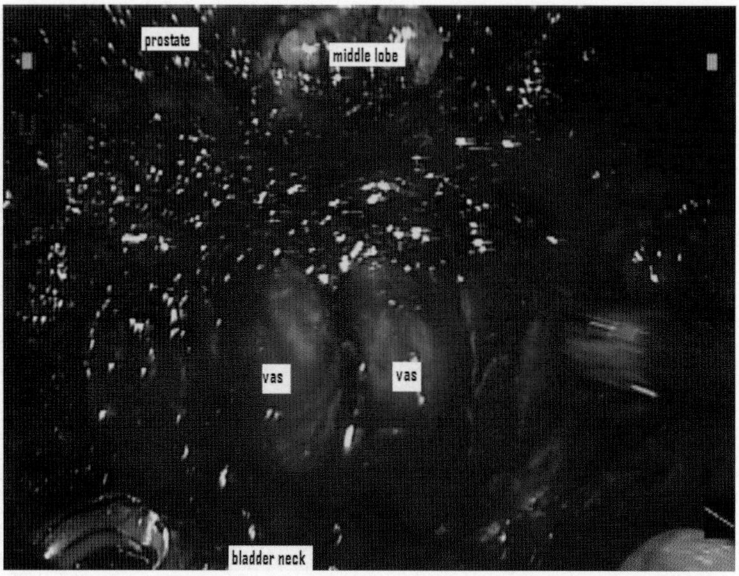

Fig. 22. The vasa are visible just behind the anterior layer of Denonvillier's fascia.

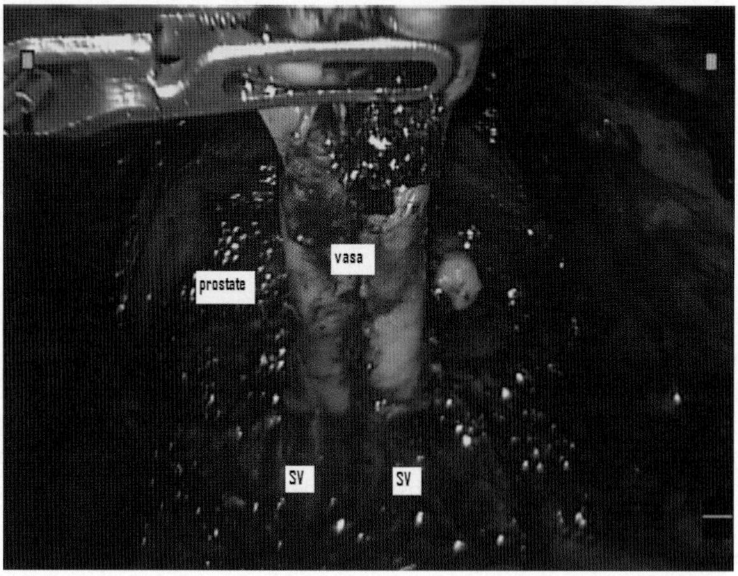

Fig. 23. Anterior traction on the vasa helps to expose the seminal vesicles.

posterior dissection proceeds down that side. Alternatively, both seminal vesicles without the vasa can be held with the Prograsp, with the vasa retracted anterior to the seminal vesicles. Dissection is carried out close to the posterior aspect of the seminal vesicles until the junction of the prostate and base of each seminal vesicle is reached. The posterior layer of Denonvillier's fascia is now exposed and is incised. This allows entry into a plane anterior to the perirectal fat, and with a minimum of cautery this avascular plane is developed distally toward the apex and laterally to the prostatic pedicles (Fig. 25).

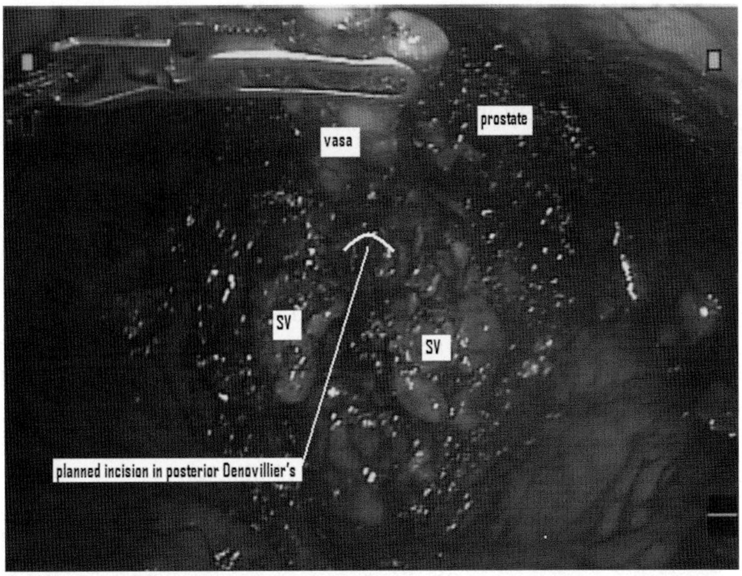

Fig. 24. Seminal vesicle dissection is complete.

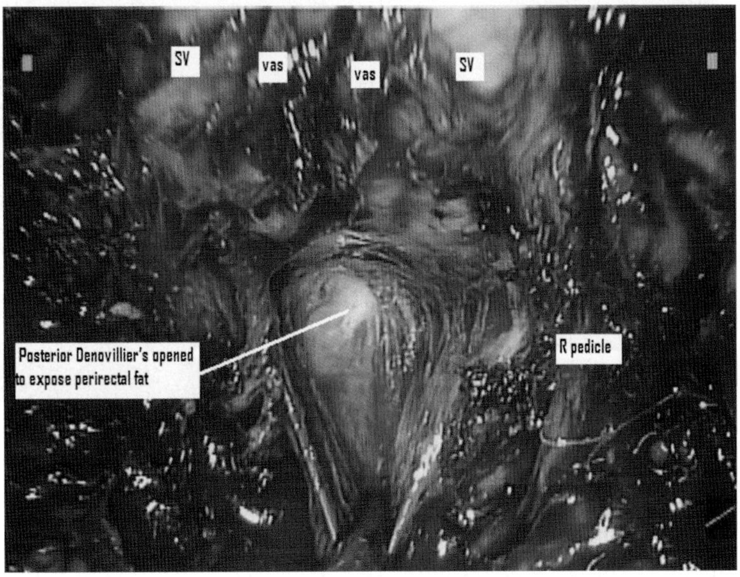

Fig. 25. The posterior layer of Denonvillier's fascia is incised and a plane developed between the prostate and the perirectal fat.

Control of the Pedicles and Nerve Sparing

After completion of the posterior dissection, the prostatic capsule can be readily identified posterolaterally. The capsule is identified as a whitish smooth structure just lateral to the base of the SV. It must now be ensured that any remaining bladder neck fibers attached to the anterolateral aspect of the prostate are divided. The fourth arm grasping the vasa and seminal vesicles retracts the prostate superomedially towards the patient's contralateral hip. The prostatic vascular pedicle can be identified as it enters the capsule of the prostate. The vessels can be individually controlled with bipolar cautery at the prostatic capsule. Alternatively thermal energy can be avoided and the vessels controlled with a 10 mm Hem-o-Lok clip (Weck) placed by the assistant or with a robotic applicator. Smaller vessels can also be controlled more precisely with titanium clips applied by the assistant. The pedicles are divided at the capsule.

Once the pedicle is divided, a plane between the NVB and the capsule of the prostate can be developed and the NVB dissected away from the prostate with blunt and sharp dissection (Fig. 26). The lateral prostatic fascia should be sharply opened on the anterolateral surface of the prostate to allow entry into the proper plane around the neurovascular pedicles and allow them to be swept posteriorly. A minimum of bipolar cautery or small clips can be used for hemostasis as the correct plane is somewhat avascular. The neurovascular tissue is separated from the prostate in continuity as the dissection proceeds distally to the apex until the posterolateral urethra is exposed (Fig. 27). Intermittent adjustment of the angle of prostate traction by the fourth arm aids in this dissection. For a nerve sacrifice procedure, a wide margin of tissue is left on the prostate as the incision of the prostatic pedicle and the previous incision of the endopelvic fascia are essentially connected.

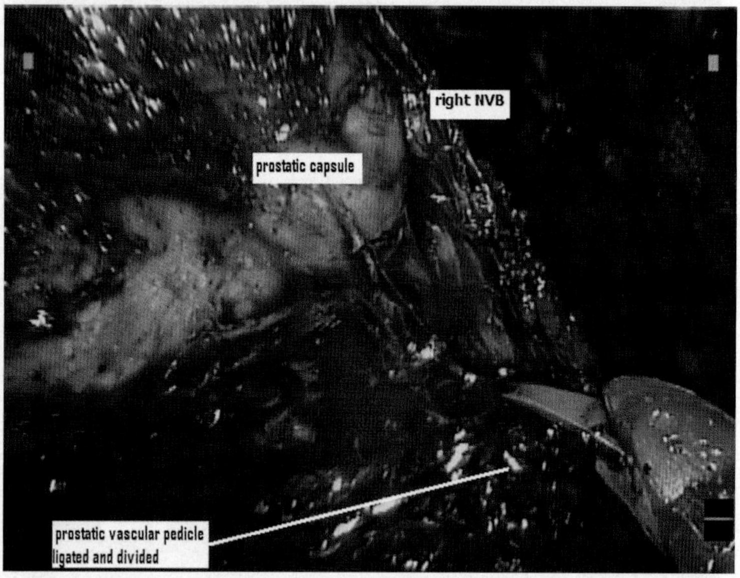

Fig. 26. The right pedicle has been ligated and divided and nerve sparing begins.

During dissection of the left prostatic pedicle and NVB the fourth arm is holding the seminal vesicles and exerting traction towards the right hip. The laparoscope and the instruments may interfere with the fourth arm. This can be avoided with the left working instrument (bipolar forceps) passed anterior to the fourth arm and the right-handed instrument (monopolar scissors) passed posterior to the fourth arm. Despite this, if there appears to be interference with the fourth arm, the assistant on the right can provide traction on the seminal vesicles and vasa instead of the fourth arm.

Apical Dissection with Division of the Dorsal Venous Complex and Urethra

Traction on the prostate with the fourth arm is now directed cranially. The Foley catheter is checked to ensure that it is in the urethra. The prostatic apex is dissected from the lateral to medial direction, by following the capsule of the prostate. Any remaining attachments to the NVBs can be sharply dissected to avoid injury to the bundles during urethral and dorsal vein transection. The dorsal vein is divided during the prostatic apical dissection, with the pneumoperitoneum increased to 20 mmHg

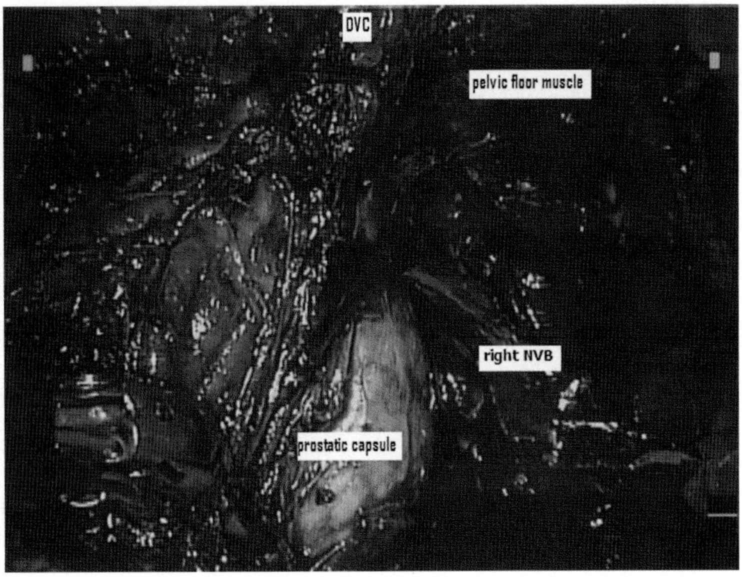

Fig. 27. Right nerve sparing continues toward the apex.

temporarily. This allows for precise apical dissection without any distortion caused by an initial DVC stitch. Bleeding from the DVC is surprisingly minimal. Selective suturing of the divided DVC with 3-0 polyglactin 910 sutures on a SH needle achieves hemostasis.

Previous dissection should have separated pelvic floor muscle fibers and neurovascular tissue from the apex and urethra (Fig. 28). Blunt dissection exposes the urethra as it enters the prostatic apex, and the anterior wall of the urethra is sharply incised without cautery (Fig. 29). The urethral length is maximized without violation of the prostate, before it is divided just distal to the prostatic apex.

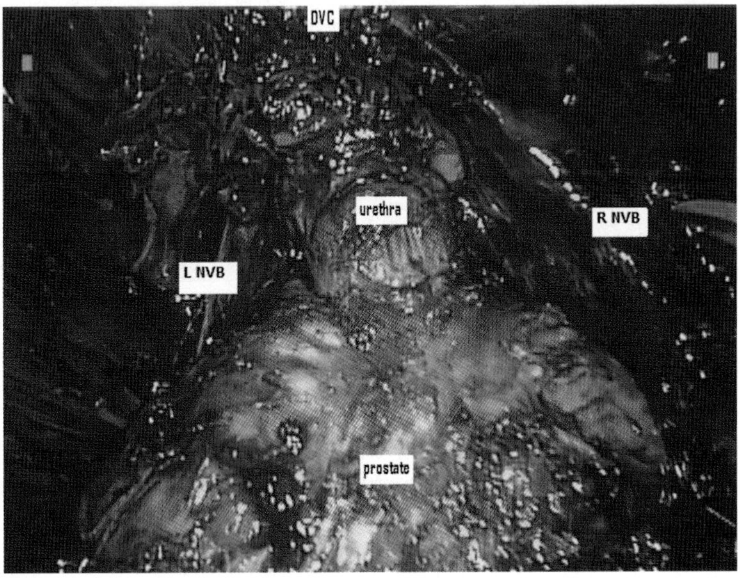

Fig. 28. The DVC has been cut and the urethra and prostatic apex exposed.

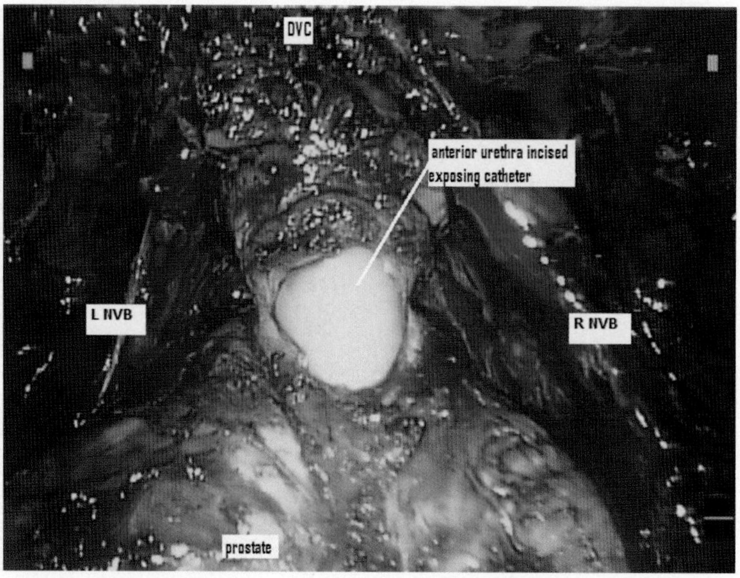

Fig. 29. The anterior urethra is incised.

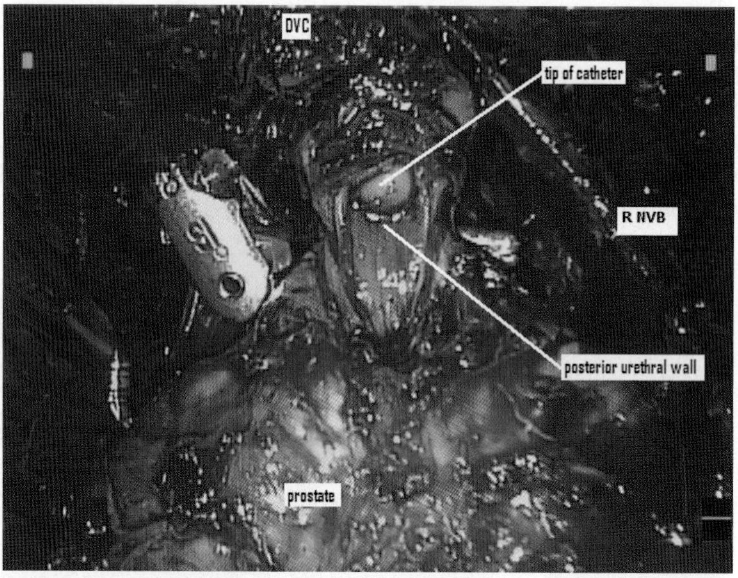

Fig. 30. The bipolar forceps are passed posterior to the urethra to prevent rectal injury during incision of the posterior urethral wall.

The Foley catheter is retracted and the posterior wall of the urethra carefully incised, taking care not to damage the rectum (Fig. 30). Any remaining attachments of the rectourethralis are sharply cut and the prostate placed into a 10 mm laparoscopic entrapment sack (Endo catch gold, Autosuture) for later removal (Fig. 31). Any bleeding in the prostatic bed is controlled with fine bipolar cautery or 3-0 sutures (Fig. 32). Clips and hemostatic agents such as Surgiflo (gelatin matrix, Johnson and Johnson) or FloSeal (gelatin granules and thrombin, Baxter) can also be used.

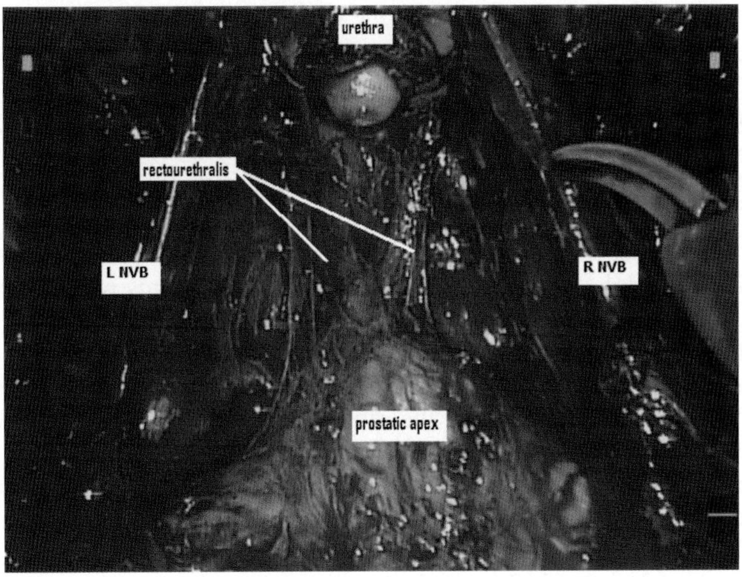

Fig. 31. The urethra and prostate are now separated, and remaining attachments to the prostate divided.

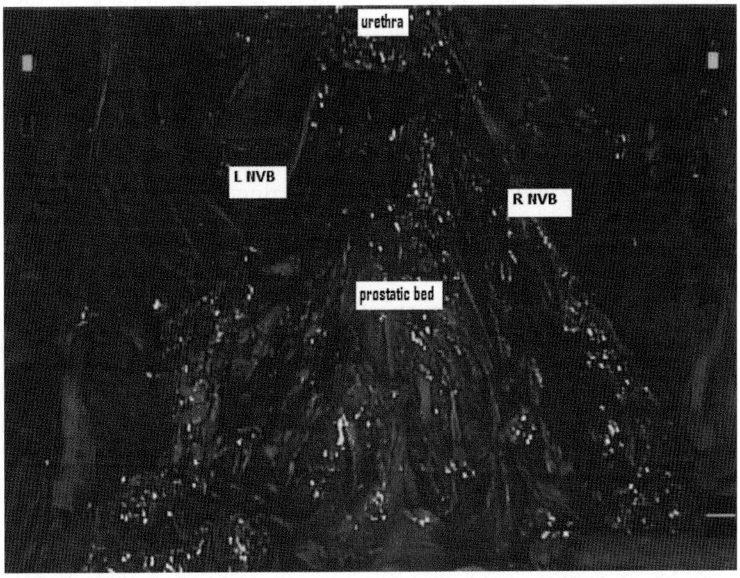

Fig. 32. The prostate is removed from the pelvis.

Bilateral Pelvic Lymph Node Dissection

For node dissection we continue to use a 0° lens, a Prograsp or Maryland bipolar forceps in the left hand, and monopolar scissors in the right hand. The external iliac vein is identified and the fibrofatty tissue lying over it retracted medially and carefully incised. The borders of this standard dissection are the external iliac vein anteriorly, the hypogastric vessels posteriorly, the pubic ramus inferiorly, the bifurcation of the iliac vein superiorly, and the pelvic side wall laterally. Small veins and large lymphatics can be ligated with bipolar cautery and divided. The fourth arm or the patient-side assistant can aid the dissection by grasping and retracting the lymphatic packet medially. The tip of the suction irrigator can also be used to gently hold the external iliac vein laterally and superiorly during the initial dissection, and the obdurator nerve medially during the later dissection, to prevent injury to either structure. After both left- and right-lymph node packets have been removed, we tag one of them with a large Hem-o-Lok clip and then place both in the specimen retrieval bag with the prostate. An extended lymph node dissection is performed in selected high risk patients.

Vesicourethral Anastomosis

For patients with large prostates or median lobe, a posterior "tennis racquet" bladder neck repair may be required. Interrupted or running sutures of 3-0 polyglactin 910 on a RB-1 or SH needle are placed posteriorly at 6 o'clock to narrow the caliber of the bladder neck. 3-0 Poliglecaprone 25 (Monocryl-Ethicon) sutrue may also be used as a continuous suture for this reconstruction. The fourth arm can hold the distal end of the suture of the running suture to ensure that the suture line remains watertight.

For the vesicourethral anastomosis we use a modification of the technique of Van Velthoven et al. *(19)* Two 3-0 poliglecaprone 25 sutures on RB-1 or SH needles are used for the anastomosis, one dyed and one undyed. Each suture is cut to 7 in. in length and their ends tied together to create a double-armed suture with a total length of 12 in. If the bladder neck is large and a parachute technique will be employed without formal reconstruction of the bladder neck, the combined suture length can be increased to 14 in.

We begin with the dyed suture by taking a bite outside-in on the bladder at the 7 o'clock position, followed by an inside-out throw at the corresponding position on the urethral stump. This is repeated once, advancing clockwise on the bladder neck and urethra. Passing the needle through the urethra is facilitated by one of the bedside assistants applying perineal pressure with a hand on the sterile drapes, and the other assistant maneuvering the catheter so that the tip moves in and out of the urethral stump. After two or three throws have been completed with the dyed suture, two throws through the bladder and urethra are performed using the undyed suture, starting at 5 o'clock and progressing slightly counter-clockwise. The bladder and urethra are now apposed by gently cinching down the dyed and

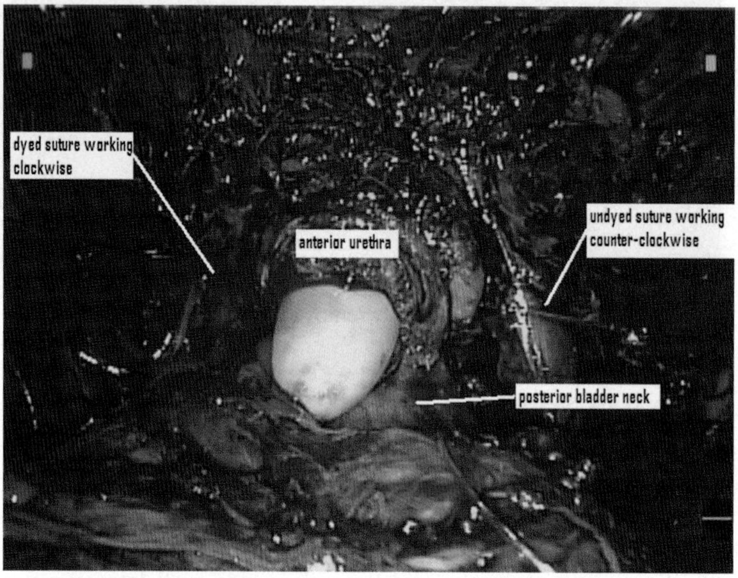

Fig. 33. The vesicourethral anastomosis is cinched down after completing two throws with each needle.

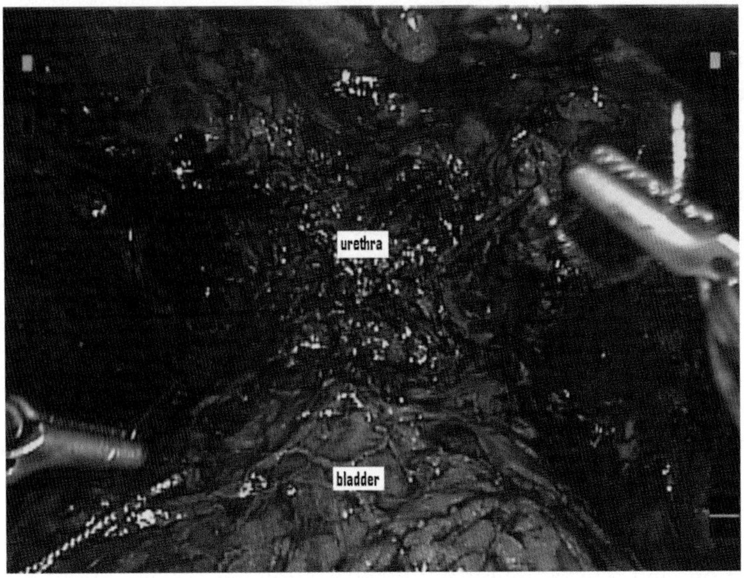

Fig. 34. The completed anastomosis.

undyed arms of the suture (Fig. 33). Suturing resumes with the dyed arm, progressing clockwise to approximately the 12 o'clock position. The undyed suture then completes the anastomosis, proceeding counterclockwise until the two arms of the suture are juxtaposed on the urethral side and a knot is tied (Fig. 34). Just prior to tying the knot, a new 18 Fr or 16 Fr Foley catheter with a 5 cc balloon is placed by the assistant and 10 cc of sterile water injected into the balloon.

After the anastomosis is complete, the catheter is pushed in so that the tip is in the dome of the bladder. The assistant inflates the bladder with 150 cc of sterile saline while the surgeon inspects the anastomosis for any evidence of leak. If no leak is visualized, we generally do not place a closed suction drain. The assistant uses a hand held laparoscopic needle driver to place the string of the specimen bag back into the abdomen through the most lateral right-sided port.

Specimen Removal and Closure

The surgeon can now leave the console and scrub to assist with specimen removal and closure. The robotic instruments and telescope are removed and the robotic arms disconnected from the trocars. The robot is then pulled away from the patient. The robotic telescope is inserted by hand into the most lateral right-sided 12 mm port. A needle driver is inserted through the center 12 mm port, grasps the end of the specimen bag string, and pulls it outside of the patient. If a drain is desired, a Jackson–Pratt or Blake drain can be inserted through the most lateral left-sided port, the trocar removed, and the drain secured to the skin with 2-0 silk. The remaining trocars are removed under laparoscopic vision. The umbilical incision is widened with bovie cautery to remove the prostate within the specimen bag. The anterior rectus fascia is then closed with a running 0-polydioxanone suture on a CT-2 needle. All incisions are then irrigated with sterile saline. We close the umbilical incision with a running subcuticular suture of 4-0 poliglecaprone 25 on a PS-2 needle. The remaining incisions are closed with a cyanoacrylate skin adhesive such as Indermil (US Surgical) or Dermabond (Ethicon), which is also used over the umbilical incision in lieu of sterile strips.

Post-operative Care

Patients are admitted overnight and receive intravenous fluid, clear liquid diet, prophylactic antibiotics, and oral analgesics. Sequential compression stockings are used for DVT prophylaxis while the patient is in bed. Ambulation is encouraged on the evening of surgery, and required on the morning after. Patients are advanced to a regular diet on the day after surgery and discharged home. Discharge medications include oral analgesics and a stool softener. They return to the office approximately 1 week after surgery for a cystogram, after which the Foley catheter is removed if no leak is detected. We now use cystograms selectively depending upon the integrity of the anastomosis.

Variations in Technique

Many different techniques have been described for both RALP and LRP. We have described a transperitoneal approach, which is currently the most popular technique for RALP. However, an extraperitoneal approach for RALP has been described, first in 2003 by Gettman and colleagues *(20)*. Advantages to extraperitoneal surgery include no contact with bowel and less ileus, no adhesiolysis required for patients with previous abdominal surgery, and a shorter distance to the operative field for obese patients. Advantages to transperitoneal surgery include a larger operative field, less risk of lymphocele formation, and a more mobilized bladder allowing for less anastomotic tension *(21)*. A large series of patients having RALP with an extraperitoneal technique show results similar to the transperitoneal technique *(22)*.

Another approach to a transperitoneal RALP is a variation of the Montsouris technique described for LRP, involving an initial posterior dissection *(23)*. The bladder is retracted anteriorly and a transverse incision made over the lower peritoneal arch. The vasa deferentia and seminal vesicles are dissected and Denonvillier's fascia incised exposing perirectal fat. When the remaining posterior dissection is complete, an inverted U-shaped peritoneal incision is made anterior to the bladder, and the remaining anterior dissection proceeds as described above. Starting with the posterior dissection may have a benefit for patients with very large prostates in whom identification of the proper plane to expose the vasa and seminal vesicles after dividing the posterior bladder neck can be difficult.

Multiple techniques have been described to improve preservation of the NVBs. Menon and colleagues have described preservation of the prostatic fascia as an important aspect of successful nerve sparing. Important steps in their "veil of Aphrodite" nerve-sparing surgery include: not ligating the DVC and not opening the endopelvic fascia to reduce traction on the nerves as the prostatic fascia is dissected off the prostatic capsule, no monopolar cautery near the NVBs or the tips of the SV, and not ligating the pedicles en masse but coagulating individual arterioles with bipolar cautery *(24)*. A similar antegrade technique, using only bipolar coagulation and avoiding clips and monopolar coagulation, has been described with comparable results *(25)*. Ahlering et al. found a significant improvement in return to erectile function by clamping the prostatic vascular pedicles with laparoscopic bulldog clamps and suturing for hemostasis rather than using bipolar coagulation *(26)*.

Adequate continence is generally the norm after both RALP and RRP. Some steps that have been suggested to improve continence after RALP include preservation of the puboprostatic ligaments, bladder neck sparing, and maintaining a long urethral stump *(27)*. However, one study of urethral stump length showed no effect on continence after RALP *(28)*. The most important steps to preserve continence are likely precise dissection of the levator ani and striated sphincter away from the urethra, avoiding monopolar coagulation, and minimizing bipolar cautery near the apex and sphincter *(21)*.

Reconstruction of the posterior musculofascial plate before the vesicourethral anastomosis has been described. This step could help improve continence rates after surgery. It includes suturing of the proximal edge of the Denonvilliers fascia and the posterior bladder wall just proximal to the bladder neck margin to the distal edge of the Denonvillier's fascia and the posterior aspect of the rhabdosphincter (posterior musculofascial plate anterior to rectum) with a running 3/0 Monocryl suture.

Table 2
Early results after robotic-assisted laparoscopic radical prostatectomy

Authors	*No. of pts.*	*EBL (ml)*	*OR time (min)*	*LOS (days)*	*Catheter (days)*	*Positive margin: all/pT2 only (%)*	*Continence*	*Intercourse*
Zorn *(4)*	300	273	282	1.4	5.9	20.9/15.1	90% 12 mo	80% 12 mo
Patel *(34)*	500	50	130	NA	6.9	9.4/2.5	95% 6 mo	NA
Kaul *(24)*	154	111	122	1.1	7.2	6.4/4.6	97% 12 mo	96% 12 mo
Borin *(28)*	200	109	NA	1.0	NA	7.5/2.8	97% 6 mo	NA

EBL, estimated blood loss; LOS, length of stay; NA, data not available mo, months.

Results

Multiple series at individual institutions comparing RALP to open RRP have shown that robotic patients have less blood loss, less pain, and a reduced length of hospitalization *(29,30)* (See Table 2). However, the increasing use of RALP has resulted in clinical pathways that have also reduced the length of hospitalization after open surgery to an equivalent duration *(31,32)*. And given that pain scores are generally low after both RALP and RRP, some authors have questioned whether the pain improvement with RALP is clinically significant *(33)*. Long-term data regarding cancer-specific and overall survival are currently unavailable for patients after RALP. However, initial results with pathological outcomes, mainly positive margin rates, seem comparable to the open RRP *(4,24,28,29,30,34)*.

There also do not seem to be any important differences between RALP and LRP when performed by a skilled surgeon *(35,36)*. The potential for improved results with RALP compared to both RRP and LRP certainly exists, though confirmation would require further study.

TAKE HOME MESSAGES

1. LRP and RALP can be safely performed with early results comparable to open surgery. However, the LRP procedure requires advanced laparoscopic skills and has a steep learning curve.
2. Intracorporeal suturing skills may be developed and refined in the pelvic trainer to help decrease operating time during the early experience.
3. Less blood loss, better pain control, shorter hospitalization, and shorter convalescence are potential advantages of laparoscopic versus open surgery.
4. Precise dissection and avoiding electrosurgical coagulation in the vicinity of the neurovascular bundles and apical/urethral dissection will give the best results regarding continence and potency.
5. Robotic assistance should be used, if available.

REFERENCES

1. Schuessler WW, Schulam PG, Clayman RV, Kavoussi LR. Laparoscopic radical prostatectomy: initial short-term experience. Urol 50: 854–857, 1997.
2. Guillonneau B, Cathelineau X, Barret E, Rozet F, Vallancien G. Laparoscopic radical prostatectomy. Preliminary evaluation after 28 interventions. Presse Med 27: 1570–1574, 1998.
3. Shrivastava A, Baliga M, Menon M. The Vattikuti Institute prostatectomy. BJU Int 99: 1173–1189, 2007.
4. Zorn KC, Gofrit ON, Orvieto MA, Mikhail AA, Zagaja GP, Shalhav AL. Robotic-assisted laparoscopic prostatectomy: functional and pathological outcomes with interfascial nerve preservation. Eur Urol: 51: 755–763, 2007.
5. Guillonneau B, Rozet F, Barret E, Cathelineau X, Vallancien G. Laparoscopic radical prostatectomy: assessment after 240 procedures. Urol Clin North Am 28: 189–202, 2001.
6. Erdogru T, Teber D, Frede T, Marrero R, Hammady A, Seemann O, et al. Comparison of transperitoneal and extraperitoneal laparoscopic radical prostatectomy using matched-pair analysis. Eur Urol 46: 312–320, 2004.
7. Bollens R, Vanden Bossche M, Roumeguere T, Damoun A, Zlotta AR, Schulam CC. Laparoscopic radical prostatectomy: analysis of the first series of extraperitoneal approach. J Urol 165 (suppl.): abstract 1354, 2001.
8. Guillonneau B, El-Fettouh H, Baumert H, Cathelineau X, Doublet JD, Fromont G, et al. Laparoscopic radical prostatectomy: oncological evaluation after 1000 cases at Montsouris Institute. J Urol 169: 1261–1266, 2003.
9. Rassweiler J, Schulze M, Teber D, Marrero R, Seemann O, Rumpelt J, et al. Laparoscopic radical prostatectomy with the Heilbronn technique: oncological results in the first 500 patients. J Urol 173: 761–764, 2005.
10. Abbou C, Salomon L, Hoznek A, Antiphon P, Cicco A, Saint F, et al. Laparoscopic radical prostatectomy: preliminary results. Urology 55: 630–664, 2000.
11. Zippe CD, Meraney AM, Sung GT, Gill IS. Laparoscopic radical prostatectomy in the USA. Cleveland Clinic experience, series of 50 patients. J Urol 165 (suppl.): abstract 1341, 2001.
12. Guillonneau B, Vallancien G. Laparoscopic radical prostatectomy: the Montsouris technique. J Urol 163: 1643–1649, 2000.
13. Bhayani SB, Pavlovich CP, Hsu TS, Sullivan W, Su LM. Prospective comparison of short-term convalescence: laparoscopic radical prostatectomy versus open radical retropubic prostatectomy. Urology 61: 612–616, 2003.
14. Rassweiler J, Seemann O, Schulze M, Teber D, Hatzinger M, Frede T. Laparoscopic versus open radical prostatectomy: a comparative study at a single institution. J Urol 169: 1689–1693, 2003.

15. Tooher R, Swindle P, Woo H, Miller J, Maddern G. Laparoscopic radical prostatectomy for localized prostate cancer: a systematic review of comparative studies. J Urol 175: 2011–2017, 2006.
16. Sulser T, Guillonneau B, Vallancien G, Gaston R, Piechaud T, Turk I, et al. Complications and initial experience with 1228 laparoscopic radical prostatectomies at 6 European centers. J Urol 165 (suppl.): abstract 615, 2001.
17. Walsh PC. The status of radical prostatectomy in the United States in 1993: where do we go from here? J Urol 152: 1816, 1994.
18. Olsson LE, Salomon L, Nadu A, Hoznek A, Cicco A, Saint F, et al. Prospective patient-reported continence after laparoscopic radical prostatectomy. Urology 58: 570–572, 2001.
19. Van Velthoven RF, Ahlering TE, Peltier A, Skarecky DW, Clayman RV: Technique for laparoscopic urethrovesical anastomosis: the single knot method. Urology 61: 699–702, 2003.
20. Gettman MT, Hoznek A, Salomon L, Katz R, Borkowski T, et al. Laparoscopic radical prostatectomy: description of the extraperitoneal approach using the da Vinci robotic system. J Urol 170: 416–419, 2003.
21. Rassweiler J, Hruza M, Teber D, Su L. Laparoscopic and robotic-assisted radical prostatectomy – critical analysis of the results. Eur Urol 49: 612–624, 2006.
22. Joseph JV, Rosenbaum R, Madeb R, Erturk E, Patel HRH. Robotic extraperitoneal radical prostatectomy: an alternative approach. J Urol 175: 945–950, 2006.
23. Wolfram M, Bräutigam R, Engl T, Bentas W, Heitkamp S, et al. Robotic-assisted laparoscopic radical prostatectomy: the Frankfurt technique. World J Urol 21: 128–132, 2003.
24. Kaul S, Savera A, Badani K, Fumo M, Bhandari A, Menon M. Functional outcomes and oncological efficacy of Vattikuti Institute prostatectomy with veil of Aphrodite nerve-sparing: an analysis of 154 consecutive patients. BJU Int 97: 467–472, 2005.
25. Chien GW, Mikhail AA, Orvieto MA, Zagaja GP, Sokoloff MH, et al. Modified clipless antegrade nerve preservation in robotic-assisted laparoscopic radical prostatectomy with validated sexual function evaluation. Urology 66: 419–423, 2005.
26. Ahlering TE. Eichel L. Skarecky D. Rapid communication: early potency outcomes with cautery-free neurovascular bundle preservation with robotic laparoscopic radical prostatectomy. J Endourol 19: 715–718, 2005.
27. Menon M, Hemal AK, Tewari A, Shrivastava A, Bhandari A. The technique of apical dissection of the prostate and urethrovesical anastomosis in robotic radical prostatectomy. BJU Int 93: 715–719, 2004.
28. Borin JF, Skarecky DW, Narula N, Ahlering TE. Impact of urethral stump length on continence and positive surgical margins in robot-assisted laparoscopic prostatectomy. Urology 70: 173–177, 2007.
29. Ahlering TE, Woo D, Eichel L, Lee DI, Edwards R, Skarecky DW. Robot-assisted versus open radical prostatectomy: a comparison of one surgeon's outcomes. Urology 63: 819–822, 2004.
30. Tewari A, Srivasatava A, Menon M. A prospective comparison of radical retropubic and robot-assisted prostatectomy: experience in one institution. BJU Int 92: 205–10, 2003.
31. Nelson B, Kaufman M, Broughton G, Cookson MS, Chang SS, et al. Comparison of length of hospital stay between radical retropubic prostatectomy and robotic assisted laparoscopic prostatectomy. J Urol 177: 929–931, 2007.
32. Kaufman MR, Smith JA, Baumgartner RG, Wells N, Chang SS, et al. Positive influence of robotically assisted laparoscopic prostatectomy on the collaborative-care pathway for open radical prostatectomy. BJU Int 97: 473–475, 2005.
33. Webster TM, Herrell SD, Chang SS, Cookson MS, Baumgartner RG, et al. Robotic assisted laparoscopic radical prostatectomy versus retropubic radical prostatectomy: a prospective assessment of postoperative pain. J Urol 174: 912–914, 2005.
34. Patel VR, Thaly R, Shah K. Robotic radical prostatectomy: outcomes of 500 cases BJU Int 99: 1019–1012, 2007.
35. Joseph JV, Vicente I, Madeb R, Erturk E, Patel HRH. Robot-assisted vs pure laparoscopic radical radical prostatectomy: are there any differences? BJU Int 96: 39–42, 2005.
36. Rozet F, Jaffe J, Braud G, Harmon J, Cathelineau X, et al. A direct comparison of robotic assisted versus pure laparoscopic radical prostatectomy: a single institution experience. J Urol 178: 478–482, 2007.

Complications of Laparoscopic Urologic Surgery

Gyan Pareek and Timothy D. Moon

INTRODUCTION

The role of laparoscopy in the field of urology has continued to evolve over the last decade with the ever increasing complexity of operations performed. This chapter will summarize reported complications and provide a concise summary and clinical pathway to prevent, identify, and manage complications associated with laparoscopic urologic surgery.

Interestingly, there is a lack of standardization for defining and categorizing complications in the urologic literature, thus making comparison of one series with another more difficult. Of the various series analyzed in this chapter some series defined major and others minor complication rates (Table 1). Some studies generalized complications, while others specified each complication. Demographic data were documented poorly, often not describing the sub-group of patients with complications. The difficulty in assimilating this non-standardized data were challenging, even though inclusion criteria were utilized to collect the data available from the series with at least a 20 case experience. Of the various series, those included in this chapter reported complications as part of their overall urologic

Table 1
Complications rates (%) by procedure type

Complications by procedure			
Procedure	*Number*	*Major comp. (%)*	*Minor comp. (%)*
LRN (15,21–25,27,29,31,37–39,42,43)	1,746	10.7	3.3
HALRN (22,25,32,33,35,38,40,50)	204	9.3	3.4
LPN (45,46)	591	21.0	2.0
HALPN (48)	30	3.3	0
LDN (18,26,28,36,47)	1,386	10.6	0.5
HALDN (17,26,30,41)	274	7.7	2.6
LNU (16,34,44,49)	133	18.8	2.3
LSN (19,20,23,37)	300	13.7	5.7
RLN (20–22,24)	195	11.3	0.5

Abbreviations: LRN, laparoscopic radical nephrectomy; HALRN, hand-assisted laparoscopic radical nephrectomy; LPN, laparoscopic partial nephrectomy; HALPN, hand-assisted laparoscopic partial nephrectomy; LDN, laparoscopic donor nephrectomy; HALDN, hand-assisted laparoscopic donor nephrectomy; LSN, laparoscopic simple nephrectomy; LNU, laparoscopic nephroureterectomy; RLN, retroperitoneal laparoscopic nephrectomy.

From: *Current Clinical Urology: Essential Urologic Laparoscopy*
Edited by: S. Y. Nakada and S. P. Hedican, DOI 10.1007/978-1-60327-820-1_19

laparoscopic experience, with the greatest experience gained from the laparoscopic renal surgery data. Complications associated with robot-assisted surgery are also summarized in this chapter. Specifically, data on robot-assisted laparoscopic radical prostatectomy (RALRP) will be the focal point as this procedure represents approximately 95% of all robot-assisted laparoscopic procedures performed.

PREOPERATIVE PLANNING

This area may be divided into anesthetic considerations, patient positioning, operative field issues, and general considerations. Clearly, the first step in treating complications is their prevention.

Patients with pulmonary dysfunction are at high risk for complications and screening with pulmonary function tests (PFT's) is important in these patients. Cardiovascular side effects may also result from pneumoperitoneum as preload volume to the right atrium may be decreased from the compressive effects of the pneumoperitoneum on the vena cava. The decreased cardiac output resulting is compounded by the increased afterload due to the compressive effects of the pneumoperitoneum on the aorta.

Knowledge of the physiologic effects of the pneumoperitoneum are paramount in preventing anesthesia-related complications. Physiological effects on the pulmonary and cardiovascular systems are especially important for the operative and anesthesia team to understand. Laparoscopy utilizes carbon dioxide (CO_2) as the insufflationary gas due to its high diffusion coefficient. Naturally some of this is absorbed, but the high solubility of CO_2 in the blood stream minimizes the risk of gas emboli. All patients who have pulmonary airway disease compromising the ability to exhale CO_2 might require consideration for surgery via another technique. Fortunately, CO_2levels are easily measured at the end of exhalation and the anesthesiologist should constantly measure these levels and adjust the ventilator to remove excess CO_2in order to prevent hypercarbia and acidosis. Additionally, pulmonary compliance is decreased and the functional residual capacity (FRC) is impaired by the pneumoperitoneum and patient positioning. Minute volume may need to be increased in order to correct the ventilation–perfusion mismatch to avoid hypercarbia and acidosis. Optimizing fluid status by preoperative intravascular volume expansion can avoid deleterious complications. Cardiac arrhythmias may also occur in 27% of patients during laparoscopy, commonly due to increased vagal tone and hypercarbia *(1)*. Decreasing CO_2 insufflation pressures and hyperventilating the patient, along with antiarrhythmic medications are used in arrhythmia management during laparoscopy. Finally, retroperitoneoscopic procedures lead to a greater risk of hypercarbia than transperitoneal surgery.

Patient Positioning

In a recent review of neuromuscular injuries from a series of 1651 patients from 15 institutions who underwent urologic laparoscopic surgery, there were 46 injuries in 45 patients (2.7%) *(2)*. Injuries were twice as common with upper abdominal procedures compared with pelvic procedures. Abdominal wall neuralgia occurred in 0.8% of patients, sensory deficits in 0.7%, and motor deficits in 0.7% *(2)*. Shoulder and back pain occurred in 0.2 and 0.1%, respectively. Rhabdomyolysis occurred in six patients (0.4%) *(2)*. This entity seems to occur in longer procedures and with heavier, more muscular male patients. The lesson to be learned from this report is that patient positioning and protective padding is extremely important and should not be delegated to others, but should at least be reviewed by the surgeon at the start of the procedure.

Many laparoscopic procedures are fairly long in duration and this is especially true when the surgeon is developing new procedures. The possibility of neuromuscular injury becomes more likely with increasing surgical duration, making it extremely important, that attention be paid to patient padding and support. Furthermore, if the patient is likely to be rotated in one direction or another during the case, new pressure points that did not exist when the patient was in the original position are created. These possibilities must be considered with appropriately padded support applied prior to the surgery. For example, when we perform laparoscopic nephrectomy in the flank position, we use a 3-in. mattress pad. The kidney rest is minimally elevated because elevation may compromise renal blood flow. Table break is limited and an axillary roll is placed. To protect the patient when rolled from side to side, we place a 6-in. gel pad behind their back for support when rolled toward their back.

Operative Field

Previous surgery does not specifically preclude a laparoscopic approach but the potential scarring and associated adhesions from prior surgery may necessitate altering one's approach. For example, if a patient has had multiple abdominal surgeries and now requires a nephrectomy, then the retroperitoneal approach might be preferred. Conversely, if the patient requires an operation to be performed by the transperitoneal route and the patient has had previous abdominal surgery, then using the Veress needle technique for abdominal insufflation may run the risk of bowel injury. As such it may be preferable to use an open "Hassan" technique to obtain access to the abdomen (see Chapter "Laparoscopic Access").

General Considerations

When transperitoneal procedures are being performed and the bowel needs to be mobilized (e.g., nephrectomy), we routinely give the patient a mechanical bowel preparation with magnesium citrate or Golytely. This seems to help postoperative recovery and also in decompressing the bowel, which avoids visual obstruction of the operative field by dilated bowel.

COMPLICATIONS OF ACCESS AND PORT PLACEMENT

The laparoscopic urologic surgeon must understand the potential complications of establishing the pneumoperitoneum and placing trocars. The most common method for abdominal insufflation is through the use of the Veress needle technique (see Chapter "Laparoscopic Access"). It is a blind technique with a reported vascular or bowel complication rate between 0.03 and 0.3% *(3)*. Crucial anatomical considerations include the location of the aorta and iliac vessels near the umbilicus, an anatomical landmark often used as the initial point of entry. Once the needle is inserted, it should be aspirated to ensure no return of visceral fluid and then injected with saline. The "drop test" will confirm that saline will flow into the peritoneal cavity. If abdominal entry becomes difficult, perhaps because of inadvertent insufflation of the abdominal wall itself, then reversion to the Hassan technique may be required (see Chapter "Laparoscopic Access"). This essentially turns a blind needle puncture into a microlaparotomy. This technique may also be chosen from the outset for patients who have had prior abdominal surgery. The first port is placed after insufflation. Historically, this has been placed blindly using bladed trocars. These trocars have two problems: first, they are placed blindly with the potential risk to abdominal contents; and second, the cutting blades may cause vascular injury and significant abdominal wall bleeding. In order to avoid these problems, we currently use Optiview trocars (Ethicon, Cincinnati, OH). These trocars have blunt plastic "blades" that separate the tissues without cutting them. Additionally, by having a clear plastic tip, the telescope and camera may be placed within the port allowing the surgeon to "look his or her way" into the abdomen. In the event that the bowel or a major blood vessel is injured at entry, immediate laparotomy will likely be required to repair the injury.

OPERATIVE COMPLICATIONS

Abdominal Surgery

Operative complications may be recognized immediately, or may be identified later, in which case they will be included as postoperative complications. Overall, the intraoperative complication rates from various contemporary series are from 2.9 to 4.5% *(4)*. Vascular injuries were the most common at 1.4% *(4–5)*. Bowel injuries were the next most common at 0.6% (0.2–0.9). Ureteral injuries were a rare but important complication at 0.3%. The conversion rate was noted to be 1.1%. The complexity of the cases included in these series was quite varied, ranging from varicocelectomy to adrenalectomy. Likewise, the total complication rates varied from 0% for simple procedures such as varicocelectomy to 13.6% for adrenal surgery *(4–7)*. Several reports have addressed specific complications. Pneumothorax has been reported at low but persistent levels (0.3%) *(5)*. The pneumothorax itself may not be recognized surgically but by anesthetic problems such as elevated ventilatory pressures and increased CO_2 levels. Pneumothoraces are most likely to be associated with upper abdominal laparoscopy. When mobilizing the liver or spleen, appropriate attention must be made to the possibility of creating a pneumothorax by diaphragmatic injury.

One of the most devastating complications that can occur is the malfunction of an Endovascular-stapling device, reported to be less than 1% *(4–9)*. Most commonly this is a preventable complication usually occurring because of stapling over clips. It is obvious from these data that care must be taken when clipping vessels when the location is in proximity to areas which will likely require vascular stapling. Other options such as merely dividing the vessel with a harmonic scalpel or ligasure device may be adequate, or even stapling the vessel if larger. Generally stapling over staples is satisfactory.

Renal Surgery

A recent metanalysis categorized complications as physiologic, access-related, intra-operative, and postoperative *(10)*. Physiologic complications occurred during prolonged pneumoperitoneum and had an effect on the cardiovascular, pulmonary, and renal systems (Tables 2 and 3). Access-related complications were rare with reported rates less than 0.5% *(10)*. Intraoperative complications in order of frequency were hemorrhage (1.4%), bowel injury (<0.5%), solid organ injury (<0.5%), diaphragmatic injury (<0.5%), and neuromuscular injury (<0.5%) *(10)*. Postoperative complications most commonly

Table 2
Types of complications (>0.5%) in various hand-assisted nephrectomy series

Type	*Number*	*Types of complications*
HALDN *(17,26,30,41)*	274	Wound infection (2.2%), arterial (1.8%), ileus (1.1%), conversion to open (0.7%), incisional hernia (0.7%), deep vein thrombosis (0.7%)
HALPN *(48)*	30	Urinoma (3.3%)
HALRN *(22,25,32,33,35,38,40,50)*	204	Venous bleeding (0.5%), arterial bleeding (1.0%), small intestinal injury (0.5%), incisional hernia (0.5%), conversion to open (2.9%), transfusion rate (2%), wound infection (1.5%), orchalgia (0.5%), ileus (2.5%), UTI (0.5%)

Abbreviations: LRN, laparoscopic radical nephrectomy; HALRN, hand-assisted laparoscopic radical nephrectomy; LPN, laparoscopic partial nephrectomy; HALPN, hand-assisted laparoscopic partial nephrectomy; LDN, laparoscopic donor nephrectomy; HALDN, hand-assisted laparoscopic donor nephrectomy; LSN, laparoscopic simple nephrectomy; LNU, laparoscopic nephroureterectomy; RLN, retroperitoneal laparoscopic nephrectomy.

Table 3
Types of complications (>0.5%) in standard laparoscopic series

Type	*Number*	*Types of complications*
LRN *(15,21–25,27,29,31, 37–39,42,43)*	1,746	Venous bleeding (1.8%), arterial bleeding (1.0%), splenic injury (0.5%), small intestinal injury (0.6%), colonic injury (1.5%), conversion to open (2.5%), transfusion rate (0.7%), ileus (1%)
LPN *(45,46)*	591	Cardiac dysrhythmias (1.5%), renal failure (1%), deep vein thrombosis (0.5%), device failure (0.5%), venous injury (0.8%), arterial injury (1.7%), conversion to open (1.9%), transfusion rate (4.4%), wound infection (0.7%), retroperitoneal hematoma (0.8%), urinoma (3.9%), ureteral injury (0.5%), reoperation rate (1.4%)
LDN *(18,26,28,36,47)*	1,386	Device failure (1.2%), vascular injury (0.9%), venous bleeding (1.7%), arterial bleeding (1.2%), splenic injury (1.3%), conversion to open (1.5%), transfusion rate (0.6%)
LNU *(16,34,44,49)*	133	Deep vein thrombosis (1.5%), visceral injury (0.8%), neural injury (0.8%), arterial bleeding (1.5%), small intestinal injury (2.3%), incisional hernia (0.8%), conversion to open (2.3%)
LSN *(19,20,23,37)*	300	Cardiac dysrhythmias (0.7%), renal failure (1%), deep vein thrombosis (0.5%), venous injury (1.7%), arterial injury (0.7%), incisional hernia (0.8%), conversion to open (3.7%), retroperitoneal hematoma (0.7%), ileus (2%), UTI (1.7%)
RLN *(20,21,22,24)*	195	Device failure (1%), venous bleeding (1.5%), arterial bleeding (1%), colonic injury (1.5%), conversion to open (1.5%), transfusion rate (0.5%), wound infection (1%), retroperitoneal hematoma (1%)

Abbreviations: LRN, laparoscopic radical nephrectomy; HALRN, hand-assisted laparoscopic radical nephrectomy; LPN, laparoscopic partial nephrectomy; HALPN, hand-assisted laparoscopic partial nephrectomy; LDN, laparoscopic donor nephrectomy; HALDN, hand-assisted laparoscopic donor nephrectomy; LSN, laparoscopic simple nephrectomy; LNU, laparoscopic nephroureterectomy; RLN, retroperitoneal laparoscopic nephrectomy.

reported were ileus (1.5%), bowel obstruction (<0.5%), herniation (<0.5%), deep vein thrombosis (0.7%), and urinary retention (<0.5%) *(10)*.

As expected, hemorrhage was the most common intraoperative complication. Interestingly, no air emboli were reported in the literature review. There was a higher complication rate associated with laparoscopic partial nephrectomy (LPN) (21%), which is possibly attributable to the steep learning curve of the procedure at the time of the study *(10)*. The significance of the difference in major and minor complication rates observed between LPN and hand-assisted laparoscopic partial nephrectomy (HALPN) is difficult to ascertain because lesion selection may have influenced the complication rate in the single available HALPN report. Furthermore, the paucity of reported minor complications in the literature limits the interpretation of the data. As data from other HALPN series emerge, complication rates may change as more surgeons perform the approach, and selection criteria changes.

Although the overall complication rates for laparoscopic radical nephrectomy (LRN) and hand-assisted laparoscopic radical nephrectomy (HALRN) are not statistically different (10.7 and 9.3%), there was a significant difference in the wound infection rate between HALRN (1.5%) and LRN (0.2%) ($p = 0.02$) *(10)*. As observed with the radical nephrectomy data, the wound infection rate was significantly higher in the hand-assisted laparoscopic donor nephrectomy (HALDN) series (2.2%) versus the laparoscopic donor nephrectomy (LDN) series (<0.5%) *(10)*. Certainly, the incision edges during hand-assisted laparoscopic surgery can undergo varying levels of injury depending on the surgeon and time required to perform the procedure. Nonetheless, this is a potential complication which should be related to the patient.

EXITING THE FIELD

As with all surgery, "drying up" before closure is an important part of the operation, and without which complications may occur. Laparoscopic procedures also require this process but with a slightly different technique from open procedures. If vascular staples/clips have been used to secure vessels, then the stumps should be inspected. Because the pneumoperitoneum itself may compress veins, it is important to lower the pressure to 5 mmHg during the several minutes of wound inspection. Port-site closure requires special attention. The original port devices all utilized cutting blades to penetrate the abdominal wall. This has the potential for two problems. First, it is possible to injure abdominal wall blood vessels, and second, the division of muscular fibers increases the risk for port-site hernias. More recently, port trocars have been introduced with plastic blades which are designed to separate the tissues rather than divide them. In their original marketing, it was suggested that formal fascial closure was not necessary. However, we have had one port-site hernia in more than 200 procedures using this device. As a result of this, and the experience of others, we recommend that all 10-mm port sites have a facial closure. To do this, we place a fascial stitch under laparoscopic guidance using one of the available closure devices (Fig. 1). After placing the stitches, $CO_2$is evacuated and the skin closed. If incisions have been made for hand assistance or specimen removal, they are closed using a standard open surgical approach.

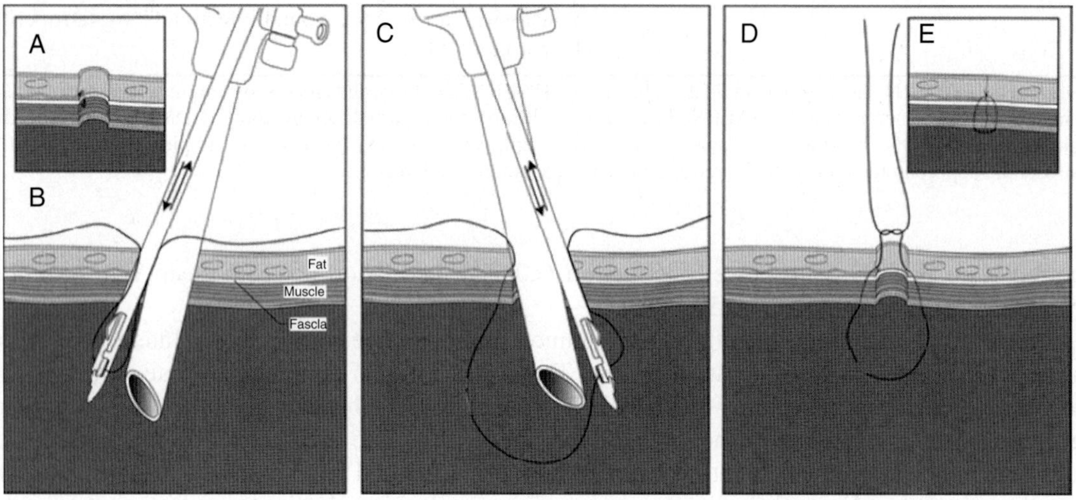

Fig. 1. (**A**) Port site showing injured blood vessel. (**B**) Placement of suture through fascia and including injured blood vessel. (**C**) Tying of knot closes port site and also ligates blood vessel.

POSTOPERATIVE COMPLICATIONS

The large series reported by Fahlenkamp et al. specifically identified that complication rates were directly linked to the complexity of the case. Simple cases like varicocelectomy had 0.8–1.3% complication rates, whereas complex cases such as adrenalectomy and nephrectomy had complication rates of 8.2–13.6% *(6)*. Likewise, reintervention rates for these groups ranged from 0 to 2.7% *(6)*.

Overall, the postoperative complication rates ranged from 1.7 to 26.1% *(6)*. Interestingly, the highest rate recorded was for the hand-assisted laparoscopic group. However, this group of authors included many items that would not be included in the complication list of other authors. Re-operation rates varied from 0.6 to 3.1% *(6)*. The group reporting a 3.1% re-operation rate did not report any other postoperative complications. Postoperative bleeding is a rare but persistent problem being reported, ranging from 0.5 to 2%. This complication emphasizes the importance of evaluating the operative field at low pressure prior to exiting the wound. Wound infections are in line with open surgery, being reported between 0.4 and 1.5% *(6)*. Nerve injuries are uncommon at up to 1%, but serve to demonstrate the importance of patient positioning and padding prior to initiating the procedure. Port-site hernias have been reported in up to 1% of cases. It is likely that this rate will decrease in the future with a greater recognition of the problem and the routine closure of 10-mm port sites (Fig. 1). Additionally, the use of non-cutting trocars will aid in reducing this problem.

POSTOPERATIVE MANAGEMENT

Over the past decade, there has been a major decrease in the postoperative hospital admission length of stay for both open and laparoscopic procedures. The major driving force for these changes has been the cost of healthcare delivery. For most of the last decade, the hospital charges associated with laparoscopy have been markedly in excess of those for open surgery. However, it has now been reported that laparoscopic nephrectomy may be more cost effective than open nephrectomy. A major part of this cost reduction has been the reduction in postoperative hospitalization. Many patients are now being hospitalized on the "23-h admission" basis. This is especially true for retroperitoneal procedures where postoperative discomfort is clearly less than for transabdominal procedures. Thus, most patients are being mobilized soon after surgery; and pain is being effectively controlled with oral analgesia. Post-operative pain is greatest after upper abdominal procedures, and least with retroperitoneal procedures. Recovery times from laparoscopic surgery are also shorter than for open surgery. Finally, because the incisions for laparoscopic procedures are either non-muscle cutting (e.g., Pfannenstiel), muscle splitting, or very small muscle cutting (5–6 cm), patients may increase their physical activities much more rapidly after these surgeries than for those open procedures with large muscle-cutting incisions.

ROBOT-ASSISTED LAPAROSCOPY

Complications associated with robot-assisted laparoscopy are prudent to mention as this technology has progressed into the mainstream of modern surgical practice. The main application for robot-assisted surgery is laparoscopic radical prostatectomy with other procedures such as laparoscopic pyeloplasty and laparoscopic renal (total or partial) nephrectomy performed less frequently. Since greater than 95% of robot-assisted surgeries are performed for laparoscopic radical prostatectomy (RALRP), the focus of complication prevention and management will be defined by experiences utilizing this technique.

Patient Positioning and Anesthesia

Principles utilized during traditional laparoscopy, mentioned earlier in this chapter, are critical to adhere to during robot-assisted surgery. The daVinci® robotic surgery system utilized to perform surgery requires proper patient positioning to accommodate the robotic system. Once the system is attached to the trocars, adjustment of the patient's position is very difficult as the robot is locked in a fixed position. During RALRP, anesthesia access with proper line placement is paramount as adjustments later in the procedure may be difficult. A gel foam mat over the operating room table helps prevent sliding of the patient during deep Trendelenburg position, a position required during RALRP.

We utilize a simple bed sheet tucking technique for the arms on the side with the elbows wrapped in gel foam or other padding, preventing ulnar or brachial plexus injury. Furthermore, shoulder straps in an X fashion are utilized to secure the upper torso, taking care not to compromise respirations. The lower extremities are always secured in the stirrups with the patient's heal serving as the pressure point. The calf area is always inspected prior to Trendelenburg position in order to prevent pressure and undue compromise of lower extremity blood flow leading to possible intra- or postoperative deep vein thrombosis. Following these maneuvers the patient's breathing patterns should be assessed in deep Trendelenburg position and attention to the possible adverse effects on the cardiac and pulmonary system caused by insufflation pressures mentioned earlier in the chapter should be avoided.

Complications of RALRP

Besides the patient positioning, anesthetic, entry, and port placement and physiologic complications of pneumoperitoneum already mentioned for laparoscopic surgery, there are few complications associated specifically with the robotic system. During RALRP, complications described in the literature are similar to those experienced with open surgery. As mentioned earlier, summarizing the non-standardized literature is difficult, but an attempt will be made to summarize complication rates based on the larger contemporary series (Table 4). Specifically rectal, thromboembolic, hemorrhagic, and anastomotic leakage complications will be highlighted as other adverse events have previously been discussed in depth.

Table 4
Complications associated with RALRP

Complication	*Brown University (unpublished) (2008)*	*Institut Montsouris (2007) (51)*	*Brigham and Womens (2006) (52)*	*Ohio State University (2006) (53)*	*UC Irvine (2006) (53)*
N	275	133	322	500	300
Rectal injury	1	0	–	2	1
Deep vein thrombosis	2	0	2	–	1
Pulmonary embolism	1	0	0	–	5
Postoperative bleeding	3	3	2	2	1
Transfusion	2	–	5	1	2
Conversion to open	1	–		–	–
Bowel injury	1	–	0	–	–
Anastomotic stricture	1	–	1	1	1

The reported rate of rectal injury during RALRP is 0–0.9% *(11)*. Two potential areas during the procedure which may potentially lead to injury include dissection distal to the vas deferens and seminal vesicles after the posterior bladder neck is divided and during dissection of the recto-urethralis muscle. Electrocautery use in these areas is discouraged as transmission of thermal injury to the rectum and other viscera may result in injury. Certainly, fibrosis and scarring and adherent tissue are likely to be present during such cases. Thus, in difficult cases intraoperative recognition and repair are key principles for a positive outcome. Most rectal injuries that occur are not sizeable and primary closure of the edges in two layers is acceptable. If there is a large defect recognized at the time of surgery with gross fecal spillage, diversion is recommended for good long-term results. In either case, intraoperative general surgical consultation should be sought and a multi-disciplinary approach to this complication should be undertaken. Testing with direct stereoscopic robotic vision along with the injection of air or saline into the rectum should be done to check the integrity of the repair.

Delayed recognition of rectal injury has also been reported. Patients presenting postoperatively with fever, leukocytosis, and peritoneal signs should undergo computed tomography examination with instillation of retrograde rectal contrast to rule out this complication. If rectal contrast extravasation is visualized, immediate general surgical consultation should be obtained for management (Fig. 2).

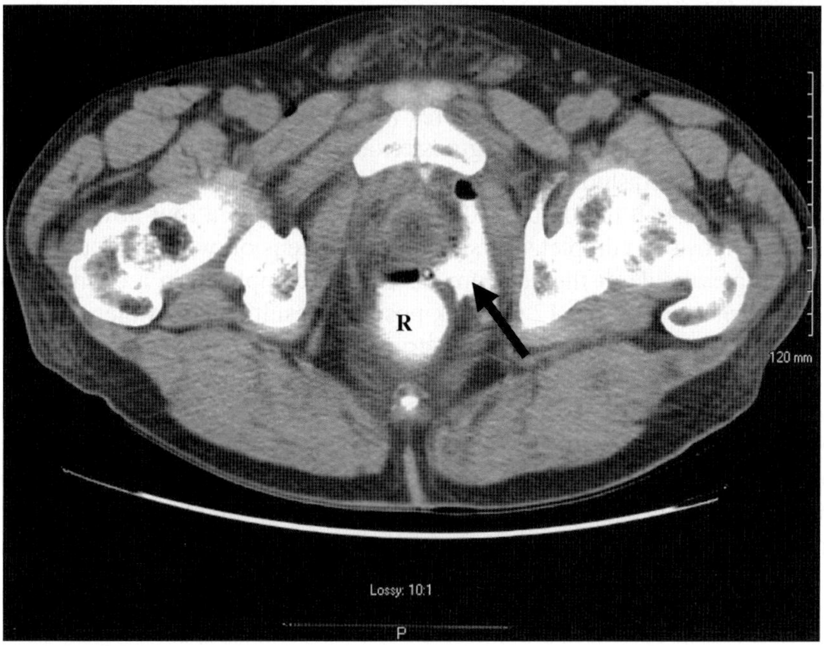

Fig. 2. Computed tomography illustrates contrast extravasation (*arrow*) through the rectum (*R*), recognized as a delayed rectal injury 5 days after RALRP.

Thromboembolic events are always of great concern while performing pelvic surgery. The reported rates of pulmonary embolism and deep vein thrombosis are 0–7.5% in large series *(12)*. During RALRP, the combination of pelvic surgery, prolonged lithotomy position and pneumoperitoneum place the patient at higher risk for such events. Albeit rare, autopsy data after RALRP have confirmed pulmonary embolism as the primary cause of immediate death. Prevention of such disastrous complications is paramount and studies reveal conflicting data on avoiding these complications. Unfractionated subcutaneous heparin preoperatively alone or in combination with compression stockings or sequential compression devices (SCD's) have been all reported to be of possible benefit. At our institution we utilize all three methods, with 5000 IU of unfractionated subcutaneous heparin given preoperatively and intraoperative use of the SCD's and compression stockings. Early ambulation is added postoperatively and has resulted in pulmonary embolism and DVT rates of 0.3 and 1%, respectively.

Significant rates of intraoperative and postoperative bleeding are rare during RALRP. Due to the extreme difficulty of assessing the amount of intraoperative hemorrhage, blood loss should be based on the surgeon's impression intraoperatively as well as intra and post operative physiologic and laboratory parameters. Transfusion rates are reported to be from 0 to 5% *(13)*. In our first 275 cases at Brown University, three patients required transfusion, representing a 1% transfusion rate. Pneumoperitoneum, along with stereoscopic vision of the prostatic anatomy contribute to the rarity of bleeding during and after the procedure. Significant bleeding usually occurs from two primary areas, including the dorsal vein complex (DVC) and epigastric vessels. Prevention, identification, and management of the latter have been discussed earlier and therefore prevention of DVC bleeding will be mentioned. DVC bleeding can be prevented with ligation or stapling (see Chapter "Laparoscopic Radical Prostatectomy").

If intense bleeding is encountered during the procedure, raising the pneumoperitoneum to 20 mmHg may help achieve adequate hemostasis. We routinely utilize bipolar cauterization and thrombin glue to achieve meticulous hemostasis after the prostate has been removed.

Anastomotic leakage can result in prolonged catheterization. We utilize a similar method of anastomosis described by Van Velthoven and collegues *(14)*, which utilizes a running suture with a single knot. The technique is described in depth elsewhere. Rarely, the water-tight closure may result in postoperative leakage with increased postoperative drain outputs. Prevention is the key for a positive outcome and some key points during the procedure are worth mentioning to prevent anastomotic leakage. At our institution, we place four initial sutures with the double armed 3-0 moncryl RB1 needles at the posterior bladder neck and corresponding posterior positions on the posterior urethra. The sutures are then pulled up in a pulley fashion. The direction of the pulling is anterior rather than cranial, avoiding tearing the sutures through the tissue. Additionally, we utilize a four arm robotic system and the left side of the anastomosis is completed first and held on tension with the fourth arm of the robotic system. The contra lateral side of the anastomosis is then completed in a counter-clockwise fashion allowing knot tying anteriorly at the 12 O'clock position, resulting in a water tight closure. Utilizing this technique, we rarely observe postoperative urinary leakage, with 99% of drains removed within 18 h of surgery. All patients have their catheter removed between postoperative day 7 and 10 without a cystogram. It is imperative at the conclusion of the procedure that the Foley catheter be observed entering the bladder. We utilize a three-step process to ensure proper catheter placement as the rare complication of urinary catheter misplacement may be avoided. After a visual confirmation of catheter placement, a balloon roll test (visualization of balloon rolling toward bladder neck with gentle traction) and catheter irrigation with saline confirm proper placement and anastomotic integrity.

SUMMARY

Laparoscopic urologic surgery has evolved to incorporate more complex reconstructive procedures, but the complications associated with these techniques are similar to those for simple procedures. Access during laparoscopy requires careful preoperative planning and knowledge of the underlying anatomy to prevent complications. Intraoperative recognition of vascular or bowel complications are a key factor for ensuring positive outcome. If a complication does occur, early recognition in the postoperative period is crucial since early intervention provides the best chance for decreasing patient morbidity. As with any surgical procedure prevention and recognition are the keys to successful management.

TAKE HOME MESSAGES

Complication rates may be minimized by:

1. Evaluating the patient carefully for appropriateness for a laparoscopic procedure.
2. Paying appropriate attention to patient positioning and padding.
3. Being aware of potential complications so that they will be recognized early (e.g., pneumothorax).
4. Carefully evaluating the operative field at the end of the procedure for hemostasis; under high- and low-insufflation pressures.

REFERENCES

1. Wolf, J.S., Jr. Pathophysiologic effects of prolonged laparoscopic operation. Semin Surg Oncol 12(2):86–95, 1996
2. Wolf, J.S., Jr., Marcovich, R., Gill, I.S., Sung, G.T., Kavoussi, L.R., Clayman, R.V., et al. Survey of neuromuscular injuries to patient and surgeon during urologic laparoscopic surgery. Urology 55:831–836, 2000

3. Shuford, M.D., McDougall, E.M., Chang, S.S., LaFleur, B.J., Smith, Jr., J.A., Cookson, M.S. Complications of contemporary radical nephrectomy: comparison of open vs. laparoscopic approach. Urol Oncol 22:121–126, 2004
4. Gill, I.S., Kovoussi, L.R., Clayman, R.V., Ehrlich, R., Evans, R., Fuchs, G., et al. Complications of laparoscopic nephrectomy in 185 patients: a multi-institutional review. J Urol 154(2):479–483, 1995
5. Permpongkosol, S., Link, R.E., Su, L.M., Romero, F.R., Bagga, H.S., Pavlovich, C.P., Jarrett, J.W., Kavoussi, L.R. Complications of 2,775 urologic laparoscopic procedures 1993 to 2005. J Urol 2007, Feb;177(2):580–585.
6. Fahlenkamp, D., Rassweiler, J., Fornara, P., Frede, T., Loening, S.A. Complications of laparoscopic procedures in urology: Experience with 2,407 procedures a 4 German centers. J Urol 162:765–771, 1999
7. Simon, S.D., Castle, E.P., Ferrigni, R.G., Lamm, D.L., Swnason, S.K., Novicki, D.E., et al. Complications of laparoscopic nephrectomy: The Mayo Clinic experience. J Urol 171:1447–1450, 2004
8. Soulie, M., Seguin, P., Richeux, L., Mouly, P., Vazzoler, N., Pontonnier, F., et al. Urologic complications of laparoscopic surgery: Experience with 350 procedures at a single center. J Urol 165:1960–1963, 2001
9. Siqueira, T.M., Kuo, R.L., Gardner, T.A., Paterson, R.F., Stevens, L.H., Lingeman, J.E., et al. Major complications in 213 laparoscopic nephrectomy cases: The Indianapolis Experience. J Urol 168:1361–1365, 2002
10. Pareek, G, Hedican, S.P., Gee, J, Bruskewitz R.C., Nakada S.Y.: Meta-Analysis of complications of laparoscopic renal surgery: comparison of procedures and techniques. J Urol April;175(4):1208–1213, 2006
11. Costello, A.J., Haxhimolla, H., Crowe, H., et al. Instillation of telerobotic surgery and initial experience of telerobotic prostatectomy, BJU Int 96:34–38, 2005
12. Bhandari, A., McIntire, L., Kaul, S.A., et al. Perioperative complications of laparoscopic radical prostatectomy after learning curve. J Urol 2005;174:915–918
13. Ahlering, T.E., Eichel, L., Edwards, R.A., et al. Robotic radical prostatectomy: a technique to reduce pT2 positive margins. Urology 64:1224–1228, 2004
14. Van Velthoven, R.F., Ahlering, T.E., Peltier, A., et al. Technique for laparoscopic running urethroviscoal anastomosis: the single knot method. Urology 61:699–702, 2003
15. Vallancien, G., Cathelineau, H., Baumert, H., Doublet, J.D., Guillonneau, B. Complications of transperitoneal laparoscopic surgery in urology: review of 1311, procedures at a single center. J Urol 168:23–26, 2002
16. Soulie, M., Salomon, L., Seguin, P., Mervant, C., Mouly, P., Hoznek, A. Multi-institutional study of complications in 1085 laparoscopic urologic procedures. Urology 58:899–903, 2001
17. Kim, F.J., Rha, K.H., Hernandez, F., Jarrett, T.W., Pinto, P.A., Kavoussi, L.R. Laparoscopic radical versus partial nephrectomy: assessment of complications. J Urol 170:408–411, 2003
18. Parsons, J.K., Varkarakis, I, Koon, R.H., Jarrett, T.W., Pinto, P.A., Kavoussi, L.R. Complications of abdominal urologic laparoscopy: longitudinal five-year analysis. Urology 63: 27–32, 2004
19. Armani, A.P., Desai, M.M., Steinberg, A.P., Ng, C.S., Area, S.C., Keokuk, J.H., et al. Complications of laparoscopic partial nephrectomy in 200 cases. J Urol 173: 42–47, 2005
20. Dunn, D.D., Portis, A.J., Shalhav, A.L., Elbahnasy, A.M., Heidorn, C., McDougall, E.M., Clayman, R.V.: Laparoscopic versus open radical nephrectomy: A 9 year experience. J Urol 164:1153–1159, 2000
21. Mcneil, S.A., Chrisofos, M., Tolley, D.A. The long-term outcome after laparoscopic nephroureterectomy: a comparison with open nephroureterectomy. BJU Int 86:619–623, 2000
22. Maartense, S., Idu, M., Bemelman, F.J., Balm, R., Surachno, S., Bemelman, W.A. Hand-assisted laparoscopic live donor nephrectomy. Br J Surg 91:344–348, 2004
23. Nogueira, J.M., Cangro, C.B., Fink, J.C., Schweitzer, E., Wiland, A., Klassen, D.K., et al. A comparison of recipient renal outcomes with laparoscopic versus open live donor nephrectomy. Transplantation 67(5):722–728, 1999
24. Rassweiler, J., Fornara, P., Weber, M., Janetschek, G., Fahlenkamp, D., Henkel, T., et al. Laparoscopic nephrectomy: The experience of the laparoscopy working group of the German Urological Association. J Urol 160(1):18–21, 1998
25. Cicco, A., Salomon, L., Hoznek, A., Saint, F., Alame, W., Gasman, D., et al. Results of retroperitoneal laparoscopic radical nephrectomy. J Endo 15:355–359, 2001
26. Gill, I.S., Schweizer, D., Hobart, M.G., Sung, G.T., Klein, E.A., Novick, A.C. Retroperitoneal laparoscopic radical nephrectomy: The Cleveland clinic experience. J Urol 163:1665–1670, 2000
27. Batler, R.A., Campbell, S.C., Funk, J.T., Gonzalez, C.M., Nadler, R.B. Hand-assisted vs. retroperitoneal laparoscopic nephrectomy. J Endo 15:899–902, 2001
28. Matin, S.F., Abreu, S., Ramani, A., Steinberg, A.P., Desai, M., Strzempkowski, B., et al. Evaluation of age and comorbidity as risk factors after laparoscopic urologic surgery. J Urol 170:1115–1120, 2003
29. Abbou, C.C., Cicco, A., Gasman, D., Hoznek, P., Chopin, D.K., et al. Retroperitoneal laparoscopic versus open radical nephrectomy. J Urol 161:1776–1780, 1999
30. Nelson, C.P., Wolf, Jr., J.S. Comparison of hand-assisted versus standard laparoscopic radical nephrectomy for suspected renal cell carcinoma. J Urol 167:1889–1994, 2002
31. Velidedeoglu, E., Williams, N., Brayman, K.L., Desai, N.M., Campos, L., Palanjian, M. Comparison of open, laparoscopic, and hand-assisted approaches to live donor nephrectomy. Transplantation, 74:169–172, 2002
32. Ono, Y., Kinukawa, T., Hattori, R., Gotoh, M., Kamihira, O., Oshima, S. The long-term outcome of laparoscopic radical nephrectomy for small renal cell carcinoma. J Urol 165:1867–1870, 2001

33. Brown, S.L., Biehl, T.R., Rawlins, M.C., Hefty, T.R.. Laparoscopic live donor nephrectomy: A comparison to the conventional open approach. J Urol, **165**:766–769, 2001
34. Portia, A.J., Yan, Y., Landman, J., Chen, C., Barrett, P.H., Fentie, D.D., et al. Long-term followup after laparoscopic radical nephrectomy. J Urol 167:1257–1262, 2002
35. Stifelman, M.D., Hull, D., Sosa, R.E., Su, L., Hyman, M.M., Stubenbord, W., et al. Hand assisted laparoscopic donor nephrectomy: a comparison with the open approach. J Urol 166:444–448, 2001
36. Ono, Y., Kotah, N., Kinukawa, T., Matsuura, O., Oshima, S. Laparoscopic radical nephrectomy: The Nagoya experience. J Urol 158(3):719–723, 1997
37. Lee, S.E., Ku, J.H., Kwak, C., Kim, H.H., Paick, S.H. Hand assisted laparoscopic radical nephrectomy: comparison with open radical nephrectomy. J Urol 170:756–759, 2003
38. Okeke, A.A., Imoney, A.G., Keeley, Jr., F.X. Hand-assisted nephrectomy: complications related to the hand-port site. BJU Int 90:364–367, 2002
39. Landman, J., Lev, R.Y., Bhayani, S., Alberts, G., Rehman, J., Pattaras, J.G., et al. Comparison of hand assisted and standard laparoscopic radical nephroureterectomy for the management of localized transitional cell carcinoma: J Urol 167:2387–2391, 2002
40. Stifelman, M.D., Handler, T., Niederm A.M., Del Pizzo, J., Taneja, S., Sosa, R.E., et al. Hand-assisted laparoscopy for larger renal specimens: a multi-institutional study. Urology 61:78–82, 2003
41. Boorjian, S., Munver, R., Sosa, R.E., Del Pizzo, J.J. Right laparoscopic live donor nephrectomy: A single institution experience. Transplantation 77:437–440, 2004
42. Fazeli-Matin, S., Gill, I.S., Hsu, T.H.S., Sung, G.T., Novick, A.C.: Laparoscopic renal and adrenal surgery in obese patients: comparison to open surgery. J Urol 162:665–669, 1999
43. Wolf, Jr., J.S., Moon, T.D., Nakada, S.Y. Hand assisted laparoscopic nephrectomy: comparison to standard laparoscopic nephrectomy. J Urol 160:22–27, 1998
44. Saika, T., Ono, Y., Hattori, R., Gottoh, M., Kamihira, O., Yoshikawa, Y., et al. Long-term outcome of laparoscopic radical nephrectomy for pathologic T1 renal cell carcinoma. Urology 62:1018–1023, 2003
45. Busby, E., Das, S., Rao Tunuguntla, H.S.G., Evans, C.P. Hand-assisted laparoscopic vs the open (flank incision) approach to radical nephrectomy. BJU Int 91:341–344, 2003
46. Wolf, Jr., J.S., Merion, R.M., Leichtman, A.B., Campbell Jr., D.A., Magee, J.C., Punch, J.D., et al. Randomized controlled trial of hand-assisted laparoscopic versus open surgical live donor nephrectomy. Transplantation 72:284–290, 2001
47. Ono, Y., Kinukawa, T., Hattori, R., Yamada, S., Nishiyama, N., Mizutani, K., et al. Laparoscopic radical nephrectomy for renal cell carcinoma: a 5 year experience. Urology 53:280–286, 1999
48. Cadeddu, J.A., Ono, Y., Clayman, R.V., Barrett, P.H., Janetschek, G., Fentie, D.D., et al. Laparoscopic nephrectomy for renal cell cancer: evaluation of efficacy and safety. A multicenter experience. Urology 52:773–777, 1998
49. Stifelman, M.D., Sosa, R.E., Andrade, A., Tarantino, A., Shichman, S.J. Hand-assisted laparoscopic nephroureterectomy for the treatment of transitional cell carcinoma of the upper urinary tract. Urology 56:741747, 2000
50. Gill, I.S., Matin, S.F., Desai, M.M., Kaouk, J.H., Steinberg, A., Mascha, E., et al. Comparative analysis of laparoscopic versus open partial nephrectomy for renal tumors in 200 patients. J Urol 170:64–68, 2003
51. Rozet, F., Jaffe, J., Braud, G. A direct comparison of robotic assisted versus pure laparoscopic radical prostatectomy: a single institution experience. J Urol 178(2): 478–482, 2007
52. Hu, J.C., Nelson, R.A., Wilson, T.G., et al. Perioperative complications of laparoscopic and robot-assisted laparoscopic radical prostatectomy. J Urol 175(2): 541–546, February 2006
53. Multi-institutional review of pathologic margins after robot-assisted laparoscopic prostatectomy (LRP). Abstract #1158 presented Tuesday., May 23, 2006 at American urological Association meeting in Atlanta, GA.

Laparoscopic Renal Ablation

Gaurav Bandi and Stephen Y. Nakada

INTRODUCTION

Nephron sparing surgery (NSS) is accepted as the treatment of choice in patients with solitary kidney, bilateral renal masses, and in patients with renal insufficiency *(1,2)*. In patients with renal tumors less than 4 cm and a normal contralateral kidney, NSS has been shown to have a decreased incidence of long-term renal insufficiency *(2)*. It has also been associated with an improved quality of life *(3,4)*. Open partial nephrectomy (OPN) is the gold standard treatment for NSS. Laparoscopic partial nephrectomy (LPN) has recently been popularized by Gill and associates *(5)*. Although LPN has been shown to have good oncologic outcomes at an intermediate follow-up *(6)*; it requires advanced laparoscopic skills and has associated perioperative morbidity *(7,8)*. A recent large multicenter retrospective study compared the perioperative outcomes between open and laparoscopic partial nephrectomy *(9)*. LPN was associated with shorter operative time, decreased operative blood loss, and shorter hospital stay. Although, the incidence of intraoperative complications was comparable in the two groups LPN was associated with longer ischemia time, more postoperative complications (particularly urological), and an increased number of subsequent procedures. Overall 25.2% of patients undergoing LPN had a postoperative complication compared to 19.8% who underwent OPN. After 3 months, renal functional outcomes for laparoscopic and open partial nephrectomy were similar.

The widespread use of cross-sectional abdominal renal imaging has led to increased detection of renal cell carcinoma *(10)*. More than 60% of renal tumors are now detected incidentally *(11,12)*. The mean age of diagnosis of renal cell carcinoma is 65 years and many of these incidental renal masses are diagnosed in elderly patients with multiple comorbidities *(12)*. These patients are at high-risk for perioperative morbidity. Less invasive ablative techniques have been developed in efforts to decrease morbidity and appropriately match cancer control. Cryoablation (CA) and radiofrequency ablation (RFA) are the most commonly used ablative techniques for the management of small renal masses. Both of them can be administered using an open, laparoscopic, or percutaneous approach. The primary goals of these ablative technologies are to achieve cancer control while preserving renal function and minimizing morbidity. We herein discuss the indications, technique, and outcomes of laparoscopic-assisted renal ablation and share our experience with laparoscopic cryoablation (LCA) for management of small renal masses.

PRINCIPLES OF CRYOABLATION

Cryosurgery was first reported by James Arnott in 1850, when he used crushed ice in salt solutions to freeze cancers of the breast and uterine cervix. Since then the instruments used in cryotherapy and

From: *Current Clinical Urology: Essential Urologic Laparoscopy*
Edited by: S. Y. Nakada and S. P. Hedican, DOI 10.1007/978-1-60327-820-1_20

equally important the instruments used to monitor cryotherapy have evolved considerably. The first renal cryosurgery performed in humans were two percutaneous renal cryoablations reported by Uchida et al. *(13)* for two patients with high-stage renal cancers *(13)*. Today, in addition to percutaneous access, cryoablation can be performed via open and laparoscopic-assisted access as well.

Cryoablation relies on the principle that temperatures below –20°C induce cell death by a variety of mechanisms. First, direct mechanical cellular injury is caused by ice crystal formation within and around the cells. One purported mechanism involves initial freezing of the extracellular fluid compartment that in turn causes osmotic dehydration of the intracellular fluid compartment *(14)*. The shift in fluid concentration creates a high concentration of solutes within the cells that is believed to cause cellular membrane injury and damage to the enzymatic activity of the cell. With further cooling, cytosol super-cools and forms intracellular ice crystals that lead to further damage of the intracellular membranes *(15)*. Secondly, secondary changes from freezing involve destruction of the microcirculation and subsequent cellular hypoxia and necrosis from vascular stasis *(16)*. Recent work has revealed the possibility of a third mechanism of cell death based on increased apoptosis in the peripheral zone of the necrotic lesion *(17)*. These mechanisms together result in a necrotic zone, which becomes apparent in 2 days after cryoablation therapy *(18)*. In order to achieve renal cell death temperatures must be below −19.4°C. For necrosis of virtually all human tissues −40°C is required *(19)*.

Renal cryoablation was initially performed with liquid nitrogen (−195.8°C). However, continued ice ball progression after halting the liquid nitrogen perfusion made controlling the ice ball size difficult. Pressurized argon gas (−185.7°C) eliminated this delay between the end of infusion and ice ball progression. Other advances in cryoablation include smaller probe sizes, larger ice ball to probe size ratios allowing for smaller probes to be used and insulated probe shafts, which limit the amount of cooling proximal to the tip. Cryoprobes currently range in size from 1.7 to 8 mm. Probe tips can be either beveled or blunt. Cryoprobes create ice ball shapes that are usually oblong, and ice ball size increases with probe diameter. Each cryoprobe has a specific isotherm, which determines the size of the ablated lesion (Fig. 1). From the edge of the ice ball (0°C) to the probe (−185.7°C) the temperatures become progressively lower making the kill zone smaller than the ice ball. Therefore, ice ball size must exceed that of the tumor in order to insure that the −20 to −40°C isotherm covers the entire lesion. *(19)*.

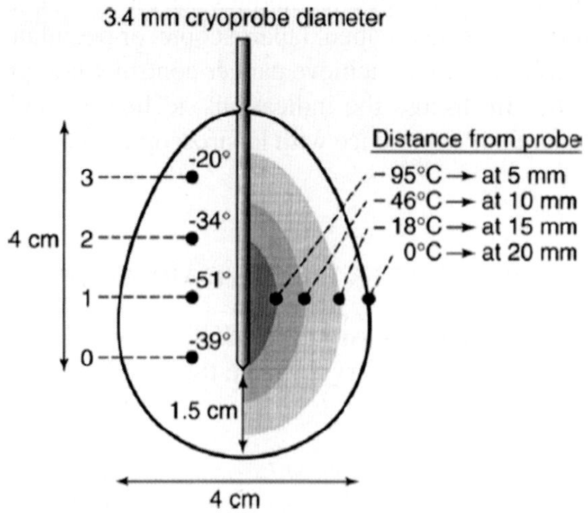

Fig. 1. Showing various isotherms of a 3.4-mm cryoprobe.

Freezing of a lesion should be done as quickly as possible, and the freeze cycle should be at least 10 min. The lesion is then thawed either passively or actively with helium gas. Animal studies have shown that the type of thaw process did not affect tissue damage *(20)*. This freeze–thaw cycle is then be repeated, as the second cycle increases the percent cell death within the original ice ball without extending the frozen margin and risking unnecessary injury to adjacent structures *(20)*. After a passive or active second thaw, the cryoprobe can be removed.

PRINCIPLES OF RADIOFREQUENCY ABLATION

RFA for renal tumors was first reported by Zlotta *(21)*. The first report on laparoscopic RFA (LRFA) by Yohannes et al. described a retroperitoneoscopic approach used to ablate a 2-cm solid mass on the anterior border of the right kidney in an elderly patient with renal insufficiency *(22)*. During RFA, radiofrequency waves are delivered to the tissues using specially designed needles. This energy is converted to heat, which leads to cell death and coagulation necrosis. The temperatures reached during RFA depend on the generator's power, tissue impedance, heat conductivity, and heat dissipation via the local circulation. The cellular and tissue effects of RFA vary with the duration of ablation and the local temperature achieved. At 50°C, proteins begin to denature, lipids melt, and irreversible tissue destruction tends to occur. At 100°C tissue coagulation, desiccation, and charring takes place *(23)*. The temperature–time dependence was elegantly shown by Bhowmick et al. in their in vitro studies that demonstrated irreversible cell injury when benign and malignant human cell lines are heated to 45°C for 60 min, 55°C for 5 min, and 70°C for 1 min *(24,25)*. Histological analysis after RFA demonstrates typical coagulative necrosis characterized by membrane disruption, protein denaturation, and vascular thrombosis *(26)*. The ablated tissue is eventually replaced by fibrosis or is re-absorbed.

Commercially available RFA units are broadly classified into temperature- or impedance-based systems. This means that the computer-controlled generator provides energy to the probe based on either the average temperature achieved at the tines or the measured impedance of the tissue during ablation. Impedance rises towards infinity when tissues are desiccated during ablation or when there is charring. Originally, ''low-energy'' ablations were accomplished with generators providing 90 W of power. These early devices have been replaced because they were ineffective. Presently, newer generators provide ''high-energy'' ablation, with power levels up to 200 W. There are a multitude of RFA probes available to the practicing urologist. RFA probes can be monopolar, with energy traveling from the probe tip to a grounding pad or bipolar with energy traveling from one probe tip to another. RFA can also be performed in a wet environment by infusing highly conductive electrolyte solutions to increase the size and speed of ablation without tissue desiccation. RFA probes can be a single electrode that controls tissue coagulation based on time and impedance feedback or may have multiple thermosensing tynes that determine the coagulation end points. Some probes are internally cooled by circulating ice cold saline around the electrode to draw away unwanted heat that is radiated back along the probe. Cooling also limits the charring around the electrode tip which can cause increased tissue impedance and decreased energy transfer to the edge of the heat ball *(23)*.

Because real-time ultrasound monitoring is not feasible with RFA, the kill zone estimation is based on minimum activated time and the deployed diameter if using thermosensing tynes. The maximum lesions size is not changed by activating the probe for longer periods of time; therefore, it is imperative that the probe be accurately placed into the center of the lesion. Once the probe is in place and the target temperature is achieved the tissue is heated for 3–8 min depending on lesion size. Probe temperatures approach 105°C in the center and diminish toward the edge as impedance increases. Heating time algorithms are dependant upon the particular electrode used as well as the electrosurgical generator which can range from 50 to 200 W. For larger lesions, a combination of longer heating times and multiple electrodes can be used to ensure adequate kill zone coverage of the tumor.

PATIENT SELECTION: INDICATIONS AND CONTRAINDICATIONS

The indications for renal tumor ablation are similar to those for partial nephrectomy. However, ablative technologies (both CA and RFA) are relatively new, with the longest follow-up reported after ablation being 5 years *(27,28)*. Until long-term outcomes become available laparoscopic-assisted ablation should be reserved for elderly patients with comorbidities, who are otherwise not candidates for partial nephrectomy. A recent study comparing patients who underwent LPN with those who underwent LCA found decreased blood loss and late complication rate in the cryoablation group, even though this group had a higher proportion of elderly patients with a high American Society of Anesthesiologists score *(29)*. Although it is technically feasible to ablate larger masses, ablation is ideal for small volume renal cortical masses less than 4 cm. Ablation can be carried out in patients with solitary kidney, transplanted kidney, renal insufficiency, Von-Hippel Lindau disease, and in patients with a normal contralateral kidney. The ability to avoid hilar vessel clamping during laparoscopic-assisted ablation also favors their use in for patients with compromised renal function.

Contraindications to renal ablation include locally advanced and / or metastatic disease and uncorrected bleeding disorders. Relative contraindications to performing laparoscopic access for ablation include prior abdominal or renal surgery and a history of renal ablation. Laparoscopic-assisted ablation should be approached cautiously in patients with renal lesions close to the renal hilum and pelvicalyceal system. Ablation of hilar lesions may be associated with heat sinking through major blood vessels leading to incomplete ablation. Injury to collecting system may be a source of urine leak in the postoperative period. Intraoperative ultrasound should be performed to rule out multicentric lesions where multiple probes or an alternative treatment modality, i.e., open or laparoscopic radical nephrectomy could be considered. Traditionally, cystic renal masses are not ideal candidates for needle-based ablation secondary to decompression of cysts, which might lead to tumor spill, instability of probes, and imperfect ablation.

Currently, no standard guidelines exist for choosing between CA and other ablative technologies such as RFA, microwave or high frequency ultrasound. Based on animal studies cryoablation is less likely to injure the renal collecting system during deep ablations when compared with RFA *(30,31)*. Although comparative experimental data suggest that almost all cryolesions resulted in complete tissue necrosis without skip lesions versus RFA *(32,26)*, the definitive tissue response may be validated only by getting strong long-term results. Recently, the group from the Cleveland Clinic compared 164 LCA versus 82 percutaneous RFA cases *(33)*. Radiologic evidence of tumor recurrence or persistence of disease was noted in three (1.8%) who underwent LCA and in nine (11.1%) who were treated with RFA. All have been successfully treated with reablation/nephrectomy, or they are currently under observation. Cancer-specific survival following cryotherapy was 98% at a median follow-up of 3 year and 100% for RFA at 1-year median follow-up. Similarly, incomplete ablation and tumor recurrence were more often seen after RFA in another multi-institution retrospective study *(34)*. Finally, in cases where real-time monitoring with imaging is necessary, CA should be used, as RFA requires contrast enhanced imaging to monitor the ablation.

There are also no guidelines for choosing between a laparoscopic versus percutaneous approach. Tumor and adjacent organ location are the most important factors which determine the access technique. Tumors on the anterior or medial aspect of the kidney are usually in close proximity to vulnerable structures such as the gall bladder, bowel, pancreas, and ureter. These organs should be dissected free from the tumor to prevent unintentional ablation which may lead to complications. Most authors believe that these lesions are better accessed with a transperitoneal laparoscopic technique *(35,33,36)*. However, in Shingleton's series 20% of the tumors ablated percutaneously were anterior *(37)*. Their use of MRI as the primary imaging modality was essential in performing anterior tumor ablations as ultrasound would be unable to monitor ice ball growth on the deep edge due to shadowing; however, lack of real-time imaging limits its use when adjacent organs are close. Tumors located on the posterior or lateral aspect of the kidney are easily accessed using a percutaneous technique. However, a retroperitoneal laparoscopic technique may provide direct access to these tumors as well. Surgeon preference and experience are crucial for choosing the optimal approach because each has advantages and limitations. The laparoscopic approach provides the surgeon direct intraoperative visualization, allowing extensive and accurate pathologic sampling. Another advantage of laparoscopic access includes the ability to perform real-time ultrasonography and visual monitoring of the ice ball formation. Although laparoscopy allows greater intraoperative control, the risk of damage to healthy tissue (e.g., renal fracture, bowel or pancreatic injury) has been reported *(38)*.

PRE-OPERATIVE PREPARATION

The pre-operative preparation for a suspected renal cell carcinoma is the same as for open or a laparoscopic approach. Thorough history and physical examination is mandatory. A complete blood count, basic metabolic panel, urine analysis, and culture are routinely performed. Metastatic evaluation usually includes a chest radiograph, abdominal CT scan, and a bone scan is reserved for patients with abnormal calcium and/or alkaline phosphatase levels. MRI is indicated in patients with a contrast allergy or renal insufficiency. Most of these patients may require pre-operative control and clearance from the internist or a specialist for their comorbidities. Patients should sign an informed consent, which includes a detailed discussion about the limitations, expectations and possible complications. Patients should be informed about the potential for performing a radical nephrectomy (laparoscopic or open) if the situation demands. We routinely perform minimal bowel preparation using 300 ml of magnesium citrate with a clear liquid diet a day prior to surgery and usually admit patients on the day of surgery. Patients are usually typed but not cross-matched for blood. Careful pre-operative planning with a radiologist who is experienced and interested in renal cryoablation regarding the approach, number, size, and placement of probes is paramount for the success of the procedure.

SURGICAL TECHNIQUE

Operating Room Set-Up

The patient position and approach depends upon the exact location of the renal mass. The patient is placed in flank position with the affected side up. The primary surgeon, first assistant, and the scrub nurse stand facing the abdomen (transperitoneal approach) or facing the spine (retroperitoneal approach). The second assistant (optional) will be on the opposite side. The monitor towers are stationed at the patient's shoulders and angled slightly towards the feet at a comfortable eye level to the operating personnel. The tower containing the laparoscopic insufflator, light source, and camera should be across the primary surgeon to facilitate monitoring of the pressure recordings. The harmonic and electrocautery generator units are at the patient's feet across the primary surgeon. The suction irrigator/aspirator system is hung on the anesthetic pole on the side of the primary surgeon at the head end of the table. The scrub nurse's mayo stand is placed directly above the patient legs and the remaining laparoscopic instruments are placed on another table in an L-shaped configuration for easy access.

Patient Positioning

The operation table is padded with two layers of foam to provide adequate padding to prevent myonecrosis. After induction of anesthesia and placement of the Foley catheter and orogastric tube, the patient is placed in semi-flank position (15–20° from vertical) for transperitoneal approach and full flank position for retroperitoneal approach with the kidney rest at the level of the 12th rib. The kidney rest is elevated minimally and the table is flexed slightly to increase the space between the rib cage and the iliac crest. The down leg is flexed and the upper leg is placed straight with three or more pillows between the legs oriented at right angles to the legs. Venodynes and stockings are routinely used to prevent deep venous thrombosis. Two arm boards are placed side by side at the level of shoulder with foam padding. A soft foam axillary roll is positioned two fingerbreadths below the axilla to prevent brachial plexopathy. Three or more pillows are placed inline between the upper extremities to support the upper arm. The safety strap is applied over the lower extremities at the level of calves. A cautery pad is strapped on the upper thigh and a 3-in. wide cloth tape is used to strap the patient from the edge of the table to the other edge of the table. The upper torso is stabilized by using 3-in. wide cloth tape from the edge of the table at the level of shoulders and is split into two strips past the elbows and is attached to either side of the arm boards. Care is taken to reposition all EKG leads, wires, and intravenous lines so that they are not under the patient at any point. A pneumatic warming device may be used on the upper torso to prevent hypothermia.

Trocar Placement

TRANSPERITONEAL APPROACH

Peritoneal insufflation is obtained by inserting a Veress needle midway between the umbilicus and the superior iliac crest just lateral to the rectus muscle. The abdomen is insufflated up to 15 mmHg pressure and then a 10- or 5-mm non-bladed trocar is passed in to the abdomen using an optiview system for the camera, depending on the surgeon's choice of using a 5- or 10-mm telescope. A second 10-mm port is placed at the lateral margin of the umbilicus and the third port is placed in a sub-costal position, just lateral to midline, half way between the xiphoid and the umbilicus. The second and third ports could be 5- or 10-mm depending on the side of the lesion and the dominant hand of the surgeon. An additional 5-mm port may be necessary on the right side to retract the inferior margin of the liver about two fingerbreadths below the costal margin in the mid-axillary line. We have a low threshold to use an open Hasson cannula technique for patients with a history of previous surgery where complicated adhesions are anticipated.

RETROPERITONEAL APPROACH

The open Hasson cannula technique is routinely used. A horizontal 2-cm incision is placed 1 cm below and lateral to the tip of the 12th rib. Then the latissimus dorsi muscle fibers are bluntly separated and the retroperitoneum is entered by opening the anterior lamella of the thoraco-lumbar fascia. Blunt finger dissection is performed to develop space by pushing the peritoneum away from the psoas major muscle. We found it is not necessary to use a balloon for formal dilatation of the retroperitoneal space. Alternatively, a trocar mounted balloon (U.S. Surgical, Norwalk, CT) may be used to develop adequate working space by instilling 800–1,000 cc. A 10-mm blunt tip trocar (U.S. Surgical, Norwalk, CT) is placed after removing the balloon dissection device and it is secured by inflating the internal retention balloon and a cinching external foam cuff. A Hassan cannula could also be used and it is tightly fixed by using fascial sutures around the trocar. Two more secondary ports are placed under vision, one 10/12-mm trocar is placed three fingerbreadths above the iliac crest in the anterior axillary line and the other 10/12-mm trocar is placed lateral to the erector spinae muscle just below the 12th rib.

Exposure of the Lesion

The camera is inserted via the lower quadrant port and the surgeon operates with the sub-costal and periumbilical ports in the transperitoneal approach. The harmonic scalpel is used to incise the line of Toldt. The colon along with the duodenum (on the right side) is reflected medially to expose the anterior surface of the kidney. Extensive mobilization of the colon, spleen, ureter, and hilum is usually not necessary. In the retroperitoneal approach, the camera is usually inserted via the middle port and the surgeon operates through the medial and lateral ports. Maintaining the orientation and identifying the psoas major muscle are very important in this approach.

We routinely use laparoscopic ultrasound to identify the lesion, determine accurate lesion depth and to exclude multicentric lesions. This is especially helpful when lesions are predominantly endophytic. Gerota's fascia can be opened to facilitate identification of the mass as well. Our technique has evolved such that we now leave Gerota's fascia intact to tamponade bleeding from the ablated site and minimize tumor spillage. Once the renal lesion is identified and well exposed, a needle biopsy of the lesion is performed under ultrasonic guidance using an 18-gauge punch biopsy gun.

Ablation Technique

CRYOABLATION

Cryoablation is performed using an argon gas-based system that operated on Joule–Thompson principle (Endocare, Irvine, CA). Various cryoprobes of different diameters are available. The number and size of probes used in a case vary depending on the size and site of the tumor. The smaller probes (1.7, 2.4, and 3.8-mm) are often passed percutaneously; the 5-mm probe can be placed percutaneously or via a laparoscopic port. Immediately after the lesion is biopsied, the tumor is punctured with an appropriate sized probe under direct laparoscopic and ultrasound guidance. The importance of placing more than one cryoprobe to achieve adequate coverage of the whole tumor could not be over emphasized. We believe most of the recurrent tumors are persistent tumors, which were missed, in the earlier freezing. We also believe that a margin of 10-mm is necessary to achieve adequate and dependable cell kill. A dual freeze–thaw cycle using argon is then performed (10 min cycles). A passive thaw is done between the freeze cycles and an active thaw is done after the second freeze. The cryolesion is monitored with real-time ultrasonography performed by a radiologist experienced in laparoscopic ultrasound. Before removal, complete thawing is allowed prior to probe removal to avoid the rare occurrence of renal fracture. Liquid thrombin and Floseal (Baxter USA, Deerfield, IL) are placed

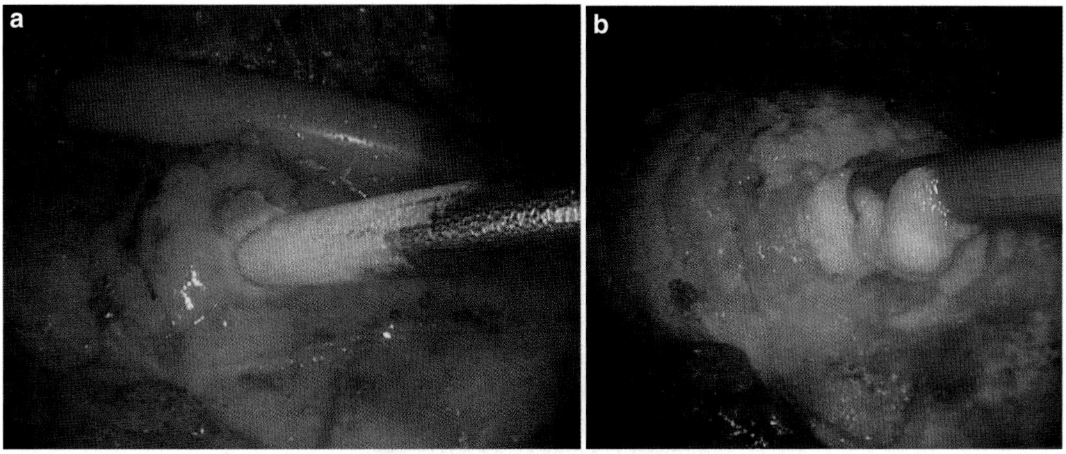

Fig. 2. Intraoperative view of laparoscopic cryoablation with laparoscopic ultrasound probe (**a**) and probe site following injection with Floseal (**b**).

into the cryoprobe defect and pressure is applied (Fig. 2a,b). It is important to observe the lesion for hemostasis for up to 20 min as delayed bleeding has been noted on some occasions. After finishing the procedure hemostasis is checked at 5 mmHg and the abdominal ports are closed using a port closure device to prevent herniation of intra-abdominal contents.

Radiofrequency Ablation

The RFA probe is introduced through the abdominal wall with the goal of placing the probe perpendicular to the tumor surface. The tines are deployed to create a zone of ablation 0.5–1 cm beyond the tumor margin. Tine deployment is confirmed with laparoscopic ultrasound before ablation is begun. The tines are hyperechoic and should be located at the periphery of the lesion before ablation is begun. The ablation is then started by activating the generator. Once the target temperature is reached, tumors requiring tine deployment <2 cm are ablated for 5 min, those requiring deployment between 2 and 3 cm for 7 min, and those requiring deployment >3 cm for 8 min. A 30-s cool-down period is followed by a second ablation cycle of identical duration. Small lesions <1 cm can be treated with a single 3- to 5-min cycle.

Ablation causes rapid tissue hyperthermia creating microbubbles that prevent accurate visualization of the tines once begun. Indeed, real-time sonographic monitoring of ablation is unnecessary during RFA because the temperatures at the margin of ablation are constantly monitored by the StarBurst probe. Large tumor biopsies may be taken after ablation using a 10-mm toothed biopsy forceps, and studies have shown that such biopsies are fully interpretable by pathologists *(39)*. Another benefit to biopsy after RFA is that the ablated tumor does not bleed even with sizable biopsies. Our approach remains pre-treatment dual core needle biopsy.

POSTOPERATIVE CARE AND FOLLOW-UP

All patients are admitted postoperatively for observation. Serum creatinine and hematocrit were measured on postoperative day 1 and patients are discharged home when they were tolerating diet with their pain well controlled on oral analgesics. Patients should be advised to avoid strenuous activity for the next 2 weeks to prevent postoperative hemorrhage.

Unlike with surgical resection, during thermal ablation therapy, the ablated renal tumor is not excised and is left in situ. Therefore, accurate assessment of ablated tumors and early postablation detection of residual or recurrent tumor is essential. This makes a rigorous follow-up protocol mandatory. Long-term surveillance imaging is essential for identifying tumor recurrence, metastatic disease, new tumors, and delayed complications after renal tumor ablation. CT is often used for postablation follow-up because of its lower cost and wider availability; however, MR imaging may be superior in some situations, such as in patients who cannot receive iodinated contrast material because of renal insufficiency (Fig. 3a,b). For patients who underwent MR imaging–guided ablation, MR imaging may be better than CT for follow-up because intraprocedural findings can be directly compared with follow-up findings. Early imaging follow-up at 1–3 months after ablation is used to establish a baseline imaging appearance, to determine if the ablation procedure was complete and to exclude complications. Rim enhancement of the ablated lesion may be seen during the first few months post-ablation, but this finding resolves gradually over time and is barely detectable after 3 months.

Patients should be evaluated periodically with medical history, physical examination, blood pressure, chest X-ray, serum electrolytes, liver function tests, and renal function tests. The ablated lesion can be followed using contrast enhanced CT scans or MRI scans every 3–4 months during the first year, every 6 months during the second year and then yearly. At follow-up examinations, successfully

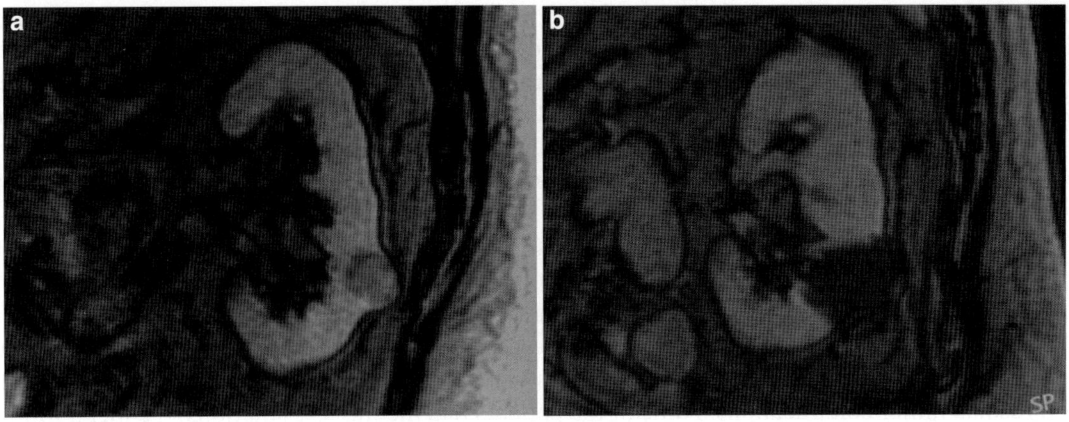

Fig. 3. MRI images pre (**a**) and post (**b**) cryoablation. Note acute nature of ablation in (**b**).

ablated renal tumors are seen as focal masses without contrast enhancement that frequently decrease in size. Presence of cresenteric or nodular enhancement and/or increase in size of the lesion is considered failure. When these findings are seen on the first post-ablative imaging, this represents residual tumor or incomplete ablation; whereas reappearance of these findings after a normal imaging on follow-up is considered recurrence.

The role of post-ablation biopsy of the treated lesion is still unclear. Serial biopsies at regular intervals are ideal but an optimal biopsy schedule is yet to be determined and biopsies are not without sampling errors and patient morbidity. Recently, Gill's group suggested that lack of enhancement on 6-mo MRI does not guarantee complete cancer cell kill following RFA of small renal tumors and may fail to detect early recurrence of persistent disease in a number of patients *(40)*. These authors recommend biopsy as an important component of patient follow-up. On the other hand, due to slow growth of some renal lesions, it may take several years before local recurrence becomes identifiable. A few studies have shown that immediate tumor excision with histological evaluation detected viable cells, for example, after RFA in 50–100% of cases *(32,41,42)*. However, the cellular changes within the ablated lesions could be delayed, up to 30 days and longer after the ablative procedure. Further collection of long-term data especially from multicenter trials along with basic research may bring better understanding of tumor destruction on a molecular level with clarification of post-ablative changes in the clinical setting.

RESULTS

Laparoscopic Radiofrequency Ablation

Early experience with LRFA was reported by Jacomides et al. *(43)* who treated 13 patients with 17 renal tumors using the RITA 1500RF 250-W generator (RITA Medical Systems, Mountain View, CA) system and Starburst XL electrodes. Mean tumor size was 1.96 cm (range, 0.9–3.6). A total of seven patients had in situ ablations, five underwent concomitant partial nephrectomy, and one with multiple tumors underwent excision of the largest tumor with the others left in situ. Mean operative times were 140 min in patients with in situ ablations and 203 min in patients who underwent partial nephrectomy. At mean follow-up of 9.8 months, no patient had radiographic evidence of recurrence and none had developed metastatic disease, despite a positive surgical margin in one patient (17%) who had undergone partial nephrectomy.

Hwang et al. *(44)* published their experience with RFA in 24 tumors in 17 patients with hereditary kidney cancer syndromes. This series included nine patients in whom 15 lesions were treated laparoscopically. Mean lesion size was 2.2 cm. Ablations were performed with use of the Valleylab 200-W Cool-tip RF system (Valleylab, Boulder, CO). A single 17-gauge electrode with a 3-cm exposed tip was positioned within the lesion for up to four 12-min ablation sessions. At a mean follow-up of 13 months, none of the laparoscopically treated lesions demonstrated enhancement suggesting recurrent disease.

The largest series on laparoscopic RFA comes from the group at the University of Texas, Southwestern. Park et al. *(45)* reported RFA of 94 tumors in 78 patients with a mean tumor size of 2.4 cm using the RITA 1500RF 250-W generator with Starburst XL probes. Of these 39 tumors (27 pathologic RCC) with a mean tumor size of 2.3 cm (range, 1–4.2) were treated laparoscopically. Mean operative time was 170 min and mean estimated blood loss was 26 ml. Four patients had major complications and three had minor complications. None of the patients had incomplete ablation. At a mean follow-up of 26 months, none of the patients had evidence of recurrent disease.

Percutaneous RFA has been more frequently utilized than LRFA. Thus the data on laparoscopic RFA are only limited to the above mentioned series. A recent article *(45)* reviewing renal RFA (both percutaneous and laparoscopic) suggests minor and major complication rate after renal RFA to be in the 5–10% range. The major complications reported in the literature include injury to the pyelocalyceal system, bowel injury, and delayed gross hematuria requiring surgical exploration or angiographic embolization. Pyelocalyceal injury can lead to either urine leakage or stricture formation. Urinomas usually resolve with ureteral stenting, whereas strictures in the collecting system may require endopyelotomy or reconstructive surgery. Minor complications include paraesthesia at the probe insertion site, self-limiting perinephric hematomas, and anesthetic-related complications. The literature demonstrates excellent renal cancer control (94.8% cancer-specific survival) after RFA of small tumors (mean size 2.4 cm), with a mean follow-up of 19.5 months. While most tumors are successfully treated after one RFA session, reablations were necessary in some. The overall renal RFA reablation rate was 8.8% in the literature. Salvage radical or partial nephrectomy is the alternative to RF reablation, and it was reported in only three cases (1.1%) after RFA.

Laparoscopic Cryoablation

Unlike RFA, renal cryoablation has been performed more often utilizing laparoscopic access. Multiple large single institution series with variable follow-up have been reported in the literature (Table 1). The clinical outcomes from the most prominent ones are described below.

Gill et al. *(46)* reported the intermediate outcome (minimum 3 years of follow-up) of cryoablation in 56 patients undergoing LCA. The mean tumor size was 2.3 cm (range, 1–5), and the mean cryolesion created was 3.6 cm. Depending on tumor location, the transperitoneal approach was used in 25% of the patients and the retroperitoneal approach in 75% of the patients. At 3 years of follow-up, 17 cryolesions (38%) had completely disappeared on follow-up MRI, and the average cryolesion size reduction was 75%. Postoperative needle biopsy found local renal tumor recurrence in two patients. In a recent update of this series, Hegarty et al. *(28)* presented data on 66 patients with a mean tumor size of 2.6 cm (range, 1–4.5) and a minimum follow-up of 60 months and reported 5-year overall and cancer-specific survival rates of 81 and 98%, respectively. Three patients (6%) developed local tumor recurrence. The results of this study indicate low local recurrence rates and good 5-year cancer specific-survival with use of LCA.

Weld et al. *(47)* reported their 3-year follow-up of LCA in 31 patients with 36 tumors. Mean tumor size was 2.1 cm (range, 0.5–4). The mean operative time was 2.9 h, with a mean estimated blood loss of 97 ml. The biopsy results revealed that 22 tumors (61%) were malignant and 14 (39%) were benign.

Table 1
Laparoscopic cryoablation clinical series

Series	*Number of patients (n)*	*Number of tumors (n)*	*Tumor size (cm)*	*Biopsy proven RCC*	*Access*	*OR time (min)*	*Conversion (%)*	*EBL (CCs)*	*Hospital stay (days)*	*Complications*	*Incomplete ablation n (%)*	*Follow-up (months)*	*Recurrence n (%)*	*Metastatic disease n (%)*	*Cancer-specific survival (%)*
Nadler et al. (2003)	15	15	2.2	10	TP 40%; RP 60%	260	0	67	3.5	2 minor	1(6.3%)	15	0	0	100
Cestari et al. *(50)*	37	37	2.6	29	TP 60%; RP 40%	194	0	165	3.8	1 major; 6 minor	0	21	1 (2.7%)	0	100
Hegarty et al. *(33)*	161	164	2.3	NA	TP 42%; RP 58%	NA	0	NA	NA	3 major; 8 minor	3(1.8%)	36	5 (3.1%)	1 (0.6%)	98
Davol et al. *(27)*	48	48	2.6	36	O 50%; TP/RP 50%	NA	0	NA	3	0 major; 7 minor	1(2.5%)	64	4 (12.5%)	1 (2%)	100
Lawatsch et al. *(51)*	59	81	2.5	27	TP 88%; RP 6%; HAL 6%	190	2	50	2	2 major; 7 minor	0	27	2 (3.3%)	0	100
Schwartz et al. (2006)	84	85	2.6	50	O 13%; TP 49%; RP 33%	NA	7	58	3	2 major; 1 minor	1(1.2%)	10	2	0	100
Weld et al. *(47)*	31	36	2.1	36	TP 71%; RP 29%	177	1	97	3	1 major	0	36	1 (3.2%)	0	100
Bandi et al. *(35)*	58	68	2.7	19	TP 63%; RP 31%; HAL 6%	247	1	64	2.5	3 major; 4 minor	2(2.9%)	22	1 (1.7%)	0	100

The 3-year cancer-specific survival rate was 100%, and no patient developed metastatic disease. One patient (2.8%) demonstrated return of abnormal enhancement within the cryolesion during follow-up, suggesting tumor recurrence.

Davol et al. *(26)* reviewed their experience with 5-year clinical follow-up on 48 patients who were treated with either open or laparoscopic renal cryoablation. The median tumor size was 2.6 cm (range, 1.1–4.6). Although the failure rate after the initial treatment was 12.5%, following retreatment the cohort achieved a cancer-free survival rate of 97.5%. The cancer-free survival rate after a single cryoablation was 87.5%, with an overall cancer-specific survival rate of 100%. This series highlights the fact that a successful cryoablation treatment might include several treatment sessions, and patients should be advised accordingly.

Our experience at the University of Wisconsin is very similar to the ones reported above. So far we have treated 58 patients with 68 renal masses using the laparoscopic technique. The mean diameter of the mass treated was 2.7 cm (range, 1–5.5). The mean operative time was 187 min and the mean estimated blood loss was 64 ml. Two patients had incomplete ablation, one of them was reablated percutaneously and the other underwent a radical nephrectomy. At a mean follow-up of 22 months, the cancer-specific and recurrence free survival were 100 and 98.3%, respectively. Our study is unique as the approach followed for cryoablation (laparoscopic or percutaneous) was selected and performed in collaboration with an uro-radiologist experienced in tumor ablation to offer the most accurate image-based therapy. Using a collaborative approach, we do offer a strong case for accurate therapies, strong patient selection, and follow-up. Other studies have reported similar short-term oncologic outcomes with the use of LCA for management of small renal masses.

LCA of renal tumors appears to be a relatively safe treatment option. Most case series have reported a low major complication rate (Table 1). This is commendable considering that mean patient age in most series is above 65 years with majority of patients being high-risk from an anesthetic standpoint. Most complications reported in these series are medical complications unrelated to the ablation itself. The incidence of urologic complications like hemorrhage, urinary stricture, and urine leak are very low and are usually related to poor patient selection (e.g., mass size greater than 4 cm, hilar lesions, mass in proximity to the collecting system). In a multi-institutional retrospective series of 271 ablative cases, the reported major complication rate was 1.8% with one death (aspiration pneumonia) that was not directly attributable to the ablation technique *(38)*. The cryoablative group of 132 cases reported a total of 20 (14.4%) complications; however, only two of these were major complications: a significant hemorrhage requiring blood transfusion following percutaneous cryoablation and an open conversion due to inability to access the tumor laparoscopically. The most common complication was pain or paraesthesia at the probe insertion site. Overall, an ablative procedure appears to be associated with minimal complications, and it may be a safer alternative to partial nephrectomy in patients with multiple comorbidities requiring a nephron-sparing surgery. The safety of cryoablation has also been assessed in other areas. Carvalhal et al. *(48)* showed that laparoscopic renal cryoablation had no deleterious effect on renal function or blood pressure when 22 patients were assessed 6 months after cessation of treatment. No increase was shown in the lithogenicity of urine at up to 2 months postoperatively *(49)*.

In 2005, Desai et al. compared the Cleveland Clinic experience with LPN versus LCA for tumors <3 cm *(29)*. A total of 78 patients were treated with LCA and 153 patients with LPN. Patients undergoing LPN were younger (mean age, 60.6 vs. 65.6 years, $p = 0.005$), healthier (American Society of Anesthesiologists class 3/4 present in 46 vs. 75%, $p = 0.001$) and a larger tumor size (2.3 vs. 2.1 cm, $p = 0.02$). Although there were no differences in operative times (190 vs. 188 min, $p = 0.77$) and hospital stay (2.3 vs. 2.1 days, $p = 0.13$), LCA was associated with lower blood loss (101 vs. 211 ml, $p = 0.000$) and a lower incidence of delayed complications after hospital discharge (2.2 vs. 16.3%, $p = 0.01$). The incidence of overall complications was also significantly lower in the LCA group (6.6 vs. 32.6%).

SUMMARY

Laparoscopy-assisted ablation is a minimally invasive treatment option for small renal masses in appropriately selected patients. It is associated with a short learning curve, decreased morbidity, and good efficacy at an intermediate term follow-up. The cytocidal effect, durability, and safety of cryoablation appear promising. However, the ideal cryogenic probe system and optimal mode of delivery have yet to be defined. Intra and extracorporeal monitoring of cryolesions is still evolving and its accuracy is dependent on the skill and experience of the operator. Compared to CA, fewer results are available for RFA, but RFA may also represent a viable clinical alternative for treating small renal masses. However, it is important to be continually critical of these technologies until more long-term follow-up is available. More data are required to provide reliable treatment of cystic lesions, larger lesions, and lesions near the collecting system and renal hilum. Until then, these technologies should still be considered developmental and offered only as an alternative to watchful waiting to patients with significant comorbidities.

TAKE HOME MESSAGES

- Laparoscopy-assisted ablation is a minimally invasive treatment option for small renal masses in appropriately selected patients.
- It has a short learning curve and is associated with low morbidity and reasonable efficacy at an intermediate-term follow-up
- As the technology and experience with renal tumor ablation continues to grow, the precise role of ablative treatments will become clear.

REFERENCES

1. Fergany AF, Hafez KS, Novick AC. Long-term results of nephron sparing surgery for localized renal cell carcinoma: 10-year followup. The Journal of Urology. 2000 Feb: **163**:442–445
2. Lau WK, Blute ML, Weaver AL, Torres VE, Zincke H. Matched comparison of radical nephrectomy vs nephron-sparing surgery in patients with unilateral renal cell carcinoma and a normal contralateral kidney. Mayo Clinic Proceedings. 2000 Dec: **75**:1236–1242
3. Clark PE, Schover LR, Uzzo RG, Hafez KS, Rybicki LA, Novick AC. Quality of life and psychological adaptation after surgical treatment for localized renal cell carcinoma: impact of the amount of remaining renal tissue. Urology. 2001 Feb: **57**:252–256
4. Shinohara N, Harabayashi T, Sato S, Hioka T, Tsuchiya K, Koyanagi T. Impact of nephron-sparing surgery on quality of life in patients with localized renal cell carcinoma. European urology. 2001 Jan: **39**:114–119
5. Moinzadeh A, Gill IS, Finelli A, Kaouk J, Desai M. Laparoscopic partial nephrectomy: 3-year followup. The Journal of Urology. 2006 Feb: **175**:459–462
6. Lane BR, Gill IS. 5-Year outcomes of laparoscopic partial nephrectomy. The Journal of Urology. 2007 Jan: **177**: 70–74; discussion 4
7. Gill IS, Matin SF, Desai MM, et al. Comparative analysis of laparoscopic versus open partial nephrectomy for renal tumors in 200 patients. The Journal of Urology. 2003 Jul: **170**:64–68
8. Ramani AP, Desai MM, Steinberg AP, et al. Complications of laparoscopic partial nephrectomy in 200 cases. The Journal of Urology. 2005 Jan: **173**:42–47
9. Gill IS, Kavoussi LR, Lane BR, et al. Comparison of 1,800 laparoscopic and open partial nephrectomies for single renal tumors. The Journal of Urology. 2007 Jul: **178**:41–46
10. Nguyen MM, Gill IS, Ellison LM. The evolving presentation of renal carcinoma in the United States: trends from the surveillance, epidemiology, and end results program. The Journal of Urology. 2006 Dec: **176**:2397–2400; discussion 400
11. Jayson M, Sanders H. Increased incidence of serendipitously discovered renal cell carcinoma. Urology. 1998 Feb: **51**:203–205
12. Luciani LG, Cestari R, Tallarigo C. Incidental renal cell carcinoma-age and stage characterization and clinical implications: study of 1092 patients (1982–1997). Urology. 2000 Jul: **56**:58–62

13. Uchida M, Imaide Y, Sugimoto K, Uehara H, Watanabe H. Percutaneous cryosurgery for renal tumours. British Journal of Urology. 1995 Feb: **75**:132–136; discussion 6–7
14. Mazur P. Freezing of living cells: mechanisms and implications. Am J Physiol. 1984 Sep: **247**:C125–C142
15. Hoffmann NE, Bischof JC. The cryobiology of cryosurgical injury. Urology. 2002 Aug: **60**:40–49
16. Daum PS, Bowers WD, Jr., Tejada J, Hamlet MP. Vascular casts demonstrate microcirculatory insufficiency in acute frostbite. Cryobiology. 1987 Feb: **24**:65–73
17. Yang WL, Addona T, Nair DG, Qi L, Ravikumar TS. Apoptosis induced by cryo-injury in human colorectal cancer cells is associated with mitochondrial dysfunction. International Journal of Cancer. 2003 Jan 20: **103**:360–369
18. Baust JG, Gage AA. The molecular basis of cryosurgery. BJU International. 2005 Jun: **95**:1187–1191
19. Chosy SG, Nakada SY, Lee FT, Jr., Warner TF. Monitoring renal cryosurgery: predictors of tissue necrosis in swine. The Journal of Urology. 1998 Apr: **159**:1370–1374
20. Woolley ML, Schulsinger DA, Durand DB, Zeltser IS, Waltzer WC. Effect of freezing parameters (freeze cycle and thaw process) on tissue destruction following renal cryoablation. Journal of Endourology/Endourological Society. 2002 Sep: **16**:519–522
21. Zlotta AR, Wildschutz T, Raviv G, et al. Radiofrequency interstitial tumor ablation (RITA) is a possible new modality for treatment of renal cancer: ex vivo and in vivo experience. Journal of Endourology/Endourological Society. 1997 Aug: **11**:251–258
22. Yohannes P, Pinto P, Rotariu P, Smith AD, Lee BR. Retroperitoneoscopic radiofrequency ablation of a solid renal mass. Journal of Endourology/Endourological Society. 2001 Oct: **15**:845–849
23. Matlaga BR, Zagoria RJ, Clark PE, Hall MC. Radiofrequency ablation of renal tumors. Current Urology Reports. 2004 Feb: **5**:39–44
24. Bhowmick P, Coad JE, Bhowmick S, et al. In vitro assessment of the efficacy of thermal therapy in human benign prostatic hyperplasia. International Journal of Hyperthermia. 2004 Jun: **20**:421–439
25. Bhowmick S, Coad JE, Swanlund DJ, Bischof JC. In vitro thermal therapy of AT-1 Dunning prostate tumours. International Journal of Hyperthermia. 2004 Feb: **20**:73–92
26. Rehman J, Landman J, Lee D, et al. Needle-based ablation of renal parenchyma using microwave, cryoablation, impedance- and temperature-based monopolar and bipolar radiofrequency, and liquid and gel chemoablation: laboratory studies and review of the literature. Journal of Endourology/Endourological Society. 2004 Feb: **18**: 83–104
27. Davol PE, Fulmer BR, Rukstalis DB. Long-term results of cryoablation for renal cancer and complex renal masses. Urology. 2006 Jul: **68**:2–6
28. Stein RJ, Kaouk JH. Renal cryotherapy: a detailed review including a 5-year follow-up. BJU international. 2007 May: **99**:1265–1270
29. Desai MM, Aron M, Gill IS. Laparoscopic partial nephrectomy versus laparoscopic cryoablation for the small renal tumor. Urology. 2005 Nov: **66**:23–28
30. Brashears JH, 3rd, Raj GV, Crisci A, et al. Renal cryoablation and radio frequency ablation: an evaluation of worst case scenarios in a porcine model. The Journal of Urology. 2005 Jun: **173**:2160–2165
31. Janzen NK, Perry KT, Han KR, et al. The effects of intentional cryoablation and radio frequency ablation of renal tissue involving the collecting system in a porcine model. The Journal of Urology. 2005 Apr: **173**:1368–1374
32. Klingler HC, Marberger M, Mauermann J, Remzi M, Susani M. ′Skipping′ is still a problem with radiofrequency ablation of small renal tumours. BJU International. 2007 May: **99**:998–1001
33. Hegarty NJ, Gill IS, Desai MM, Remer EM, O′Malley CM, Kaouk JH. Probe-ablative nephron-sparing surgery: cryoablation versus radiofrequency ablation. Urology. 2006 Jul: **68**:7–13
34. Matin SF, Ahrar K, Cadeddu JA, et al. Residual and recurrent disease following renal energy ablative therapy: a multi-institutional study. The Journal of Urology. 2006 Nov: **176**:1973–1977
35. Bandi G, Wen CC, Hedican SP, Moon TD, Lee FT, Jr., Nakada SY. Cryoablation of small renal masses: assessment of the outcome at one institution. BJU International. 2007 Oct: **100**:798–801
36. Park S, Anderson JK, Matsumoto ED, Lotan Y, Josephs S, Cadeddu JA. Radiofrequency ablation of renal tumors: intermediate-term results. Journal of Endourology / Endourological Society. 2006 Aug: **20**:569–573
37. Shingleton WB, Sewell PE, Jr. Percutaneous renal tumor cryoablation with magnetic resonance imaging guidance. The Journal of Urology. 2001 Mar: **165**:773–776
38. Johnson DB, Solomon SB, Su LM, et al. Defining the complications of cryoablation and radio frequency ablation of small renal tumors: a multi-institutional review. The Journal of Urology. 2004 Sep: **172**:874–877
39. Margulis V, Matsumoto ED, Lindberg G, et al. Acute histologic effects of temperature-based radiofrequency ablation on renal tumor pathologic interpretation. Urology. 2004 Oct: **64**:660–663
40. Hegarty NJ, Kaouk J, Remer EM, O′Malley CM, Novick AC, Gill IS. Lack of enhancement on 6-month MRI does not guarantee complete cancer cell kill following radiofrequency ablation of small renal tumors. The Journal of Urology. 2006: **175 (Suppl)**:552
41. Michaels MJ, Rhee HK, Mourtzinos AP, Summerhayes IC, Silverman ML, Libertino JA. Incomplete renal tumor destruction using radio frequency interstitial ablation. The Journal of Urology. 2002 Dec: **168**:2406–2409; discussion 9–10

42. Rendon RA, Kachura JR, Sweet JM, et al. The uncertainty of radio frequency treatment of renal cell carcinoma: findings at immediate and delayed nephrectomy. The Journal of Urology. 2002 Apr: **167**:1587–1592
43. Jacomides L, Ogan K, Watumull L, Cadeddu JA. Laparoscopic application of radio frequency energy enables in situ renal tumor ablation and partial nephrectomy. The Journal of Urology. 2003 Jan: **169**:49–53; discussion
44. Hwang JJ, Walther MM, Pautler SE, et al. Radio frequency ablation of small renal tumors: intermediate results. The Journal of Urology. 2004 May: **171**:1814–1818
45. Park S, Cadeddu JA. Outcomes of radiofrequency ablation for kidney cancer. Cancer Control. 2007 Jul: **14**:205–210
46. Gill IS, Remer EM, Hasan WA, et al. Renal cryoablation: outcome at 3 years. The Journal of Urology. 2005 Jun: **173**:1903–1907
47. Weld KJ, Figenshau RS, Venkatesh R, et al. Laparoscopic cryoablation for small renal masses: three-year follow-up. Urology. 2007 Mar: **69**:448–451
48. Carvalhal EF, Gill IS, Meraney AM, Desai MM, Schweizer DK, Sung GT. Laparoscopic renal cryoablation: impact on renal function and blood pressure. Urology. 2001 Sep: **58**:357–361
49. Ng CS, Gill IS. Impact of renal cryoablation on urine composition. Urology. 2002 Jun: **59**:831–834
50. Cestari A, Guazzoni G, dell'Acqua V, Nava L, Cardone G, Balconi G, Naspro R, Montorsi F, Rigatti P. Laparoscopic cryoablation of solid renal masses: intermediate term followup. J Urol. 2004 Oct: **172**(4 Pt 1):1267–70
51. Lawatsch EJ, Langenstroer P, Byrd GF, See WA, Quiroz FA, Begun FP. Intermediate results of laparoscopic cryoablation in 59 patients at the Medical College of Wisconsin. J Urol Apr: **175**(4):1225–9

Index

From: *Current Clinical Urology: Essential Urologic Laparoscopy*
Edited by: S. Y. Nakada and S. P. Hedican, DOI 10.1007/978-1-60327-820-1

S

Springer